T0280384

Handbook of Infectious Disease Data Analysis

Chapman & Hall/CRC
Handbooks of Modern Statistical Methods

Series Editor: Garrett Fitzmaurice, Department of Biostatistics, Harvard School of Public Health, Boston, MA, U.S.A.

The objective of the series is to provide high-quality volumes covering the state-of-the-art in the theory and applications of statistical methodology. The books in the series are thoroughly edited and present comprehensive, coherent, and unified summaries of specific methodological topics from statistics. The chapters are written by the leading researchers in the field, and present a good balance of theory and application through a synthesis of the key methodological developments and examples and case studies using real data.

For more information about this series, please visit: https://www.crcpress.com/go/handbooks

Handbook of Infectious Disease Data Analysis

Edited by

Leonhard Held
University of Zurich, Zurich, Switzerland

Niel Hens
Hasselt University, Hasselt, Belgium and University of Antwerp
Antwerp, Belgium

Philip O'Neill
University of Nottingham, Nottingham, UK

Jacco Wallinga
Leiden University, Leiden, the Netherlands

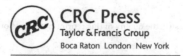

CRC Press
Taylor & Francis Group
Boca Raton London New York

CRC Press is an imprint of the
Taylor & Francis Group, an **informa** business

A CHAPMAN & HALL BOOK

CRC Press
Taylor & Francis Group
6000 Broken Sound Parkway NW, Suite 300
Boca Raton, FL 33487-2742

First issued in paperback 2021

© 2020 by Taylor & Francis Group, LLC
CRC Press is an imprint of Taylor & Francis Group, an Informa business

No claim to original U.S. Government works

ISBN 13: 978-1-03-208735-1 (pbk)
ISBN 13: 978-1-1386-2671-3 (hbk)

This book contains information obtained from authentic and highly regarded sources. Reasonable efforts have been made to publish reliable data and information, but the author and publisher cannot assume responsibility for the validity of all materials or the consequences of their use. The authors and publishers have attempted to trace the copyright holders of all material reproduced in this publication and apologize to copyright holders if permission to publish in this form has not been obtained. If any copyright material has not been acknowledged please write and let us know so we may rectify in any future reprint.

Except as permitted under U.S. Copyright Law, no part of this book may be reprinted, reproduced, transmitted, or utilized in any form by any electronic, mechanical, or other means, now known or hereafter invented, including photocopying, microfilming, and recording, or in any information storage or retrieval system, without written permission from the publishers.

For permission to photocopy or use material electronically from this work, please access www.copyright.com (http://www.copyright.com/) or contact the Copyright Clearance Center, Inc. (CCC), 222 Rosewood Drive, Danvers, MA 01923, 978-750-8400. CCC is a not-for-profit organization that provides licenses and registration for a variety of users. For organizations that have been granted a photocopy license by the CCC, a separate system of payment has been arranged.

Trademark Notice: Product or corporate names may be trademarks or registered trademarks, and are used only for identification and explanation without intent to infringe.

Publisher's Note
The publisher has gone to great lengths to ensure the quality of this reprint but points out that some imperfections in the original copies may be apparent.

**Visit the Taylor & Francis Web site at
http://www.taylorandfrancis.com**

**and the CRC Press Web site at
http://www.crcpress.com**

Contents

Editors

Leonhard Held is Professor of Biostatistics at the University of Zurich.

Niel Hens is Professor of Biostatistics at Hasselt University and the University of Antwerp.

Philip O'Neill is Professor of Applied Probability at the University of Nottingham.

Jacco Wallinga is Professor of Mathematical Modelling of Infectious Diseases at the Leiden University Medical Center.

Contributors

Steven Abrams
Center for Statistics
Interuniversity Institute of Biostatistics
and Statistical Bioinformatics
Hasselt University
Hasselt, Belgium

and

Global Health Institute
Department of Epidemiology and
Social Medicine
University of Antwerp
Antwerp, Belgium

Benjamin Allévius
Department of Mathematics
Stockholm University
Stockholm, Sweden

Daniela De Angelis
MRC Biostatistics Unit
School of Clinical Medicine
University of Cambridge
Cambridge, United Kingdom

and

Statistics, Modelling and Economics
Department
National Infection Service
Public Health England
London, United Kingdom

Marc Baguelin
Department of Infectious Disease
Epidemiology
School of Public Health
Imperial College London

and

Faculty of Epidemiology and Population
Health
London School of Hygiene & Tropical
Medicine
London, United Kingdom

Ottar N. Bjørnstad
Center for Infectious Disease Dynamics
Pennsylvania State University
University Park, Pennsylvania

Maciej F. Boni
Department of Biology
Center for Infectious Disease Dynamics
Pennsylvania State University
University Park, Pennsylvania

Tom Britton
Department of Mathematics
Stockholm University
Stockholm, Sweden

Ewan Cameron
Big Data Institute
Nuffield Department of Medicine
University of Oxford
Oxford, United Kingdom

Caroline Colijn
Department of Mathematics
Simon Fraser University
Burnaby, British Columbia, Canada

Benjamin J. Cowling
School of Public Health
The University of Hong Kong
Hong Kong

Emanuele Del Fava
Carlo F. Dondena Centre for Research on
    Social Dynamics and Public Policy
Bocconi University
Milan, Italy

and

Max Planck Institute for Demographic
    Research
Rostock, Germany

Xavier Didelot
School of Life Sciences
University of Warwick
Coventry, United Kingdom

Peter J. Diggle
Lancaster Medical School
Lancaster University
Lancaster, United Kingdom

and

Health Data Research UK
London, United Kingdom

Tracy Qi Dong
University of Washington
Department of Biostatistics
Seattle, Washington

Susan Hahné
Centre for Infectious Diseases, Epidemiology
    and Surveillance
National Institute for Public Health
    and the Environment (RIVM)
Bilthoven, the Netherlands

M. Elizabeth Halloran
Vaccine and Infectious Disease Division
Fred Hutchinson Cancer Research Center
and
Department of Biostatistics
School of Public Health
University of Washington
Seattle, Washington

Leonhard Held
Epidemiology, Biostatistics and
    Prevention Institute
University of Zurich
Zurich, Switzerland

Niel Hens
Center for Statistics
Interuniversity Institute of Biostatistics
    and Statistical Bioinformatics
Hasselt University
Hasselt, Belgium

and

Centre for Health Economic Research
    and Modelling Infectious Diseases
Vaccine and Infectious Disease Institute
University of Antwerp
and
Epidemiology and Social Medicine
University of Antwerp
Antwerp, Belgium

Michael Höhle
Department of Mathematics
Stockholm University
Stockholm, Sweden

Nicholas P. Jewell
Department of Medical Statistics
London School of Hygiene & Tropical
    Medicine
London, United Kingdom

Jan van de Kassteele
Department of Statistics, Informatics and
    Mathematical Modeling
National Institute for Public Health and the
    Environment (RIVM)
Bilthoven, the Netherlands

Eben Kenah
Division of Biostatistics
College of Public Health
Ohio State University
Columbus, Ohio

Don Klinkenberg
Centre for Infectious Diseases,
    Epidemiology and Surveillance
National Institute for Public Health
    and the Environment (RIVM)
Bilthoven, the Netherlands

Karen A. Krogfelt
Department of Virus and Microbiological
    Special Diagnostics
Statens Serum Institut
Copenhagen, Denmark

and

Department of Science and Environment
Roskilde University
Roskilde, Denmark

Theodore Kypraios
School of Mathematical Sciences
University of Nottingham
Nottingham, United Kingdom

C. Jessica E. Metcalf
Department of Ecology and Evolutionary
    Biology
Princeton University
Princeton, New Jersey

Sebastian Meyer
Institute of Medical Informatics, Biometry,
    and Epidemiology
Friedrich-Alexander-Universität
    Erlangen-Nürnberg
Erlangen, Germany

Vladimir N. Minin
Department of Statistics
University of California
Irvine, California

Kåre Mølbak
Division of Infectious Diseases Preparedness
Statens Serum Institut

and

Department of Veterinary and Animal
    Sciences
Faculty of Health and Medical Sciences
University of Copenhagen
Copenhagen, Denmark

Peter J. Neal
Department of Mathematics and Statistics
Lancaster University
Lancaster, United Kingdom

Angela Noufaily
Warwick Medical School
University of Warwick
Coventry, United Kingdom

Philip D. O'Neill
School of Mathematical Sciences
University of Nottingham
Nottingham, United Kingdom

Richard Pebody
Respiratory Diseases Department
Public Health England
London, United Kingdom

Anne M. Presanis
MRC Biostatistics Unit
School of Clinical Medicine
University of Cambridge
Cambridge, United Kingdom

Ziv Shkedy
Center for Statistics
Interuniversity Institute of Biostatistics
    and Statistical Bioinformatics
Hasselt University
Hasselt, Belgium

Theresa Stocks
Department of Mathematics
Stockholm University
Stockholm, Sweden

Jon Wakefield
University of Washington
Departments of Statistics and Biostatistics
Seattle, Washington

Jacco Wallinga
Department of Biomedical Data Sciences
Leiden University Medical Center
Leiden, the Netherlands

and

Centre for Infectious Diseases, Epidemiology
    and Surveillance
National Institute for Public Health
    and the Environment (RIVM)
Bilthoven, the Netherlands

Laura F. White
School of Public Health
Boston University
Boston, Massachusetts

Amy K. Winter
Johns Hopkins Bloomberg School
    of Public Health
Johns Hopkins University
Baltimore, Maryland

Jessica Y. Wong
School of Public Health
The University of Hong Kong
Hong Kong

Part I

Introduction

1

Introduction

Leonhard Held, Niel Hens, Philip D. O'Neill, and Jacco Wallinga

CONTENTS

1.1 Aims and Scope of This Handbook

The purpose of this handbook is to provide an overview of modern statistical methods which have been developed specifically to analyze infectious disease data. The reader is assumed to have a background in mathematics and statistics, but no specialist knowledge of infectious diseases is assumed. Since the topic of this book is an enormous one, we do not claim to provide a comprehensive coverage of all existing methods. However, we will describe many of the key approaches, and throughout there will be many examples and case studies.

The key approaches are presented here in a series of chapters that each address a specific topic or provide a specific perspective. The chapters serve the complementary purpose of introducing graduate students and others to the field of infectious disease data analysis, acting as a reference for researchers in this field, and helping practicing statisticians and infectious disease epidemiologists to choose an appropriate method to solve a particular infectious disease data problem.

1.2 Historical Development of Infectious Disease Data Analysis

Historically, infectious disease data analysis is one of the oldest areas of statistics, and the work on infectious diseases has resulted in several concepts, methods, and algorithms in the general field of statistics [1, 2].

Infectious disease data analysis dates its origin to 1760 when Daniel Bernoulli presented a paper on smallpox [3]. In his time, it was realized that inoculation of young children with smallpox material protected them against infection with smallpox. But inoculation was a dangerous affair. Bernoulli calculated the long-term benefits of inoculation, in terms of increase in life expectancy when the risk of dying from smallpox would be eliminated. Unfortunately for Bernoulli he was more than 200 years ahead of his time. His approach was criticized by other scientists and had little impact. In retrospect, this work is seen as a pioneering paper in statistics, as it introduced the concept of competing risks in survival analysis. And of course this work is seen as a pioneering paper in the field of infectious disease data analysis as it is among the first publications that use statistical analysis of infectious disease data to assess the effect of infection control.

In 1926, McKendrick published an article entitled "Applications of mathematics to medical problems" which analyzed data on a cholera outbreak. He estimated an infection rate when the observed data do not distinguish between those individuals who were not susceptible to the infection and those who were susceptible but do not develop symptoms [4]. His approach to dealing with this partially observed data was later defined and popularized as the Expectation-Maximization algorithm, an algorithm that often is used in statistics. In 1927, McKendrick, together with Kermack, published an article called "A contribution to the mathematical theory of epidemics" [5]. They introduced theory that captures the transmission of infection. They used this theory to address the conditions that are required for epidemics to occur, the time course of the number of new infections, and the final number of infections that will have occurred when the epidemic is over, and they applied their theory to data on an outbreak of plague in Bombay. Their theoretical approach is very general, and it introduced the standard compartmental models of disease transmission that are still in use today.

Around 1956, Bartlett published a series of papers on the mathematical epidemiology of infectious diseases [6–8]. He focused on counts of measles cases in the Welsh district of Ffestiniog and several other towns in England and Wales, and considered the conditions that are required for measles epidemics to die out, and the conditions that are required for measles to persist. In his work there is a central role for chance events, for stochasticity. He was the first to use computer simulations to help understand the observed patterns in infectious disease epidemics. Bartlett is perhaps best known to statisticians for his work on stochastic processes and his seminal work on estimating power spectra in time series analysis.

Since then, much of the statistical analysis of infectious disease has been geared towards estimating model parameters from infectious disease data. The development of mathematical models of disease transmission is marked by the seminal books "Mathematical Theory of Infectious Diseases" by Bailey [9] and "Infectious diseases of humans: dynamics and control" by Anderson and May [10]. Various books capture further developments in this field, emphasizing stochastic modelling [11], mathematical modelling [12], or public health relevance [13], and including infectious diseases in animal populations [14]. These models are now of interest to a broad range of scientists, and also to policy makers who wish to prevent or control epidemics of infectious diseases. In some countries, the outcome from modelling studies are now a politically acceptable contribution to the decision-making process on public health policy. Examples include the quantitative assessment of the effectiveness of proposed control measures, and the evaluation of the effectiveness of control measures as actually used. Given their role in policy making, it is crucial that these transmission models are informed by the available infectious disease data.

The title of the present handbook echoes the title of the 1989 monograph "Analysis of Infectious Disease Data" by N.G. Becker [15]. This excellent monograph offers mathematical approaches to tackle the difficulties that arise in analyzing infectious disease data. Over the past decades these mathematical approaches have been supplemented by more algorithmic approaches. A factor that has greatly contributed to the increased attention to algorithmic approaches is the advent of substantially greater and accessible computational power. As in many other areas of statistics, analysis of datasets on infectious disease outbreaks now can be performed using computationally intensive statistical methods such as Markov chain Monte Carlo (MCMC) methods (see, e.g., [16–18]).

Taken together, the increased engagement with public health policy and the advent of computationally intensive statistical methods have stimulated an increased enthusiasm for analyzing infectious disease data over the past decades. The increased enthusiasm also has led to a large number of publications on the topic in a wide variety of scientific journals. This handbook aims to bring these modern statistical methods together.

1.3   Infectious Disease Data

What sets infectious disease data apart from other data, and non-infectious disease data in particular, is that the data are usually highly dependent, and usually only partially observed. Here we give brief remarks about these aspects.

Infectious disease data such as daily or weekly numbers of infectious disease counts are dependent, and so any statistical analysis should take this into account. It is possible to fit models containing dependencies, such as multilevel models or time series models. But we know quite a bit about how the dependency comes about: each infection is the result of another infection, which in turn is caused by another infection. This dependency structure can be captured by a model of disease transmission. The appeal of using transmission models is that the resulting model parameter estimates are usually meaningful in an epidemiological or biological sense. This, in turn, provides a motivation for relying on such models to interpret observed epidemics, and to assess proposed control measures for public health policy makers. The focus of the statistical methods described in this handbook is towards understanding the transmission process that generated the data. However, we also discuss methods for outbreak detection and prediction, which may require fitting the data to a more standard statistical model.

Infectious disease data are partial in the sense that the actual events of infection, and the moments of transmission, are not observed. This situation is almost invariably the case for human infectious diseases, when the onset of symptoms is usually the first sign that an individual has been infected. Even in situations where there are frequent diagnostic tests, uncertainty about the precise moment of transmission remains. There are other senses in which the data are partial: infected individuals are not included in a dataset because they did not show typical symptoms, or they did not seek medical attention, or they were simply not reported. A related issue is that the population of susceptibles at risk of infection may not be known precisely, both in the sense that some individuals might have prior immunity due to vaccination or previous exposure to infection, that some individuals might not have been exposed to infection, or in the sense that individuals who enter or leave the study population were not recorded. In addition to these issues, there might be uncertainty about the diagnosis. An infected individual may not meet the strict case definition, and a diagnostic test for infection or past infection may produce equivocal results. In a statistical analysis of infectious disease data, the partial availability of observations should be taken into account.

1.4   The Structure of This Handbook

1.4.1   Basic concepts

Part II of this handbook will briefly introduce the reader to basic concepts of infectious disease data analysis. Here we focus on the dynamics of the number of infections in a population, and the resulting dependency structure of the observations. There is a similar focus on dependency structures in the fields of demography (the dynamics of number of human individuals in a population) and population biology (the dynamics of the number of organisms in a population). To some extent, we may characterize infectious disease dynamics as the population biology of pathogens [19]. As a consequence, several of the basic concepts in infectious disease data analysis are entirely standard within the field of epidemiology, and some other basic concepts are shared with the fields of population biology and demography.

Rather than introducing concepts chapter by chapter, we will provide in each chapter a different perspective on the same basic concepts. First, we take a biological perspective to see how the dependencies in the data arise. We provide an epidemiological background on the infectious disease data, how they are collected, and typical data types and data structures. We introduce the key variables in infectious disease analysis that are familiar from statistical epidemiology, such as incidence, prevalence, and hazard rates. We introduce the key variables in infectious disease data analysis that are familiar from demography and population biology, such as the reproduction number, the generation interval, contact rates, the epidemiological growth rate, and the required control effort. Once these concepts are in place, we offer a basic outline of the epidemic models that describe the dependency structure inherent to the infectious disease data. Throughout, the objective of Part II is to reveal the coherence of the basic concepts.

1.4.2   Analysis of outbreak data

Part III of this handbook is concerned with outbreak data, i.e., data that are collected during a specific outbreak of infectious disease. Such data typically consist of times at which cases are detected and also may feature covariate information such as the age, location, or vaccination status of each case. An appealing aspect of outbreak data is the level of detail typically present, with a clear focus on a particular population of individuals. This aspect, in turn, provides an opportunity for relatively detailed modelling. Conversely, the specific nature of any one outbreak can make it hard to generalize the results of any analysis to a broader context.

The focus of Part III is on fitting stochastic models of disease transmission to the data at hand. Historically, several approaches have been taken, many of which are described in [9] and [15], some of which we now briefly recall. First, in simple situations it may be possible to calculate the likelihood of the observed data directly, from which maximum likelihood estimates can be obtained, usually by numerical optimization. Examples include data from household studies, where population sizes are small and there are relatively few possible outcomes to consider. Second, models that are Markov processes are often amenable to analysis, which can make it possible to compute the likelihood of a partially observed outbreak. Third, models can contain simplifying assumptions to make analysis possible, one example being the assumption that individuals are infected at a fixed non-random time period before they are detected as cases. Fourth, martingale methods can be used to analyze some Markov models, the key idea being to construct suitable martingales from which estimating equations can be derived.

Although such historical approaches remain valid and useful in many situations, there are three limitations that often apply to these methods. The first limitation is that they usually are not easy to adapt to situations involving missing data, particularly if the underlying transmission model is not simplistic. This fact is relevant because, as mentioned, transmission is rarely observed in infectious disease outbreaks. The second limitation is that several of the methods implicitly require Markov process epidemic models. This limitation is a practical drawback, since many real-life infectious diseases do not adhere to the assumptions of Markov processes, such as the appearance of exponentially distributed times between events. The final limitation is that the methods are rarely useful in a Bayesian setting.

The methods we describe in Part III of the book make progress in addressing all of these limitations. As might be anticipated, they typically require intensive computation, and many of the methods have arisen as a direct consequence of the advances in computational statistics, particularly in the Bayesian framework, since the early 1990s.

1.4.3 Analysis of seroprevalence data

In the past few decades population immunity has been assessed primarily based on cross-sectional serosurvey collections. This approach has been shown to be a particular useful for those pathogens for which the antibody test (e.g., ELISA) correlates well with the level of immunity.

Next to monitoring the immune status of populations, although to a lesser extent, serological serosurveys have been used to inform transmission modeling studies in pre-vaccination and post-vaccination settings. One typically relies on assumptions of time homogeneity to estimate key parameters such as the reproduction number from a single cross-sectional serosurvey in pre-vaccination settings, whereas in post-vaccination settings, or more generally in time-heterogeneous settings [20], a single cross-sectional serosurvey only provides a snapshot of the immune status of the population and therefore is typically only used to validate models. To truly inform transmission modelling studies repeated cross-sectional serosurveys are needed, the use of which has gained noticeable attention in the past decade, i.e., following the A(H1N1)v2009 pandemic. Whereas it is apparent that there are still major methodological gaps to be filled in, there has been a considerable development in both the methods used and the range of questions that can be asked from such data including estimating loss of immunity over time for which the best source of information are longitudinal studies that are, however, rare and challenging to implement over a suitable time period.

Given that serological surveys provide the most direct measurement to define the landscape of population immunity, setting up a systematic collection of serum banks combined with targeted testing would fill in an important gap to better understand and control infectious diseases at both national and global levels [21]. Whereas countries would greatly benefit from such a system, even at the national level, systematically collecting data from serosurveys is rarely done. One of the reasons, aside budgetary and logistic constraints, might be the lack of widespread methodology to design and analyze such data. We hope that the contributions in Part IV of this book will contribute to filling in this gap and eventually will help in establishing serosurveillance as a standard surveillance apparatus.

1.4.4 Analysis of surveillance data

The continuous collection, examination, and analysis of infectious disease data is often called surveillance. Many countries have implemented surveillance systems for a number of notifiable diseases. A typical task of such surveillance systems is to detect sudden increases in incidence. Clustering of infectious diseases may occur in time but also in space [2].

Surveillance data usually are reported as the number of new cases in a particular region and time interval, usually weeks or days. Additional stratification by age group and gender is also quite common. Individual information on cases is usually rare, in particular for humans where data protection plays an important role.

Many authors have discussed the shortcomings of surveillance data, [1, 22]. Typical problems include reporting delays, underreporting, and errors in diagnosis. However, surveillance systems have improved considerably in recent years. Electronic reporting, today the standard in such systems, had a clear impact on the reduction of reporting delays. Furthermore, currently many surveillance systems are based on lab-confirmed and not just symptomatic cases, increasing drastically the sensitivity. However, problems still remain in the temporal and particular spatial resolution, where usually the administrative area of residence is taken is a proxy for the spatial location of case, even if the case may have been infected elsewhere and was perhaps traveling across different areas during the time of infection. Furthermore [1] points out that public health control actions, such as vaccination or school closures, are rarely taken into account in the analysis of surveillance data.

The statistical analysis of surveillance data dates back to traditional methods for the identification of cluster in space and space-time and simple time series methods. However, advanced statistical modelling makes it possible to analyze the spread of infectious diseases across space and time in a more detailed fashion. Control actions can be taken into account as explanatory variables and predictions of future disease incidence can be derived, which then may be used to implement appropriate public health response. Furthermore, modern statistical methods can be used to integrate different sources of surveillance data to ensure timely delivery of real-time epidemic assessments. In Part V of this handbook we aim to describe the current state-of-the-art in the analysis of surveillance data.

1.5   Outlook

Infectious disease data analysis is a highly active and fast growing field of research. Over the past decades, we have seen several new types of data being introduced. These data range from social contact data to biomarkers for susceptibility to infection, and from the genetic sequence of a pathogen in an infected individual to serological panels that test for a range of specific antibodies in a single blood sample. Furthermore, there is a strong push to digitize large historical datasets and make datasets that have been collected with public funding available to the research community. The public health relevance of infectious disease data analysis provides a strong push to offer reliable statistical analyses of data as fast as possible, even as data collection is ongoing during an outbreak. The linkage of data from electronic surveillance systems makes it possible to have larger and more detailed data than before. We believe this collective push will shift the field of infectious disease data analysis.

What direction will the field of infectious disease analysis take in the future? We hope to provide the readers with a sufficient background to explore any direction they like, and with a necessary background to overcome the challenges along the way.

References

[1] Klaus Dietz. Biometric advances in infectious disease epidemiology. In Peter Armitage and Herbert A. David, eds., *Advances in Biometry*, pp. 319–338. John Wiley & Sons, New York, 1996.

[2] C. Paddy Farrington. Communicable diseases. In *Encyclopedia of Biostatistics*, pp. 995–1017. John Wiley & Sons, Chichester, UK, 2nd ed., 2005.

[3] Daniel Bernoulli. Essai d'une nouvelle analyse de la mortalité causée par la petite vérole, et des avantages de l'inoculation pour la prévenir. *Histoire de l'Acad., Roy. Sci.(Paris) avec Mem*, 1–45, 1760.

[4] Anderson G McKendrick. Applications of mathematics to medical problems. *Proceedings of the Edinburgh Mathematical Society*, 44(834):98–130, 1926.

[5] William Ogilvy Kermack and Anderson G McKendrick. A contribution to the mathematical theory of epidemics. *Proceedings of the Royal Society of London A*, 115(834):700–721, 1927.

[6] Maurice S Bartlett. Measles periodicity and community size. *Journal of the Royal Statistical Society. Series A (General)*, 120(1):48–70, 1957.

[7] Maurice S Bartlett. Deterministic and stochastic models for recurrent epidemics. In *Proceedings of the Third Berkeley Symposium on Mathematical Statistics and Probability*, University of California Press, Berkeley, CA, vol. 4, p. 109, 1956.

[8] MS Bartlett. Monte Carlo studies in ecology and epidemiology. In *Proceedings of the Fourth Berkeley Symposium on Mathematical Statistics and Probability*, University of California Press, London, UK, vol. 4, pp. 39–55, 1961.

[9] Norman TJ Bailey. *The Mathematical Theory of Infectious Diseases and its Applications*. Charles Griffin & Company Ltd, New York, 1975.

[10] Roy M Anderson and Robert M May. *Infectious Diseases of Humans: Dynamics and Control*. Oxford University Press, Oxford, UK, 1992.

[11] Daryl J Daley and Joe Gani. *Epidemic Modelling: An Introduction*. Cambridge University Press, Cambridge, UK, 1999.

[12] Odo Diekmann, Hans Heesterbeek, and Tom Britton. *Mathematical Tools for Understanding Infectious Disease Dynamics*. Princeton University Press, Princeton, NJ, 2012.

[13] Emilia Vynnycky and Richard White. *An Introduction to Infectious Disease Modelling*. Oxford University Press, Oxford, UK, 2010.

[14] Matt J Keeling and Pejman Rohani. *Modeling Infectious Diseases in Humans and Animals*. Princeton University Press, Princeton, NJ, 2008.

[15] Niels G Becker. *Analysis of Infectious Disease Data, volume 33 of Monographs on Statistics and Applied Probability*. Chapman & Hall, London, UK, 1989.

[16] Kari Auranen, Elja Arjas, Tuija Leino, and Aino K Takala. Transmission of pneumo-coccal carriage in families: A latent Markov process model for binary longitudinal data. *Journal of the American Statistical Association*, 95(452):1044–1053, 2000.

[17] Gavin J Gibson and Eric Renshaw. Estimating parameters in stochastic compartmental models using Markov chain methods. *Mathematical Medicine and Biology: A Journal of the IMA*, 15(1):19–40, 1998.

[18] Philip D O'Neill and Gareth O Roberts. Bayesian inference for partially observed stochastic epidemics. *Journal of the Royal Statistical Society: Series A (Statistics in Society)*, 162(1):121–129, 1999.

[19] Roy M Anderson and Robert M May. Population biology of infectious diseases: Part I. *Nature*, 280(5721):361, 1979.

[20] Niel Hens, Ziv Shkedy, Marc Aerts, Christel Faes, Pierre Van Damme, and Philippe Beutels. *Modeling Infectious Disease Parameters Based on Serological and Social Contact Data: A Modern Statistical Perspective*. Springer, New York, 2012.

[21] C Jessica E Metcalf, Jeremy Farrar, Felicity T Cutts, Nicole E Basta, Andrea L Graham, Justin Lessler, Neil M Ferguson, Donald S Burke, and Bryan T Grenfell. Use of serological surveys to generate key insights into the changing global landscape of infectious disease. *The Lancet*, 388(10045):728–730, 2016.

[22] Johan Giesecke. *Modern Infectious Disease Epidemiology*. Hodder Arnold, London, UK, 2nd ed., 2002.

Part II

Basic Concepts

2

Population Dynamics of Pathogens

Ottar N. Bjørnstad

CONTENTS

2.1 Introduction

Population dynamics of pathogens is the description of how incidence of infectious agents varies in space and time, and the host and pathogen factors responsible for this variation. "Pathogens" is a catch-all term for small, typically the size of a single cell or smaller, organisms with a parasitic life-style that cause sickness and/or death of its host and requires onwards transmission for continued persistence. Some pathogens — the "directly transmitted" — achieve this by moving directly from host to host without any specialized transmission stages, either via a respiratory, fecal-oral, or sexual route. Others — the "vector-borne" — have complicated life-cycles involving biting arthropods to complete the infection cycle. Pathogens further differ with respect to host tropism. Some appear only able to infect a single host species while others have a wide host range [1]. Given that parasitism is arguably the most common consumer strategy across the tree of life [2], pathogen population ecology is a vast area of study. Moreover, because of the great importance of pathogens in history, economics, food production, public health, and human/animal well-being, students of this topic use tools from a variety of disciplines including statistics and mathematics. The purpose of this chapter is to give an introduction to the diverse dynamics of infectious disease agents and visit on some of the mathematical and statistical methods used to characterize and understand these. Much of what is sampled here is the detailed focus of other chapters in this handbook.

2.2 Patterns of Endemicity

Pathogens — regardless of taxonomic grouping: bacterial, protozoan, fungal, or viral — show an extremely diverse range of dynamic interaction within the host and, as a consequence, at the population level. Some, like human immunodeficiency virus (HIV), hepatitis B, and various herpes viruses, cause persistent infections. Others, like influenza, measles, and pertussis, cause transient infection followed by clearance. Of such acute infections, some leave life-long immunity upon recovery such as the various vaccine-preventable childhood infections. Others are non-immunizing, or provide transient immunity. Immune-evasion may be due to rapid evolution; the influenza A virus, for example, evolves by mutation and recombination at a rate where past immunity is typically not effective for more than 5 years or so [3, 4]. Others, like the bacteria that cause gonorrhea (*Neisseria gonorrhea*) or some of the protozoans responsible for malaria (e.g., *Plasmodium falciparum*), evade past immunity by having very wide "antigenic repertoires": an ability to express a wide range of similarly functioning surface proteins that are antigenically distinct, and thus not cross-reactive from infection cycle to infection cycle [5, 6]. It turns out these in-host subtleties are critical determinants of population-level patterns of disease dynamics because of the way they shape the pathogens' "Susceptible-Infected" (SI) compartmental flows (i.e., how hosts move between the susceptible, infected and removed classes).

Compartmental models are the bread-and-butter for modeling directly transmitted infections [7]. The simplifying idea is that a host population may be thought of as consisting of individuals that can be classified according to their infection status such as Susceptible, Exposed (infected, but not yet infectious), Infectious and Removed (recovered with immunity or dead), or some variation on this theme, giving rise to some version of the SEIR (Susceptible-Exposed-Infectious-Recovered) model:

$$\frac{dS}{dt} = \mu(N - S) - \frac{\beta I S}{N} + \omega R, \qquad (2.1)$$

$$\frac{dE}{dt} = \frac{\beta I S}{N} - (\mu + \sigma)E, \qquad (2.2)$$

$$\frac{dI}{dt} = \sigma E - (\mu + \gamma)I, \qquad (2.3)$$

$$\frac{dR}{dt} = \gamma I - (\mu + \omega)R. \qquad (2.4)$$

In the above incarnation μ is the birth/death rate, β is the transmission rate, $1/\omega$ is the average duration of immunity, $1/\sigma$ is the average latent period, and $1/\gamma$ is the average infectious period. The logic of the transmission term is that β is the contact rate among hosts times the probability of infection given a contact. The I infectious individuals in the population will by assumption contact some random number of other individuals, a fraction $s = S/N$ of which will be susceptible (or equivalently the S susceptibles will contact some number of individuals a fraction I/N of which will be infectious).

The literature on compartmental models in epidemiology is vast, and cannot fully be retold in a chapter. We can, however, use this simple model to illustrate how the different in-host dynamics lead to contrasting patterns at the population level. We use the deSolve-package in R to integrate the differential equations assuming (i) a persistent infection ($\gamma = 0$; SI dynamics), (ii) recovery leads to sterilizing immunity ($\omega = 0$; SIR dynamics), (iii) there is no immunity ($\omega = \infty$; in the below we instead use a large number; SIS dynamics), or (iv) immunity is transient (SIRS dynamics). The following R-code defines the "gradient-functions" for the system of ordinary differential equations (ODEs) and numerically integrates them to generate Figure 2.1.

```
> seirmod=function(t, y, parms){
+    S=y[1]
+    E=y[2]
+    I=y[3]
+    R=y[4]
+
+    with(as.list(parms),{
+    dS = mu * (N  - S)  - beta * S * I / N + omega*R
+    dE = beta * S * I / N - (mu + sigma) * E
+    dI = sigma * E - (mu + gamma) * I
+    dR = gamma * I - mu * R - omega*R
+    res=c(dS, dE, dI, dR)
+    list(res)
+    })
+    }

> require(deSolve)
> times  = seq(0, 10, by=1/52)
> start = c(S=0.999, E=0, I=0.001, R = 0)
> paras1  = c(mu = 1/10, N = 1, beta =  500, sigma = 365/8,
+             gamma = 0, omega=0)
> si = as.data.frame(ode(start, times, seirmod, paras1))
> plot(si$time, si$I, type="l", log="y", ylim=c(1E-5, 1),
+     ylab="prevalence", xlab="year")
> paras2  = c(mu = 1/10, N = 1, beta =  500, sigma = 365/8,
+             gamma = 365/5, omega=0)
> sir = as.data.frame(ode(start, times, seirmod, paras2))
> lines(sir$time, sir$I, type="l", col=2)
> paras3  = c(mu = 1/10, N = 1, beta =  500, sigma = 365/8,
+             gamma = 365/5, omega=100)
> sis = as.data.frame(ode(start, times, seirmod, paras3))
> lines(sis$time, sis$I, type="l", col=3)
> paras4  = c(mu = 1/10, N = 1, beta =  500, sigma = 365/8,
+             gamma = 365/5, omega=2)
> sirs = as.data.frame(ode(start, times, seirmod, paras4))
> lines(sirs$time, sirs$I, type="l", col=4)
> legend("bottomright", c("SI", "SIR", "SIS", "SIRS"),
          col=c(1,2,3,4), lty=rep(1, 4))
```

The SI-flow model yields several important insights: (i) Persistent infections are predicted to exhibit "stable endemism" and may reach very high prevalence. A number of lesser known chronic herpes viruses, for example, are estimated to infected upward of 90 percent of all humans [8]. (ii) Fully immunizing infections have a propensity for exhibiting recurrent epidemics (though they will not be sustained in the absence of some form of external forcing; see section on Seasonality below). Moreover, the "virgin" epidemic (the invasion) wave can be very violent, and followed by such deep post-epidemic troughs that the chain-of-transmission can easily break. (iii) Acute non-immunizing infections, in contrast, are predicted to show a pattern of stable endemicity around their epidemic equilibria. The contrasting predictions are borne out in the reported incidence of measles and gonorrhea in,

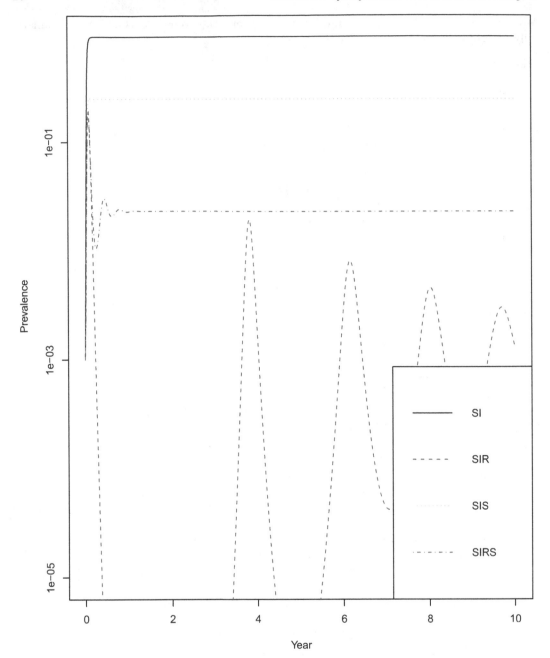

FIGURE 2.1
Predicted invasion dynamics of pathogens governed by SI, SIR, SIS, and SIRS-like flows.

for example, Pennsylvania (Figure 2.2). Measles shows violent recurrent epidemics, with an almost 10,000-fold difference in incidence between peak and trough week, characteristic of the SIR flow. Gonorrhea shows fuzzy variability around a slowly drifting endemic equilibrium characteristic of pathogens with SIS flow.

There is, however, a "problem of persistence" for highly transmissible, acute, immunizing infection [9, 10]. They can invade a susceptible host population quickly, but the

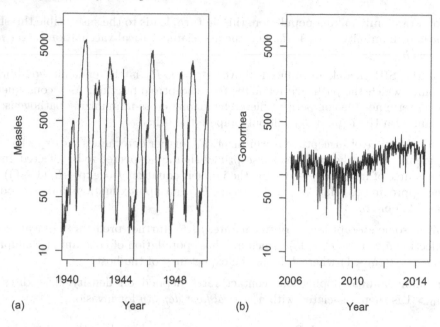

FIGURE 2.2
Reported weekly incidence of (a) measles (with a SIR-like flow) and (b) gonnorhea (with a SIS-like flow) in Pennsylvania.

post-epidemic troughs are very deep so the chain of transmission may easily break in all but very large host populations. Measles, for example, requires the recruitment of somewhere between 100 and 200 susceptibles every week for sustained transmission, leading to Bartlett's [11] classic observation of a *critical community size* for measles of some 250,000–500,000 people. Similarly, phocine distemper virus (the "measles of seals") invaded harbor seals along the Northern European coastline twice, in 1988 and 2002 [12, 13]. The virus caused havoc in both instances killing around half of all the seals, and probably infecting more than 90 percent, only to go regionally extinct after less than a year of circulation.[1]

2.3 Reproductive Ratio

The basic reproductive ratio, R_0, of a pathogen — by definition the expected number of secondary cases from an average primary case in a completely susceptible population — is such a central quantity, it deserves its own section in any chapter on pathogen population dynamics. The literature on R_0 is enormous, so here, I will just enumerate a handful of important theoretical results pertaining to the dynamics of immunizing infectious diseases in randomly mixing host populations.

- Most celebrated is the threshold quantity $R_0 > 1$ which determines whether a pathogen can invade a host population.

---

[1] Evidence suggest a reservoir for the virus is the much larger harp seal populations in the high arctic [12].

- For a randomly mixing population, this, in turn, leads to the susceptible threshold for herd immunity, $s^* = 1/R_0$, and the associated critical vaccination target $p_c = 1 - 1/R_0$.

- For the SIR model, introduced above, $s^* = 1/R_0$ is the endemic equilibrium around which the pathogen regulates the susceptible fraction. As a consequence, R_0 determines the competitive hierarchy among cross-immunizing pathogens; the strain with the highest R_0 will outcompete the others.

- In the absence of susceptible recruitment, R_0 further determines the expected final epidemic size — the fraction of susceptibles that are expected to be infected during the course of infection — given by the implicit equation $f = \exp(-R_0(1-f))$ and the approximate relation $f \simeq 1 - \exp(-R_0)$, an approximation that is good for $R_0 > 2.5$ or so.

- Given some susceptible recruitment rate, μ, R_0 further predicts the mean age of infection $\bar{a} \simeq 1/(\mu(R_0 - 1))$, which in a host population of constant size simplifies to $\bar{a} \simeq L/(R_0 - 1)$ where L is the life expectancy of the host.

- In many animal populations contact rates depend on density. The threshold $R_0 > 1$ is then associated with a *critical host density* for invasion.[2]

Because of the importance of R_0, a number of approaches and methods have been proposed for its quantification.[3] For the lack of a better classification, we may roughly think of them as (i) "analytical," (ii) "initially exponential," and (iii) "more elaborate." The analytical uses an appropriate mathematical model with best bet parameters to calculate the expected number of secondary cases. For example, for a pathogen approximated by the SEIR flow, the expected number of secondary cases is the probability of becoming infectious following infection times the average infectious period times transmission rate assuming all N individuals are susceptible. From eqs. 2.1 through 2.4 (assuming $\omega = 0$) we get $R_0 = (\sigma/(\sigma + \mu)) \times (1/(\gamma + \mu)) \times \beta N/N = \frac{\sigma}{\sigma+\mu}\frac{\beta}{\gamma+\mu}$. With known latent period $(1/\sigma)$, infectious period $(1/\gamma)$, and birth rate (μ) we can thus calculate R_0 for a range of relevant transmission rates.

The "initially exponential" method arise from the observation that initially during invasion into a susceptible host population the infection will spread exponentially at a rate $(R_0 - 1)/\tau$, where τ is the serial interval. The serial interval is the time taken for the secondary cases to be infected once the primary case is infected (see Chapter 5). The epidemic is thus initially expected to double after $\tau \log(2)/(R_0 - 1)$ time units. Hence, if a pathogen with a mean serial interval of 10 days doubles in 3 weeks, R_0 is estimated to be 1.3. Alternatively we can regress log(cumulative incidence) on time to estimate the rate of exponential increase by the slope, ρ, and calculate $R_0 = \tau\rho + 1$ or some version thereoff [14]. The "initial exponential" approach is detailed in Chapter 5.

As an example of the "more elaborate" models, we can use Ferrari et al.'s [15] maximum likelihood removal method for estimating R_0 based on the so-called "chain-binomial" model of infectious disease dynamics. The chain-binomial model, originally proposed by Bailey [16], is a discrete-time, stochastic alternative[4] to the continuous-time, deterministic SIR model discussed previously. In contrast to the S(E)IR models, the chain-binomial assumes that

---

[2] It is worth stressing that the critical host density — estimated around 1 fox / km^2 for rabies [17] and around 20 mice / ha for *Sin nombre* hantavirus — is very different from the previously introduced concept of a critical community size. The former is to do with disease invasion, while the latter is to do with long-term persistence of highly transmissible, immunizing infections.

[3] Or the effective reproductive ratio (R_E); the expected number of secondary cases in a partially immune population, $R_E = sR_0$, where s is the fraction of the population that is susceptible.

[4] This model also forms the foundation for the TSIR model [18, 19] which will be discussed below.

an epidemic is formed from a succession of discrete generations of infectious individuals in a coin-flip fashion. Just like in the SIR model, we assume that infectious individuals exert a force of infection on susceptibles, $\beta I/N$. In a generation, t, of duration given by the serial interval (which we use as the basic time unit), the probability that any given susceptible will escape any infectious contacts will be $exp(-\beta I/N)$. The converse outcome will happen with a probability $1 - exp(-\beta I/N)$. Thus, if there are S_t susceptibles, we expect $S_t(1 - \exp(-\beta I_t/N))$ new infecteds in generation $t+1$. Since we assume that contacts happen at random, the simple stochastic chain-binomial model is

$$I_{t+1} \sim \text{Binomial}(S_t, 1 - \exp(-\beta I_t/N)),$$

$$S_{t+1} = S_t - I_{t+1} = S_0 - \sum_{i=1}^{t} I_i. \qquad (2.5)$$

If we ignore observational error, we have two unknown parameters: the initial number of susceptibles, S_0, and the transmission rate, β. The reproductive ratio is a composite of these two $R = S_0(1 - \exp(-\beta/N))$, which for large populations is approximately $\beta S_0/N$. Thus β is approximately the (effective) reproductive ratio at the beginning of the epidemic. The removal method estimates β and S_0 from a sequence of binomial likelihoods.

We can employ a standard recipe for doing a maximum likelihood analysis (see [20] for an excellent ecological discussion of this). The first step is to write a function for the likelihood. Conditional on some parameters, the function returns the negative log-likelihood of observing the data given the model. The R function to calculate a binomial likelihood is dbinom. We can thus define a likelihood-function for the chain-binomial model:[5]

```
> llik.cb = function(S0,beta,I){
+     n = length(I)
+     S = floor(S0-cumsum(I[-n]))
+     p = 1-exp(-beta*(I[-n])/S0)
+     L = -sum(dbinom(I[-1],S,p,log=TRUE))
+     return(L)
+ }
```

For illustration consider the data from reporting center 1 in Niamey, Niger, from the 2003 outbreak of measles [21] aggregated in 2-week intervals (crudely the serial interval of measles).

```
> niamey=c(22,27,64,84,116,172,173,651,786,1041,842,903,745, 211,
           83, 11)
```

There were 5931 cases during the epidemics, so S_0 needs to be at least that number. We minimize the negative log-likelihood using the mle2-function in the bbmle-package [20] to find maximum likelihood estimates and confidence intervals.

```
> require(bbmle)
> fit=mle2(llik.cb, start=list(S0=7085, beta=2.3),
+          method="Nelder-Mead",data = list(I = niamey))
> summary(fit)
```

Maximum likelihood estimation

---

[5] We use the floor-function for the vector of S's because dbinom requires the denominator and numerator to be integers. The [-x] subsetting in R means "drop the x'th observation"; thus the [-n] and [-1] makes sure that adjacent pairs of observations are aligned correctly.

```
Call:
mle2(minuslogl = llik.cb, start = list(S0 = 7085, beta = 2.3),
    method = "Nelder-Mead", data = list(I = niamey))

Coefficients:
        Estimate Std. Error z value      Pr(z)
S0    7.6920e+03 1.1887e+02  64.711 < 2.2e-16 ***
beta  1.9116e+00 3.7077e-02  51.557 < 2.2e-16 ***
---
Signif. codes:
0 *** 0.001 ** 0.01 * 0.05 . 0.1   1


-2 log L: 871.6747

> confint(fit)

            2.5 %      97.5 %
S0    7473.590563 7943.63539
beta     1.839656    1.98491
```

So the joint maximum likelihood estimate (MLE) estimates are $S_0 = 7692$ (CI: 7473, 7943) and $\beta = 1.91$ (CI: 1.83, 1.98). In this case, β is an estimate of the *effective* reproductive ratio because of pre-existing immunity due to vaccination and previous outbreaks.

There are some benefits to using the "more elaborate" models. In addition to providing statistical power and confidence intervals, they can provide a closer link between "patterns" and "process." For example, the chain-binomial which forms the basis of the R_0 removal estimator is also a model (albeit a relatively simple one) for stochastic disease dynamics. The stochastic simulator is the probabilistic mirror of the likelihood:

```
> sim.cb=function(S0, beta, I0){
+ I=I0
+ S=S0
+ i=1
+ while(!any(I==0)){
+ i=i+1
+ I[i]=rbinom(1, size=S[i-1], prob=1-exp(-beta*I[i-1]/S0))
+ S[i]=S[i-1]-I[i]
+ }
+ out=data.frame(S=S, I=I)
+ return(out)
+ }
```

To illustrate this concept, we can superimpose 100 stochastic chain-binomial simulations on the observed epidemic (Figure 2.3).

```
> plot(niamey, type="n", xlim=c(1,18),
+       ylab="Observed and simulated", xlab="Generation")
> for(i in 1:100){
+ sim=sim.cb(S0=floor(coef(fit)["S0"]),
+            beta=coef(fit)["beta"], I0=8)
+ lines(sim$I, col=grey(.5))
+ }
> points(niamey, type="b", lwd=2)
```

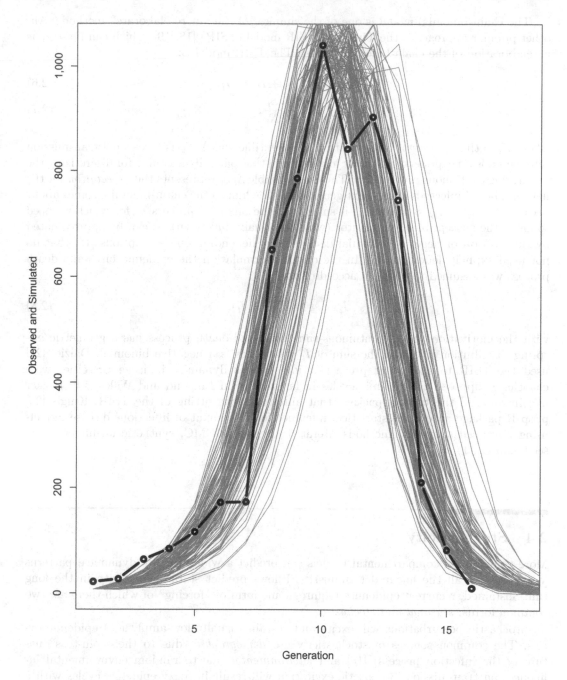

FIGURE 2.3
Observed (black) and 100 simulated (grey) epidemics using the chain-binomial model and
mle-parameters for S_0 and β from Niamey's district 1 data.

The chain-binomial model is one of the simplest of the "more elaborate" methods. Another popular approach is the Time series SIR model (TSIR) [18, 19], which can be seen as an elaboration of the chain-binomial model. The TSIR model is:

$$S_{t+1} = S_t + B_t - I_t, \qquad (2.6)$$

$$\lambda_{t+1} = \beta_u \frac{S_t}{N_t} I_t^\alpha \qquad (2.7)$$

where B_t is the number of births (into the susceptible class), β_u is a seasonal transmission rate, and α is an exponent (normally just under 1) that partially accounts for discretizing the underlying continuous process [22]. The final variable λ_{t+1} represents the *expectation* for the new number of infecteds in the next generation. The link to the chain-binomial comes about because $1 - exp(-\phi) \approx \phi$, when ϕ is small, and the binomial process — for which we need to know the susceptible denominator (which is usually unknown) — can be approximated by the Poisson or negative binomial distributions depending on assumptions [18] that do not need explicit denominators. In the original formulation the epidemic birth-and-death process was assumed to play out according to:

$$I_{t+1} \sim \text{NegBin}(\lambda, I_t), \qquad (2.8)$$

with the motivation that a continuous-time birth-and-death process has a geometric off-spring distribution [23], and the sum of I_t geometrics is a negative binomial. Dalziel [24] used the TSIR to show that prevaccination measles dynamics in large US cities were chaotic, as opposed to the limit cycles in large cities in England and Wales [14]. Becker [25] introduced the `tsiR` R-package that automates the fitting of the TSIR. King's [26] `pomp` R package automates statistical inference for the gamut of infectious disease models using advanced statistical methods (iterated filtering, MCMC, synthetic likelihoods, etc; see Chapter 11).

2.4   Stochasticity

More complicated compartmental models can predict a wide range of dynamical patterns [e.g., 27], but all the linear deterministic SI-flows predict stable endemicity in the long run. Sustained, recurrent epidemics requires some form of "forcing" of which there are two common forms: *seasonal* and *stochastic*.

Stochastic perturbations will excite and sustain (usually low-amplitude) epidemic cycles. The common sources of stochasticity are *demographic* (due to the "coin-toss" nature of the infection process) [16] and *environmental* due to random environmental influences on transmission. Stochastic excitation will result in fuzzy epidemic cycles with a frequency related to the damping period of the underlying epidemic clockwork. Thus, the period will depend on properties of the pathogen and host. For example, for the SIRS model sometimes used to model influenza dynamics [3], the period is approximately [7] $4\pi/\sqrt{(4(R_0 - 1)/(G_I G_R) - ((1/G_R) - (1/A))^2)}$, where A is the mean age of infection, G_I is the infectious period $(1/\gamma)$, and G_R is the average duration of immunity $(1/\omega)$.

More generally, the period can be calculated for any particular SI-like flow from the eigenvalues of the Jacobian of the linearized system evaluated at the endemic equilibrium. When the endemic equilibrium is a "focus" (i.e., the transient is dampened oscillations), the dominant eigenvalues will be a pair of complex conjugates, $a \pm bi$, and the damping period is $2\pi/b$. As a practical illustration, we can use the R-language to work through an example for the SIR model:

$$\frac{dS}{dt} = \mu(N - S) - \frac{\beta IS}{N} \tag{2.9}$$

$$\frac{dI}{dt} = \frac{\beta IS}{N} - (\mu + \gamma)I \tag{2.10}$$

$$\frac{dR}{dt} = \gamma I - \mu R, \tag{2.11}$$

The equilibria occur when dS/dt, dI/dt, and dR/dt all equal zero. For simplicity we set $N = 1$ (i.e., model the fraction of the population in each compartment). The disease-free equilibrium is $s^* = 1$, $i^* = 0$, and $r^* = 0$, and the endemic equilibrium is $s^* = (\gamma + \mu)/\beta = 1/R_0$, $i^* = \mu(R_0 - 1)/\beta$, and $r^* = 1 - i^* - s^*$. Thus, for a given set of parameters (e.g., life-expectancy of 50 years, infectious period of 5 days, and $R_0 = 15$), the endemic equilibrium is:

```
> N=1
> gamma=365/5
> beta=1095.3
> mu=1/50
> Istar=mu*(beta/(gamma+mu)-1)/beta
> Sstar=(gamma+mu)/beta
```

where all the rates are per year.

The R-compartment of the SIR model does not affect dynamics. So for this analysis we only need to consider the S and I equations, when we calculate and evaluate the Jacobian. The Jacobian is the matrix of partial derivatives of the gradient-equation with respect to the state variables. The Jacobian is very useful because its eigenvalues describe the dynamical behavior in the vicinity of the equilibrium.

```
>    dS = expression(mu * (1  - S)  - beta * S * I / 1)
>    dI = expression(beta * S * I / 1 - (mu + gamma) * I)
>    j11 = D(dS, "S"); j12 = D(dS, "I")
>    j21 = D(dI, "S"); j22 = D(dI, "I")
```

We define a list of parameters and steady states for the endemic equilibrium, and then piece together the Jacobian matrix:

```
> vals  = list(mu = mu, N = N, beta =  beta, gamma = gamma,
            S=Sstar, I=Istar)
> J=with(vals,
+      matrix(c(eval(j11), eval(j12),
+      eval(j21), eval(j22)),  ncol=2, byrow=T))
> eigen(J, only.values=TRUE)


$values
[1] -0.15+4.519192i -0.15-4.519192i
```

The eigenvalues are a pair of complex conjugates with negative real parts, thus the equilibrium is a stable focus with damping period (in years) of

```
> 2*pi/Im(eigen(J)$values[1])
```

```
[1] 1.390334
```

2.5   Seasonality: Resonance, Dissonance and Exotica

Some level of seasonality is very common in infectious diseases and is usually reflected in seasonal cycles in incidence (even for persistent infections for which prevalence may remain relatively stable[6]) [28]. Influenza is the poster child for seasonality in infection risk in the public eye [e.g., [29]]. Figure 2.4a shows the mean weekly influenza-related deaths in Pennsylvania between 1972 and 1998. The pronounced winter-peaked seasonality of these respiratory viruses are not fully understood, but are thought to be linked to how weather conditions — notably absolute humidity [30] — affect transmissibility of the virus, so the effective reproductive ratio (R_E) only peaks above 1 during winter in temperate regions.

Seasonality arises from a variety of causes depending on the mode of transmission of the pathogen: air-borne (like influenza), vector-borne, or water/food-borne. Lyme's disease, for example, is caused by vector transmitted bacteria in the genus *Borrelia*. Vectors are a variety of tick species whose activity and development is strongly temperature dependent. Figure 2.4b shows the sharply seasonal incidence of human cases of Lyme's in Pennsylvania between 2006 and 2014. Most mosquito-vectored pathogens, such as the *Plasmodium* protozoans causing malaria and dengue virus, also show strong seasonality because of the temperature and precipitation dependence of the vector life cycle. The seasonality of cholera infections, caused by the *Vibrio cholerae*, is possibly the most studied among water-borne pathogens. The seasonality in southeast Asia is caused by rainfall variation associated with the monsoon season [31]. However, less known water-borne diseases like giardiasis caused by amoebae in the genus *Giardia* can also show marked seasonality (Figure 2.4c). Finally, human (or any host) behavior can cause seasonality in exposure. Childhood disease dynamics, for example, are often shaped by "term-time" forcing: increased transmission when schools are open. Weekly average pre-vaccination incidence of measles in Pennsylvania, for instance, collapse as school closes for the summer only to resume robust circulation after the vacation (Figure 2.4d).

Seasonality can be thought of as periodic annual perturbations to the disease dynamics. Complicated dynamics can arise in immunizing infections when the internal periodic clockwork discussed in the previous section is subject to seasonal forcing. The best studied example of this phenomenon is pre-vaccination measles. The SIR-model (eqs. 2.9 through 2.11) in the previous section was parameterized with roughly measles-like parameters to show that in a nonseasonal environment, this pathogen has a propensity to cycle with a roughly 1.4 year period. However, historical transmission was concentrated to school-age children and, thus, subject to strong term-time forcing. Rich data from big cities (above the critical community size) [9] reveal that measles exhibited annual, biennial, or erratic triennial outbreaks [24]. In London (and most large UK cities), for instance, measles exhibited

---

[6] *Prevalence* is the number (or fraction) of infected individuals at a given time, while *incidence* is the number of new case; see Chapter 4.

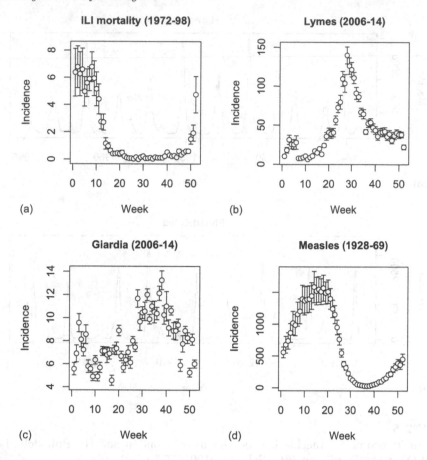

FIGURE 2.4

Mean (± 1 SD) weekly incidence of (a) deaths due to influenza like illness, (b) Lyme's disease, (c) giardiosis, and (d) prevaccination measles in Pennsylvania. (Reprinted from Bjørnstad, O.N., *Epidemics: Models and Data using R.* Springer, Berlin, Germany, 2018.)

annual outbreaks in the late 1940s initiated at the end of each new school year, that gave way to biennial outbreaks with a major outbreak in each odd year and a minor outbreak every even year (Figure 2.5a). In Philadelphia (and many other US cities), in contrast, annual outbreaks were more irregular in amplitude but with a tendency towards a 3-year periodicity (Figure 2.5b). These conspicuous dynamic differences are due to subtle changes in the interaction between the internal clockwork of the disease dynamics and the external term-time forcing.

Seasonally forced epidemics tend to lock onto the period of the forcing function or a multiple thereof. The post–World War II baby boom resulted in a 30 percent increase in birth rates, accelerating the internal clock 2-3 months closer to an annual cycle. Susceptible recruitment was thus sufficient to fuel an epidemic every school year. As the birth rates dropped, this was no longer the case and the system bifurcated to a biennial cycle [19, 33] with odd-year major epidemics throughout England except a small enclave around Norwich with even-year epidemics [34]. With stronger seasonality — for example, due to the comparatively longer summer breaks in USA compared to UK — there may not be

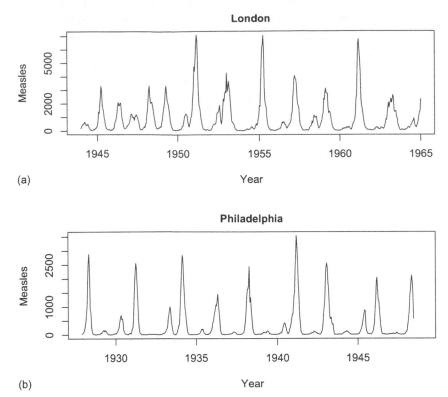

FIGURE 2.5

Biweekly incidence of pre-vaccination measles in (a) London and (b) Philadelphia. (From Dalziel, B.D. et al., *PLoS Comput. Biol.*, 12, e1004655, 2016.)

an easy compromise between the period of the internal clockwork and the external forcing function, giving rise to quasiperiodic chaotic epidemics [24]; the statistical 3-year period being a hallmark of chaos [35].

More elaborate mathematical models of infectious diseases predict a range of more complicated ("exotic") dynamics including chaotic transients ("repellors") [36], "almost attractors" [37] and coexisting attractors with intertwined basins of attraction [27, 33].

Inspired by Rand and Wilson's [36] mathematical analysis, Rohani et al. [38] studied whooping cough dynamics during the transient following introduction of mass-vaccination in UK in 1958. Whooping cough is caused by an airborne bacteria in the genus *Bordetella* that leads to pneumonia. Pre-vaccination, whooping cough was a leading cause of death of children under 5 years and exhibited a variety of dynamics from low-amplitude annual to 3–4 year cycles [39]. Rohani et al. [38] concluded that the post-vaccination multi-annual cycles were most likely due to an unstable "almost attractor". Lavine et al. [40] used a similar approach of combining wavelet time series analysis with mathematical models to study a curious run of violent 3-year cycles in pre-vaccination whooping cough dynamics in Copenhagen; again concluding that the most likely explanation was the coexistence of a low-amplitude annual attractor and high-amplitude cyclic "almost attractors".

2.6 Wavelet Analysis

The classic tool to study periodicity in time series is the periodogram (an estimate of the spectral density of a time series). This method, however, assumes unchanging dynamical patterns over time and is thus not the best method to use for the study of disease dynamics because changes in host demography or vaccine cover (or environmental changes, or pathogen evolution) often lead to changes in dynamic behavior [34]. Wavelet analysis [41] — a method that also estimates the power spectrum of a time series, but allows this spectrum to change over time — has therefore become a popular tool in the study of pathogen dynamics.

The classical ("Schuster") periodogram will automatically estimate the spectrum of a time series (of length T) at the following $T/2$ frequencies: $\{\frac{1}{T}, \frac{2}{T}, \ldots, \frac{T/2}{T}\}$ (or equivalently periods: $\{T, \frac{T}{2}, \ldots, 2\}$ where the time unit of the period is the sampling interval). Wavelets, in contrast, do not have such "canonical" periods for decomposition. If we use the *Morlet* wavelet [which is, for example, provided by the cwt-function of the Rwave package for R [42], we need to specify the periods we wish to consider through specifying the number of octaves, no, and voices, nv. With eight octaves the main periods will be $\{2^1, 2^2, \ldots, 2^8\}$ $= \{2, 4, \ldots, 256\}$. The number of voices specifies how many subdivisions to estimate within each octave. With four voices the resultant periods will be $\{2^1, 2^{1.25}, 2^{1.5}, 2^{1.75}, 2^2, 2^{2.25}, \ldots\}$. Various algorithms have been proposed to identify ridges in a wavelet spectrum. Lavine et al. [40] used the "crazy climber" ridge finding algorithm [42] to identify transitions in dynamics. The practicalities of the Copenhagen whooping cough analysis is as follows (Figure 2.6b):

```
> require(Rwave)
> pertcop = read.csv("pertcop.csv")
> no=8 #set number of octaves
> nv=16 #set number of voices
> #calculate associated periods
> a=2^seq(1, no+1-1/nv, by=1/nv)
> #continous wavelet transform
> wfit=cwt(sqrt(pertcop$cases), no, nv, plot=FALSE)
> wspec = Mod(wfit)
> par(mfrow=c(2,1), mar=c(2,4,2,1))
> layout(matrix(c(1,1,2,2,2), ncol=1))
> plot(as.Date(pertcop$date), pertcop$cases, type="l",
+      ylab="Cases")
> image(x=as.Date(pertcop$date), wspec,
+      col=gray((30:10)/32),
+      y=a/52, ylim=c(0,5), ylab="Period (years)", main="",
+      xlab="Year")
> contour(x=as.Date(pertcop$date), wspec,
+ y=a/52, ylim=c(0,5), zlim=c(0.7, max(wspec)), add=T)
```

The wavelet analysis reveals a burst of power with a 3-year periodicity between 1914 and 1923. Lavine et al. [40] combined this with an analysis of a seasonal compartmental model involving susceptible, infected, immune, waining, and resuceptible individuals and concluded that the dynamics is most consistent with the trajectory transiently following a periodic trajectory that is nearly stable (a periodic "almost attractor") [37].

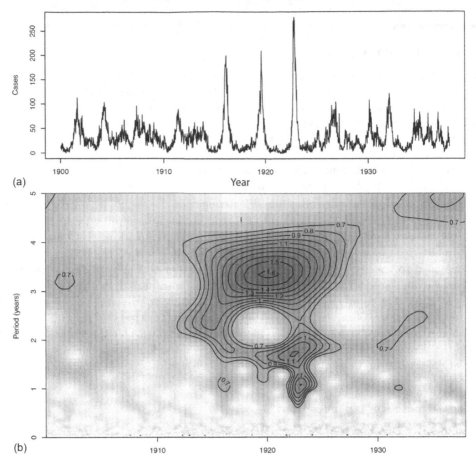

(a)

(b)

FIGURE 2.6

(a) Incidence of pre-vaccination whooping cough in Copenhagen. (b) Wavelet spectrum.
(From Lavine, J.S. et al., *PLoS One*, 8, e72086, 2013.)

2.7   Further Heterogeneities: Age

Despite the apparent success of simple SEIR-like models in capturing the dynamics of
many infections (in big host communities), many host heterogeneities are known to be
critically important for disease dynamics. Woolhouse et al. [43] studied several vector-borne,
water-borne, and sexually transmitted diseases and proposed the "20/80"-rule: 20 percent
of infecteds account for 80 percent of the force of infection (FOI). "Superspreaders" —
individuals that contribute to transmission in a statistically outlying fashion — are known
to be important in the emergence of recent human pathogens such as severe acute respiratory
syndrome (SARS) and HIV [44]. Superspreaders can arise because of host behavior (such
as promiscuity and the spread of sexually transmitted diseases (STDs)) or physiology (such
as asymptomatic, longterm carriage).

Age is an obvious and important heterogeneity shaping transmission for several reasons.
For one, young and old hosts are often more susceptible; The young because immune-
memory has not yet fully built up; The old because of physiological and immunological

senescence. Moreover, contact rates are often age-dependent and age-stratified (see Chapter 6). Mossong et al. [45], for example, carried out a big diary-based study across countries in Europe. They showed that on average school-aged children have contact with almost twice as many other people than pre-school children and 50 percent more than work-age adults. In addition, most contacts are among like-aged people (with a secondary contact ridge along the intergenerational age gap). As a consequence, both susceptibility and exposure of many pathogens are age-structured. The matrix governing contact rates among host groups is called the WAIFW (Who-Aquires-Infection-From-Whom) matrix. The hazard rate (per time unit) at which susceptibles in a particular age-group contracts infection is called the age-specific force of infection (FOI) in mathematical epidemiology. Age-seroprevalence curves — the fraction of individuals that shows evidence of past exposure (and are thus antibody positive) to a particular pathogen — can be important data for estimating the overall FOI in a host population, and also how the FOI is age-stratified. If $\phi(a)$ is the age-specific FOI, then the integrated FOI up to age a is $\int_0^a \phi(a)da$; thus, the probability of not being infected by age a is $\exp(-\int_0^a \phi(a)da)$ and the probability of being infected on or before age a is (see Chapter 4)

$$p(a) = 1 - e^{-\int_0^a \phi(a)da}. \tag{2.12}$$

This is the catalytic model introduced by [46]. In the simplest case, if we assume that the FOI is independent of both age and time, the probability of being infected by age a is $1 - \exp(-\phi a)$, for which we can use a standard generalized linear model ($\texttt{glm}$) framework to work with. Let us assume we test some n_a individuals of each age a and find from serology that i_a individuals have been previously infected. Inferring ϕ from this data is a standard binomial regression problem: $p(a) = 1 - \exp(-\phi a)$ is the expected fraction infected (or seropositive) by age a. Thus $\log(-\log(1 - p(a))) = \log(\phi) + \log(a)$, so we can estimate a constant log-FOI as the intercept from a $\texttt{glm}$ with binomial error, a complimentary log-log link and log-age as a regression "offset".[7] The R call will be of the form

```
> glm(cbind(inf, notinf) ~ offset(log(a)),
+ family=binomial(link="cloglog"))
```

Black [47] carried out a measles antibody study of some 300 people in pre-vaccination Connecticut. The age-seroprevalence profile is typical of pre-vaccination childhood diseases: High seroprevalence of the very young due to the presence of maternal antibodies that wanes through the first year, followed by rapid build-up of immunity to almost 100 percent seroprevalence by age 20 (Figure 2.7). There is perhaps some evidence of loss of immunity in the elderly. We use the binomial regression scheme on the 1–40 year old groups, and compare predicted and observed seroprevalence by age (2.7):

```
> black=read.csv("black.csv")
> b2=black[-c(1,8,9),] #subsetting age brackets
> fit=glm(cbind(pos,neg)~offset(log(mid)),
+           family=binomial(link="cloglog"), data=b2)
> phi=exp(coef(fit))
> curve(1-exp(-phi*x), from=0, to=60, ylab="Seroprevalence",
+           xlab="Age")
> points(black$mid, black$f, pch="*", col="red")
> exp(fit$coef)

(Intercept)
  0.1653329
```

---

[7] An offset is a covariate that has a fixed coefficient of unity in a regression.

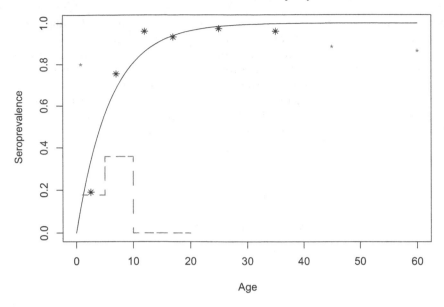

FIGURE 2.7
Seroprevalence-by-age from the measles antibody study of [47] from pre-vaccination Connecticut. The solid line is the predicted age-prevalence curve for the subset of the data used for estimation (black stars) assuming a constant FOI. The step-function is the piecewise constant FOI estimated using the method of [49]. The smaller stars are data excluded from the analysis due to maternal antibodies or possibly waning titres. Data are centered on the midpoints of each age-bracket.

The estimated FOI is 0.16/year, giving a predicted mean age of infection of 6 years. Age-specificity in ϕ requires more elaborate estimation schemes (like the general likelihood framework used in the removal estimator discussed previously). Common functions used are the piecewise constant and the log-spline function [48, 49]. Figure 2.7 also shows the piecewise constant FOI showing evidence of peak FOI in the 5–9 year olds reflecting dominance of circulation among primary school children. Analyses of serological data is the focus of Chapter 14.

2.8 Spatial Dynamics

The previous sections focus largely on pathogens whose local chains-of-transmission remains unbroken. However, a number of particularly acute, immunizing infections persist in "consumer-resource metapopulation" where the infection depletes the susceptible pool so deeply that frequent extinctions occur. Persistence is only secured through spatial coupling among asynchronous locally non-persistent chains-of-transmission. In disease ecology, a metapopulation is the setting where the host population is subdivided into many connected sub-populations (e.g., multiple cities). Influenza in non-tropical areas typify this behavior. Mass-vaccination has pushed the persistence of many childhood diseases such as mumps and measles from local to metapopulation. The spatial dynamics of infectious disease is therefore of great basic and applied importance.

Disease invasion in animal host-species often takes a characteristic wave-like shape with range expansion happening through local movement of susceptible and infected individuals. Rabies is a prime example. In the late 1970s, some raccoons from Southeastern USA were relocated to an area in Virginia/West Virginia at least one of which was infected with rabies [50]. This sparked an invasion wave predominantly in a northeasterly direction at a rate of 30–45 kilometers per year (km/yr) that reached Canada in 1999 [51]. Following invasion, rabies established endemically through the area.

Phocine distemper virus has twice invaded Norse sea seal populations over the last 50 years [13]. First in 1988 and then in 2002. For unclear reasons, the epicenter of both invasions was a seal colony on the small Danish island of Anholt in the Kattegat strait between Denmark and Sweden. Both instances resulted in radial spread to seal colonies in Netherlands, Sweden, Norway, and the UK, decimating the seal populations during the span of around 9 months, only to go regionally extinct at the end of each invasion event. In these, and many other zoonoses, a distance-dependent spatial risk "kernel" sometimes modified by landscape heterogeneities [52] or shortest sea-route distance [12] reliably predict the spatial invasion. In disease ecology (and population ecology more generally), a spatial kernel denotes the probability density distribution of movement between any two locations i and j. On homogenous landscapes, exponential, Gaussian, or Bessel-K(0) kernels are all theory-motivated choices depending on the assumptions made with respect to the process of spatial contagion [53].

The invasion wave of fox rabies across Europe from the 1940s is mathematically one of the most studied case studies of zoonotic disease invasion [53–55]. Starting from an epicenter in Poland, rabies spread at around 30–60 km/yr. Appropriate models for spatial spread of infection depends on the nature of the spatial transmission process ("distributed contacts" vs. "distributed infecteds") [56]. Van den Bosch et al. [53] assumed that rabies transmitted among foxes with relatively stable home ranges (and thus a distributed contacts scenario), and derived an approximate formula for the expected wave speed: $c = \frac{d}{\tau}\sqrt{2 \log R_0}$, where d is the standard deviation of the spatial transmission kernel (in this case related to the size of each home range) and τ is the serial interval. With a serial interval of about 33 days and a typical home range size (which is assumed to be density-dependent), Van den Bosch et al. [53] predicted a wave speed of 45 km/yr (at low densities), and 30 km/yr (at high densities) as long as the fox density is above the "critical host density" [see footnote 2] of around 1/km^2. Using a "dispersing infecteds" scenario — assuming foxes diffuse randomly across the landscape during the course of infection, so d is related to the movement of foxes — Murray et al. [54] predicted wave-like spread of rabies at a rate $c = \frac{d}{\tau}\sqrt{2(R_0 - 1)}$ [44]. Murray et al. [54] predicts a wave speed of around 50 km/yr. In contrast to [53], the latter model predicts spread to increase with fox density. Mollison [55] provides a discussion of different spread formulations, in general, and rabies (and other) case studies, in particular.

Pathogens also spread among humans both within and between local communities. Regional spread of human pathogens, however, rarely spread in a simple diffusive pattern because human mobility patterns are more complex. Movement may be distant dependent, but overall flow between any two communities also typically depends on the size (and desirability) of both "donor" and "recipient" location [58, 59]. Grenfell et al. [34], for example, showed that the spatiotemporal dynamics of measles across all cities and villages in pre-vaccination England and Wales exhibited "hierarchical waves," in which the timing of epidemics relative to the big urban conurbations (the donors) depended negatively on distance but positively on the size of the recipient. Xia et al. [60] subsequently showed that a metapopulation TSIR-model where movement among communities followed a "generalized gravity model" could approximate the dynamic patterns; The "gravity model" is a model of mobility/transportation from transportation science that posits that transportation volume between two communities depends inversely on distance, d, but bilinearly on size, N [58, 59].

In particular, Xia et al. [60] proposed that $c_{ij} \propto N_i^{c_1} N_j^{c_2} / d_{ij}^{c_3}$, where the c's are coefficients. Gravity models have since been applied to study the spatial dynamics of a variety of other human infections [e.g., [61, 62]].

2.9   Data

There are many wonderful reasons to study infectious disease dynamics: its importance for public health, food production, economics, geopolitics, elegant nonlinear mathematics, and exciting statistical challenges. One final reason is the abundance of high-quality data [63]. Causes of, particularly human, mortality and morbidity have been recorded through time first by priests and doctors and then more systematically by public health officials, such as the World Health Organization, the Registrar General in the UK and the Centers for Disease Control and Prevention in the USA. Project Tycho (http://www.tycho.pitt.edu) is a recent effort to digitize and make publicly available such historical data [64]. Much of the data used in this introductory chapter was downloaded from Tycho.

Acknowledgment

Odo Diekmann, Jess Metcalf, and Jacco Wallinga provided valuable comments on early drafts of this chapter.

References

[1] Grant McFadden. Poxvirus tropism. *Nature Reviews Microbiology*, 3(3):201–213, 2005.

[2] Kevin D Lafferty, Stefano Allesina, Matias Arim, Cherie J Briggs, Giulio De Leo, Andrew P Dobson, Jennifer A Dunne, Pieter TJ Johnson, Armand M Kuris, David J Marcogliese et al. Parasites in food webs: The ultimate missing links. *Ecology Letters*, 11(6):533–546, 2008.

[3] Jacob Bock Axelsen, Rami Yaari, Bryan T Grenfell, and Lewi Stone. Multiannual forecasting of seasonal influenza dynamics reveals climatic and evolutionary drivers. *Proceedings of the National Academy of Sciences*, 111(26):9538–9542, 2014.

[4] Katia Koelle, Sarah Cobey, Bryan Grenfell, and Mercedes Pascual. Epochal evolution shapes the phylodynamics of interpandemic influenza A (H3N2) in humans. *Science*, 314(5807):1898–1903, 2006.

[5] Sunetra Gupta, Neil Ferguson, and Roy Anderson. Chaos, persistence, and evolution of strain structure in antigenically diverse infectious agents. *Science*, 280(5365):912–915, 1998.

[6] Herve Tettelin, Nigel J Saunders, John Heidelberg, Alex C Jeffries, Karen E Nelson, Jonathan A Eisen, Karen A Ketchum, Derek W Hood, John F Peden, Robert J Dodson

et al. Complete genome sequence of *Neisseria meningitidis* serogroup B strain MC58. *Science*, 287(5459):1809–1815, 2000.

[7] Matt J Keeling and Pejman Rohani. *Modeling Infectious Diseases in Humans and Animals*. Princeton University Press, Princeton, NJ, 2008.

[8] Herbert W Virgin, E John Wherry, and Rafi Ahmed. Redefining chronic viral infection. *Cell*, 138(1):30–50, 2009.

[9] Bryan Grenfell and John Harwood. (Meta)population dynamics of infectious diseases. *Trends in Ecology and Evolution*, 12(10):395–399, 1997.

[10] Aaron A King, Sourya Shrestha, Eric T Harvill, and Ottar N Bjørnstad. Evolution of acute infections and the invasion-persistence trade-off. *The American Naturalist*, 173(4):446–455, 2009.

[11] Maurice S Bartlett. The critical community size for measles in the United States. *Journal of the Royal Statistical Society. Series A (General)*, 123(1):37–44, 1960.

[12] Jonathan Swinton, John Harwood, Bryan T Grenfell, and Chris A Gilligan. Persistence thresholds for phocine distemper virus infection in harbour seal Phoca vitulina metapopulations. *Journal of Animal Ecology*, pages 54–68, 1998.

[13] Karin Harding, Tero Härkönen, and Hal Caswell. The 2002 European seal plague: Epidemiology and population consequences. *Ecology Letters*, 5(6):727–732, 2002.

[14] Marc Lipsitch, Ted Cohen, Ben Cooper, James M Robins, Stefan Ma, Lyn James, Gowri Gopalakrishna, Suok Kai Chew, Chorh Chuan Tan, Matthew H Samore et al. Transmission dynamics and control of severe acute respiratory syndrome. *Science*, 300(5627):1966–1970, 2003.

[15] Matthew J Ferrari, Ottar N Bjørnstad, and Andrew P Dobson. Estimation and inference of R-0 of an infectious pathogen by a removal method. *Mathematical Biosciences*, 198(1):14–26, 2005.

[16] Norman T J Bailey. *The Mathematical Theory of Epidemics*. Griffin, London, UK, 1957.

[17] Roy M Anderson, Helen C Jackson, Robert M May, and Anthony M Smith. Population dynamics of fox rabies in Europe. *Nature*, 289:765–771, 1981.

[18] Ottar N Bjørnstad, Bärbel F Finkenstadt, and Bryan T Grenfell. Dynamics of measles epidemics: Estimating scaling of transmission rates using a time series SIR model. *Ecological Monographs*, 72(2):169–184, 2002.

[19] Bryan T Grenfell, Ottar N Bjørnstad, and Bärbel F Finkenstadt. Dynamics of measles epidemics: Scaling noise, determinism, and predictability with the TSIR model. *Ecological Monographs*, 72(2):185–202, 2002.

[20] Benjamin M. Bolker. *Ecological Models and Data in R*. Princeton University Press, Princeton, NJ, 2008.

[21] Rebecca F Grais, Andrew JK Conlan, Matthew J Ferrari, Ali Djibo, Philippe J Le Menach, Ottar N Bjørnstad, and Bryan T Grenfell. Time is of the essence: exploring a measles outbreak response vaccination in Niamey, Niger. *Journal of the Royal Society Interface*, 5(18):67–74, 2008.

[22] Kathryn Glass, Yincun Xia, and Bryan T Grenfell. Interpreting time-series analyses for continuous-time biological models—measles as a case study. *Journal of Theoretical Biology*, 223(1):19–25, 2003.

[23] David G Kendall. Stochastic processes and population growth. *Journal of the Royal Statistical Society. Series B (Methodological)*, 11(2):230–282, 1949.

[24] Benjamin D Dalziel, Ottar N Bjørnstad, Willem G van Panhuis, Donald S Burke, C Jessica E Metcalf, and Bryan T Grenfell. Persistent chaos of measles epidemics in the prevaccination United States caused by a small change in seasonal transmission patterns. *PLoS Computational Biology*, 12(2):e1004655, 2016.

[25] Alexander D Becker and Bryan T Grenfell. TSIR: An R package for time-series susceptible-infected-recovered models of epidemics. *PLoS One*, 12(9):e0185528, 2017.

[26] Aaron A King, Dao Nguyen, and Edward L Ionides. Statistical inference for partially observed markov processes via the R package pomp. *Journal of Statistical Software*, 69(12):1–43, 2016.

[27] Jennie S Lavine, Aaron A King, and Ottar N Bjørnstad. Natural immune boosting in pertussis dynamics and the potential for long-term vaccine failure. *Proceedings of the National Academy of Sciences*, 108(17):7259–7264, 2011.

[28] Sonia Altizer, Andrew Dobson, Parviez Hosseini, Peter Hudson, Mercedes Pascual, and Pejman Rohani. Seasonality and the dynamics of infectious diseases. *Ecology Letters*, 9(4):467–484, 2006.

[29] Ottar N Bjørnstad and Cecile Viboud. Timing and periodicity of influenza epidemics. *Proceedings of the National Academy of Sciences*, 13(46):12899–12901, 2016.

[30] Jeffrey Shaman and Melvin Kohn. Absolute humidity modulates influenza survival, transmission, and seasonality. *Proceedings of the National Academy of Sciences*, 106(9):3243–3248, 2009.

[31] Diego Ruiz-Moreno, Mercedes Pascual, Menno Bouma, Andrew Dobson, and Benjamin Cash. Cholera seasonality in Madras (1901–1940): Dual role for rainfall in endemic and epidemic regions. *EcoHealth*, 4(1):52–62, 2007.

[32] Ottar N Bjørnstad. *Epidemics: Models and Data Using R*. Springer, Berlin, Germany, 2018.

[33] David JD Earn, Pejman Rohani, Benjamin M Bolker, and Bryan T Grenfell. A simple model for complex dynamical transitions in epidemics. *Science*, 287(5453):667–670, 2000.

[34] Bryan T Grenfell, Ottar N Bjørnstad, and Jens Kappey. Travelling waves and spatial hierarchies in measles epidemics. *Nature*, 414(6865):716–723, 2001.

[35] Tien-Yien Li and James A Yorke. Period three implies chaos. *The American Mathematical Monthly*, 82(10):985–992, 1975.

[36] David A Rand and Howard B Wilson. Chaotic stochasticity: A ubiquitous source of unpredictability in epidemics. *Proceedings of the Royal Society of London B: Biological Sciences*, 246(1316):179–184, 1991.

[37] JP Eckmann and David Ruelle. Ergodic theory of chaos and strange attractors. *Reviews of Modern Physics*, 57(3):617, 1985.

[38] Pejman Rohani, Matthew J Keeling, and Bryan T Grenfell. The interplay between determinism and stochasticity in childhood diseases. *The American Naturalist*, 159(5):469–481, 2002.

[39] Hélene Broutin, Jean-François Guégan, Eric Elguero, François Simondon, and Bernard Cazelles. Large-scale comparative analysis of pertussis population dynamics: Periodicity, synchrony, and impact of vaccination. *American Journal of Epidemiology*, 161(12):1159–1167, 2005.

[40] Jennie S Lavine, Aaron A King, Viggo Andreasen, and Ottar N Bjørnstad. Immune boosting explains regime-shifts in prevaccine-era pertussis dynamics. *PLoS One*, 8(8):e72086, 2013.

[41] Christopher Torrence and Gilbert P Compo. A practical guide to wavelet analysis. *Bulletin of the American Meteorological Society*, 79(1):61–78, 1998.

[42] René Carmona, Wen-Liang Hwang, and Bruno Torresani. *Practical Time-Frequency Analysis: Gabor and Wavelet Transforms, with an Implementation in S*, vol. 9. Academic Press, Orlando, FL, 1998.

[43] Mark EJ Woolhouse, C Dye, J-F Etard, T Smith, JD Charlwood, GP Garnett, P Hagan, JLK Hii, PD Ndhlovu, RJ Quinnell et al. Heterogeneities in the transmission of infectious agents: Implications for the design of control programs. *Proceedings of the National Academy of Sciences*, 94(1):338–342, 1997.

[44] James O Lloyd-Smith, Sebastian J Schreiber, P Ekkehard Kopp, and Wayne M Getz. Superspreading and the effect of individual variation on disease emergence. *Nature*, 438(7066):355, 2005.

[45] Joël Mossong, Niel Hens, Mark Jit, Philippe Beutels, Kari Auranen, Rafael Mikolajczyk, Marco Massari, Stefania Salmaso, Gianpaolo Scalia Tomba, Jacco Wallinga et al. Social contacts and mixing patterns relevant to the spread of infectious diseases. *PLoS Medicine*, 5(3):e74, 2008.

[46] Hugo Muench. *Catalytic Models in Epidemiology*. Harvard University Press, Cambridge, MA, 1959.

[47] Francis L Black. Measles antibodies in the population of New Haven, Connecticut. *Journal of Immunology*, 83:74–83, 1959.

[48] Bryan T Grenfell and Roy M Anderson. Pertussis in England and Wales: An investigation of transmission dynamics and control by mass vaccination. *Proceedings of the Royal Society of London B: Biological Sciences*, 236(1284):213–252, 1989.

[49] Gráinne H Long, Divya Sinha, Andrew F Read, Stacy Pritt, Barry Kline, Barry T Harvill, Peter J Hudson, and Ottar N Bjornstad. Identifying the age cohort responsible for transmission in a natural outbreak of bordetella bronchiseptica. *PLoS Pathogens*, 6(12):e1001224, 2010.

[50] Andy Dobson. Raccoon rabies in space and time. *Proceedings of the National Academy of Sciences*, 97(26):14041–14043, 2000.

[51] Marta A Guerra, Aaron T Curns, Charles E Rupprecht, Cathleen A Hanlon, John W Krebs, and James E Childs. Skunk and raccoon rabies in the eastern United States: Temporal and spatial analysis. *Emerging Infectious Diseases*, 9(9):1143, 2003.

[52] David L Smith, Brendan Lucey, Lance A Waller, James E Childs, and Leslie A Real. Predicting the spatial dynamics of rabies epidemics on heterogeneous landscapes. *Proceedings of the National Academy of Sciences*, 99(6):3668–3672, 2002.

[53] Frank van den Bosch, Johan AJ Metz, and Odo Diekmann. The velocity of spatial population expansion. *Journal of Mathematical Biology*, 28(5):529–565, 1990.

[54] James D Murray, E Ann Stanley, and David L Brown. On the spatial spread of rabies among foxes. *Proceedings of the Royal Society of London. Series B, Biological Sciences*, 229(1255):111–150, 1986.

[55] Denis Mollison. Dependence of epidemic and population velocities on basic parameters. *Mathematical Biosciences*, 107(2):255–287, 1991.

[56] Timothy C Reluga, Jan Medlock, and Alison P Galvani. A model of spatial epidemic spread when individuals move within overlapping home ranges. *Bulletin of Mathematical Biology*, 68(2):401–416, 2006.

[57] Roy M Anderson, Helen C Jackson, Robert M May, and Anthony M Smith. Population dynamics of fox rabies in Europe. *Nature*, 289:765–771, 1981.

[58] Sven Erlander and Neil F Stewart. *The Gravity Model in Transportation Analysis: Theory and Extensions*, vol. 3. VSP, Zeist, the Netherlands, 1990.

[59] A Stewart Fotheringham. Spatial flows and spatial patterns. *Environment and Planning A*, 16(4):529–543, 1984.

[60] Yingcun Xia, Ottar N Bjørnstad, and Bryan T Grenfell. Measles metapopulation dynamics: A gravity model for epidemiological coupling and dynamics. *The American Naturalist*, 164(2):267–281, 2004.

[61] James Truscott and Neil M Ferguson. Evaluating the adequacy of gravity models as a description of human mobility for epidemic modelling. *PLoS Computational Biology*, 8(10):e1002699, 2012.

[62] Cécile Viboud, Ottar N Bjørnstad, David L Smith, Lone Simonsen, Mark A Miller, and Bryan T Grenfell. Synchrony, waves, and spatial hierarchies in the spread of influenza. *Science*, 312(5772):447–451, 2006.

[63] Pejman Rohani and Aaron A King. Never mind the length, feel the quality: The impact of long-term epidemiological data sets on theory, application and policy. *Trends in Ecology & Evolution*, 25(10):611–618, 2010.

[64] Willem G Van Panhuis, John Grefenstette, Su Yon Jung, Nian Shong Chok, Anne Cross, Heather Eng, Bruce Y Lee, Vladimir Zadorozhny, Shawn Brown, Derek Cummings et al. Contagious diseases in the United States from 1888 to the present. *The New England Journal of Medicine*, 369(22):2152, 2013.

3

Infectious Disease Data from Surveillance, Outbreak Investigation, and Epidemiological Studies

Susan Hahné and Richard Pebody

CONTENTS

3.1 Introduction

Before deciding the most appropriate analytical method and then applying it to infectious disease data, a thorough understanding of the different types of data which are available, the way in that they are collected, and the limitations inherent to them is essential. This knowledge will influence the approach you might take and then what conclusions you may or may not be able to draw from your analyses.

In this chapter, we first provide a general introduction to the available types of data on infectious diseases, which we divide into two kinds: epidemiological and microbiological data. 'Big data' does not necessarily fall into these two categories and is discussed in the context of surveillance (Section 3.3). Subsequently, in Sections 3.3 and 3.4, we address the main methods of how data on infectious diseases can be collected: by surveillance, outbreak investigation and by dedicated studies. In these sections, more details on specific types of data derived from these methods will be provided. Examples of the kinds of data and study designs are given throughout the text.

The overall aim of the current chapter is to provide the reader with a sense of the types of data available on infectious diseases, how they are generated, their strengths and limitations, and to guide readers towards where data may be obtained.

3.2   Infectious Disease Data: General Aspects

3.2.1   Epidemiological data

Basic epidemiological data on infectious diseases in individuals or populations includes information on (possible) exposure to infectious agents, other determinants of infection (risk factors), the occurrence of symptoms and microbiological evidence of an infection, demographic characteristics of the host, and, in cohort studies, on the time of follow up of individuals in the study and the reasons for loss to follow up. More specific epidemiological data such as contact pattern data are discussed elsewhere (in Chapter 6).

In infectious disease epidemiology, it is important to realize that the definition of what constitutes an exposure to an infectious agent varies depending on the pathogen, and what is known about its routes of transmission and infectiousness. An individual who has been present in a room with an infectious case of measles can be classified as exposed to measles, whereas merely being present in a room with a person who is infected with hepatitis B does not indicate exposure to hepatitis B. The definition of what constitutes an effective exposure may change over time when more knowledge of the pathogen becomes available. The concept of exposure is central to the definition of what constitutes an epidemiological link: An individual can be classified as having an epidemiological link if exposed to a person in whom the infection is diagnosed. Establishing whether a person has an epidemiological link needs to take into account the characteristics of the pathogen, including its infectiousness and routes of transmission and having detailed information on the exposure of the individual.

Data on the presence of determinants for infection other than exposure to a pathogen is usually also collected in epidemiological studies, e.g., to study the association between these determinants and an outcome or to assess the representativeness of the study population. Determinants can include behavioral, environmental, and demographic characteristics, and information on these determinants often is collected through questionnaires that are completed through an interview or by participants to a study. The quality of the questionnaire and the way it is completed is a main determinant of the validity and usefulness of the resulting data. On-line questionnaires completed by the study participant avoid the need for data entry by the research team but can of course also contain data entry errors. When data is entered from paper questionnaires, double data entry is good practice to limit this.

A central step in the generation of epidemiological data on infectious diseases is to decide which individuals are classified as infected. This classification is most systematically done by a priori agreeing on a case definition. Case definitions in infectious disease epidemiology usually consist of a set of clinical, epidemiological, and/or microbiological criteria. The clinical criteria in a case definition usually consist of the typical symptoms of the disease. The epidemiological criteria are defined by what constitutes an epidemiological link (see above) while microbiological criteria are defined by laboratory testing (see Section 3.2.2). International organizations such as the World Health Organization (WHO) the European Center for Disease Prevention and Control (ECDC), and the Brighton Collaboration have established case definitions to aid standardized data collection. The importance of case definitions for surveillance and outbreak investigations is outlined in Section 3.3 and 3.4, respectively.

3.2.2   Microbiological data

Exposure to micro-organisms (bacteria, viruses, fungi, or parasites) of an individual can result in a symptomatic or asymptomatic infection, which, for certain pathogens (such as human immunodeficiency virus (HIV) or hepatitis B), can result in a carrier status. Exposure to certain pathogens may also merely lead to colonization, in which the pathogen is present in certain non-sterile body compartments such as the skin or mucosa. Infection, carriage and colonization all may result in transmission to others.

For most infections, a definitive conclusion on whether it has occurred in an individual depends on confirmatory testing in a microbiology laboratory. There are only a few pathogens in which certain clinical symptoms are thought to be pathognomonic of infection. An example of this is measles, characterized by fever and rash, whereby the appearance of so-called Koplik spots on the patient's oral mucosa is highly specific for the diagnosis. Since Koplik spots only occur in about 70 percent of measles cases and are often not recognized, the sensitivity of this symptom is only moderate: many measles cases will be missed if only cases with Koplik spots are considered true cases.

Data on microbiology testing aiming to diagnose an infection typically consists of the type of test that was used (e.g., polymerase chain reaction (PCR)), the type of sample which was tested (e.g., a nose swab), and the test result. The latter can be qualitative (e.g., positive, negative, equivocal), semi-quantitative (e.g., intensity of a result), or quantitative (a numerical value). Some laboratory tests can only provide a qualitative test result. An example of this is culture of pathogens, which only indicates whether or not a certain pathogen is present in a sample. Quantitative test results can be transformed into qualitative data by using thresholds for what constitutes a negative, equivocal, or positive result. These thresholds often are defined by the manufacturer of the test, reflecting a specific aim of testing, e.g., diagnosing infection with a high degree of specificity. This aim may differ from the needs of a specific study, and hence pre-defined kit thresholds may not be optimal. Therefore, it is preferable to use quantitative data when available.

Laboratory testing to diagnose an infection can further be distinguished into two types: tests aimed at detecting the pathogen (e.g., PCR) and tests to identify the immunological reactions generated by the body upon encountering a pathogen (e.g., serological tests). The sensitivity of these methods highly depends on the timing of sampling relative to the onset of symptoms. To detect pathogens in acute infections, samples need to be taken relatively soon after onset of symptoms, while full characterization of immunological reactions requires later samples.

After diagnosing a pathogen at the genus level (e.g., Salmonella), further characterization at the species and subspecies level can be done by applying specific methods. Determination of, e.g., strains, clones, and sequence types currently usually requires characterizing part of the pathogen's genome by sequencing it. Recent advances in sequencing methods have reduced the time and costs needed for this greatly, and hence genomic data, including whole genome sequencing (WGS) data is becoming increasingly available. A relatively new area of molecular microbiology, metagenomics, involves characterization of the entire genomic content of a biological sample. High-throughput sequencing methods, labeled as next generation sequencing (NGS) are needed for this purpose. Metagenomics is applied to studying microbiomes, which can be defined as the population of microorganisms that inhabit a certain location (e.g., the nasopharynx or the gut). Characterizing such populations requires methods which do not depend on culturing micro-organisms, since many pathogens cannot be grown in culture yet. In addition to assessing their genomic content, microbiomes also can be characterized by studying small molecules or proteins present in the sample [1].

A separate area of microbiological testing is aimed at documenting indirect evidence of infection by assessing the body's immunological response to it. These methods also are used to assess vaccine induced immunity. The immune response to infection (and vaccination) usually consists of two different mechanisms: a cellular and a humoral response. In the cellular response, immune cells directly attack the pathogen, while the humoral response acts through antibodies. Microbiological tests aimed at diagnosing infections by assessing the immune response are focused mostly on testing the presence of humoral rather than cellular immunity, since standardized assays for the latter are lacking. Data resulting from microbiological tests of humoral immunity can give qualitative and quantitative results about the presence of antibodies specific for a certain pathogen. It also can give an indication of when the infection was acquired by performing avidity testing, which is used in e.g. HIV diagnosis and surveillance [2].

In addition to diagnosing infections and characterizing pathogens, microbiological testing also can provide other data relevant from a public health perspective. This includes data to assess the infectiousness of an infected individual and whether the pathogen causing the infection is resistant to antimicrobial drugs. Assessing infectiousness can be done by determining the pathogen load (e.g., the viral load, which represents the number of copies of the virus present in the sample). Testing for antimicrobial resistance can be done by microbiological tests in which cultured bacteria or fungi are exposed to a panel of antimicrobial agents to assess their effect on growth of the bacteria. Applying certain clinical breakpoint criteria when assessing pathogen growth results in a qualitative test result (e.g., 'resistant'). The internal and external validity of results depends on the quality of the laboratory procedures and on the use of standard clinical breakpoint criteria. The presence of antimicrobial resistance in micro-organisms also can be detected by genotypic methods sequencing genes coding for resistance traits. However, the presence of such genes does not necessarily indicate the presence of resistance since this also depends on the level of gene expression.

3.2.3   Data errors and bias

When analyzing data, it is important to be aware of potential errors which may be inherent, since ignoring these may lead to incorrect conclusions. Errors in epidemiological or laboratory data can be classified into two main categories: those arising from random errors and those arising from systematic errors. Random errors are due to chance driven variation in measurements or sampling. The size of random error can be reduced by increasing the sample size of a study, which will increase the precision of the measurement. Systematic errors in data can result from non-representative sampling procedures (e.g., working with self-selected participants who are likely to differ from randomly selected participants) and from systematic measurement errors. Increases in sample size will not reduce the size of systematic errors.

Systematic data errors only lead to bias when they are differential, i.e., when the extent of it depends on study participants' characteristics and their outcomes. Bias is defined as a systematic deviation of results or inferences from truth [3]. In general, we can try to avoid bias by having an optimal design, collection, analysis, interpretation, and reporting of a study. Bias in epidemiological studies can arise in many ways, and dozens of types of biases have been described. The two major types of bias we will describe here are selection bias and information bias. We will not discuss confounding bias, since it is mainly a problem with epidemiological interpretation of results of studies into effects of determinants, while selection bias and information bias are also applicable to broader use of data.

Selection bias occurs when the chances of individuals to be included (or stay) in the study population are related to their level of exposure and the occurrence of the outcome of interest. When selection bias is present, study participants differ from non-participants (who are eligible for the study) in terms of the relation between the exposure and the outcome. An example of selection bias distorting a vaccine effectiveness study is when vaccinated cases who have become ill are more likely to participate than vaccinated individuals who have not become ill. This bias would result in an underestimate of vaccine effectiveness.

Information bias refers to flaws in measuring exposure, covariate, or outcome variables that result in different accuracy of information between comparison groups [3]. Invalid information can lead to misclassification of the exposure status of individuals. When the study aim is to assess the effect of an exposure on an outcome, it is of key importance to assess whether this misclassification is differential (i.e., differing between cases and non-cases) or non-differential. Non-differential misclassification results in underestimating an effect, while differential misclassification can lead to over- or underestimating effects. In a vaccine effectiveness study, information bias can arise when cases of the infection of interest are more likely to remember that they were vaccinated than people who have not become ill. This would result in an underestimation of the protective effect of vaccination.

Systematic errors in microbiological data can result from biased (non-representative) sampling procedures, systematic mistakes in handling of samples, and laboratory procedures (e.g., poor quality growth medium). It is key to understand the sensitivity and specificity of testing, and whether cross-reactions occur, to interpret test results well. The application of different testing algorithms or expert rules also can result in biased results. If e.g. antimicrobial susceptibility testing for antimicrobial agent B is only performed when the pathogen is resistant against agent A, test results for agent B are not representative of the entire population.

3.3 Data from Surveillance of Infectious Diseases

3.3.1 Introduction

Surveillance was first used in public health in the 14th century in southern Europe, when it was carried out to detect cases of plague among people who had been placed in quarantine, usually after travel abroad. Early detection of cases and their subsequent isolation was a direct tool to control the spread of infectious diseases. It is used still in a similar fashion currently as the main method to control serious infectious diseases such as ebola, for which until recently no effective vaccine existed. Surveillance of diseases rather than of individuals was first systematically performed by John Graunt (1620–1674), who analyzed the London Bills of Mortality to understand patterns of death and in particular to understand the extent of the problem with plague. This work was further developed by William Farr (1807–1883), a statistician who introduced a certificate for cause of death and used mortality data to understand the course of infectious disease epidemics in order to identify opportunities for control [4]. In the 1950s, Alexander Langmuir, generally considered the father of modern surveillance, defined disease surveillance as "the continued watchfulness over the distribution and trends of incidence through the systematic collection, consolidation and evaluation of morbidity and mortality reports and other relevant data together with the timely and regular dissemination to those who need to know" [5]. In 1968 the World Health Assembly summarized this definition as "surveillance is information for action" [6]. Surveillance is, together with outbreak investigation and epidemiologic studies, a main tool of applied infectious diseases epidemiology. It is aimed at generating evidence to support infectious disease prevention and control by identifying trends and outbreaks, aiding public health prioritization of disease control and evaluating interventions. It also can be used to generate hypotheses for further research.

The aim of this section is to provide a general overview of surveillance methods, examples of surveillance data, and information on where it may be accessed. The sections on surveillance methods do not aim to instruct the reader on how to set up, perform, or evaluate surveillance systems, but rather to aid access to and appropriate interpretation of the data that is generated by such systems. Liaising closely with surveillance and disease control experts at an early stage when considering using surveillance data is important to ensure optimal data is obtained and to avoid misinterpretation.

3.3.2   The population under surveillance

To understand the data resulting from an infectious disease surveillance system, it is important to know what was defined as the population covered by the system. In national, population-based surveillance, the population under surveillance is usually the entire population of a country. However, in many instances this type of comprehensive surveillance may not be feasible or necessary. An alternative to comprehensive surveillance is sentinel surveillance, whereby data is coming from a selection of hospitals or general practitioner (GP) practices only (see Section 3.3.4.1). In this situation the size and characteristics of the population under surveillance are important to understand to ensure, e.g., that accurate age-specific incidence rates can be calculated. In the surveillance of zoonoses, animals may be the population under surveillance. To be able to interpret surveillance data, its representativeness for the population under surveillance needs to be carefully assessed: are population subgroups such as undocumented migrants included? Is there a bias towards reporting cases in certain age groups or with certain (more severe) disease manifestations? To assess this is usually problematic, since a gold standard dataset often is not available. It requires close liaison and discussion with surveillance and disease experts.

3.3.3   The use of case definitions in surveillance

Infectious disease surveillance systems usually aim to identify people or animals infected with a certain pathogen in order to assess the incidence rate of the infection of interest in a population. Since asymptomatic infections are difficult to detect unless serological assessment is undertaken of a probabilistic sample of the entire population, this means in practice identifying people or animals with disease symptoms that may be caused by the infection. To allow comparison of the incidence rate in one population with the rate in other populations, consistent use of the same criteria to decide who is a case is a prerequisite. The set of criteria used to define a case is called a case definition. Case definitions are not only essential in surveillance, but in many epidemiologic studies including outbreak investigations.

Case definitions in infectious disease epidemiology usually consist of a set of clinical, epidemiological, and/or microbiological criteria, a description of the population that is being studied, and, particularly in outbreak investigations, a point in time from which onwards cases are counted. International organizations such as ECDC and the WHO and many countries have established a set of standard case definitions which aid standardized data collection. An example of this is the European Union (EU) case definition for measles (see Box 3.1).

BOX 3.1 EU CASE DEFINITION FOR MEASLES

Clinical Criteria: Any person with fever AND Maculo-papular rash AND at least one of the following three: Cough, Coryza, Conjunctivitis

Laboratory Criteria: At least one of the following four: Isolation of measles virus from a clinical specimen, Detection of measles virus nucleic acid in a clinical specimen, Measles virus specific antibody response characteristic for acute infection in serum or saliva, Detection of measles virus antigen by DFA in a clinical specimen using measles specific monoclonal antibodies. (DFA = direct fluorescence antibody)

Epidemiological criteria: An epidemiological link by human to human transmission

Case Classification

- Possible case: Any person meeting the clinical criteria

- Probable case: Any person meeting the clinical criteria and with an epidemiological link

- Confirmed case: Any person not recently vaccinated and meeting the clinical and the laboratory criteria

Source: `https://ecdc.europa.eu/en/infectious-diseases-public-health/surveillance-and-disease-data/eu-case-definitions`

The design of a case definition for surveillance purposes needs to consider the level of sensitivity, specificity, and positive predictive value required to achieve the aim of the surveillance. It also needs to reflect the diagnostic practices and health care seeking behaviour in a certain setting. If microbiological testing is rarely performed for a certain condition, a surveillance case definition including only microbiological criteria is inappropriate. An example of this is influenza, the incidence of which is usually assessed by counting the number of people presenting with influenza like illness (ILI) in primary care, irrespective of any microbiological diagnosis.

To allow some flexibility in the sensitivity, specificity, and positive predictive value of a case definition, often layered, hierarchical definitions are proposed for suspected and confirmed cases (see Box 3.1). The criteria for a suspected case usually include only a set of clinical symptoms, while confirmed cases have a higher degree of certainty to have the disease of interest. This certainty can be based on the results of microbiologic testing and/or on epidemiologic information increasing the likelihood that the symptoms of disease are due to a certain infection (see information on epidemiologic link in Section 3.2).

3.3.4   Data for surveillance of infectious diseases

The data sources used in surveillance of a particular disease are determined by the aim of the surveillance, which data sources are (routinely) available, the required quality of the data, the resources required to implement the system, and the feasibility of running the surveillance system. For the system to be sustainable, the requirements for those contributing the data and maintaining the system need to be as simple as possible. This usually compromises the quality of the data, leading to suboptimal timeliness, completeness, or accuracy. To compensate for this, it is useful to include several data sources in a surveillance system, so that by triangulation the number and validity of conclusions that can be drawn from the surveillance can be enhanced (see Box 3.2 and Figure 3.1). Below, main data sources used in infectious disease surveillance are discussed.

BOX 3.2 USE OF MULTIPLE DATA SOURCES FOR THE SURVEILLANCE OF ROTAVIRUS IN THE NETHERLANDS

Rotavirus (RV) causes acute gastro-enteritis (AGE), which is in most cases short-lived and does not lead to health-care visits. RV infection is not notifiable in the Netherlands. The main source of data for RV surveillance in the Netherlands is the weekly reporting of the number of RV diagnoses by a number of virological laboratories. This system does not yet fully capture the number of laboratory tests performed. A decrease in the number of RV diagnosis can therefore reflect a genuine decrease in transmission of the virus, but also a decrease in how frequent cases with AGE are tested for RV. Considering an additional, independent data source such as the frequency of general practitioner (GP) visits for AGE facilitates drawing conclusions on the incidence of RV infection. The absence of a clear RV peak in winter 2014 observed in data from the virologic laboratories was confirmed by data from GP surveillance [6]. See Figure 3.1.

3.3.4.1 Data generated in the health service

Health service providers are an important source of data for infectious disease surveillance because they routinely record health events which may be of interest to public health.

Notifiable diseases. Almost every country has a list of infectious diseases which clinicians and/or laboratories are obliged by law to report to their public health authorities.

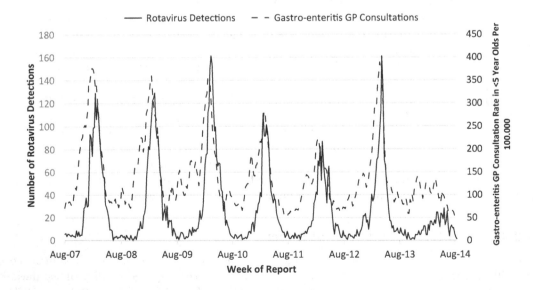

FIGURE 3.1

Number of rotavirus detections by a number of virological laboratories and frequency of GP visits for acute gastro-enteritis in <5 year olds by week, The Netherlands, August 2007 – August 2014. (Adapted from Hahné, S. et al., *Eurosurveillance*, 19, 20945, 2014.)

These notifiable diseases are usually severe with a potentially large impact on public health. Together with the report of the diagnosis of the disease, minimal information that is usually collected includes the date of onset, sex, age, place of residence of the patient, and some information on risk factors for infection such as recent travel history. The usefulness of data on notifiable diseases first depends on whether a clear and practicable case definition was applied when selecting which patients are notified. When the case definition is only based on clinical symptoms, its likelihood to indicate a true case of a certain infectious disease (i.e., the positive predictive value) depends on the prevalence of the disease in the population. Second, the usefulness of notification data depends on the completeness of reporting. Usually, notified cases represent only the tip of the iceberg of all patients with the notifiable condition, since not all patients consult health care, and reporting by health care providers is usually also incomplete. This may not necessarily be a problem for public health decision making, depending on how constant and representative the reporting is. Changes in completeness of reporting over time can be caused by changes in the health care seeking behavior of patients (e.g., due to media coverage of an outbreak) or by changes in diagnostic practices or the availability of a new test. Completeness of reporting of notifiable diseases can be improved by obliging microbiological laboratories to report patients with a notifiable disease, since for most notifiable diseases a confirmation by microbiological testing is part of the case definition. This reporting can be potentially supported by automated extractions from laboratory information management systems. Timeliness is another attribute of surveillance data which influences its usefulness for public health decision making. In rapidly emerging outbreaks, delays in the time between onset of the infection and notification can make it difficult to assess whether the outbreak is ongoing or subsiding. Using techniques to adjust for such reporting delays and to create thresholds based on historical incidence, it is possible to create automated alerts when significantly more notifications are being seen than expected. This is the basis for further investigations to determine whether the increase is real and what might be explaining it. In addition to compulsory notification, voluntary reporting of health events by health care providers and/or microbiological laboratories can be organized through reporting schemes.

Sentinel surveillance. For infectious diseases which are common and which do not require a public health response for every case (such as influenza), reporting of all cases in a country usually is not necessary for public health decision making. In these situations it may be more efficient to establish a sentinel surveillance system where only a selection of health service providers or laboratories report cases. Having only a subset of health service providers or laboratories involved in reporting can make it feasible to improve the quality of data through training of data providers and to enhance the data by collecting additional information or laboratory testing of cases, as outlined earlier. An example of sentinel surveillance established by many countries is the GP sentinel influenza surveillance, where GPs report patients consulting with acute ILI and take a respiratory swab from a sample of patients to test in a laboratory for influenza. This type of surveillance has proved invaluable to monitor the intensity of influenza transmission, the dominant circulating strains, and to act as a platform for vaccine effectiveness studies to measure the performance of seasonal influenza vaccine and inform optimal selection of vaccine strains by the annual WHO Vaccine composition meeting.

Routinely recorded health care and mortality data. Routinely recorded health service data on medical encounters (i.e., electronic health records) also can be a useful source of data for infectious diseases surveillance. This data includes the routine registration of health events in primary care, specialist care (e.g., sexually transmitted infection (STI) clinics), hospitals, by health insurance companies, and death registration (see Box 3.3). It also includes pharmacotherapeutical data, e.g. on the number of prescriptions of antibiotics in a certain population.

Routine health service data is most useful when information on health events is coded, e.g. using the International Classification of Diseases (ICD) developed by the WHO. An overview of coding systems is available from https://www.nlm.nih.gov/research/umls/sourcereleasedocs/#.

Most coding systems do not require or include information on laboratory confirmation, which limits the specificity and therefore usefulness of the data for infectious disease surveillance and research. Furthermore, there may be regional and temporal differences and changes in the way that coding is undertaken. Another limitation of routinely collected health data is that there often are significant delays between the occurrence of the health event and the availability of the data, although methods are available to adjust for this.

BOX 3.3 ROUTINELY RECORDED MORTALITY DATA FOR PUBLIC HEALTH SURVEILLANCE

In Europe, a project for monitoring of excess mortality for public health action (EuroMOMO) assesses weekly 'real-time' all-cause age-specific excess mortality in countries in Europe. By using a standardised approach, results can be pooled. Through this monitoring a significant peak in mortality in adults >65 years of age in 2014/2015 was detected [7]. See Figure 3.2.

Surveillance using data on only clinical symptoms is an example of syndromic surveillance. The main advantage of syndromic surveillance is its timeliness, since it uses data which may be available before microbiologic diagnoses are established. It can include a wide range of health data such as GP or emergency room consultation data, telephone consultation data, and data on medical purchases (e.g., over the counter drugs). It also can include non-health-data, as outlined in 3.3.4.2. An example of syndromic surveillance data is provided in Box 3.3 and Figure 3.2.

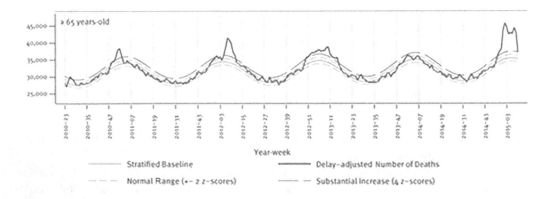

FIGURE 3.2
Number of deaths by week and modelled baseline in persons >65 years of age, obtained from pooled analysis of data from EuroMOMO countries, week 23, 2010 – week 9, 2015 ($n = 14$ countries). (Adapted from Mølbak, K. et al., *Eurosurveillance*, 20, 2015.)

Laboratory surveillance. Obtaining data on infections in humans directly from microbiological laboratories for surveillance purposes is attractive since a laboratory diagnosis is usually highly specific and data is often electronically available. Laboratory surveillance is the key method for surveillance of antimicrobial resistance. Data from laboratory surveillance may include basic demographic information such as age, gender, and date of sample and results of individual patients' microbiological tests. More information on the types of laboratory data that may be available is provided in Section 3.2.2. The interpretation of laboratory data for infectious disease surveillance purposes is greatly facilitated if, in addition to data on the number of positive tests in a certain period of time, also data on the number of tests that were performed in that period is available. This information allows disentangling whether any observed changes in the incidence of an infection are due to increased testing (such as following the introduction of near-patient testing) or likely to reflect a genuine increase in the number of infected individuals.

The validity and precision of laboratory data first depends on the quality and type of laboratory test used. Random errors in the data can result from measurement variation. Systematic errors can result from certain decisions during the collection, processing, and analyses of the laboratory data (3.2.3). Limitations of laboratory data include that usually information on the symptoms of the patient and the clinical outcome are not available. Another difficulty can be that results of repeat testing of the same patient are included, which makes it difficult to distinguish separate infection episodes. Many systems have developed approaches to de-duplicate such repeats. However to optimize comparability it is important that standard approaches are employed.

Surveillance of zoonoses. Surveillance of zoonoses (infections which can spread between vertebrate animals and humans) usually requires dedicated surveillance in not only humans, but also animal reservoirs, vectors and sometimes the environment (so called one health surveillance). Birds are an important reservoir for a large number of influenza viruses. Some of these viruses occasionally take on the ability to spread from birds to humans, and occasionally then from person to person (which can then develop into a pandemic). Early detection of viruses that may have acquired the potential for spread from bird to human is important as part of pandemic preparedness. A recent example is A(H7N9), which is currently circulating in poultry flocks in China, and has acquired the ability to spread from bird to human. Avian surveillance has been important to detect if the virus has spread elsewhere in China and to neighboring countries.

International surveillance. The importance of international surveillance is being increasingly recognized, as infectious diseases do not respect borders and can easily spread as was seen with SARS in 2003. The International Health Regulations are a surveillance tool whereby countries are compelled to report events of international public health importance at the earliest possible stage. The sharing of such information at an early stage helps to support control and prevention efforts as was well illustrated with emergence of Middle East Respiratory Syndrome-Corona Virus (MERS-CoV) in 2011. International organizations such as WHO and ECDC have international surveillance as one of their main tasks.

Surveillance pyramid. The previously listed sources of data generated in the health service can be visualized in the form of the surveillance pyramid (Figure 3.3). To understand the validity of data resulting from surveillance, it is necessary to understand to what extent individuals in a certain level of the pyramid are representative of the individuals in a lower level. Since surveillance data is derived from real-life situations rather than dedicated studies, the determinants of why certain individuals go from one level of the pyramid to the next are usually not random, and this can result in important biases. When only severely ill people are tested and the severity of the infection varies by age, the age distribution of laboratory positive cases is not representative of all individuals with the infection of interest.

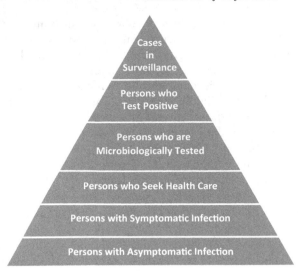

FIGURE 3.3
The surveillance pyramid.

When many cases with an infection die at home before reaching health care and diagnostic facilities, the burden of disease and case fatality may be underestimated.

3.3.4.2   Non-health data for the surveillance of infectious diseases

Denominator data. A key source of non-health data which is important for surveillance is demographic data on population denominators. In many countries this is collected and made available by a national statistics bureau, either derived from a population census or, in some countries, from a population register. Denominator data is crucial to be able to calculate incidence rates and to assess how representative surveillance data is of the general population.

Citizen science. The growing use of the internet has enabled a form of surveillance where members of the public are encouraged to report certain health issues. Examples of this are the tick bite radar in the Netherlands (www.tekenradar.nl) and the Flusurvey in the UK (https://flusurvey.org.uk/). Data often is presented on-line to provide feedback to the population. These surveys can be tailored to rapidly answer acute questions. These initiatives can be classified as citizen science, a phrase which encompasses a wide range of research involving active citizen participation. Biases in data generated by citizen science may arise since the data is generated by a self-selected part of the population, which is generally better educated and younger. Whether any biases are important for the interpretation of the study results depends mainly on the study question.

Big data. The availability of digital data has enormously increased in the past 15 years or so, mainly due to growing use of the internet, social media, and mobile phones. This data often labeled as "big data," a term which is applied to data of large volume, rapid availability (velocity), and large variety, with some other "V" words being added to this description (veracity validity, value, volatility). The use of big data for public health surveillance lagged behind its use for, e.g., marketing purposes, but is increasingly recognized. It includes analyses of data generated through the use of search engines on the internet, such as Google. The advantages include the fast availability of the data, and that it includes information from individuals who have not consulted formal health care. However, there are many potential biases that need to be borne in mind consequent upon the way that the population interact with the internet and algorithms are fitted. For example, Google's "Flu and Dengue Trends" initiatives were ceased after results were disappointing, due to reasons including overfitting of the underlying algorithms. In general, it also is important to realize that disease-related internet search queries or messages in social media Twitter or Facebook may reflect a variety of situations which are unrelated to the real occurrence of infections.

3.3.5   Confidentiality and privacy in surveillance

In most countries, laws exist which grant special rights to public health authorities to collect data on infectious diseases in humans, animals, and institutions for public health surveillance. Unlike research, the data collection for the purpose of public health surveillance usually is not overseen by an ethical review board, and does not involve obtaining informed consent from participants. This arrangement creates ethical questions since it infringes on the privacy of individuals. To protect privacy, public health organizations, therefore, are bound by laws on how data should be handled in a confidential manner. A key measure to improve confidentiality is to remove personal identifying information wherever this is possible. However, some personal identifiers remain necessary, especially at local levels, to obtain follow-up information or to de-duplicate data. To improve confidentiality, surveillance data at national level is usually anonymized. However, by linking data sources (e.g., by probabilistic linkage methods), the usefulness of the data may be much increased but at the same time individuals may become identifiable. Linking data, therefore, is a controversial area in surveillance. Professionals involved in surveillance are usually bound by certain rules of conduct aimed at further improving confidentiality.

The release of surveillance data is in some countries also governed by dedicated laws, e.g., granting the public access to all information which was collected by using collective funds. This again may infringe on privacy, so personally identifiable surveillance data is usually exempt from this. Surveillance data should be made available to the public in such a way that individuals cannot be identified even through deductive disclosure. The rules for this, the minimum number of people in cells of tabulated data, are becoming increasingly well defined.

When data collection is done for research purposes, ethical guidelines usually require a review by an ethical review board and often involve obtaining informed consent from participants [8]. The informed consent procedure should include at least a clear explanation of the purposes of the data collection, what it will be used for, who can access the data, and how long it will be stored.

3.3.6   Where to access surveillance output and data?

Typically, public health departments responsible for infectious disease surveillance routinely produce reports presenting surveillance indicators such as incidence and prevalence of a selected group of infectious diseases or syndromes, aggregated by demographic variables, risk factors, or geographical regions. These reports contain aggregate data, usually without detailed information on age, sex, or location of the patient. These reports are regularly shared with stakeholders contributing data, public health policy makers, and often with a wider audience.

More basic outputs of surveillance, such as the weekly number of notified cases of infectious diseases, usually is available also from public health institutes' websites. This data is usually still in aggregated form, often in a pdf which cannot directly be used for data analyses.

Researchers usually require more detailed, disaggregated data for analyses, ideally available in an electronic format which is directly useable. The availability of this type of data is increasing, as a result of specific projects (e.g., Project Tycho (http://www.tycho.pitt.edu/) and efforts of public health institutes (e.g., the German 'survstat' https://survstat.rki.de/default.aspx, the English Fingertips project http://fingertips.phe.org.uk/profile/health-profiles/data#page/0, and the European Atlas of Infectious Disease https://ecdc.europa.eu/en/surveillance-atlas-infectious-diseases). Availability of disaggregated data is further increased by the requirement of an increasing number of scientific journals authors to make it available upon publication of a research article. Despite these efforts, unfortunately, many barriers to sharing health data remain.

3.4   Data from Observational Epidemiological Studies and Outbreak Investigations of Infectious Diseases

3.4.1   Introduction

Epidemiology is the study of the occurrence and distribution of health-related states or events in specified populations, including the study of determinants influencing such states, and the application of this knowledge to control the health problems [3]. Epidemiological studies can be experimental or observational. Examples of experimental studies are clinical trials used to study the effects, safety, and impact of pharmaceutical treatments or vaccination.

In this section, we focus mainly on observational epidemiological studies, in which the researcher does not interfere with the conditions or determinants that are studied. Surveillance as a specific type of observational epidemiological study is discussed in 3.3. Observational studies can be used to generate or test hypotheses. The former is usually done by descriptive epidemiology while testing hypotheses requires analytical epidemiological designs and methods. Analytic epidemiological studies can have individuals or populations as the unit of observation. For the study of individuals, three main study designs exist: cohort (prospective) studies, case-control studies, and cross-sectional studies. Observational studies in which populations rather than individuals are studied are called ecological studies. All of these study designs, except the cross-sectional design, can be applied both prospectively and retrospectively, depending on whether the exposure measurement occurs before or after the disease occurrence.

In this section, we will describe the designs and methods used in these different types of observational epidemiological studies. In the last sections, we will discuss methods of the investigation of outbreaks and of emerging diseases, both particularly relevant for the epidemiological study of infectious diseases. Throughout the text, we will provide examples of data derived from some of these epidemiological study designs. The main aim of this section is to provide background information about where and how epidemiological data may be generated and inherent limitations which may be arising from this.

3.4.2   Cohort studies

Of all epidemiological observational study designs, the cohort study is the main design to make inferences on causality, since it follows people over time from exposure(s) to outcome(s) and hence provides information on the temporal relation between these two. In a cohort study, a group of people, who differ in the extent to which they are exposed to a potential determinant of the disease(s) of interest, is followed up in time whereby ascertaining the occurrence of health outcome(s) of interest and, ideally, the duration of time of follow-up and reasons for drop-out. People who are lost to follow-up no longer contribute to the data, and are called censored observations: their disease outcome status remains unknown. When analyzing a cohort study in real-time (at several moments when the cohort progresses in time), the outcome for many individuals in the cohort may be yet unknown and these then are classified also as censored observations. In a cohort study, the association between exposure and health outcome is quantified by calculating a measure of association which compares the occurrence of the health outcome between groups of individuals with a certain exposure status. The measure of association can be a relative risk (not taking the time of follow-up into account), a rate ratio (taking the duration of follow-up into account) or a hazard-ratio (taking both the duration of follow-up and the timing of the health event into account).

Data of cohort studies typically contains individual information on certain exposures, other determinants influencing the risk of certain health outcomes (confounders which may be adjusted for in the analysis), the occurrence and timing of certain health outcomes, the time of follow-up, and reasons for droping-out of the study.

In this described design of cohort studies, individuals are typically included in the cohort irrespective (i.e., unconditional) of their exposure to an infection of interest. In epidemiological studies of infectious diseases, study designs can be used in which cohorts are followed up which are more or less uniformly exposed to a certain infection. These studies are called conditional on exposure and are, of course, only ethical when effective post-exposure prophylaxis and/or treatment are made available to participants. The main advantage of this type of study is that efficiency is increased (the incidence of infection is higher in these cohorts). An example of a cohort study design conditional on exposure is the household follow-up study, in which household members of cases of an infectious disease are followed-up over time whereby ascertaining new cases of the infection of interest in household members. Household studies are a specific type of a contact-tracing study. In contact tracing studie, individuals who have an epidemiological link to a case (see Section 3.2.1), i.e., contacts, are included as study participants. Data from contact tracing studies typically includes individual data on age, gender, infection status (and, in case of a symptomatic infection, the disease onset date), some identification of the most likely source, date(s) of exposure, and exposure duration [9].

Bias in data from cohort studies can occur in several ways. First, when people who are lost to follow-up differ in terms of determinants or characteristics from those who remain in the study, the resulting data is not representative of the initial cohort. This outcome can lead to a biased assessment of the effects of a certain determinant, when the loss to follow-up is related to both to the determinant and the outcome of interest. A second cause of bias can result from unequal assessment of health outcome status between exposed and unexposed individuals, or, vice versa, from unequal assessment of the disease status between exposed and non-exposed individuals. Another important source of bias occurs when the exposure status of study participants is dependent on factors which also are related to the health outcome of interest (confounding by indication, e.g., frailty bias in influenza vaccine studies). Other sources of bias, e.g. those discussed in 3.2.3, can also occur in cohort studies.

3.4.3 Case-control studies

In a traditional case-control study, cases of a certain disease are compared to controls (non-diseased individuals) in terms of their exposure to a certain determinant. The major advantage over cohort methods is the efficiency achieved by the reduction in sample size. However, choosing suitable controls, which should be representative of the population that gave rise to the cases, can be problematic and may introduce bias. The measure of association which is calculated in case-control studies is the odds ratio, comparing the odds of exposure between cases and controls. Depending on the sampling method, the odds ratio can be directly interpreted as a risk of rate ratio [10].

Ideally controls should meet two criteria – first, their exposures should be representative of the population from which the cases arise and second assessment of determinants, e.g., vaccine status, in both cases and controls should be the same. The key principal to avoid bias in case-control studies is to ensure that cases and controls are derived from the same source population. Biased estimates of the odds ratio occur when cases systematically differ from controls in characteristics, that are related to both the exposure and health outcome of interest.

Different sources of controls can be used (e.g., from the community or other persons admitted to hospital), but it is often challenging to meet these two requirements. In attempts to reduce the occurrence of bias in case-control studies, alternatives to selecting healthy individuals as controls are being used. The test-negative design (TND) is a specific form of a case-control study design in which controls are individuals who present with the same clinical syndrome (e.g., influenza-like illness) but who have a negative microbiologic test result for the infection of interest. The main advantage of the TND is that biases arising from different health care seeking behavior (propensity to consult) between cases and controls is reduced [11]. Another variant of the traditional case-control study, is the case-case study. Here, the referent group consists of patients of another (form) of the disease.

Data generated during case-control studies is similar to that in cohort studies (see previous) except for that time of follow-up and censoring are not relevant. In addition to biases mentioned previously, biases listed in 3.2.3 also may apply.

3.4.4   Cross-sectional studies

In a cross-sectional epidemiological design, a group of individuals is studied by ascertaining exposures and outcomes at the same point in time. A prevalence study is an example of a cross-sectional study which aims to estimate the prevalence of a certain health status. In analyses of cross-sectional studies, groups of individuals with a different status regarding their exposure to determinants of infections can be compared in terms of their prevalence of infection. Alternatively, the odds of exposure can be compared between cases and non-cases. An important limitation of cross-sectional studies is that the sequence in time between a potential determinant and the outcome of interest is unknown, unless historical information is ascertained, without such longitudinal data it is not possible to ascertain a causal relationship. Biases occurring in cross-sectional study data can arise through overrepresentation of cases with a long duration of illness.

An example of a cross-sectional study design is a serological survey (see Box 3.4). This type of survey can be used in the evaluation of a vaccination program. It also can be used to study risk factors for infection, provided the infection gives rise to long-lasting antibodies (see Chapter 16) [12, 13]. Modeling approaches with underlying assumptions can be used to make estimates of incidence from such prevalence surveys. Biases in data from serological studies can arise due to the sampling of individuals who may not be representative of the population of interest. Cross-sectional seroprevalence data often is studied by age. When doing so, it is important to realize that an increase in seroprevalence by age can reflect both an ongoing and a decreasing risk of infection over time, representing an age and cohort effect, respectively. In one-off cross-sectional studies, it is impossible to disentangle these effects (Figure 3.4).

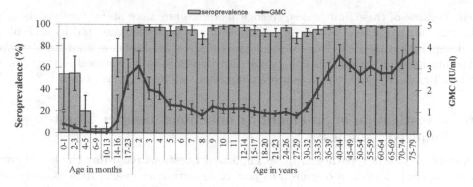

FIGURE 3.4

Weighted age-specific seroprevalence and geometric mean concentrations (GMC) of measles IgG antibody (with 95% confidence intervals) in the general population. (Adapted from Mollema, L. et al., *Epidemiol Infect.*, 42, 1100–1108, 2014.)

BOX 3.4 AN EXAMPLE OF A CROSS-SECTIONAL STUDY: MEASLES SEROPREVALENCE IN THE NETHERLANDS

Measles virus infection gives rise to an immune reaction, which includes the generation of antibodies that persist for life. This outcome also holds for measles vaccination, although a small proportion of vaccinated persons does not respond to the vaccine and antibodies wane over time. Measles virus specific antibodies can be quantified in serum, and when a threshold level is applied, the seroprevalence of measles antibodies can be assessed in a population [14].

In the Netherlands, a large survey of was undertaken in 2006/2007 which was used to assess measles immunity in the general population [14]. Over 6,000 individuals participated by giving blood and filling out a questionnaire. Serum samples were tested for measles virus specific IgG, and seroprevalence and geometric mean concentrations (GMC) calculated. Results are displayed in Figure 3.4 showing a gap in immunity in infants below the age of the first dose of measles containing vaccine (MCV) (14 months), a decline in antibody levels after MCV-1, and relatively high GMCs in older adults. The GMC and seroprevalence results by age need to be interpreted in the context of (historic) measles vaccination schedules, their uptake, and information on the incidence of measles virus infection over time.

3.4.5 Ecological studies

Studies in which the units of observation are groups of people rather than individuals are called ecological (or aggregate) studies. Data collected in ecological studies are measurements averaged over individuals, e.g., an incidence of an infectious disease in the population or the prevalence of uptake of preventive measures. Importantly, the degree of association between these population averages of disease and exposure may differ from the associations between the two assessed at an individual level. An oversight of this phenomenon is referred to as the ecological fallacy. Ecological studies also are prone to confounding, since populations studied are likely to differ in many factors potentially related to the disease being studied. Because of these limitations, ecological studies are more useful for hypothesis generation than for hypothesis testing. An example of a hypothesis generated by an ecological study design is that the zika virus caused microcephaly: this idea came from the observation that the incidence of both microcephaly and zika virus infection increased at the same time in 2015 in Brazil. To prove the causal relation, other studies were necessary.

3.4.6   Investigation of an emerging infectious disease: "First-few-hundred" studies

The emergence of a new pathogen raises important questions regarding the key characteristics of the newly identified organism as part of severity assessment, such as its transmissibility to close contacts and the likelihood that someone who is infected will developed symptoms and suffer more severe consequences. First-few-hundred studies are longitudinal cohorts that involve the follow-up of the first cases and their close household and other contacts together with gathering clinical and biological data to ascertain whether there is serological or virological evidence of infection. These data can be used to derive parameters such as the secondary household attack rate, the reproductive number, the incubation period, and the proportion symptomatic [15].

Differential follow-up depending on key exposures or outcomes has the potential to introduce significant bias in this type of study. Furthermore, results of first-few-hundred studies are highly dependent on the characteristics of the selected patients, their region and, e.g., their economic status. Results based on studies of a relatively small number of patients from specific regions may not be representative of results on a global scale. An example of this occurred when a new pandemic influenza strain emerged in 2009 in Mexico. This influenza virus was first thought to cause relatively severe disease, based on an initially small sample of infected patients.

3.4.7   Outbreak investigation

A key characteristic of many infectious diseases is that they can cause outbreaks. Outbreaks can occur due to infections which are communicable (i.e., with a capacity to spread from person-to-person). Non-communicable pathogens, such as, e.g., Legionella, can also cause outbreaks, typically in the form of a common source outbreak where people are exposed to a common source that is contaminated. When this common source is limited to a certain geographical location and was present only for a short period of time, a point source outbreak can result. When the source of infection continues to be contaminated and people continue to be exposed, an ongoing common source outbreak can be the result. Depending on whether the pathogen is communicable, common source outbreaks can be propagated by subsequent person-to-person spread. Descriptive epidemiological data can be used to distinguish these types of outbreaks (see Chapter 23).

The words outbreak and epidemic are synonymous. The definition of an outbreak is "the occurrence in a community of region of cases of an illness, specific health-related behaviour, or other health-related events clearly in excess of normal expectancy" [3]. The implication of this definition is that in order to declare an outbreak, one needs to have information on what the normal frequency of the occurrence of the illness is.

From a public health perspective, the primary aim of investigating outbreaks is to document evidence for interventions to stop the outbreak, limit its impact, and prevent the occurrence of similar ones in the future. An additional aim can be to find evidence for early identification of cases to allow appropriate treatment (i.e., secondary prevention). Investigating outbreaks also can aid in detecting gaps in health programs aimed at preventing and controlling infectious diseases. In addition to these aims directly related to outbreak control and secondary prevention, the investigation of outbreaks can help to increase knowledge about the pathogen, about, e.g., risk factors for transmission, host-related risk factors, the natural course of disease, and effectiveness of interventions. Outbreaks can be considered as natural experiments, providing an opportunity to document evidence by performing an outbreak investigation.

Outbreak investigation refers to the context of the epidemiological study, rather than to a distinct epidemiological design or method. Epidemiological outbreak investigations for disease control are usually done following a number of specific steps [16]. After the outbreak is confirmed and a representative sample or all cases has been identified, descriptive epidemiological analyses are a key step to generate hypotheses. Descriptive epidemiology in outbreak investigation and surveillance require identical analyses: a description of cases by time, place, person, and type. A description of cases by time, i.e. the "epidemic curve" can be particularly informative to hypothesize whether the outbreak is due to a point source. Hypotheses testing about the cause of the outbreak usually requires an analytical epidemiological study, e.g., a cohort, case-control, cross-sectional, or ecological design (see previous discussion).

References

[1] GM Weinstock. Genomic approaches to studying the human microbiota. *Nature*, 489(7415):250, 2012.

[2] G Murphy and JV Parry. Assays for the detection of recent infections with human immunodeficiency virus type 1. *Eurosurveillance*, 13(36):18966, 2008.

[3] M Porta. *A Dictionary of Epidemiology*. Oxford: Oxford University Press, 2008.

[4] S Declich and AO Carter. Public health surveillance: Historical origins, methods and evaluation. *Bulletin of the World Health Organization*, 72(2):285, 1994.

[5] AD Langmuir. The surveillance of communicable diseases of national importance. *New England Journal of Medicine*, 268(4):182–192, 1963.

[6] S Hahné, M Hooiveld, H Vennema, A Van Ginkel, H De Melker, J Wallinga, W Van Pelt, and P Bruijning-Verhagen. Exceptionally low rotavirus incidence in the Netherlands in 2013/14 in the absence of rotavirus vaccination. *Eurosurveillance*, 19(43):20945, 2014.

[7] K Mølbak, L Espenhain, J Nielsen, K Tersago, N Bossuyt, G Denissov, A Baburin, M Virtanen, A Fouillet, T Sideroglou, et al. Excess mortality among the elderly in European countries, December 2014 to February 2015. *Eurosurveillance*, 20, 2015.

[8] World Health Organization, Council for International Organizations of Medical Sciences et al. *International Ethical Guidelines for Health-Related Research Involving Humans*. Geneva, Switzerland: Council for International Organizations of Medical Sciences, 2016.

[9] L Soetens, D Klinkenberg, C Swaan, S Hahné, and J Wallinga. Real-time estimation of epidemiologic parameters from contact tracing data during an emerging infectious disease outbreak. *Epidemiology*, 29(2):230–236, 2018.

[10] MJ Knol, JP Vandenbroucke, P Scott, and M Egger. What do case-control studies estimate? Survey of methods and assumptions in published case-control research. *American Journal of Epidemiology*, 168(9):1073–1081, 2008.

[11] EW Orenstein, G De Serres, MJ Haber, DK Shay, CB Bridges, P Gargiullo, and WA Orenstein. Methodologic issues regarding the use of three observational study designs to assess influenza vaccine effectiveness. *International Journal of Epidemiology*, 36(3):623–631, 2007.

[12] H Wilking, M Thamm, K Stark, T Aebischer, and F Seeber. Prevalence, incidence estimations, and risk factors of toxoplasma gondii infection in Germany: A representative, cross-sectional, serological study. *Scientific Reports*, 6:22551, 2016.

[13] TB Hallett, J Stover, V Mishra, PD Ghys, S Gregson, and T Boerma. Estimates of HIV incidence from household-based prevalence surveys. *AIDS (London, England)*, 24(1):147, 2010.

[14] L Mollema, GP Smits, GA Berbers, FR Van Der Klis, RS Van Binnendijk, HE De Melker, and SJM Hahné. High risk of a large measles outbreak despite 30 years of measles vaccination in the Netherlands. *Epidemiology & Infection*, 142(5):1100–1108, 2014.

[15] E McLean, RG Pebody, C Campbell, M Chamberland, C Hawkins, JS Nguyen-Van-Tam, I Oliver, GE Smith, C Ihekweazu, S Bracebridge, et al. Pandemic (h1n1) 2009 influenza in the UK: Clinical and epidemiological findings from the first few hundred (ff100) cases. *Epidemiology & Infection*, 138(11):1531–1541, 2010.

[16] Outbreak investigations. https://wiki.ecdc.europa.eu/fem/w/wiki/387.outbreak-investigations. Accessed: 16 March 2018.

4

Key Concepts in Infectious Disease Epidemiology

Nicholas P. Jewell

CONTENTS

4.1 Introduction

This chapter introduces key population concepts that describe qualitatively and quantitatively the evolution of both acute infectious disease outbreaks and the current state of endemic scenarios, and variation in such across key population subgroups. Such concepts include the incidence proportion, attack rate, secondary attack rate, and the hazard function (or force of infection). We briefly note how these key quantities might be numerically estimable from population or sample data.

4.2 Incidence

Broadly speaking, the risk of a disease is "the probability that an individual without disease will develop disease over a defined age or time interval" (Gail, 1999) [1]. For a fixed finite population, this quantity often is referred to as the *incidence proportion* associated with the disease in question over that time interval. We say more in the following discussion as to why the definition refers to a probability and the quantity to a proportion. Unpacking this definition requires careful thought and precise descriptions including (1) an accurate definition of what constitutes the occurrence of a disease (and the description of a test to detect infection), (2) the delineation of an appropriate timescale and the window (or interval) of time when disease is recorded, and (3) the definition of the population at risk of disease development. This definition of risk sometimes is referred to as cumulative risk since it counts all disease occurrences accumulating over the specified time period.

For an infectious disease, the ideal answer to the first of these definitional questions is a definitive confirmatory test of infection, preferably one that can be obtained non-invasively with a rapid return of results. Practically speaking, such tests almost always are subject to misclassification and it is important to address the specificity and sensitivity of test results (reflecting the probability of false positives and false negatives) when estimating and interpreting estimates of incidence proportions. Dependency on symptoms to identify infection is almost always unacceptably unreliable except in unusual circumstances, in part because this approach may only capture severe cases of infection and thereby miss a substantial number of individuals who may be less affected by infection but still remain infectious at least for some period of time.

The second question, regarding the interval over which incidence should be assessed depends on the context and the nature of the infection process. Ideally, it makes sense to have individuals at risk of infection over the entire time interval in question, thus suggesting an appropriate start and end of the risk period. In this sense, we would start an individual's risk interval at the beginning of exposure to risk and end it when no risk is believed to remain. However, using intervals that vary across individuals over chronological time is often cumbersome and not feasible with aggregate population data. In these cases, it often is implicitly assumed that some individuals will necessarily be at risk only over the majority of the defined interval—this is of little consequence to a proportion estimate so long as all individuals are exposed to risk in a reasonably homogeneous way over the risk interval.

Even picking the origin of the time interval in question requires careful thought. For epidemics, the time origin is usually the beginning of the outbreak. If the epidemic lasts for a substantial amount of time, then various incidence proportions may be considered over different time periods to assess dynamic changes in incidence as the epidemic evolves—this is discussed further in this chapter. In endemic settings, there is no natural beginning, and time is usually measured in terms of age, so that the incidence proportion at time t captures the probability of infection by age t.

For convenience, the timescale for considering infections is usually chronological time but need not be so. Use of standard time in this way assumes that risk is somewhat equivalent from individual to individual if they are exposed for a common interval. On the other hand, for certain infection transmission routes, this may not be reasonable. For example, with regard to sexually transmitted infectious diseases, such as HIV, a more appropriate timescale might be the number of unprotected sexual contacts. Clearly, here, there is no risk of infection for those with no sexual contacts no matter how much time elapses, and so it does not make sense to assume any risk over such chronological time periods. For example, Jewell and Shiboski (1990) [2] used data on partners of HIV infected individuals to estimate the cumulative incidence proportion for intervals that counted specific sexual contacts between partners as the timescale of interest, defining the incidence proportion for a partner over intervals that commenced with the original infection of the other partner (the index case).

Many investigators refer to an Incidence Proportion as an *attack rate*, particularly in outbreak investigations where the risk periods are short. Technically speaking, the quantity is not a rate, but a proportion, since the denominator does not involve individual time at risk. The *secondary attack rate*, or SAR, focuses this concept on individuals exposed to a *known* infected or some other source of infection. The SAR is defined as the proportion (or probability) of individuals who are infected through contact with a specified infectious person (during their relevant infectious period—see following). Again, this number is technically not a rate. The SAR often is used in examining the frequency of infections in small sub-populations, for example, household members exposed to a single infected in their homes (the latter being infected from a source outside the household). School classrooms provide another example. In other applications, known contacts with an infected individual are captured through contact tracing with each such contact observed to ascertain subsequent infection. A household SAR often is used to assess a vaccine's efficacy, particularly for infections transmitted by direct close contact between a susceptible and an infected. Halloran (2005) [3] describes an example of an early use of the SAR in this fashion due to Kendrick and Eldering (1939) [4] in a study of pertussis vaccines.

4.2.1 Sampling interpretation of the incidence proportion, attack rate, and secondary attack rate

What does the probability (in the previous definitions) refer to when an incidence proportion (or attack rate) of 30 percent is claimed for a specific infectious disease? The interpretation is not based on any assumption that the outcome in question occurs at random. In fact, disease development may be almost entirely deterministic, albeit according to an infection mechanism not yet well understood or measurable. What is meant by such a statement is that the risk definition refers to the probability that a *randomly sampled* individual will experience the outcome (infection) in the appropriate interval according to the necessary precise definition. Here, the randomness in the probability statement arises from sampling and not the disease mechanism. With this interpretation, it immediately follows that the risk is simply the fraction of the population who experience the event subject to the relevant definitional conditions.

4.2.2 Dependence of incidence on cofactors

Usually, it is valuable to divide populations at risk into subgroups and determine and compare the incidence proportion over these smaller subpopulations. Most commonly, age and sex may be used to define subgroups and any resulting variation of incidence across these groups may yield insight into the mode of transmission and/or infection or particular susceptible subgroups. Such subgroup incidence proportions allow for estimation of relative comparisons (the relative risk, the ratio of two incidence proportions) or absolute comparisons (the excess risk, the arithmetical difference in two incidence proportions).

The population age at incidence distribution for an infectious disease is of particular interest since it may suggest patterns of spread and where interventions may be most effective. For acute infectious diseases with complete ascertainment and accurate confirmatory diagnostic testing, this distribution is straightforward to estimate. Using ideas from case-only studies (Greenland, 1999) [5], this distribution also allows for estimation of the Relative Risk of infection across different age categories so long as the total population age distribution is known and there is complete case ascertainment. See McKeown and Jewell (2011) [6] for a discussion of this approach with application to laboratory confirmed cases of H1N1 influenza during the 2009 epidemic.

In less acute situations where, in addition, infection may be a silent phenomenon due to the absence of overt clinical symptoms, the latter strategy may not be useful. In such cases, population screening data where diagnostic tests can detect the presence of (prior) infection, may still be used to estimate the age at incidence distribution under certain assumptions. Such data often is referred to as seroprevalence data where the test involves detection of viral antibodies indicating previous infection. Statistically, this involves survival analysis techniques applied to what is known as *current status data* (here the current infection status of an individuals is measured at a known age); see Jewell and Emerson (2013) [7] and Hens et al. (2010) [8]. Necessary assumptions for unbiased estimation require that infected individuals are not removed from the population at greater rates (due to increased mortality, e.g.), that there is no chronological drift in the age at incidence distribution, and that detectable seropositivity persists after its first appearance following infection. An example of this method applied to Hepatitis A data in Bulgaria is given in Keiding (1991) [9]. Petito and Jewell (2017) [10] present an application to estimation of the age at incidence of Hepatitis C for non-Hispanic white women of childbearing age based on maternal testing at birth using the publicly available 2014 U.S. Birth Data File, also extending the methodology to allow for group tested seroprevalence data. This idea for estimating an age at incidence distribution dates back as far as Muench (1934) [11] who applied simple versions of the technique to data on yellow fever in South America, and also on whooping cough and tuberculosis in the United States.

4.3 Prevalence

Referring to the same risk interval underlying an incidence proportion, the (point) prevalence is the proportion of the population observed at risk that are currently infected at time t (within the interval). The interval, or period, prevalence for the entire interval $[0, T]$ is the proportion of the population at risk that were infected at any point during the interval. For example, the adult prevalence of HIV infection worldwide (ages 15–49) was 0.8 percent in 2015 (http://www.who.int/gho/hiv/en/), although this prevalence varies markedly across continents. For example, the same prevalence was 4.4 percent in Africa.

Point prevalence (P) and incidence proportion (I) are closely related concepts. When incidence is constant over time, and D is the duration of infection (the length of time from original infection until disease expression, typically death or immunity), a common relationship prevails: $P = I \times D$. However, these conditions are unusual and never occur during an outbreak or epidemic. Nevertheless, the relationship illustrates a general phenomenon that restricts the value of prevalence in understanding infection dynamics, namely that it not only depends on infection rates but also on disease duration. It is not, therefore, immediately apparent—for factors that influence prevalence—whether the relationship arises because of effects on incidence, duration, or both. In some cases, the prevalence of an infection can increase even though incidence is declining when progress is made in extending disease duration—this has often occurred, for example, in population HIV prevalence. In general, changes in prevalence lag changes in incidence, constraining the value of prevalence as a metric of progress in reducing infections. Despite these etiologic limitations, prevalence remains useful for determining the burden of disease in a population as a basis for resource planning and allocation. Keiding (1991) [9] provides a much more general and nuanced discussion of the relationship between prevalence and incidence.

4.4 The Hazard Rate

If the risk interval discussed previously is long, then several challenges arise in both estimating and interpreting the incidence proportion. Principal among these is that individuals may not be at risk over the entire time interval for a variety of reasons, or they may not be observed over the entire interval. Some individuals may only enter observation during the time period, and would not have been observed had they contracted infection before their surveillance began (the issue of delayed-entry or left truncation). More commonly, individuals may be lost to surveillance after a period of time (often referred to as right censoring).

If such patterns of incompleteness in the observation period systematically differ across subgroups, observed variations in incidence may be misleading. A simple solution to some of these vagaries of surveillance involves the calculation of an average *incidence rate* over the interval. The numerator of the incidence rate is the same as for an incidence proportion (the number of observed infections) but the denominator is replaced by the cumulative time at risk for all individuals under surveillance (allowing for the possibility that not all individuals are observed for the entire risk interval). The latter term is often referred to loosely as "person years at risk." Note that with this definition, an incidence rate refers to an average both over the population and the time interval; that is, it does not differentiate between risk at the beginning of an interval from that at the end. In some cases, the incidence rate is not constant over the interval, and thus this average may mask interesting infection dynamics over time.

A simpler way of tracking variation in incidence over a time interval, or the problem of a population that is unstable in that there is substantial immigration and emigration to and from the population at risk, is to simply divide the risk interval into multiple shorter time periods, and estimate the average incidence rate for each of these in turn. Typically, there will be less variation in both the population and their risk over smaller time intervals. Assuming that sufficient data is available, it would then be possible to plot the average incidence rate for a time interval against the midpoint, for example, of the interval in question. Such a plot would display infection risk dynamics. In the limit—where the lengths of the intervals get increasingly smaller—this plot reveals the *hazard rate*, which thus often is referred to as the instantaneous incidence rate over time (or historically, the *force of infection*).

The hazard function is necessarily always positive. The simplest form of a hazard function is when it is constant over the time interval—this corresponds to the time to infection being exponentially distributed. More complex hazard functions can be described using more flexible distributions that can allow the hazard function to increase or decrease over time or do both within the same interval. The area under the hazard curve is known as the *cumulative hazard function*.

During an outbreak, the hazard function will generally increase over time (since the beginning of the outbreak) before peaking and declining as the epidemic runs its course. The specifics of the growth of the hazard function over time depend critically on the value of the *reproductive number*, R_0, that describes the average number of new infections induced by one infected individual. When R_0 is large, the hazard function grows rapidly from the beginning of an outbreak, in comparison to situations with smaller values. For endemic infection risks, interest generally focuses on how the hazard function varies with age; Farrington (1990) [12] discusses estimates of the hazard function as a function of age for measles, mumps, and rubella—prior to the availability of vaccines—all of which display a rapid increase followed by a slow decline.

The hazard function, denoted by $h(t)$, is closely related to the incidence proportion over varying time intervals at risk. If the time period is denoted by $[0, t]$ with corresponding incidence proportion given by $I(t)$, then

$$h(t) = \frac{\frac{dI(t)}{dt}}{(1 - I(t))},$$ (4.1)

assuming a closed population. The denominator of $h(t)$ often is referred to as the survival function $S(t)$, as it denotes the proportion of the population at risk that does not acquire infection by time t, the 'survivors.' Over the same interval, the hazard function and survival function contain identical information in that we can solve (4.1) for $S(t)$ in terms of $h(t)$, yielding

$$S(t) = \exp\left(-\int_0^t h(t)\right).$$ (4.2)

Note that if the length of the time interval is essentially infinite, $S(t)$ will tend to a finite limit that represents the proportion of the population that is ultimately uninfected. This is only greater than zero if the cumulative hazard function, $\int_0^t h(t)$, remains finite as t tends to ∞.

4.5   Estimation of Incidence Proportion and Rates

Classic methods of estimating an incidence proportion require either (1) systematic follow-up of a defined cohort of individuals subject to infection with the ability to detect incident infections at any point in the defined risk interval or (2) accurate population ascertainment of cumulative infection counts supplemented with population demographic information regarding the size of the population at risk. For general estimation of the hazard function, cohort data is necessary including information on the times of infection for each case. As noted previously, with aggregate data, an average incidence rate can be estimated if the total number of individual time at risk is reported together with cumulative infection counts; in some cases, approximations of the time at risk total can be obtained by standard demographic techniques. Relative comparison of incidence proportions and hazard functions also can be obtained through case-control studies where a random sample of infecteds are compared to a random sample of individuals who remain infection free at the end of the risk interval (or with variants of control sampling associated with incidence density methods and case-cohort studies). Case-control strategies often are used to investigate acute infectious outbreaks (see Wheeler et al. [13] for an example linking consumption of green onions to infection with the Hepatitis A virus). Halloran, Preziosi, and Chu (2003) [14] describe methods to quantify vaccine efficacy based on estimated SARs. Infectious disease incidence data differ from that for most chronic non-infectious diseases in that there may be correlation among susceptibles in the same study, particularly when using SARs. Appropriate estimation of the variability of statistical estimators must account for this correlation (see, for example, Dunson and Halloran (1996) [15]).

Incidence estimates from population data necessarily depend critically on complete surveillance (equivalently the absence of underreporting) and rapid availability of test results. For the latter scenario, reporting delay is a common phenomenon that can significantly impact the accuracy of incidence estimation. Both of these phenomena are particularly adverse when the rates of underreporting and/or reporting delay systematically differ across population subgroups, thereby compromising natural comparative analysis of incidence patterns across the same groups.

Planning intervention studies to reduce infections requires some knowledge of recent infection rates to allow adequate sample sizes to be selected to detect efficacy. Accurately quantifying recent incidence rates for long-term infectious diseases like HIV remains a significant challenge and methods are rapidly evolving together with advances in the technology of diagnostic testing. Currently two general approaches are largely in use, either separately or in combination. The first uses mathematical models to derive recent incidence rates from series of prevalence estimates (see Hallett (2011) [16] for discussion). The second approach exploits data on contemporaneous assays applied to cross-sectional survey information. In brief, one version of this technique exploits a sensitive test of recent infection; in the case of HIV, early examples of this method employed tests of p24 antigenemia that can detect infection at a time when HIV antibodies cannot yet be measured. Rates of such positive tests, along with separate knowledge of the length of the period where p24 antigens can be detected but HIV antibodies cannot, are used to estimate recent HIV infection rates

(Brookmeyer and Quinn, 1995) [17]. Janssen et al. (1998) [18] noted that the value of this approach was limited due to the briefness of the period noted, and suggested a similar strategy based on a combination of sensitive and non-sensitive antibody tests. Both of these estimation methods depend on variants of the prevalence equals incidence times duration relationship. Challenges include the often substantial between-individual variation in responses to biomarker assays (undermining the value of a mean duration of the recent infection period), and quantification of the so-called false recent rate (FRR) that captures the fraction of long-term infecteds who are classified as recent infections.

4.6   Outcomes Other than Infection

Previously, we focused attention on incidence of infection, that is, when the disease process begins. Other key events in the natural history are also of substantial interest and key to understanding the development and impact of epidemics. For example, the time between infection and the onset of clinical symptoms is known as the *incubation period*. Likely, the length of incubation will randomly vary across individuals so that a population incubation distribution is required. In the early stages of the HIV epidemic, knowledge of the incubation distribution allowed observable counts of AIDS diagnoses to form the basis of estimated incidence counts and patterns (Brookmeyer and Gail, 1986) [19] through a technique known as back-calculation. For HIV, the effectiveness of back-calculation was sensitive to assumptions about the incubation period and whether it changed over calendar time as the epidemic progressed both before, and as, treatments were available to delay symptom onset (Bacchetti et al., 1993) [20].

Closely related to the incubation period is the *latent period* which measures the time from infection to when an infected individual becomes infectious (and can thus transmit the infection to others). Often, the beginning of these time periods are determined by the time of exposure to an infectious agent since this time may be hard to distinguish from the occurrence of infection. Similarly, the end of the latent period often coincides approximately with the onset of symptoms so that the latent and incubation periods may be very similar. Incubation periods differ substantially for many common viral infections, ranging from a few days for influenza to around a week for dengue infection, 1 to 2 months for mononucleosis, and a decade or more for HIV. The length of the latent period is crucial in determining the risk of the spread of an infection, and infected individuals may not be ascertained during this time period (whereas interventions to limit infectiousness are available once symptoms are apparent).

After infection, there is often substantial interest in how the associated disease is expressed, often by full recovery (and potential future immunity) or death. With acute infectious diseases, these represent the only two possible outcomes, and the *case fatality ratio* (CFR) is defined as the proportion of infected individuals who die from the disease. (The associated hazard function associated with time from infection to death is often referred to as the force of mortality.) During an epidemic, counts on both recovered individuals and deaths may be recorded and such data (and times to these events) can be analyzed using competing risk methods to estimate the CFR. A crucial challenge to this approach is the availability of an accurate diagnostic test that rapidly identifies infected individuals in a population (so that here, as for assessing infection rates, underreporting and reporting delay must be addressed in estimation). In the early stages of an epidemic, only infections and deaths may be counted with the CFR estimated by the fraction of deaths among the total number of infected. This estimator, however, underestimates the CFR, and it often is better to consider the fraction of deaths among infected individuals whose outcomes are fully determined. For examples and discussions of these issues associated with the CFR for severe acute respiratory syndrome (SARS); see Donnelly et al. (2003), Galvani, Lei & Jewell (2003), and Jewell et al. (2007) [21–23]. Lipsitch et al. (2015) [24] provide a broad discussion of biases that may affect estimation of the CFR during outbreaks. Knowledge of how the CFR varies across geographic regions, and over the course of an epidemic, may provide insight into the evolution of the virulence of infection; Galvani, Lei & Jewell (2003) [22] discuss these points for SARS.

4.7 Discussion

Estimation of quantities such as the hazard function and incubation period distribution, for example, depend on prior information (that may suggest parametric forms for these quantities) and available data. As with all such concepts defined here, the structure and granularity of available data constrain and suggest various estimation strategies. The existence of selection bias, misclassification of diagnostic test information, and missing data present serious challenges to accurate quantification in the field. In many examples, interest focuses not only on population estimates of infection rates, incubation, and case fatality information, but also on exactly how certain cofactors influence such quantities. Regression models have been developed widely to address these demands. A gentle introduction of the use of survival analysis techniques with infectious disease data is given by Cole and Hudgens (2010) [25].

References

[1] Mitchell H Gail. Risk. In Peter Armitage and Theodore Colton, editors, *Encyclopedia of Biostatistics*, pp. 3837–3838. John Wiley & Sons, Chichester, UK, 1999.

[2] Nicholas P Jewell and Stephen C Shiboski. Statistical analysis of HIV infectivity based on partner studies. *Biometrics*, 46:1133–1150, 1990.

[3] M Elizabeth Halloran. Secondary attack rate. In Peter Armitage and Theodore Colton, editors, *Encyclopedia of Biostatistics*, pages 4025–4029. John Wiley & Sons, Chichester, UK, 1998.

[4] Pearl Kendrick, Grace Eldering. A study in active immunization against pertussis. *American Journal of Hygiene*, 29:133–153, 1939.

[5] Sander Greenland. A unified approach to the analysis of case-distribution (case-only) studies. *Statistics in Medicine*, 18(1):1–15, 1999.

[6] Karen McKeown and Nicholas P Jewell. The usefulness of age-standardized measures of attack rates based on confirmed disease cases. Technical report, Preprint, University of California, Berkeley, CA, Department of Biostatistics, 2012.

[7] Nicholas P Jewell and R Emerson. Current status data: An illustration with data on avalanche victims. In John P Klein, Hans C Van Houwelingen, Joseph G Ibrahim, and Thomas H Scheike, editors, *Handbook of Survival Analysis*, pages 391–412. CRC Press, Chichester, UK, 2013.

[8] Niel Hens, Marc Aerts, Christel Faes, Ziv Shkedy, O Lejeune, P Van Damme, and P Beutels. Seventy-five years of estimating the force of infection from current status data. *Epidemiology & Infection*, 138:802–812, 2010.

[9] Niels Keiding. Age-specific incidence and prevalence: A statistical perspective. *Journal of the Royal Statistical Society. Series A (Statistics in Society)*, 371–412, 1991.

[10] Lucia C Petito and Nicholas P Jewell. Misclassified group-tested current status data. *Biometrika*, 103(4):801–815, 2016.

[11] Hugo Muench. Derivation of rates from summation data by the catalytic curve. *Journal of the American Statistical Association*, 29(185):25–38, 1934.

[12] C Paddy Farrington. Modelling forces of infection for measles, mumps and rubella. *Statistics in Medicine*, 9(8):953–967, 1990.

[13] Charlotte Wheeler, Tara M Vogt, Gregory L Armstrong, Gilberto Vaughan, Andre Weltman, Omana V Nainan, Virginia Dato et al. An outbreak of hepatitis a associated with green onions. *New England Journal of Medicine*, 353(9):890–897, 2005.

[14] M Elizabeth Halloran, Marie Pierre Préziosi, and Haitao Chu. Estimating vaccine efficacy from secondary attack rates. *Journal of the American Statistical Association*, 98(461):38–46, 2003.

[15] David B Dunson and M Elizabeth Halloran. Estimating transmission blocking efficacy of malaria vaccines. Technical report, Technical Report 96-16, Emory University, Department of Biostatistics, Atlanta, GA, 1996.

[16] Timothy B Hallett. Estimating the HIV incidence rate–recent and future developments. *Current Opinion in HIV and AIDS*, 6(2):102–107, 2011.

[17] Ron Brookmeyer and Thomas C Quinn. Estimation of current human immunodeficiency virus incidence rates from a cross-sectional survey using early diagnostic tests. *American Journal of Epidemiology*, 141(2):166–172, 1995.

[18] Robert S Janssen, Glen A Satten, Susan L Stramer, Bhupat D Rawal, Thomas R O'brien, Barbara J Weiblen, Frederick M Hecht et al. New testing strategy to detect early HIV-1 infection for use in incidence estimates and for clinical and prevention purposes. *JAMA*, 280(1):42–48, 1998.

[19] Ron Brookmeyer and Mitchell H Gail. Minimum size of the acquired immunodeficiency syndrome (AIDS) epidemic in the United States. *The Lancet*, 328(8519):1320–1322, 1986.

[20] Peter Bacchetti, Mark R Segal, Nancy A Hessol, and Nicholas P Jewell. Different AIDS incubation periods and their impacts on reconstructing human immunodeficiency virus epidemics and projecting AIDS incidence. *Proceedings of the National Academy of Sciences*, 90(6):2194–2196, 1993.

[21] Christl A Donnelly, Azra C Ghani, Gabriel M Leung, Anthony J Hedley, Christophe Fraser, Steven Riley, Laith J Abu-Raddad et al. Epidemiological determinants of spread of causal agent of severe acute respiratory syndrome in Hong Kong. *The Lancet*, 361(9371):1761–1766, 2003.

[22] Alison P Galvani, Xiudong Lei, and Nicholas P Jewell. Severe acute respiratory syndrome: Temporal stability and geographic variation in death rates and doubling times. *Emerging Infectious Diseases*, 9(8):991, 2003.

[23] Nicholas P Jewell, Xiudong Lei, Azra C Ghani, Christl A Donnelly, Gabriel M Leung, Lai-Ming Ho, Benjamin J Cowling, and Anthony J Hedley. Non-parametric estimation of the case fatality ratio with competing risks data: An application to severe acute respiratory syndrome (sars). *Statistics in Medicine*, 26(9):1982–1998, 2007.

[24] Marc Lipsitch, Christl A Donnelly, Christophe Fraser, Isobel M Blake, Anne Cori, Ilaria Dorigatti, Neil M Ferguson et al. Potential biases in estimating absolute and relative case-fatality risks during outbreaks. *PLoS Neglected Tropical Diseases*, 9(7):e0003846, 2015.

[25] Stephen R Cole and Michael G Hudgens. Survival analysis in infectious disease research: Describing events in time. *AIDS (London, England)*, 24(16):2423–2431, 2010.

Key Parameters in Infectious Disease Epidemiology

Laura F. White

CONTENTS

5.1   Introduction

Epidemiologists often are interested in understanding the population level impact of a disease and effective approaches to limit its pathological impact on a population. Parameters are valuable tools that characterize populations and diseases in meaningful, quantifiable ways. These parameters can determine what interventions and control measures are most appropriate to contain a disease and predict how it might impact a population. Estimates of these parameters are derived from available data using statistical or mathematical models. In this chapter, we use the term parameter to refer to the true unknown quantities. We explicitly use the term estimated parameter to refer to the numeric summaries that are derived from data.

We are familiar with many parameters and use them frequently. For example, a mean is a parameter that is an attempt to understand the central tendency of a population (e.g., average BMI among adults in a particular location, mean CD4 count among an HIV infected population, etc.). The estimated mean is calculated by taking information from a sample of

n individuals, intended to represent the population being studied. We sum the individual values of the characteristic of interest (e.g., BMI or CD4 count) and divide by the total number surveyed, n. A proportion is a type of mean that is used to summarize a dichotomous attribute. In this case, we are considering the likelihood of one of the two possible responses (e.g., vaccinated versus unvaccinated). The sample proportion is calculated in the same way as a sample mean. We assign those with the attribute (for instance being vaccinated) a 1 and the rest a 0. Then we can sum these and divide by the sample size, n. Calculation of these estimated parameters is a familiar practice.

In infectious disease epidemiology there are many parameters that are commonly used to better characterize and understand infectious diseases and their (potential) impact on a population. These parameters most frequently aim to characterize the transmission, burden, and severity of a disease. There are also many parameters that are used to quantify the impact of interventions on a disease, for example, those pertaining to vaccine efficacy, herd immunity, and test characteristics of diagnostics.

There are many reasons to estimate parameters in an infectious disease setting. Parameters are useful inputs in modeling exercises to prepare and plan for disease outbreaks. They guide our understanding of how to best contain current infectious diseases. Parameters are useful for understanding the impact that therapies and interventions may have. When an outbreak occurs there is great interest in determining how severe the disease is, how fast it is spreading, the interventions that will be most effective, and the most vulnerable populations.

In this chapter we describe commonly used infectious disease epidemiology parameters and statistical approaches to their estimation. We focus on parameters relevant to the progression of disease, transmission, and severity.

5.2 Key Infectious Disease Intervals

We first discuss estimation of several intervals that are relevant to understanding the dynamics of an infectious disease. We define them here and then discuss statistical methods for their estimation in this section.

- **Generation Interval**: Time between infection events in an infector-infectee pair
- **Serial Interval**: Time between symptom onset in an infector-infectee pair
- **Incubation Period**: Time from infection until onset of symptoms
- **Latent Period**: Time from infection to infectiousness
- **Infectious Period**: Time an individual is infectious

The relationship between these intervals is shown in Figure 5.1. The generation interval is very useful in modeling transmission of a disease in a population and understanding the speed with which it will spread. However, its endpoints are unobservable, making the serial interval a desireable surrogate. In fact, the serial interval is an unbiased estimate of the generation interval if the incubation periods are independent of one another [1]. The serial interval and generation interval contain information that is critical to describing the speed at which an epidemic will unfold. For example, the mean serial interval of influenza is estimated to be around 2 days [3]; however, for tuberculosis, this quantity has been estimated to be as long 3.5 years, though it is possible it is even longer, [4] leading to dramatically different population and individual level dynamics. When used with the reproductive number, as will be shown, this provides valuable information about the rapidity with which a disease

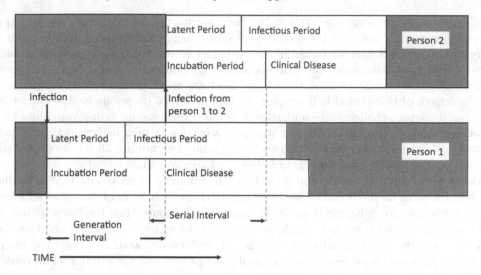

FIGURE 5.1
Schematic of key infectious disease intervals. (Adapted from [2].)

will spread, as well as interventions that will likely be most effective. Severe Acute Respiratory Syndrome (SARS), which has a reproductive number that is similar in magnitude to influenza, was effectively contained by use of quarantine measures due to its relatively long serial interval of 8–10 days [5, 6] and lack of asymptomatic transmission [7].

The incubation distribution plays an important role in public health, including determining appropriate quarantine periods, the source of an infection, and the relationship between transmission and infectiousness [8]. Several reviews of this quantity have been published, for example, for gastroentiritis [9], acute respiratory infections [10], and influenza [8]. In non-sexually transmitted diseases, the point at which infection occurs is typically difficult to ascertain, often leading to the time of infection being best described by an interval where contact with an infectious individual occurred. Contact tracing studies (such as those conducted in households) are frequently used to define transmission events. Incorrect ascertainment of infector-infectee pairs, discrete data, and ambiguity on the exact timing of the start and end point of this interval are challenges in working with this data, as they are for serial interval data. Many have approached estimation of the latent period by eliminating observations that are too long (or short) and assuming a fixed, known point of exposure as the starting point and summarizing observed intervals, with no adjustment for any of the data issues [11, 12]. Kuk and Ma [13] describe a rigorous approach to estimating this interval from contact tracing data and using the serial interval.

Estimation of the latent period is similar to that of the incubation period. The only difference is that we must determine when an individual becomes infectious, rather than diseased. In many diseases, it is assumed that these coincide; however, this is not always the case, such as in influenza [14], in polio where most infections are asymptomatic, but infectious, or, as a more complicated setting, and in HIV where individuals can be highly infectious despite being completely asymptomatic for a short period immediately following infection followed by a dramatic decline in infectivity [15]. However, the tools used in the estimation of the serial interval distribution and incubation period distribution are applicable once endpoints, or intervals for the endpoints, have been defined for the latent period.

The infectious period has the greatest paucity of statistical methods described for its estimation, but is of extreme public health importance. It often is determined from viral shedding data (see, for example, [16]) or by observing bacterial loads. However, infectiousness is dependent on not only the quantity of pathogen in an infected individual, but the ability of the infected host to transmit the pathogen to others. For example, it is widely accepted that extrapulmonary tuberculosis, unlike its pulmonary form, is not transmissible from an infected host because there is no mechanism for transmission. So, examining only the length of this period is inadequate to fully describe its public health importance. There are numerous challenges to understanding infectiousness, including variability in the virulence and infectiousness of differing strains of a pathogen, host behaviors that influence transmission (social connectedness, hygiene, etc.), and determining all modes of transmission (for example, sexual transmission of ebola and zika was unexpected).

As the serial interval, incubation period, and latent interval have data that is similarly collected, the same methods can be used to estimate them with, at most, minor modification. When individuals are only infectious at the onset of symptoms, then the latent period and incubation period are equivalent. Unique estimation tools for the latent period are only required when the onset of infectiousness is not understood well. However, the interval censoring tools used for estimation of the incubation period and the serial interval could be applied.

These intervals are used commonly to parameterize mathematical models, though occasionally mathematical models are used to obtain estimates of these intervals (for example, Cori et al. [17] obtained estimates of the SARS latent and infectious periods using viral shedding data in an SEIR model). Many mathematical models assume exponential distributions for these intervals, which simplifies the models but leads to incorrect inferences for the reproductive number [18] and frequently oversimplifies the true dynamics of the disease. More recent work has been done using alternative and more flexible parametric distributions, such as the Gamma distribution.

When data is collected on these intervals, they appear skewed. Because of this, Log-normal distributions have been used historically to summarize these distributions [19]. The Log-normal distribution is convenient to work with. In fact, we can log transform the observed intervals and run a regression model that is then equivalent to an accelerated failure time model [20]. The advantage of this approach is that it allows for the inclusion of covariates in the estimation of the interval. However, it is now recognized that other parametric and nonparametric distributions should be considered since the Log-normal distribution often provides an inadequate or inferior fit to the data.

These intervals are often summarized in the literature by their mean or median and standard deviation or range. In the case of the incubation distribution the 95th or 99th quantile are used to determine the length of quarantine. These summary statistics are helpful for parameterizing models, determining policy, and succinctly summarizing a disease, but being able to provide good summary statistics hinges on the accuracy with which the underlying distribution is estimated. For example, if a Log-normal distribution is assumed, then the resulting mean estimate would likely be different than if a Gamma distribution is used. This could result in inaccuracies in reproductive number estimates, the ideal quarantine time, and treatment and containment procedures.

Estimates of these intervals are based on observed data. This data often comes from contact tracing studies where sick individuals are identified and then those in close proximity to them are contacted to determine if they infected or were infected by the initial case. In the case of the serial interval, the time between symptom onset is recorded and it is generally assumed that negative serial intervals are not possible. In this case, intervals are often reported in days (or weeks for diseases with longer latency, such as tuberculosis or HIV). The discrete nature of the data must be accounted for in the estimation of the serial interval distribution. It also is possible that individuals might be erroneously identified as an infector-infectee pair.

In the remainder of this section we discuss methods that are appropriate to estimate infectious disease intervals. These methods are broadly applicable to any of the intervals specified previously, assuming adequate data is collected. Specifically we describe methods to

1. Estimate continuous parametric distributions from discretely collected data,

2. Accommodate uncertainty around the start and end point of the interval,

3. Account for truncation in the data collected, and

4. Allow for uncertainty in the transmission chain.

5.2.1   Parametric estimation

Observed interval data, whether for the serial interval, incubation distribution, or latent period, tend to be skewed and nonnegative. Sartwell [19] proposed the use of the Log-normal distribution to describe this data. However, the Gamma and Weibull distributions also have been suggested as appropriate distributions. We describe the probability density function (pdf) and cumulative density function (CDF) by $f(x_i|\theta)$ and $F(x_i|\theta)$, respectively. In the case of the Log-normal distribution, θ is composed of the location and scale parameters, μ and σ. If the intervals we observe are denoted by $x_1, \ldots, x_n$, then we can use straightforward maximum likelihood estimation (MLE) to obtain estimates of θ. In other words, we differentiate the log likelihood with respect to θ and solve to obtain maxima. The log likelihood is given by

$$l = \sum_i log(f(\theta|x_i)). \tag{5.1}$$

For the Log-normal distribution, closed form solutions for $\theta = (\mu, \sigma^2)$ are given by

$$\hat{\mu} = \frac{1}{n}\sum_i^n \log(x_i), \qquad \hat{\sigma}^2 = \frac{1}{n}\sum_i^n (\log(x_i) - \hat{\mu})^2. \tag{5.2}$$

When closed form solutions for the parameters of the distribution are not available (such as for the Gamma and Weibull distributions), numerical optimization tools, such as the Newton Raphson approach, can be used. Akaike information criterion (AIC) can be used to choose the best fitting parametric distribution. Alternatively, Bayesian approaches are appropriate to obtain posterior distributions of the parameters.

5.2.2   Discrete data adjustment

The methods in the previous section assume that the x_i are continuously observed. This would mean that we observe the exact moment in which an individual is infected, symptomatic, etc. Typically this data is observed in discrete intervals, such as days or weeks. We will later describe how treating this as interval censored data can account for this issue. First, we describe an alternative approach that assumes a discrete probability distribution (typically a multinomial distribution) parameterized by a continuous distribution [21].

We let $g(t)$ be a discrete probability mass function describing the probability of an interval of length t. We observe n_t intervals of length t ($N = \sum_t n_t$), then a log likelihood is given by

$$l = \sum_{t=1}^{D_{max}} n_t log(g(t)), \tag{5.3}$$

where D_{max} is the maximal serial interval assumed. In influenza, this interval often is set to 7–10 days but could be appropriately adjusted for other diseases. We can assume a parametric distribution to describe the $g(t)$ such as a multinomial distribution. For a distribution that assumes continuous time, we can take the discretely observed serial intervals (for example, in days, rather than in continuous time) and define $g(t)$ as

$$g(t) = \frac{[F(t + 0.5) - F(t - 0.5)]}{[F(D_{max} + 0.5) - F(0.5)]}. \tag{5.4}$$

In this case $\sum_{t=1}^{D_{max}} g(t) = 1$. Again, we can use the typical distributional assumptions for $F(t|\theta)$ which include the Gamma, Log-normal, and Weibull distributions. In this case, the log likelihood will be maximized over the parameters of the assumed parametric distribution. AIC criteria can be used to select the best-fitting distribution. In their study of several sources of influenza data, Donnelly et al. estimate the serial interval to be 2.9 days (95% CI, 2.63.3 days) assuming a Weibull distribution [21].

An alternative approach is described by Hens et al. [22] and is designed for data grouped into transmission clusters, for example, households. This approach allows for missing links in the transmission chain (as will be described following) [23]. As before, the discreteness that they describe is a result of using a continuous time distribution for estimation when the times are measured discretely (in the case of influenza, in days). For their example, this means that cases that are reported 1 day apart from each other could have occurred anywhere between 0–48 hours apart, which is the level of detail needed to more accurately fit a continuous parametric distribution. This latter issue is accommodated in a likelihood by using a triangle distribution. The triangle distribution is defined by $h(x|s)$, where s is the mode of the triangular distribution. The triangular distribution is given by

$$h(x|s) = \begin{cases} x - s + 1, & \text{for } s - 1 \leq x < s \\ -x + s + 1, & \text{for } s \leq x \leq s + 1 \\ 0, & \text{otherwise.} \end{cases} \tag{5.5}$$

The likelihood of observing an interval, such as a serial interval, of s days is given by

$$p(s|\theta) = \int_{s-1}^{s+1} h(x|s) f(x|\theta) dx \tag{5.6}$$

where $f(x|\theta)$ is the parametric pdf, such as a Gamma distribution.

5.2.3   Censoring

A separate approach to dealing with the uncertainty in either the start and/or end point of the observed data is to use interval censoring techniques from survival analysis [24]. In this case, the data we observe are described by intervals, rather than exact x_i. These intervals can be longer and more variable in length than the discrete intervals described in Section 5.2.2. We define (L_i, R_i) such that the true time of the event, X_i is within this interval, i.e., $L_i < X_i < R_i$. We also allow that not all data might be censored and let $\delta_i = 1$ if the data is exactly observed. Then the likelihood for θ is given by

$$L(\boldsymbol{\theta}|x_1, \ldots, x_N) = \prod_i f(x_i|\boldsymbol{\theta})^{\delta_i} (F(R_i|\boldsymbol{\theta}) - F(L_i|\boldsymbol{\theta}))^{1-\delta_i}. \tag{5.7}$$

We can proceed by using a numerical optimizer or Bayesian approach for estimation of $\boldsymbol{\theta}$.

Reich et al. [25] also describe interval censoring techniques for the estimation of the incubation distribution. They approach the problem of doubly interval-censored data where both the start and end point are assumed to be interval-censored. They use techniques for doubly interval-censored data and then a more simple data reduction approach. In the latter, they calculate the longest possible interval and the smallest possible interval. They then treat this as a single interval-censored problem. The latter approach, although inferior in simulation, is realistic in many settings when data is only reported as an interval and it is not clear if the ambiguity on the interval is at the start or end point.

5.2.4 Truncation

Cowling et al. [24] describe an approach to estimate the serial interval using statistical tools for time-to-event data that accounts for both interval censoring and truncation. This approach is broadly applicable to incubation periods, as well [20].

Left truncation of the data was present in their study because individuals included in the study who had been symptomatic at least 1 day result in observed serial intervals that would be at least 1 day long. We denote the lower bound induced by truncation by ν_i. Then the likelihood function is modified to be

$$L(\theta|x_1,\dots,x_N) = \prod_i \left(\frac{f(x_i|\theta)}{1 - F(\nu_i|\theta)} \right)^{\delta_i} \left(\frac{F(R_i|\theta) - F(L_i|\theta)}{1 - F(\nu_i|\theta)} \right)^{1-\delta_i}. \tag{5.8}$$

Cowling et al. [24] have an excellent e-Appendix including code provided to implement this approach as well as Turnbull's nonparametric estimator, described following.

In Cowling et al.'s example using data from a household contact study of 122 index cases and their 350 household contacts during the 2007 influenza season in Hong Kong, they determined a Weibull distribution with mean 3.6 days (95% CI: 2.9–4.3 days) fit the data from 14 pairs best using AIC criteria.

5.2.5 Nonparametric estimation

Turnbull [26] and Peto [27] derived a nonparametric estimator for the survival curve (which can be used to describe the distribution of the intervals of interest) that accommodates interval censored data. Lindsey and Ryan [28] describe an algorithm for implementing this method that has been used to estimate the serial interval of influenza [24] and the incubation distribution of SARS [20] and avian influenza [29]. The approach accounts for data that is observed in intervals, rather than exact time points. For instance, we would report (L_i, R_i) as the observed data, when it is known that the event of interest occurred between time point L_i and R_i, $L_i \leq R_i$. If there is no censoring, then $L_i = R_i$.

The L_i and R_i is ordered and intervals that start with an L and end with an R are called equivalence sets. Only in equivalence sets can the survival curve jump. More details on this approach are provided in the papers by Turnbull [26], Lindsey and Ryan [28], and Cowling et al. [24]. The package Icens in R can be used to implement this method and Cowling et al. [24] provides code and an example of this approach.

5.2.6 Uncertain transmission links

Typically the serial, latent, and incubation intervals are estimated through detailed contact investigations and then summarizing the observed intervals between assumed infector-infectee pairs [5, for example]. These studies often are performed within households or schools, with the assumption that most transmission occurs between individuals who have substantial contact with one another. It also is assumed typically that serial intervals are non-negative. There is potential for misspecifying transmission links with this study design. As an alternative approach, Ten Asbroek et al. [30] proposed using genetic data to determine the transmission chain in tuberculosis. However, determining how to link cases of infectious disease using genetic data is challenging and complicated by the need to determine the pathogen specific mutation rate and determination of the impact of the bottleneck created by transmission [31, 32].

It often is not feasible to determine definitively whether two individuals have transmitted disease to one another, even if they are in close proximity and have had sustained contact with one another. For instance, there is potential that an intermediary host, such as a shared household member, infected both of them, but they developed symptoms at different times, creating the illusion that one infected the other. Vink et al. [3] provide a systematic review of existing estimates of the serial interval for infectious diseases and propose a likelihood based approach that uses a mixture distribution to allow for observed links to be between cases that are co-primary, primary-secondary, primary-tertiary, or primary-quaternary. This approach uses the Expectation-Maximization algorithm to obtain estimates from a likelihood that is a mixture of the four potential types of links between the cases. The technical appendix in [3] provides the R-code for this method. We do not detail this method here, but recognize this as a useful tool in concert with the following methods we describe. Most of the statistical developments in serial interval estimation have been motivated by influenza, although these approaches could potentially be applicable to other diseases with similar attributes, including person-to-person transmission.

te Beest et al. [33] and Hens et al. [22] describe an approach to account for uncertainty in transmission links using structured data, such as that from a household, such that there are n_c individuals coming from c households. Transmission is assumed to have occurred within households. The likelihood is

$$l(\theta|x) = \sum_c \sum_i f(t_{ci} - t_{c\eta(i)}|\theta). \tag{5.9}$$

In the case of te Beest et al. [33] they use the description given in (5.6). t_{ci} and $t_{c\eta(i)}$ are the times of symptom onset for an infector-infectee pair. The authors describe a Markov chain Monte Carlo (MCMC) approach for obtaining estimates of the parameters of $f()$, θ, which they assume is Gamma distributed. In their approach they use data collected early in the 2009 H1N1 influenza pandemic in the Netherlands. The data comes from transmission clusters in schools, workplaces, households, camps, and other social settings. They found differences in the serial interval estimates between the types of transmission clusters, with the longest average serial interval in schools (3.4 days, 95% CI: 2.5–4.5 days) and the shortest estimated in households (2.1 days, 95% CI: 1.6–2.9 days). A similar approach was used by the same author to estimate the serial interval for pertussis in infants [33]. Again, the method was used to account for uncertainty in some of the transmission links and to determine important strata for presenting the serial interval. The authors found that the serial interval varied, depending on whether the infector was the fathers or sibling as opposed to a mother infecting the infant.

5.2.7 Case Study: 2009 H1N1 pandemic influenza in South Africa

We illustrate how to use a parametric approach to estimate the serial interval with data collected during the 2009 H1N1 influenza pandemic in South Africa. In this example, we show how to account for discretely observed data. Archer et al. [34] describe a detailed analysis of the first 100 reported cases of pandemic influenza in South Africa. Contact

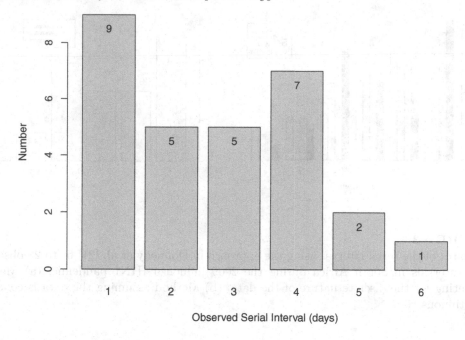

FIGURE 5.2
Observed time, in days, between symptom onset in 29 primary and secondary case pairs of pandemic H1N1 influenza in South Africa.

tracing was performed for these individuals and of 158 susceptible contacts, 29 instances of transmission were observed. Figure 5.2 summarizes the time between symptom onset in the primary and secondary cases. Data are reported in days, with no interval censoring or issues with truncation indicated. Therefore, we illustrate how to account for discrete data. The authors provide a summary of the mean and standard deviation of the data as 2.7 days (SD = 1.5). We fit this data using a parametric approach and account for the discreteness in the data. Table 5.1 and Figure 5.3 give the estimates for the serial interval assuming either a Gamma, Weibull, or Log-normal distribution with and without the adjustment for the discreteness of the data. The data collected was discrete and thus we would tend to favor the results using a likelihood that accounted for discreteness in the data. In this case, the AIC criteria suggests that the Weibull distribution provides the best fit to the data.

TABLE 5.1
Estimates of the serial interval using the approach in Donnelly et al. [21] fit to 29 observed serial intervals in South Africa during the 2009 Influenza H1N1 pandemic

| Distribution | Discrete | | | Continuous | | |
	Mean	Standard deviation	AIC	Mean	Standard deviation	AIC
Gamma	2.69	1.53	101.1	2.68	1.54	104.50
Weibull	2.69	1.50	100.9	2.70	1.44	104.25
Lognormal	2.71	1.57	101.5	2.73	1.85	105.41
Raw data				2.70	1.50	

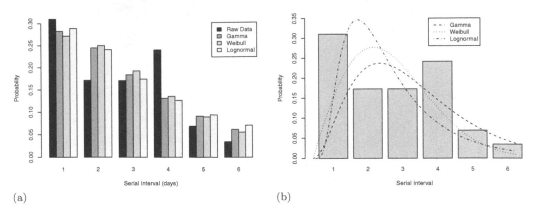

(a)   (b)

FIGURE 5.3

Estimates of the serial interval using the approach in Donnelly et al. [21] fit to 29 observed serial intervals in South Africa during the 2009 influenza H1N1 pandemic. (a) Method accounting for the discrete nature of the data. (b) Method assuming the data is collected is continuous.

The code required to fit the Gamma versions of these models is provided here. The Lognormal and Weibull models follow closely.

```
time.data <- c(9,5,5,7,2,1)

# log likelihood for the Gamma, assuming continuous data
gamma.log.like.cont <- function(parameters,times){
  # function to get the log likelihood of the gamma distribution
  # assume shape and rate parameterization
  # assume the data is continuous

  k <- exp(parameters[1])
  lambda <- exp(parameters[2])

  l.lik <- 0
  for(i in 1:length(times)){
    l.lik <- log(dgamma(times[i],k,1/lambda))+l.lik
  }
  return(-l.lik)
}
# log likelihood for the Gamma assuming discrete data
gamma.log.like.D <- function(parameters,times,Dmax){
  # function to get the log likelihood of the gamma distribution
  # assume shape and rate parameterization
  # assume the data is discrete

  k <- exp(parameters[1])
  lambda <- exp(parameters[2])

  # get unique set of times
  times.num <- table(times)
```

```
len.t <- length(times.num)
times.u <- as.numeric(names(times.num))

# get p_i's and log lik
ps <- NULL
l.lik <- 0
denom.ps <- pgamma(Dmax+0.5,k,1/lambda)-pgamma(0.5,k,1/lambda)
for(i in 1:len.t){
    ps[i] <- (pgamma(times.u[i]+0.5,k,1/lambda)
    -pgamma(times.u[i]-0.5,k,1/lambda))/denom.ps
    l.lik <- times.num[i]*log(ps[i])+l.lik
}

return(-l.lik)
}

# estimate the mean and SD assuming discrete data #
######################################################
# obtaining Maximum likelihood estimates #
gamma.est <- optim(par=c(1,1),fn=gamma.log.like.D,times=time.data,
Dmax=6,method="L-BFGS-B",lower=c(-Inf,-Inf),upper=c(Inf,Inf))
shape.gamma <- exp(gamma.est$par[1])
scale.gamma <- exp(gamma.est$par[2])
gamma.denom <- pgamma(6.5,shape.gamma,1/scale.gamma)-
pgamma(0.5,shape.gamma,1/scale.gamma)
# daily SI probabilities
gamma.ps <- (pgamma(c(1:6)+0.5,shape.gamma,1/scale.gamma)
             -pgamma(c(1:6)-0.5,shape.gamma,1/scale.gamma))/gamma.denom
gamma.mean <- sum(gamma.ps*c(1:6))
gamma.sd <- sqrt(sum((c(1:6)^2)*gamma.ps)-gamma.mean^2)

# estimate the mean and SD assuming continuous data #
######################################################
gamma.est <- optim(par=c(1,1),fn=gamma.log.like.cont,times=time.data,
       method="L-BFGS-B",lower=c(-Inf,-Inf),upper=c(Inf,Inf))
gamma.mean <- exp(gamma.est$par[1])*exp(gamma.est$par[2])
gamma.sd <- sqrt(exp(gamma.est$par[1]))*exp(gamma.est$par[2])
```

5.3   Reproductive Numbers

The reproductive number is a commonly used parameter to quantify the transmission potential of a disease. The parameter is meant to describe the average number of infections caused by an infectious individual. There are multiple versions of this parameter, the most commonly referenced being the basic reproductive number, R_0, defined as the reproductive number in an entirely susceptible population. While the condition of having an entirely susceptible population is seldom achieved, this parameter is extremely useful for planning purposes, as well as designing interventions and determining vaccine coverage necessary to achieve herd immunity [35]. In this setting, our goal is to determine what interventions are needed to drive this value below its critical threshold of one.

In the most simple setting assuming the population is closed to people moving in or out and homogeneity in mixing patterns, R_0 is intuitively defined as the product of the contact rate, the probability of infection for any given contact, and the length of time one is infectious. See the calculation of R_0 for compartmental models, such as the susceptible-infected-recovered (SIR) model, see Chapters 2 and 7. Many extensions of this follow, such as allowing for heterogeneity in mixing patterns, time varying infectivity probabilities, and migration in and out of the population. In fact, assuming a single reproductive number for a large population is unrealistic, given our expectation that the factors that lead to transmission of a disease can vary dramatically over a population due to such issues as sanitation and population density.

The time dependent effective reproductive number, $R(t)$, considers the presence of individuals in the population who are not susceptible to infection, effectively eliminating a portion of the contacts an individual makes from being eligible for infection and lowering the estimate of the reproductive number relative to the basic reproductive number. As an outbreak unfolds and individuals recover and build immunity or control measures are implemented this number is most relevant. Again, we are interested in determining measures to drive this number below 1.

Mathematical models are a useful tool to study the impact of a broad spectrum of policies on the reproductive number. These models, with their many disease and setting specific assumptions, allow for estimation of the reproductive number and careful study of the impact of policies on transmission. [36] provide excellent detail on these approaches and the mathematical theory underpinning their derivation. These models require specification of a compartmental structure and parameterization of the model transitions. Data or previously calculated parameters are typically used to parameterize the model.

After the SARS outbreak of 2003, infectious disease modelers recognized a need for tools to estimate key infectious disease parameters, in particular the reproductive number, in real time with data that is routinely available in an outbreak. The most common source of data is a line list, containing information on each reported case of disease. This information includes a date of diagnosis and often includes basic demographics, date of symptom onset, as well as lab results or clinical information pertaining to the course of disease (e.g., hospitalization and mortality data). In this section, we describe approaches to estimation of reproductive numbers, both R_0 and R_t, using information obtained from a line list. From the line list, we obtain the number of new cases reported each data by $N_0, N_1, \ldots, N_T$ and show how this information is used in estimation.

5.3.1   Estimation of R_0

The basic reproductive number, R_0, is appropriate to estimate in a population that is naive to a pathogen. This estimate is particularly relevant when there has been a substantial shift in influenza strains or the emergence of a new pathogen, such as SARS and ebola. This parameter is useful in understanding the potential threat a new pathogen poses. We illustrate two approaches for its estimation during the initial stages of an outbreak.

5.3.1.1   Branching processes

A fairly basic approach to estimating the basic reproductive number has its origins in demography. This measure was originally used to determine the probability of a particular family line going extinct. The birth process method has a clear analogue in infectious disease where a birth is an infection event creating successive generations of infected individuals. If the reproductive number is greater than 1, then the population of individuals who have been infected will grow exponentially; if it is less than 1, then the numbers of diseased individuals will dwindle to extinction. This method is applicable only during the initial phase of an infectious disease epidemic, when we assume exponential growth of cases and wish to estimate the basic reproductive number.

This method makes use of the line list and an estimate of the serial interval, $g(t)$ or $f(t)$. The estimate of the serial interval is used to group the data into generations. For diseases with a longer serial interval that shows very little variability, this is fairly straightforward to do [37], (e.g., with measles). If the average length of the serial interval is μ then on day t of the outbreak, we will have observed $G = t/\mu$, generations and would expect to see $N_0 R_0^G$ cases, where N_0 are the initial number of cases. In this case we group the $\mathbf{N} = N_1, \ldots, N_T$ into generational data, denoted by $\mathbf{M} = M_1, \ldots, M_G$. The estimate for the R_0 is given by

$$\hat{R}_0 = \frac{\sum_{s=1}^{G} M_s}{\sum_{s=1}^{G} M_{s-1}}. \tag{5.10}$$

This mathematical construct allows for the derivation of several helpful quantities. For example, we can derive the probability of having a large outbreak, or in other words, an outbreak that would grow exponentially if there were an infinite number of susceptible individuals. If the infectious period is exponentially distributed, then this is given by

$$\pi = 1 - 1/R_0. \tag{5.11}$$

Similar derivations are available for infectious periods with other distributional assumptions [37].

5.3.1.2 White and Pagano

An alternate approach that allows for use of the full serial interval distribution in estimation of R_0 is described by White and Pagano [38]. We also can obtain estimates of the serial interval using this approach. This likelihood based method makes two probabilistic assumptions: (1) the reproductive number follows a Poisson distribution and (2) the serial interval can be described by a multinomial distribution. In essence, we assume that an individual infects r individuals, where $r \sim \text{Poisson}(R_0)$. Then the r cases distribute in time according to a multinomial distribution with parameters k and $\mathbf{p} = \{p_1, \ldots, p_k\}$, where k is the maximum length of the serial interval. In reality, the serial interval can be parameterized by any continuous distribution, $f()$, and then discretized into the multinomial distribution as described in 5.2.2. The log likelihood is given by

$$l(R_0, \mathbf{p}|\mathbf{N}) \propto \sum_{t=1}^{T} N_t log(\mu_t) - \mu_t, \tag{5.12}$$

where $\mu_t = R_0 \sum_{j=1}^{min(k,t)} p_j N_{t-j}$. In a frequentist framework, we can obtain MLEs for R_0 and $\mathbf{p}$ using a numeric optimizer. Bayesian approaches using MCMC can improve estimates through the inclusion of prior information on the serial interval [39]. If a reliable estimate of the serial interval exists, then the estimator for R_0 using all data available up to day T, during the exponential growth phase of an outbreak, can be obtained algebraically from (5.12), as

$$\hat{R}_0 = \frac{\sum_{t=1}^{T} N_t}{\sum_{t=1}^{T} \sum_{j=1}^{min(k,t)} p_j N_{t-j}}. \tag{5.13}$$

We can choose any parametric form for the serial interval, such as a Gamma, Weibull, or Log-normal distribution and then discretize the distribution into (for example, daily) probabilities, p_j, that are a function of θ.

5.3.2 Estimation of R_t

As an outbreak unfolds or a pathogen persists in a population, the effective reproductive number is useful for monitoring the impact of interventions and the ability of the disease to persist in a population. Modeling studies often consider interventions needed to bring R_t below 1.

5.3.2.1 Wallinga and Teunis

Wallinga and Teunis [40] propose a method to estimate daily effective reproductive numbers for SARS from the line list of cases, using a estimate of the serial interval distribution and assuming that the entire outbreak has been observed. This latter assumption renders this method less effective as a real-time tool, but, as we show, modifications are available to improve its real-time performance. In this method, the number of new cases on day t is denoted by N_t and the probability of a serial interval of length x is given by $g(x)$. We first define the relative probability that a case j who is symptomatic on day t_j has been infected by a case i who was symptomatic on day $t_i < t_j$ as

$$p_{ij} = \frac{g(t_j - t_i)}{\sum_{j \neq i} g(t_j - t_i)}. \tag{5.14}$$

Then the effective reproductive number for case i is given by

$$R_i = \sum_j p_{ij}. \tag{5.15}$$

If $t_i = t_k$ then it follows that $R_i = R_k$. This method is sensitive to right censoring in the data, for example, if the entire outbreak has not been observed. Cauchemez et al. [41] presented a Bayesian modification of this approach to allow for real time estimation and showed that as one attempts to estimate R_t as t approaches the current time, the precision of the estimates decreases.

5.3.2.2 EpiEstim tools

An alternative approach to estimating R_t was first described by Fraser [42] and elaborated on by Cori et al. [43]. In this approach, they model transmission assuming a Poisson process, where the number of cases that an individual infected on day $t - s$ infects s days after becoming infectious is given by $R_t w_s$, where R_t is the reproductive number on day t and w_s describes the infectiousness s days after infectiousness begins. In this case the w_s sum to one. With this framework and the incidence data, $N_1, \ldots, N_t$, the likelihood is given by

$$L(N_t|N_1, \ldots, N_{t-1}, w, R_t) = \frac{(R_t \Lambda_t)^{N_t} e^{-R_t \Lambda_t}}{N_t!} \tag{5.16}$$

where $\Lambda_t = \sum_{s=1}^{t} N_{t-1} w_s$. If we assume that transmission is constant during fixed time windows defined by τ, then this likelihood can be simplified to estimate the $R_{t,\tau}$ in a Bayesian framework. We show that if a Gamma prior distribution with parameters α and β is used for $R_{t,\tau}$, such that the mean is $\alpha\beta$ and the variance is $\alpha\beta^2$, then the posterior distribution of $R_{t,\tau}$ is Gamma with parameters $\left(\alpha + \sum_{s=t-\tau+1}^{t} N_s, \frac{1}{1/\beta + \sum_{s=t-\tau+1}^{t} \Lambda_s}\right)$. The technical appendix in [43] provides more detail on the suitable choice of τ and when in the course of the epidemic reliable estimates of $R_{t,\tau}$ can be obtained. Their approach is easily implemented through an R package EpiEstim or using a spreadsheet provided in [43]. The EpiEstim package in R also implements the Wallinga and Teunis method.

5.3.3 Case study: 2009 H1N1 pandemic influenza in the United States

We illustrate these techniques using data from the United States during the 2009 H1N1 influenza pandemic [44]. In brief, analyses are based on the first 1,368 confirmed and probable cases with a date of report on or before May 8, 2009. Among these, 750 had a date of symptom onset reported. The epidemic curve is shown in Figure 5.4a.

We first describe approaches to account for missing data. This came in three forms: (1) missing onset dates, (2) data not yet reported, due to reporting delays, and (3) cases never reported. An imputation approach, using a loglinear regression model was used to impute missing onset times. The regression models the lag between the report date and the date of symptom onset as a function of the report date and an indicator of recent travel to Mexico. Results from the imputation are shown in Figure 5.4a.

Another anomaly in the data is the decrease in reported cases after April 27. This decrease is not because the outbreak was in decline at this time, but is attributable to delays in reporting cases. Using the reporting delay distribution created for the imputation, we can augment the data to be a closer representation of true case burden. We do this by estimating that the true number of cases on day t is given by $M_t = N_t / \sum_{j=1}^{\min T-t,l} q_j$, where q_j is the probability of a delay in reporting of j days, l is the length of the reporting delay distribution, and N_t is the observed number of reports on day t.

Finally, we note that the degree to which cases were reported varied during this time period. As providers became aware of the situation, they were more likely to test and report cases. Assuming that severity of influenza was consistent, then the percent of (unknown) influenza infected individuals who are hospitalized should be consistent. We can use hospitalization rates in our observed data to determine the reporting fraction. Of the cases reported during the month of April, we observe that the rate of hospitalization declined by approximately 10 percent each day. This decline would indicate that the ratio of observed cases on consecutive days was 90% of the ratio of true cases. From this we estimate that the reporting fraction was 0.15 until April 13 and thereafter decreased to 0.11, implying that only a small fraction of cases are reported to the Center for Disease Control and Prevention (CDC). The impact of accounting for these latter two issues in the data is shown in [44].

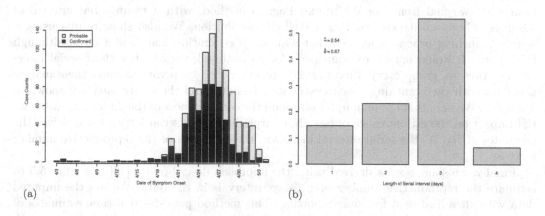

(a)   (b)

FIGURE 5.4
Analysis of 2009 H1N1 influenza outbreak in the United States. (a) Epidemic curve data collected by the first week of May. Data shown are confirmed and probable cases, as well as the number of cases added from imputing the missing disease onset dates. (b) Serial interval estimates obtained using confirmed and probable cases data ending 4/27.

TABLE 5.2
Estimates of the reproductive number during the initial phase of the influenza H1N1 pandemic in the United States

Approach	SI assumption	RF	$\hat{R}_0$ Original	$\hat{R}_0$ Imputed	$\hat{R}_0$ Augmented
WP	Estimated	N	$1.59(1.12, 1.66)$	$2.36(1.51, 2.94)$	$2.51(1.51, 2.88)$
WP	Estimated	Y	$1.40(0.93, 1.39)$	$1.75(1.42, 2.17)$	$1.84(1.48, 2.29)$
WP	$\mu = 3.6$	N	$2.87(2.55, 3.06)$	$3.83(3.46, 4.12)$	$4.11(3.74, 4.42)$
WP	$\mu = 3.6$	Y	$2.25(2.04, 2.46)$	$2.78(2.69, 3.23)$	$2.97(2.88, 3.45)$
Branching process	$\mu = 3$	N	2.69	3.50	3.86
Branching process	$\mu = 3$	Y	2.01	2.48	2.70

Note: WP refers to the White and Pagano method, RF denotes reporting fraction, and indicates if an adjustment was made for the estimated underreporting of cases in the analysis. We do not show confidence intervals for the branching process estimates, as analytical estimates are not readily calculated.

We first use the White and Pagano method to simultaneously estimate the basic reproductive number, R_0, and serial interval using data up to and including April 27. We varied the maximal serial interval length, k, between 4 and 7 and find, using an AIC-like criteria that setting $k = 4$ provides the best fit to the data. Figure 5.4b shows the estimated serial interval using a multinomial parameterization. Here the mean is estimated to be 2.54 days (SD = 0.67 days) with a modal value of 3 days. The estimates for R_0 from this same model fit are shown in Table 5.2 along with estimates obtained from using the augmented and imputed data sets. Estimates accounting for the incomplete reporting also are shown. This method also accounts for imported cases, as described in [44].

Alternatively, we use an estimate of the serial interval given by Cowling et al. [24] from household contact studies of influenza patients. Using this serial interval, we only estimate the reproductive number using (5.13). Cowling el al. estimated serial interval slightly longer than what we find from the White and Pagano method, with a mean serial interval of 3.6 days (SD = 1.6 days) assuming a Weibull distribution. We also show results using a simple branching process approach that assumes a generation length of 3 days, although this approach would not be recommended for an outbreak with such a short serial interval. For this, we group every 3 days of data together into "generations" and then analyze this data with the branching process estimator. Results from these estimates are shown in Table 5.2. We note that the assumptions around the completeness of the data had a substantial impact on the estimates we obtain. Not surprisingly, the serial interval also drives the estimates of R_0. As the serial interval increases, the estimates of the reproductive number increase.

Finally, we show results derived using the approach described by [43] in Figure 5.5 to estimate the reproductive number over 7-days intervals in the data. We use the imputed data without adjustment for underreporting. This method provides real-time estimates of the reproductive number. Averaging these estimates over the period of epidemic growth yields an estimate of R_0 that is 2.45. This estimate is close to the White and Pagano estimates of 2.36 obtained with the same data, but less than the estimate 3.83 that is obtained when using the same assumed serial interval.

We provide code for the implementation of the White and Pagano method, as well as the branching process estimator. EpiEstim can be used for the other results described.

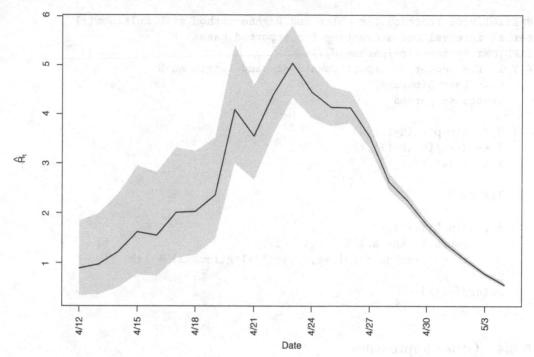

FIGURE 5.5
Estimates of R_t using the approach describe by Cori et al. [17] and EpiEstim tools.

```
a.daily.cts.2 <- c(1,0,1,0,0,0,1,3,1,1,0,0,1,0,1,2,1,1,2,1,4,3,8,25,
9,52,79,85,153,254, 251,149,296,129,43,39,14,3)

# branching process estimates #
##############################
# imputed data #
# clump into generations of 3 #
gen.cts <- cumsum(a.daily.cts.2[1:30])
[3*c(1:(length(a.daily.cts.2[1:30])/3))]
gen.cts <- c(gen.cts[1],diff(gen.cts))
sum(gen.cts[1:10])/sum(gen.cts[1:9])
# [1] 3.497462

# White and Pagano method on imputed data with k=4 #
tmp <- constrOptim(rep(1.2,k),likN.MNi,N=a.daily.cts[1:27],
Y=i.daily.cts[1:27],ui=diag(1,k),ci=rep(0,k),
method="Nelder-Mead")
ps.tmp <- tmp$par/sum(tmp$par) #multinomial p's
R0.est <- sum(tmp$par) #estimate of R0
# mean of SI
SI.mean <- sum(ps.tmp*c(1:length(ps.tmp)))
# sd of the SI
SI.sd <- sum(ps.tmp*(c(1:length(ps.tmp))^2)) - pars.t[17,i-3]^2
log.lik <- tmp$value #log likelihood value
```

```
# likelihood function for White and Pagano method with multinomial
serial interval and accounting for imported cases  #
likN.MNi <- function(params,N,Y){
# Y is the vector of import counts of same length as N
    k <- length(params)
    thetas <- params

    N <- c(rep(0,(k-1)),N)
    Y <- c(rep(0,(k-1)),Y)
    l <- length(N)

    lik <- 0

    for(i in k:(l-1)){
        lambda <- thetas%*%N[i:(i-k+1)]
        lik <- -lambda + (N[i+1]-Y[i+1])*log(lambda) + lik
    }
    return(-lik)
}
```

5.3.4   Other approaches

The approaches we have discussed are most relevant to person-to-person transmissible diseases. Malaria and other vector born diseases pose many challenges in the estimation of the reproductive number. Many have approached this using mathematical modeling, incorporating the vector into the model [45]. An alternative approach proposed by Churcher et al. [46] proposes simply testing the hypothesis that the reproductive number is greater than 1, due to the complexity and lack of information needed to obtain a specific estimate. In this way, programs can determine if control measures are driving transmission below the critical threshold.

Ebola, particularly the outbreak in 2014, exposed great challenges in estimating the reproductive number. The data quality was poor, limiting our ability to obtain reliable estimates. There were some early papers using relatively simple approaches to estimate the reproductive number; however, the reliability of these estimates is questionable due to gross underreporting and irregularities in the observed data [47, 48].

5.4   Parameters for Disease Severity

We have described parameters that characterize how a disease will spread through a population. It is additionally important to understand how severe a disease is, as well as how many individuals it is likely to impact. For example, a disease that can infect a large portion of the population, but causes minimal morbidity and mortality, such as the common cold, is not a high public health priority. However, a disease with high mortality, but that impacts a relatively small portion of the population, such as ebola, is likely to be considered a major public health concern. In 2009, this was a critical question for the H1N1 influenza pandemic, which was poised to infect a large portion of the global population, but it was not clear how severe the disease would be in terms of mortality and the burden placed on healthcare facilities (for example, the number who require hospitalization). We can use attack rates, prevalences, and incidence to estimate the number infected. A critical parameter to understanding severity is the case fatality ratio (CFR), which describes the probability of death among those infected. The case hospitalization rate (CHR), which describes the probability of hospitalization, and similarly the case intensive care unit (ICU) rate (CIR), are important for determining the impact of a disease on the healthcare system. We focus on estimation of the CFR and the attack rate/prevalence in this section, although many of the ideas we describe apply to the other measures of severity.

In their most simple forms, the CFR and attack rate (AR) are described by simple ratios: $AR = N/M$ and $CFR = n/N$, where n is the number who die out of the N who are infected or diseased in a population of M individuals. There are challenges in estimating both n and N for most diseases. For example, surveillance systems likely will miss cases of disease, leading to underestimation of N. In the ebola outbreak in West Africa in 2014, it is unknown how many cases were not reported due to many challenges, including poor infrastructure and distrust of public health officials [49]. In influenza outbreaks, many cases go unreported because lab testing is not common and most who are sick do not seek medical attention. It is also possible to overestimate N by using a less specific syndromic case definition. Estimating the number who die, n, is complicated by several factors, including the time that it takes for individuals to die, as well as ambiguity over defining the cause of death. For example, individuals with influenza often die from pneumonia or some other complication (or combination of complications) resulting from their influenza.

Estimating the total number of individuals impacted by an infectious disease is a challenging problem and tools used for this vary depending on the illness and the data available. We briefly describe two approaches here. The first is to use capture recapture methods. This approach is borrowed from ecology, where the interest is in estimating the total number of animals in a geographic region. In this approach, at least two data sources that pull from the same population are necessary and it is required that we are able to link individuals between the data sources. As an example, we might have reportable disease data and mortality records and devise a way to determine the individuals who appear in both data sets and those who only appear in one source. Using basic probability rules and assumptions, such as independence in the data sources and homogeneity of the probability of being in either source, the Lincoln-Peterson estimator provides an approximation of the entire population, including those who are not in either data source. When more than one data source is available, loglinear models or multinomial models are used and it is possible to relax some of the assumptions required for the Lincoln-Peterson estimator. This approach has been used in many public health settings, including to estimate total case burden for ebola [49], HIV [50], and tuberculosis [51]. Many examples of this approach exist in the literature, as well as excellent tutorials, such as [52].

A second approach to estimate the case burden is the use of multipliers. This approach is based on assuming that the number of cases that ultimately get reported is a fraction of the total cases. We can describe the attrition between the total cases and observed cases through a series of steps as depicted in Figure 5.6. For example, many individuals never seek healthcare and for those who do, many are never tested to obtain a definitive diagnosis. By understanding the probability of each of these steps occurring, we can create multipliers, which are the reciprocal of the proportion that complete each step in the process. Reed et al. [53] used this approach to estimate the number of pandemic influenza H1N1 cases in the United States in 2009. Using surveys, information on the sensitivity of influenza lab tests and other sources of information on reporting practices, they created multipliers to expand the number of cases that ultimately get reported to the CDC to the total estimated number of cases in the United States. The multipliers were drawn from uniform distributions with upper and lower limits to define reasonable levels of uncertainty around the estimated proportions. The procedure was performed repeatedly to get an estimate of the variability. They derive a multiplier of 79 (90% range: 47−148), indicating that for every

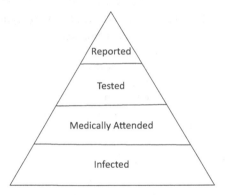

FIGURE 5.6
Basic depiction of reporting triangle.

case of influenza reported to the CDC, there were 79 additional cases that went unreported. Similar approaches have been used elsewhere, for example in estimating the incidence of tuberculosis among children [54].

Estimates of the CFR are extremely important for justifying interventions in a disease; however, their calculation can be very challenging. For example, in 2003 as the SARS pandemic was unfolding, the World Health Organization (WHO) initially estimated the CFR to be around 6−7 percent. Eventually, more sophisticated statistical analyses estimated a much higher CFR of 13.2 percent (9.8−16.8) for patients under 60 years of age and 43.3 percent (35.2−52.4) for those at least 60 years old [55]. The main reason for the difference in the estimates was that individuals took time to die, so the basic estimate derived from the ratio of the number reported dead to the number reported ill underestimated the number who ultimately would die among those who were reported ill. In [55] they derive an estimator for the CFR that incorporates time delay between admission into a healthcare facility and death or discharge. In this setting, all SARS patients reported were admitted so the distributions beginning from admission are appropriate. The CFR is given by π_F and the distributions describing the time to death and discharge are defined as $F()$ and $G()$, respectively. We can construct a likelihood function to estimate the parameters of $F()$ and $G()$, as well as the CFR, π_F. The likelihood for those who die t days after admission is $\pi_F(F(t+1) - F(t))$; for patients who are discharged t days after admission the likelihood is $(1 - \pi_F)(G(t+1) - G(t))$; and patients who have neither died nor been discharged t days post admission the likelihood is $\pi_F(1 - F(t)) + (1 - \pi_f)(1 - (t))$. We also used a modified Kaplan-Meier survival curve to estimate the CFR.

Estimating the CFR during the 2009 H1N1 pandemic was very challenging and proved critical in the interpretation of the significance of the pandemic. Initial estimates from Mexico were very high and alarming; however, with time the CFR was estimated to be much lower than initially presumed. The scope of this pandemic, which resulted in millions being infected with influenza, but only a small fraction of those cases likely reported posed substantial challenges for estimating the CFR. Additionally, Influenza often is not implicated as a cause of death, when it may have been the driving factor of mortality, for example in an individual who contracts fatal pneumonia as a result of Influenza. Presanis et al. [56] described an approach to estimating CFRs using a Bayesian synthesis model. Similar to the multiplier method described for estimating the AR, this approach assumes a triangle similar to Figure 5.6, but with mortality as the peak of the triangle. They use numerous data sources, such as surveys, to describe the probabilities of transitioning between each level of the triangle. The authors provide the technical details of the construction of their model and then fit this model using a Bayesian MCMC approach. They report age-specific symptomatic CFRs (as well as CHR and CIR) and show that the highest CFR was among those $18 - 64$, a common observation in pandemic influenza settings. The overall estimated CFR of 0.048 percent (0.026%–0.096%) which was lower than estimates derived during the same time period using the delay distribution approach [57]. A key difference between these estimates was that Presanis et al. estimated the CFR for symptomatic individuals only, which likely explains at least a portion of the discrepancy in between the estimates.

5.5 Conclusion

We have provided a summary of data driven approaches to estimating some of the most common epidemiological parameters for infectious diseases. This chapter is a not a comprehensive summary of available methods, but rather a summary of highly cited and relevant methods to estimating these parameters from data that is often available. The approaches here are applicable to some of the most publicized infectious diseases, where most of the methodological work has been done. However, modifying these tools or developing more applicable tools for existing or emerging infectious diseases should be a high priority. We have purposely focused on methods that are relevant to diseases as they are emerging or re-emerging. The constant threat of new outbreaks, bioterrorist events, and re-emergence of infectious diseases requires that we are prepared to rapidly estimate parameters that are relevant to transmission and severity with the aim of responding appropriately and in a timely manner.

References

[1] Åke Svensson. A note on generation times in epidemic models. *Mathematical Biosciences*, 208:300–311, 2006.

[2] Johan Giesecke. *Modern Infectious Disease Epidemiology*, Hodder Arnold, London, UK, 2nd ed., 2002.

[3] Margaretha Annelie Vink, Martinus Christoffel, Jozef Bootsma, and Jacco Wallinga. Systematic reviews and meta-and pooled analyses serial intervals of respiratory infectious diseases: A systematic review and analysis. *American Journal of Epidemiology*, 180(9):865–875, 2014.

[4] Ellen Brooks-Pollock, Mercedes C. Becerra, Edward Goldstein, Ted Cohen, and Megan B. Murray. Epidemiologic inference from the distribution of tuberculosis cases in households in Lima, Peru. *Journal of Infectious Diseases*, 203:1582–1589, 2011.

[5] Marc Lipsitch, Ted Cohen, Ben Cooper, James M. Robins, Stefan Ma, Lyn James, Gowri Gopalakrishna et al. Transmission dynamics and control of severe acute respiratory syndrome. *Science*, 300(5627):1966–1970, 2003.

[6] Laura Forsberg White and Marcello Pagano. Transmissibility of the influenza virus in the 1918 pandemic. *PLoS One*, 3(1):e1498, 2008.

[7] Stéphane Le Vu, Yazdan Yazdanpanah, Dounia Bitar, Julien Emmanuelli, Isabelle Bonmarin, Jean-Claude Desenclos. Absence of infection in asymptomatic contacts of index SARS case in France. *Eurosurveillance*, 11(1):9–10, 2006.

[8] Hiroshi Nishiura. Early efforts in modeling the incubation period of infectious diseases with an acute course of illness. *Emerging Themes in Epidemiology*, 4:2, 2007.

[9] Rachel M. Lee, Justin Lessler, Rose A. Lee, Kara E. Rudolph, Nicholas G. Reich, Trish M. Perl, and Derek At Cummings. Incubation periods of viral gastroenteritis: A systematic review. *BMC Infectious Diseases*, 13:446, 2013.

[10] Justin Lessler, Nicholas G. Reich, Ron Brookmeyer, Trish M. Perl, Kenrad E. Nelson, and Derek A. T. Cummings. Incubation periods of acute respiratory viral infections: A systematic review. *The Lancet Infectious Diseases*, 9(5):291–300, 2009.

[11] Tomislav Svoboda, Bonnie Henry, Leslie Shulman, Erin Kennedy, Elizabeth Rea, Wil Ng, Tamara Wallington et al. Public health measures to control the spread of the severe acute respiratory syndrome during the outbreak in Toronto. *New England Journal of Medicine*, 350(23):2352–2361, 2004.

[12] Monali Varia, Samantha Wilson, Shelly Sarwal, Allison McGeer, Effie Gournis, Eleni Galanis, and Bonnie Henry. Investigation of a nosocomial outbreak of severe acute respiratory syndrome (SARS) in Toronto, Canada. *Canadian Medical Association Journal*, 169(4):285–292, 2003.

[13] Anthony Y. C. Kuk and Stefan Ma. The estimation of SARS incubation distribution from serial interval data using a convolution likelihood. *Statistics in Medicine*, 24(16):2525–2537, 2005.

[14] Eleni Patrozou and Leonard A. Mermel. Does influenza transmission occur from asymptomatic infection or prior to symptom onset? *Public Health Reports*, 124:193–196, 2009.

[15] William C. Miller, Nora E. Rosenberg, Sarah E. Rutstein, and Kimberly A. Powers. Role of acute and early HIV infection in the sexual transmission of HIV. *Current Opinion in HIV and AIDS*, 5(4):277–282, 2010.

[16] Joseph Sriyal Peiris, Chung-Ming Chu, Vincent Chi-Chung Cheng, Paul K. S. Chan, Ivan Hung, Leo L. M. Poon, Kin-Ip Law, et al. Clinical progression and viral load in a community outbreak of coronavirus-associated SARS pneumonia: A prospective study. *The Lancet*, 361(9371):1767–1772, 2003.

[17] Anne Cori, Alain-Jacques Valleron, Fabrice Carrat, Gianpaolo Scalia Tomba, Gilles Thomas, and Pierre-Yves Boëlle. Estimating influenza latency and infectious period durations using viral excretion data. *Epidemics*, 4:132–138, 2012.

[18] Helen J. Wearing, Pejman Rohani, and Matt J. Keeling. Appropriate models for the management of infectious diseases. *PLoS Medicine*, 2(7):e174, 2005.

[19] Philip E. Sartwell. The distribution of incubation periods of infectious disease. *American Journal of Hygiene*, 51:310–318, 1952.

[20] Benjamin J. Cowling, Matthew P. Muller, Irene O. L. Wong, Lai-Ming Ho, Marie Louie, Allison McGeer, and Gabriel M. Leung. Alternative methods of estimating an incubation distribution. *Epidemiology*, 18(2):253–259, 2007.

[21] Christl A. Donnelly, Lyn Finelli, Simon Cauchemez, Sonja J. Olsen, Saumil Doshi, Michael L. Jackson, Erin D. Kennedy et al. Serial intervals and the temporal distribution of secondary infections within households of 2009 pandemic influenza A (H1N1): Implications for influenza control recommendations. *Clinical Infectious Diseases : An Official Publication of the Infectious Diseases Society of America*, 52(Suppl 1): 123–130, 2011.

[22] Niel Hens, Laurence Calatayud, Satu Kurkela, Teele Tamme, and Jacco Wallinga. Robust reconstruction and analysis of outbreak data: Influenza A(H1N1)v transmission in a school-based population. *American Journal of Epidemiology*, 176(3):196–203, 2012.

[23] Dennis E. te Beest, Jacco Wallinga, Tjibbe Donker, and Michiel van Boven. Estimating the generation interval of influenza A (H1N1) in a range of social settings. *Epidemiology*, 24(2):244–250, 2013.

[24] Benjamin J. Cowling, Vicky J. Fang, Steven Riley, Joseph Sriyal Peiris, and Gabriel M. Leung. Estimation of the serial interval of influenza. *Epidemiology (Cambridge, Mass.)*, 20(3):344–347, 2009.

[25] Nicholas G. Reich, Justin Lessler, Derek A. T. Cummings, and Ron Brookmeyer. Estimating incubation period distributions with coarse data. *Statistics in Medicine*, 28(15):1982–1998, 2009.

[26] Bruce W. Turnbull. The empirical distribution function with arbitrarily grouped, censored and truncated data. *Journal of the Royal Statistical Society, Series B*, 38(3):290–295, 1976.

[27] Richard Peto. Experimental survival curves for interval-censored data. *Source Journal of the Royal Statistical Society. Series C (Applied Statistics)*, 22(1):86–91, 1973.

[28] Jane C. Lindsey and Louise M. Ryan. Tutorial in biostatistics methods for interval-censored data. *Statistics in Medicine*, 17(2):219–238, 1998.

[29] Victor Virlogeux, Ming Li, Tim K. Tsang, Luzhao Feng, Vicky J. Fang, Hui Jiang, Peng Wu et al. Practice of epidemiology estimating the distribution of the incubation periods of human avian influenza A(H7N9) virus infections. *American Journal of Epidemiology*, 182(8):723–729, 2015.

[30] Augustinus H. A. Ten Asbroek, Martien W. Borgdorff, Nico Nagelkerke, Maruschka M. G. G. Šebek, Walter Devillé, Jan D. A. Van Embden, and Dick van Soolingen. Estimation of serial interval and incubation period of tuberculosis using DNA fingerprinting. *International Journal of Tuberculosis and Lung Disease*, 3(5):414–420, 1999.

[31] Colin J. Worby, Philip D. O'Neill, Theodore Kypraios, Julie V. Robotham, Daniela De Angelis, Edward J. P. Cartwright, Sharon J. Peacock, and Ben S. Cooper. Reconstructing transmission trees for communicable diseases using densely sampled genetic data. *The Annals of Applied Statistics*, 10(1):395–417, 2016.

[32] Colin J. Worby, Marc Lipsitch and William P. Hanage. Within-host bacterial diversity hinders accurate reconstruction of transmission networks from genomic distance data. *PLoS Computational Biology*, 10(3):e1003549, 2014.

[33] Dennis E. te Beest, Donna Henderson, Nicoline A. T. Van Der Maas, Sabine C. De Greeff, Jacco Wallinga, Frits R. Mooi, and Michiel Van Boven. Estimation of the serial interval of pertussis in Dutch households. *Epidemics*, 7:1–6, 2014.

[34] Brett N. Archer, Geraldine A. Timothy, Cheryl Cohen, Stefano Tempia, Mmam-pedi Huma, Lucille Blumberg, Dhamari Naidoo, Ayanda Cengimbo, and Barry D. Schoub. Introduction of 2009 pandemic influenza A virus subtype H1N1 into South Africa: Clinical presentation, epidemiology, and transmissibility of the first 100 cases. *Journal of Infectious Diseases*, 206(suppl 1):S148–S153, 2012.

[35] Paul Fine, Ken Eames, and David L. Heymann. Herd immunity: A rough guide. *Clinical Infectious Diseases*, 52(7):911–916, 2011.

[36] Odo Diekmann, Hans Heesterbeek, and Tom Britton. *Mathematical Tools for Understanding Infectious Disease Dynamics*. Princeton University Press, Princeton, NJ, 2013.

[37] Niels G. Becker. *Analysis of Infectious Disease Data*. Chapman and Hall, London, UK, 1989.

[38] Laura Forsberg White and Marcello P. Pagano. A likelihood-based method for real-time estimation of the serial interval and reproductive number of an epidemic. *Statistics in Medicine*, 27(16):2999–3016, 2008.

[39] Carlee B. Moser, Mayetri Gupta, Brett N. Archer, and Laura F. White. The impact of prior information on estimates of disease transmissibility using Bayesian tools. *Plos One*, 10(3):e0118762, 2015.

[40] Jacco Wallinga and Peter Teunis. Different epidemic curves for severe acute respiratory syndrome reveal. *American Journal of Epidemiology*, 160(6):509–516, 2004.

[41] Simon Cauchemez, Pierre Yves Boëlle, Christl A. Donnelly, Neil M. Ferguson, Guy Thomas, Gabriel M. Leung, Anthony J. Hedley, Roy M. Anderson, and Alain Jacques Valleron. Real-time estimates in early detection of SARS. *Emerging Infectious Diseases*, 12(1):110–113, 2006.

[42] Christophe Fraser. Estimating Individual and household reproduction numbers in an emerging epidemic. *Plos One*, 2(8):e758, 2007.

[43] Anne Cori, Neil M. Ferguson, Christophe Fraser, and Simon Cauchemez. A new framework and software to estimate time-varying reproduction numbers during epidemics. *American Journal of Epidemiology*, 178(9):1505–1512, 2013.

[44] Laura Forsberg White, Jacco Wallinga, Lyn Finelli, Carrie Reed, Steven Riley, Marc Lipsitch, and Marcello Pagano. Estimation of the reproductive number and the serial interval in early phase of the 2009 influenza A/H1N1 pandemic in the USA. *Influenza and Other Respiratory Viruses*, 3(6):267–276, 2009.

[45] David L. Smith, F. Ellis Mckenzie, Robert W. Snow, and Simon I. Hay. Revisiting the basic reproductive number for malaria and its implications for malaria control. *PLoS Biology*, 5(3):e42, 2007.

[46] Thomas S. Churcher, Justin M. Cohen, Joseph Novotny, Nyasatu Ntshalintshali, Simon Kunene, and Simon Cauchemez. Measuring the path toward malaria elimination. *Science*, 344(6189):1230–1232, 2014.

[47] David Fisman, Edwin Khoo, and Ashleigh Tuite. Early epidemic dynamics of the West African 2014 Ebola outbreak: Estimates derived with a simple two-parameter model. *PLoS Currents*, 6, 2014.

[48] Sherry Towers, Oscar Patterson-Lomba, and Carlos Castillo-Chavez. Temporal variations in the effective reproduction number of the 2014 West Africa Ebola outbreak. *PLoS Currents*, 6, 2014.

[49] Etienne Gignoux, Rachel Idowu, Luke Bawo, Lindis Hurum, Armand Sprecher, Mathieu Bastard, and Klaudia Porten. Use of capture-recapture to estimate underreporting of Ebola virus disease, Montserrado County, Liberia. *Emerging Infectious Diseases*, 21(12):2265–2267, 2015.

[50] Pascale Bernillon, Laurence Lievre, Josiane Pillonel, Anne Laporte, and Dominique Costagliola. Record-linkage between two anonymous databases for a capture-recapture estimation of underreporting of AIDS cases: France 1990–1993. *International Journal of Epidemiology*, 29(1):168–174, 2000.

[51] World Health Organization. Global Tuberculosis Report 2015. Technical report, Geneva, Switzerland, 2015.

[52] Ernest B. Hook and Ronald R. Regal. Completeness of reporting: Capture recapture methods in public health surveillance. In *Monitoring the Health of Populations*, pages 341–360. Oxford University Press, Oxford, UK, 2003.

[53] Carrie Reed, Frederick J. Angulo, David L. Swerdlow, Marc Lipsitch, Martin I. Meltzer, Daniel Jernigan, and Lyn Finelli. Estimates of the prevalence of pandemic (H1N1) 2009, United States, April–July 2009. *Emerging Infectious Diseases*, 15(12):2004, 2009.

[54] Helen E. Jenkins, Arielle W. Tolman, Courtney M. Yuen, Jonathan B. Parr, Salmaan Keshavjee, Carlos M. Pérez-Vélez, Marcello Pagano, Mercedes C. Becerra, and Ted Cohen. Incidence of multidrug-resistant tuberculosis disease in children: Systematic review and global estimates. *Lancet (London, England)*, 383(9928):1572–1579, 2014.

[55] Christl A. Donnelly, Azra C. Ghani, Gabriel M. Leung, Anthony J. Hedley, Christophe Fraser, Steven Riley, Laith J. Abu-Raddad et al. Epidemiological determinants of spread of causal agent of severe acute respiratory syndrome in Hong Kong. *Lancet*, 361(9371):1761–1766, 2003.

[56] Anne M. Presanis, Daniela De Angelis, Angela Hagy, Carrie Reed, Steven Riley, Ben S. Cooper, Lyn Finelli et al. The severity of pandemic H1N1 influenza in the United States, from April to July 2009: A Bayesian analysis. *PLoS Medicine*, 6(12):e1000207, 2009.

[57] Tini Garske, Judith Legrand, Christl A. Donnelly, Helen Ward, Simon Cauchemez, Christophe Fraser, Neil M. Ferguson, and Azra C. Ghani. Assessing the severity of the novel influenza A/H1N1 pandemic. *BMJ*, 339:b2840, 2009.

6

Contact Patterns for Contagious Diseases

Jacco Wallinga, Jan van de Kassteele, and Niel Hens

CONTENTS

6.1 Introduction

Transmission of infection requires proximity between an infectious individual and a susceptible individual. The two individuals being proximate constitutes a "contact event." Rates of such contact events are used in epidemic models to determine the rate at which infections will spread among individuals within a population. The contact rates between any pair of individuals may vary, depending on the demographic characteristics of the two individuals. The precise pattern of contact rates for all pairs of individuals in the population critically determines the predicted risk of infection in the population, the predicted impact of interventions, and the predicted optimal allocation of intervention measures. Getting the pattern of contact rates right, therefore, is a key element in infectious disease modeling for public health. This chapter provides an introduction into the observation, the statistical analysis, and the use of estimated rates for such contact events.

Early efforts in modeling infectious disease transmission relied on the assumption of random mixing or homogeneous mixing [24]. This assumption implies that the rate of contact between any pair of individuals is the same within a population, and that infectious individuals choose others to be contacted at random, without any preference for any specific characteristic of the contacted individual. The assumption of random mixing runs counter to our everyday experience where many contacts are made repeatedly with relatively few individuals, and most other individuals in the population are hardly ever contacted. However, modeling results that rely on the assumption of random mixing tend to agree qualitatively with observations of infection dynamics. The effectiveness of the random mixing assumption can be understood, at least in part, from the observation that in a population where individuals have local contacts, the large-scale dynamic behavior shifts from typical for local contacts towards typical for random contacts by adding only a few random contacts [2]. That is, we often only need a few random contacts for the assumption of random mixing to provide good approximations.

For many infectious diseases, observations on incidence and prevalence of cases are stratified by sex and age. This stratification of the population into groups allows a bit more sophistication than random mixing: we can assume that contacts are made at random within and between each of the groups, and that the contact rates for any pair of individuals is determined by the groups that these individuals belong to. If the population is stratified by sex and age into n groups, this will require a number of $n \times n$ parameters to define the contact rates within and between those groups. With this stratification we will have n data points. This leaves us with an identifiability problem, as we have to infer more parameter values than there are data points.

One obvious approach to deal with such an identifiability problem is to impose a model for the possible values that the contact rates can take, and to constrain this model such that no more than n parameters have to be estimated. For example, we could allow for each group to have a different rate for making contacts, regardless of whom is contacted (this assumption is termed stratified random mixing or proportionate mixing [3]). Alternatively, we could assign each of the $n \times n$ contact rates to one out of only n parameters that are to be estimated (such an assignment is termed the "Who Acquired Infection from Whom matrix" (WAIFW) [4]). Whatever the specific model constrains we impose, after fitting the model predictions to observed incidence or prevalence we should carefully inspect the inferred contact rates for plausibility.

An alternative approach to deal with the identifiability problem is to use more data, of a different kind: we can use information from social behavior surveys to estimate the contact rates. This use should be done with great care, as information from behavior surveys can be subject to difficulties associated with nonresponse bias, insufficient number of participants, and untruthful answers by respondents. The use of surveys on sexual behavior to inform contact rates in models for sexually transmitted infections, such as infections with gonorrhea and HIV, dates back to the 1990s [5, 6]. The development of social contact behavior surveys to inform contact rates for models of close contact infections or airborne droplet infections, such as measles and influenza, is more recent [1, 7, 8].

An additional advantage of informing contact rate patterns by social contact survey data is that it allows for an assessment of the contact rates at a fine-scale stratification by age, sex, location, or any other variable we wish to include. If we would push this refinement to its limits, we would capture the rate of contact events between each pair of individuals in the population. This method offers us a social contact network where the nodes represent individuals and links represent social contacts between individuals. A seminal study by Rapoport and Horvath [9] identified a social contact network in a junior high school population by asking the pupils to name their best friends in school. The study also showed how an epidemic would spread if any infected individual would infect his or her two best friends. Yet such detailed datasets on social contact networks are rare, and they do not exist for large populations.

In this chapter, we will describe the social contact data that is used to infer contact rate patterns. We introduce the statistical approaches that are available to infer contact rate patterns from social contact data, and we will briefly indicate how these contact rate patterns can be used in models for infectious disease transmission. We have chosen to frame most of our exposition around a case study that is relevant to understanding the spread of close contact infections, such as measles, pertussis, or influenza.

6.2   Definition of Contact

A precise definition of a contact event is elusive, but for the purpose of this chapter, we will use the following definition:

A contact event is an event involving two individuals, such that infection would have been transmitted had the contacting individual been infectious and had the contacted individual been susceptible.

This definition allows us to talk about contact events between two individuals, regardless of the epidemiological status (susceptible, infected, or immune) of each of those two individuals. And if we have additional information that one individual involved in the contact event is infectious and the other is susceptible, we know that this contact event will lead to transmission of infection from one to the other. This definition is reminiscent of the informal definition of the basic reproduction number of an infection; the basic reproduction number can be thought of as the total number of different individuals that have had a contact event with one typical infectious individual during its infectious period. The trouble with contact events in this definition is that, in most cases, they are not observable. This method makes contact events a poor subject for statistical analysis, and that is why we invoke proxy measures.

A good proxy measure for contact events should be an observable quantity that can be elucidated from behavioral surveys or other data sources. The choice of an appropriate proxy measure depends on the transmission route of the infection of interest. Some examples are provided below.

- When the pathogen is transmitted by sexual contact, such as chhlamydia, the proxy measure could be the number of different sex partners in the past year as reported by a survey participant.

- When the pathogen spreads by close contacts or airborne droplets, such as influenza, the proxy measure could be the number of different individuals having a direct face-to-face conversation on a given day as reported by a survey participant.

- When the pathogen spreads predominantly in a hospital setting, such as Methicillin-resistant *Staphylococcus aureus* (MRSA), the proxy measure could be the number of different hospitals that a patient had been admitted to according to a patient healthcare database.

- When the pathogen spreads by the vector-borne route, such as yellow fever, the proxy measure could be a composite of the number of different individuals in close spatial proximity and the number of mosquito bites on a given day as reported by a survey participant.

We hypothesize that the rate of proxy contact events is proportional to the actual contact events for the infection of interest. This hypothesis (the "social contact hypothesis") should be tested against data, for example, by checking whether the resulting contact rate patterns offers a good prediction of actual transmission events.

6.3 Case Study: Contact Patterns Relevant to Spread of Close Contact Infections

6.3.1 Social contact survey

We illustrate the statistical analysis of social contact patterns by age and sex using survey data collected within the POLYMOD study [1]. In this study participants were recruited in eight European countries (Belgium, Germany, Finland, Great Britain, Italy, Luxembourg, The Netherlands, and Poland). The survey set-up of the multi-country study is presented in [1]. The survey protocol varied slightly between countries. We choose to focus only on the data collected in the Netherlands. The complete data set for the Netherlands was presented in the publication of [13].

In the Netherlands, the participants were selected using stratified randomized selection from population records (first a random selection of municipalities, then a random selection of individuals within municipalities). Only individuals from 0 to 80 years old were selected. The selected individuals were invited to participate over the years 2006 and 2007. The age and sex of the participants were obtained from their population records.

The participants were asked to complete a questionnaire on one assigned day. There were three different types of diaries: one for children (age 0–8), which was completed by their parents; one for teens (age 9–17); and one for adults (age 18+). Participants were asked to report the number of different persons they contacted. A contact was defined as either skin-to-skin contact such as a kiss or handshake (a physical contact), or a two-way conversation with three or more words in the physical presence of another person but no skin-to-skin contact (a nonphysical contact). Participants also were asked to provide information about the age and sex of each contact person. In total, 825 participants recorded characteristics of 11,225 other individuals they had contacted.

6.3.2 Data cleaning

If the age of a contact individual was not known precisely, participants could indicate an age range. Multiple imputation was used to replace the reported age range by a uniformly sampled age from that range (10 times). From age 20 onward, the reported age of contacts suggested a digit preference bias, a tendency for participants to record ages that end with a zero or five. Multiple imputation was used to remove this digit preference bias, by replacing excess reports by a uniform sampling from an age range from 2 years younger to 2 years older (10 times).

The survey questionnaire allowed for a maximum number of 45 different individuals to be contacted. Because only 22 out of 825 participants reached that maximum, possible right censoring of the number of different individuals was ignored. Records with missing age or sex of participants or contacted individuals were excluded from analysis. Records on contacted individuals that were older than 80 years were excluded. In total 53 out of 825 participants and 1,037 out of 11,225 contacted individuals were excluded.

6.3.3   Notation

We use subscripts j as an index for a participant's age, and i as an index for a contacted individual's age. Both indices i, j take integer values from 0 to 80. We take s as an index for a participants's sex, and r as an index for a contacted individual's sex. Both indices r, s are binary and refer to either male or female. Together, these indices are used to describe $81 \times 2 = 162$ possible combinations of age and sex for the participants, an equal number of combinations of age and sex for their contacts, and $162 \times 162 = 26,244$ possible combinations of ages and sexes to characterize the reported social interactions in this survey.

We take the following observables from the social contact survey and from census data:

- $w_{j,s}$, the number of individuals in the Dutch population of age j and sex s, according to the national census bureau (Statistics Netherlands, StatLine (2015),with reference date January 1, 2007);

- $T_{j,s}$, the number of participants of age j and sex s in the survey;

- $Y_{i,r\leftarrow t,j,s}$ the number of different individuals of age i and sex r that were contacted by the tth participant of age j and sex s in the survey, t is an index for participants that runs from 1 to $T_{j,s}$;

- $m_{i,r\leftarrow j,s}$ is the mean number of individuals with age i and sex r that are contacted by a participant of age j and sex s. That is, $m_{i,r\leftarrow j,s} = E(Y_{i,r\leftarrow t,j,s})$. The elements m make up a 162×162 matrix $\mathbf{M}$, which is called the "social contact matrix";

- $c_{i,r\leftarrow j,s}$ is the per capita contact rate with others of age i and sex r by participants of age j and sex s. That is, $c_{i,r\leftarrow j,s} = m_{i,r\leftarrow j,s}/w_{i,r}$. The elements c make up a 162×162 matrix $\mathbf{C}$, which is called the "contact rate matrix."

Notation alert: publications may differ in the order of indexes for participants and the contacted individuals. To stress the direction from participant to contacted individuals we have included an arrow.

6.4   Reciprocity of Contacts

We have a reciprocal proxy measure for contact events in this case study: having a conversation and touching are reciprocal events. On the individual level this means that if John has had a conversation with Mary, Mary must have had a conversation with John; if John has touched Mary, Mary must have touched John. On the population level this means that the total number of contacts that exist from age i and sex r with others of age j and sex s must equal the total number of contacts that exist from age j and sex s with others of age i and sex r. This can be stated in the notation that we have just introduced:

$$m_{i,r\leftarrow j,s} w_{j,s} = m_{j,s\leftarrow i,r} w_{i,r}. \tag{6.1}$$

From the definition of contact rates it follows that

$$m_{i,r\leftarrow j,s} = c_{i,r\leftarrow j,s} w_{i,r}. \tag{6.2}$$

Substituting this equation 6.2 into 6.1, and dividing both sides by $w_{i,r} w_{j,s}$ reveals that contact rates should be symmetric with respect to the groups i and j:

$$c_{i,r\leftarrow j,s} = c_{j,s\leftarrow i,r}. \tag{6.3}$$

Reciprocity of the proxy measure implies a diagonal symmetry of the contact rate matrix.

6.4.1   A visual inspection of the contact data

Reciprocity allows us to answer an important question in the analysis of self-reported sociological information: can the participants' self-reported behavior be confirmed by others [12, 17]? We check for accuracy by comparing reports of participants in one group with reports of participants in another group on the contact rate between the two groups. We calculate crude age- and sex-specific contact rates,

$$\tilde{c}_{i,r \leftarrow j,s} = \frac{1}{w_{i,r}} \frac{1}{T_{j,s}} \sum_{t=1}^{T_{j,s}} y_{i,r \leftarrow t,j,s}, \tag{6.4}$$

where y is the reported number of different contacts per participant. The outcome is shown in Figure 6.1.

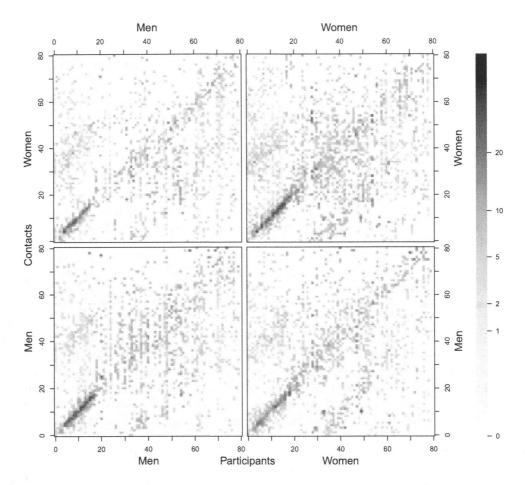

FIGURE 6.1
Crude age and sex-specific contact rates according to a social contact survey in the Netherlands, 2006–2007. The reported social contacts are categorized as male-to-male in the bottom left panel, female-to-female in the bottom right panel, male-to-female in the top left panel, and female-to-female in the top right panel. The horizontal axis of each panel indicates the age of the participants and the vertical axis indicates the age of the individuals they contacted. The colour indicates the relative value of the contact rate, light colours indicate low rates and dark colours indicate high rates.

These crude contacts rates reveal a tendency for the self-reported data to be symmetric along the diagonal, which means that participants in different age classes agree on the number of contacts between them. We note that the symmetry is not exact; the age of the contacted individuals (vertical axes) is bit more blurred than the age of the participant (horizontal axes). This can be explained because we have precise knowledge of the age of participants, but have to rely on reported age, sometimes as age ranges, of their contacts. The intensity of contacts for infants as reported by their parents is not precisely in line with the number of contacts that other age groups report with infants. That is because the proxy measure of having a face to face conversation is poorly defined for an infant, and it might be interpreted and remembered differently by the infant's parents and the contacted person. Overall, the impression is that the crude contact rates are symmetric along the diagonal, which means that participants in different age classes agree on the number of contacts between them.

Figure 6.1 also makes clear that the data is sparse. We have 825 randomly selected participants, and it is not obvious that these will cover all 162 different combinations for age and sex for our participants combination: there are no male participants of age 25 and 80, and no female participants of age 80. We have a total number of 11,225 reported social interactions in the survey, and it is clear that these do not cover all of the 26,244 possible combinations. As a consequence, the values of the crude contact rates fluctuate, and often are equal to 0. Before they can be used to inform contact rates in epidemic models, we need to deal with the sparseness of the data.

6.5 Statistical Analysis of the Contact Data

6.5.1 Piecewise constant contact rates

One approach to deal with the sparseness of the data is to pool the data into wider bins. This approach to estimating contact rate patterns was introduced by [8]. Here we illustrate this approach by ignoring sex and by aggregating the age of participants and their contacts into 5-year age bins.

We model the number of contacted individuals of one participant as a negative binomial distribution with mean $m_{i \leftarrow j}$ and dispersion parameter $k_{i \leftarrow j}$ such that the variance is $m_{i \leftarrow j} + m_{i \leftarrow j}^2 / k_{i \leftarrow j}$:

$$Y_{i,r \leftarrow j,s} \sim NegBin(m_{i \leftarrow j}, k_{i \leftarrow j}). \tag{6.5}$$

Because we have reciprocity, we can invoke equation 6.2 and express the number of contacts reported by age group i with age group j $m_{i \leftarrow j}$ in terms of the contact rate as $c_{i \leftarrow j} w_i$. We can do the same with the number of contacts reported by age group j with age group i, and express the number of contacts $m_{j \leftarrow i}$ in terms of contact rate as $c_{j \leftarrow i} w_j$. And because of the symmetry in contact rates (equation 6.3), this term equals $c_{i \leftarrow j} w_j$. This method allows us to infer the contact rate $c_{i \leftarrow j}$ from the reported number of contacts from group i to group j and from the reported number of contacts from group j to group i.

The log likelihood function for the contact rate $c_{i \leftarrow j}$ given data y is

$$\ell(c_{i \leftarrow j}, k_{i \leftarrow j}, k_{j \leftarrow i} | y) = \sum_{t=1}^{T_j} \log NegBin(y_{t, i \leftarrow j}; c_{i \leftarrow j} w_j, k_{i \leftarrow j})$$

$$+ \sum_{t=1}^{T_i} \log NegBin(y_{t, j \leftarrow i}; c_{i \leftarrow j} w_i, k_{j \leftarrow i}). \tag{6.6}$$

We look for the contact rates $c_{i \leftarrow j}$ and the dispersion parameters $k_{i \leftarrow j}, k_{j \leftarrow i}$ that maximize the log likelihood. Repeating this for all values of i and all values of j gives us the maximum likelihood estimates (MLEs) $c_{i \leftarrow j}$ for piecewise constant contact rates.

6.5.2   Bivariate smoothing

A second approach uses bivariate smoothing to estimate contact patterns by age of respondent and contact. This approach was used first by [14]. This approach allows us to study contact pattern at a finer scale than the piecewise constant approach. Here, we use 1 year age intervals for age and we still ignore sex. We assume that the contact counts $Y_{i \leftarrow j}$ are independently distributed, according to a negative binomial distribution with mean $m_{i \leftarrow j}$, and a single overall dispersion parameter k such that the variance is $m_{i \leftarrow j} + m_{i \leftarrow j}^2 / k$.

$$Y_{i,r \leftarrow j,s} \sim NegBin(m_{i \leftarrow j}, k). \tag{6.7}$$

In contrast to the piecewise constant approach, the overdispersion parameter k is assumed constant for all combinations of age groups.

We model the logarithm of the mean number of contacts as a tensor-product smooth with thin plate regression splines:

$$\log m_{i \leftarrow j} = \sum_{u=1}^{K} \sum_{v=1}^{K} \beta_{uv} b_u(i) a_v(j). \tag{6.8}$$

β_{uv} are unknown parameters, and b_u and a_v are basis functions for the marginal smoothers. The exact number of basis functions K is not crucial. However, if it is too small, then we will oversmooth and if it is too large, then the computation will be slower; a typical value would by $K = 10$ [14]. The smoothing can be performed in R with the `gam` function from the `mgcv` package [15]. The result is a set of smoothed estimates of the number of contacts $m_{i \leftarrow j}$.

Finally, we obtain the contact rates between two groups from the smoothed estimates of the number of contacts between those groups while accounting for the reciprocal nature of contacts:

$$c_{i \leftarrow j} = \frac{1}{2} \frac{m_{i \leftarrow j}}{w_i} + \frac{1}{2} \frac{m_{j \leftarrow i}}{w_j}. \tag{6.9}$$

Because we use smoothed estimates of the number of contacts, the resulting estimates for the contact vary smoothly with age whenever the numbers of individuals w_i and w_j vary smoothly with age (Figure 6.2).

6.5.3   Hierarchical Bayesian modeling of contact rates

A third approach uses a hierarchical Bayesian model to smooth contact rates while allowing for reciprocity. This approach was used first by [11]. This approach allows us to study contact patterns at an even finer scale than the bivariate smoothing approach. Here, we use 1 year age intervals for age and we include sex. The hierarchical Bayesian model has three levels:

- At the first level the number of contacts of any age and sex-specific combination in the dataset is described by a Negative Binomial distribution

$$Y_{i,r \leftarrow t,j,s} \sim NegBin(m_{i,r \leftarrow j,s}, k); \tag{6.10}$$

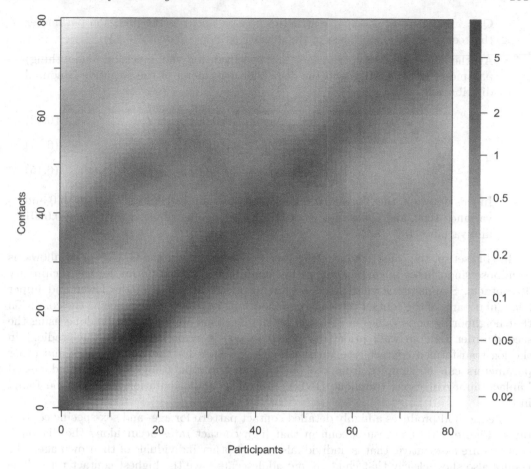

FIGURE 6.2
Estimated constant contact rates by age using a bivariate smoothing approach to analyze data from a social contact survey in the Netherlands, 2006–2007. The horizontal axis indicates the age of the participants and the vertical axis indicates the age of the individuals they contacted. The colour indicates the relative value of the contact rate, light colours indicate low rates and dark colours indicate high rates. The legend gives absolute values for the contact rates per million.

- At the second level, the mean of the total number of contacts is described as

$$\log m_{i,r\leftarrow j,s} = \log w_{i,r} + \log c_{i,r\leftarrow j,s} \tag{6.11}$$

$$\log c_{i,r\leftarrow j,s} = \beta + x_{i,r\leftarrow j,s}, \tag{6.12}$$

where we can interpret β as a mean for the log-transformed contact rates and $x_{i,r\leftarrow j,s}$ as deviations from this mean. These deviations $x_{i\leftarrow j}$ have a smooth and symmetric structure. Here, we model it as a realization of a zero mean two-dimensional Gaussian Markov Random Field (GMRF) over the ages i and j and both sexes (a GMRF is a random field following a multivariate Normal distribution with conditional independence assumptions [10]). The conditional independence relations are specified by a precision matrix

$\mathbf{Q} = \tau\mathbf{R}$, where $\mathbf{R}$ is a sparse structure matrix and τ is the precision parameter that controls the smoothness of the deviations $x|\tau \sim Normal(0, \mathbf{Q})$.

- At the third level, hyper priors are specified for the precision (smoothing) parameter of the GMRF and the dispersion parameter of the Negative Binomial distribution

$$\beta \sim Normal(0, 0.001), \tag{6.13}$$

$$\tau \sim Gamma(1, 0.0001), \tag{6.14}$$

$$\log k \sim Normal(0, 0.001). \tag{6.15}$$

In this notation, the $Normal(0, 0.001)$ is a Gaussian distribution with mean 0 and variance 1000, and $Gamma(1, 0.0001)$ is a Gamma distribution with mean 0.0001 and variance 10^8.

In this setup, the construction of the precision matrix $\mathbf{Q}$ of the GMRF prior allows us to impose smoothness in contact rates while simultaneously accounting for the reciprocity of contacts. Symmetry is guaranteed by forcing identical values in the lower and upper triangular parts of the contact rate matrix. Smoothing is achieved by imposing the condition that neighboring node values of x should be similar. This approach can be done using the second order random walk prior [10], which reflects a prior belief that the gradient in the log-transformed contact rate varies smoothly. Values for the contact rates and other parameters can be sampled from the posterior distribution using the integrated nested Laplace approximations technique (INLA) [16]. The implementation in R can be found in [13].

The method produces a highly detailed contact pattern for age- and sex-specific contact rates (Figure 6.3). The results confirm that high contact rates occur along the diagonal: contacts are assortative, that is, individuals contact other individuals of their own age. The results also show clearly that children and adolescents have the highest contact rates. The results reveal that children and adolescents contact other children and adolescents of their own sex, whereas adults contact other adults regardless of their sex. We detect only a few other exceptions to the overall assortative pattern: children have more contact with adults who are approximately 30 years older than with other adults, and women have more contact with children than men do.

6.6 Summary Measures

The resulting age-specific contact matrices reveal a much higher contact rate between individuals of the same age as compared to individuals. We can summarize and quantify this tendency by using a measure of disassortativeness [18]. The basic idea is to quantify the second moment along the diagonal of the age distribution, normalized by the variance of the age distribution:

$$I_s^2 = \frac{1}{2\sigma^2} E_c(i-j)^2, \tag{6.16}$$

where j refers to the age of participants and i tot the age of contacts, σ^2 is the variance of the age distribution, and E_c is the expectation with respect to the density of contact pairs

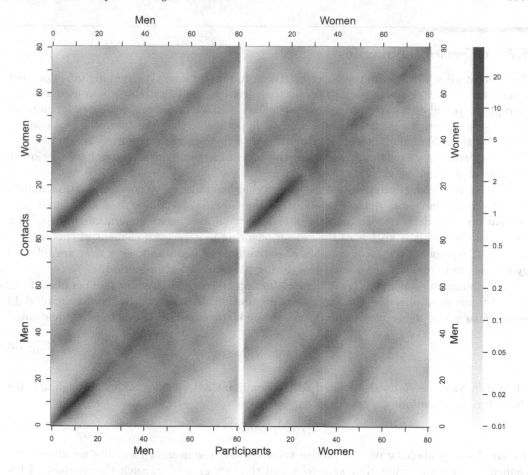

FIGURE 6.3

Estimated contact rates by age and sex using a hierarchical Bayesian approach to analyze data from a social contact survey in the Netherlands, 2006–2007. The estimated social contact rates are categorized as male-to-male in the bottom left panel, female-to-female in the bottom right panel, male-to-female in the top left panel, and female to female in the top right panel. The horizontal axis of each panel indicates the age of the participants and the vertical axis indicates the age of the individuals they contacted. The colour indicates the relative value of the contact rate, light colours indicate low rates and dark colours indicate high rates. The legend gives absolute values for the contact rates per million.

in the population, $\frac{w_i c_{i \leftarrow j} w_j}{\sum_i \sum_j w_i c_{i \leftarrow j} w_j}$. An attractive property of this measure is that it takes the value of $I_s^2 = 0$ when the contact pattern reflects completely assortative mixing and $I_s^2 = 1$ when the contact pattern reflects homogenous mixing.

When we apply this measure of disassortativeness for the contact matrices by age and sex as estimated by the hierarchical Bayesian approach (Figure 6.3) we get a value of $I_s^2 = 0.51$ (95 percent CI: 0.49–0.53). This outcome is in agreement with the range of values 0.44–0.52 found for self-reported social contacts obtained in several European countries with respect to age [18]. All values deviate from 1, the value expected for homogeneous mixing, which provides statistical evidence against a null-hypothesis of homogeneous mixing.

6.7   Infection Dynamics

We explore what the age- and sex-specific risk would be for a newly emerging infection that is transmitted via close contacts or respiratory droplets, and that spreads in a completely susceptible population. We convert the estimated contact rates into estimates for number of contacts per capita using equation 6.2. We hypothesize that the rate of actual contact events for the infection of interest is proportional to the rate of rate of proxy contact events. The proportionality constant q measures the ratio of actual contact rates for infection to contact rates for proxy events.

The matrix $q\mathbf{M}$ is often called the "reproduction matrix." The reproduction matrix provides a fundamental characterization of transmission dynamics in a structured host population. For deterministic models it is known as the "next generation matrix," for stochastic models it is known as the "mean offspring matrix." An element of this matrix, $qm_{i,r\leftarrow j,s}$, represents the mean number of individuals of age i and sex r that are infected by a single individual of age j and sex s during its entire infection period.

The dominant eigenvalue R_0 of the reproduction matrix $q\mathbf{M}$ gives the number of contacts made by a typical infective in a structured population. It is related to the dominant right eigenvector $\mathbf{w}_1$ of the reproduction matrix through the standard characteristic equation:

$$q\mathbf{M}\mathbf{w}_1 = R_0\mathbf{w}_1. \tag{6.17}$$

The top eigenvalue R_0 is also related to the dominant left eigenvector $\mathbf{v}_1$ through another characteristic equation:

$$\mathbf{v}_1^T q\mathbf{M} = R_0\mathbf{v}_1^T. \tag{6.18}$$

To avoid any ambiguity on the precise values of the eigenvector elements we choose the elements of $\mathbf{w}_1$ such that they sum to 1 and the elements of $\mathbf{v}_1$ such the product of left and right eigenvectors equals 1. The eigenvectors $\mathbf{w}_1$ and $\mathbf{v}_1$ are completely determined by $\mathbf{M}$ and do not depend on q. If the social contact matrix $\mathbf{M}$ is primitive, a condition that is met when all its elements are positive, the existence of unique real positive values of the elements of the associated eigenvectors $\mathbf{w}_1$ and $\mathbf{v}_1$ are guaranteed via the Perron-Frobenius Theorem (see [19]).

The dominant eigenvalue of the reproduction matrix $q\mathbf{M}$ is interpreted as the basic reproduction number R_0 [19]. The corresponding normalized left and right eigenvectors also have a clear epidemiological interpretation: the right eigenvector $\mathbf{w}_1$ can be interpreted as the observed number of infections over a given time interval in each group; the left eigenvector $\mathbf{v}_1$ can be interpreted as the per susceptible risk of being infected during a given observation interval ("force of infection") [20]. The latter interpretation hinges on the underlying contact matrix being symmetric.

Here we calculate the dominant left eigenvector of the social contact matrix $\mathbf{M}$ that corresponds to the contact rate pattern as estimated. The results show that the expected infection risk increases at a young age, from a relatively low risk for infants to a high risk for teenagers. For young adults the infection risk drops, and there is a small increase in risk around the age of 40. At older ages the risk decreases again (Figure 6.4). Between ages 18 and 38 women have a significantly higher infection risk than men, and between ages 50 and 65 women have a lower risk than men.

The value of the proportionality constant q (that is, the ratio of actual contact rates for infection to contact rates for proxy events) can be calibrated such as to achieve a specific value for the basic reproduction number. The value of the proportionality constant q can

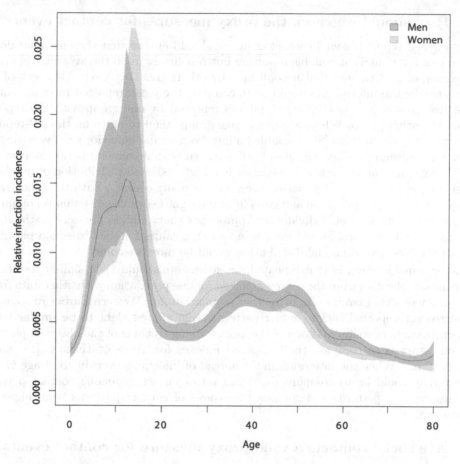

FIGURE 6.4
Predicted risk of infection in the initial phase of an epidemic. A new respiratory pathogen spreads via social contacts as presented in Figure 6.3 in a completely susceptible population. The lines indicate the median risk, the shaded area the 95 percent credibility interval, the darker colour indicates risk for men, the lighter colour indicates the risk for women.

also be estimated by fitting model predictions to serological data, assuming this data is collected in an endemic equilibrium [8, 14], or proportion of population infected per group over an epidemic [8].

6.8 Perspective

Epidemic modeling studies increasingly rely on contact patterns that are based on observed behavior, and an increasing amount of social contact data is becoming available. So far, there are relatively few statistical methods available to analyze these contact data and to infer the contact parameters required for modeling. This leaves much room for advancing the statistical analysis of social contact data. Here, we highlight four areas with unresolved problems.

6.8.1   How should we check the proxy measures for contact events?

When using self-reported social contact data, we should ensure that the outcomes do not depend on an individual's unreliable reporting but rest firmly upon the average response of a large group of participants that is confirmed by others [12, 17]. A sensible check of self-reported sociological information would be to compare the mean reported rates of contacts between two groups by contrasting the rate as reported by one group with the reported rate from the other group. Whereas different age groups tend to agree on the self-reported social contacts between them [8], a reliable finding from sexual behavior surveys is that the different sexes disagree about the rate of self-reported sexual contacts between them [21]. A possible explanation for such a discrepancy is a highly skewed distribution of number of contacts per person, where a few persons account for many contacts with the other group. This requires accurate description and good fit of the right tail of the distribution of number of contacts to capture those individuals. Approaches that provide fine-scale estimates of contact rates while allowing for different group-specific values for the dispersion parameter $k_{i,r \leftarrow j,s}$ of the Negative Binomial distribution would be most welcome.

Another sensible check is that repeated measurements should yield similar results. We should compare the data from the survey reported for one population with other data from a similar survey of a comparable size in another population. For Western European countries, the reported self-reported social contact patterns seem at first sight to be similar [1]. As the assortativeness of contacts is one of the most striking features of the observed patterns, an obvious start is to compare the computed indexes for disassortativeness [18] among contact patterns. When the interest is in the spread of infections over different age groups, an alternative would be to compare the dominant eigenvectors among contact patterns. Comparing contact patterns and summary measures of contact patterns is an important open problem.

6.8.2   Are social contacts a valid proxy measure for contact events?

In the case study, we presented a social contact event as a proxy measure for an infectious contact event. The question is whether this proxy measure results in a better description of epidemiological data than using *a priori* assumptions such as random mixing and stratified mixing that do not require the use of additional social contact data. This analysis can be done by comparing observed serological data to predictions [8, 14]. In such a test, we could allow for the proportionality constant q to vary over groups to check our assumption that this variable is a constant.

A closely related issue is the comparison between alternative proxy measure for an infection of interest. In our case study we presented the number of self-reported physical contacts (touching) and non-physical contacts (conversation) of any duration during one particular day, but we could have chosen to work with only physical contacts (touching) of a duration longer than 15 minutes. The social contact studies have more information on the duration of contact, the type of contact, and the setting of the contact (at home, at work, at school, leisure, and other). The observations can be included to form better proxy measures that are more informative of actual transmission. Taking full advantage of the information that is gathered in the sociological surveys is an important open problem.

6.8.3   How should we move from contact rates between groups
to spatially explicit contact networks?

The social contact questionnaires can be extended to ask about the spatial coordinates of a participant's residence and the place of contact [22]. Information on the spatial distance would inform models for the spatial spread of infection. Currently, most spatial epidemic models are based on assumptions how individuals travel, such as the gravity model [23]. A statistical approach towards analyzing displacement of contacts is currently being explored.

For some infections, such as sexually transmitted infections, the use of contact rate patterns is insufficient to model transmission. We might interpret contacts as relationships, and we need information on the number of different relationships during an infectious period, the order in which subsequent relationships are formed, and the concurrency of relationships. As a start, the social contact questionnaires also can be extended to ask which of the contacted individuals make contact with the other. This information would allow us to quantify a degree of clustering in the contact network [22]. Even though this is an important step forward, it still leaves us with local, small-scale properties of the contact network ("ego networks" in the parlance of social network analysis). Other study designs, different from the social contact surveys discussed here, are required to collect information on large-scale properties of the contact network.

6.8.4 What are the determinants of contact patterns?

The general approach to studying contact patterns has been entirely descriptive. If we would have a better understanding of the demographic and cultural determinants of the social contact network, we might be able to predict a social contact pattern for any population where such determinants are known. This information would allow us to use contact patterns and epidemic models for populations where survey data are unavailable, to report on infection risks for entire continents while allowing for heterogeneity in contact patterns between regions, and to make long-term projections for incidence and prevalence of infectious diseases while accounting for demographic change over such long time frames. Such long-term projections are crucial for public health policy making. Finding determinants requires a lot of data. Fortunately, an increasing amount of contact data is being recorded and published, for different population with different demographics and different cultural backgrounds [11]. A substantial part of these contact data are made available. This situation leaves it up to the statisticians to develop the statistical methods for detecting the determinants that shape the contact patterns we see.

References

[1] WO Kermack and AG McKendrick. A contribution to the mathematical theory of epidemics. *Proceedings of the Royal Society of London A*, 115(772):700–721, 1927.

[2] DJ Watts and SH Strogatz. Collective dynamics of 'small-worls' networks. *Nature*, 393 (6684):440, 1998.

[3] HW Hethcote. Modeling heterogeneous mixing in infectious disease dynamics. In V Isham and G Medley, editors, *Models for Infectious Human Diseases: Their Structure and Relation to Data*, Publications of the Newton Institute, p. 215–238. Cambridge, UK: Cambridge University Press, 1996.

[4] RM Anderson and RM May. *Infectious Diseases of Humans: Dynamics and control.* Oxford, UK: Oxford University Press, 1992.

[5] S Haraldsdottir, S Gupta, and RM Anderson. Preliminary studies of sexual networks in a male homosexual community in Iceland. *Journal of Acquired Immune Deficiency Syndromes*, 5(4):374–381, 1992.

[6] GP Garnett and RM Anderson. Contact tracing and the estimation of sexual mixing patterns: The epidemiology of gonococcal infections. *Sexually Transmitted Diseases*, 20 (4):181–191, 1993.

[7] WJ Edmunds, CJ O'callaghan, and DJ Nokes. Who mixes with whom? A method to determine the contact patterns of adults that may lead to the spread of airborne infections. *Proceedings of the Royal Society of London B: Biological Sciences*, 264(1384): 949–957, 1997.

[8] J Wallinga, P Teunis, and M Kretzschmar. Using data on social contacts to estimate age-specific transmission parameters for respiratory-spread infectious agents. *American Journal of Epidemiology*, 164(10):936–944, 2006.

[9] J Mossong, N Hens, M Jit, P Beutels, K Auranen, R Mikolajczyk, M Massari et al. Social contacts and mixing patterns relevant to the spread of infectious diseases. *PLoS Medicine*, 5(3):e74, 2008.

[10] A Rapoport and WJ Horvath. A study of a large sociogram. *Systems Research and Behavioral Science*, 6(4):279–291, 1961.

[11] J van de Kassteele, J van Eijkeren, and J Wallinga. Efficient estimation of age-specific social contact rates between men and women. *The Annals of Applied Statistics*, 11(1): 320–339, 2017.

[12] S Wasserman and K Faust. *Social Network Analysis: Methods and Applications*, vol. 8. Cambridge, UK: Cambridge University Press, 1994.

[13] T Smieszek, EU Burri, R Scherzinger, and RW Scholz. Collecting close-contact social mixing data with contact diaries: Reporting errors and biases. *Epidemiology & Infection*, 140(4):744–752, 2012.

[14] N Goeyvaerts, N Hens, B Ogunjimi, M Aerts, Z Shkedy, P Van Damme, and P Beutels. Estimating infectious disease parameters from data on social contacts and serological status. *Journal of the Royal Statistical Society: Series C (Applied Statistics)*, 59(2): 255–277, 2010.

[15] SN Wood. *Generalized Additive Models: An Introduction with R*. Boca Raton, FL: CRC Press, 2017.

[16] H Rue and L Held. *Gaussian Markov Random Fields: Theory and Applications*. Boca Raton, FL: CRC Press, 2005.

[17] H Rue, S Martino, and N Chopin. Approximate Bayesian inference for latent Gaussian models by using integrated nested laplace approximations. *Journal of the Royal Statistical Society: Series B (Statistical Methodology)*, 71(2):319–392, 2009.

[18] CP Farrington, HJ Whitaker, J Wallinga, and P Manfredi. Measures of disassortativeness and their application to directly transmitted infections. *Biometrical Journal*, 51 (3):387–407, 2009.

[19] O Diekmann, H Heesterbeek, and B Britton. *Mathematical Tools for Understanding Infectious Disease Dynamics*. Princeton, NJ: Princeton University Press, 2012.

[20] J Wallinga, M van Boven, and M Lipsitch. Optimizing infectious disease interventions during an emerging epidemic. *Proceedings of the National Academy of Sciences*, 107 (2):923–928, 2010.

[21] DD Brewer, JJ Potterat, SB Garrett, SQ Muth, JM Roberts, D Kasprzyk, DE Montano, and WW Darrow. Prostitution and the sex discrepancy in reported number of sexual partners. *Proceedings of the National Academy of Sciences*, 97(22):12385–12388, 2000.

[22] L Danon, JM Read, TA House, MC Vernon, and MJ Keeling. Social encounter networks: Characterizing Great Britain. *Proceedings of the Royal Society Series B*, 280(1765): 20131037, 2013.

[23] Y Xia, ON Bjørnstad, and BT Grenfell. Measles metapopulation dynamics: A gravity model for epidemiological coupling and dynamics. *The American Naturalist*, 164(2): 267–281, 2004.

[24] T Hoang, P Coletti, A Melegaro, J Wallinga, C Grijalva, J Edmunds, P Beutels, and N Hens. A systematic review of social contact surveys to inform transmission models of close contact infections. *Epidemiology*, 30(5):723–736, 2019.

7

Basic Stochastic Transmission Models and Their Inference

Tom Britton

CONTENTS

7.1 Introduction

The current chapter aims to present some basic stochastic models for the spread of infectious diseases in human or animal populations and also to describe how to perform inference about important model parameters, such as the basic reproduction number R_0 and the critical vaccination coverage v_C. Naturally, there is some overlap, but also differences, between the current chapter and other overview papers, in particular two chapters by the same author. However, Britton [1] has more focus on the stochastic analysis of models and only briefly touches upon inference procedures, and Britton and Giardina [2] describe briefly many different inferential aspects with extensive references to the literature. In the current chapter we focus on basic models and try to be more self-contained, more complex and realistic models are treated in later chapters of the book. There are, of course, numerous papers dealing with this type of inference. Two recent books on the topic are Becker [3] and Deskman et al. [4], the latter also is more theoretical and provides extensive modeling.

The mathematical/statistical models describe the spread of a transmittable disease. What makes such diseases different from other diseases, regarding the mathematical analysis and reality, is that transmittability implies that the health status of different individuals will be *dependent*, as opposed to other diseases where the occurence of diseases in different individuals happen independently. These dependencies make the mathematical treatment, as well as the statistical analysis, more involved, as we will see. We will present some simple models and only briefly discuss extensions towards more realistic models, and the presented inference procedures will focus on estimation of basic parameters.

The rest of this chapter is structured as follows. In Section 7.2, we define the basic models to be used, and in the next section we discuss some model extensions. In Section 7.4, we present the main inference procedures for a couple of different types of data. In Section 7.5, we study effects of preventive measures put in place before or during an outbreak, and how such effects may be estimated from previous outbreak data.

7.2 The Standard Stochastic SIR Epidemic Model

The class of models we analyze are where individuals may be classified into three classes: Susceptibles (individuals who have not experienced the disease but who are susceptible to infection), Infectives (individuals who have been infected and may transmit the disease onwards), and Recovered (individuals who can no longer transmit the disease and who are immune to the disease). Such models are called SIR models from the three classes and how individuals may move between the three states. If individuals who get infected first enter a latent state before becoming infectious, the models are called SEIR model where 'E' stands for Exposed but not yet infectious. If immunity is not permanent but wanes, the model would be called an SIRS model indicating the non-transient nature of such a model.

We consider a population of size n, where approximations/limit results rely on n being large. When we look at short-term outbreaks we consider a fixed population of size n, whereas later, when considering endemic diseases, we let n denote the average population size in a community in which individuals die and new individuals are born.

7.2.1 Definition: the standard stochastic SIR epidemic

We now define what we call the *standard stochastic SIR epidemic* in a fixed and closed community. Consider a community of size n in which an SIR epidemic spreads. Initially all individuals are susceptible except one index case who is infectious. Individuals who get infected remain infectious for a random period I, having mean $E(I) = \iota$, and then recover. Infectious individuals have infectious contacts at rate β, each time with a uniformly chosen individual in the community. An infectious contact with a susceptible individual implies that the latter gets infected whereas other contacts have no effect. The epidemic goes on (infectious individuals having infectious contacts until they recover) until the first time T when no one is infectious. Then the epidemic stops.

We let $S(t), I(t)$, and $R(t)$, respectively, denote the number of susceptible, infectious and recovered, at time t measured from the start of the epidemic. Since the population is fixed and closed we have $S(t) + I(t) + R(t) = n$ for all t. The corresponding fractions are denoted $\bar{S}(t) = S(t)/n$ and similarly. Whenever the dependence on n is important, we equip the quantities with an n-index. As regards to parameters, we have the infectious contact rate β and the duration of the infectious period I being a random variable. Of fundamental importance is $R_0 := \beta E(I) = \beta\iota$, and called the basic reproduction number. This value is hence the average number of infectious contacts an infectious individual has during the individual's infectious period. In the beginning of the outbreak and assuming a large community, all such contacts will be with distinct and susceptible individuals with high probability, so R_0 is the expected number of individuals an infected person infects in the beginning. It should hence not come as a surprise that a big (or major) outbreak can only happen if $R_0 > 1$.

7.2.2   The general stochastic epidemic

Two specific choices of infectious periods I have received special attention in the literature. The first is where $I \sim Exp(\gamma)$ (so $\iota = 1/\gamma$). This model is often called the *general stochastic epidemic* (or the Markovian epidemic) and its main reason for receiving attention is that the model then becomes Markovian thus having mathematically tractable properties. In the limit as $n \to \infty$, this model corresponds to the (deterministic) *general epidemic model* defined by the differential equations:

$$s'(t) = -\beta s(t) i(t)$$
$$i'(t) = \beta s(t) i(t) - \gamma i(t) \qquad (7.1)$$
$$r'(t) = \gamma i(t).$$

For this model $R_0 = \beta/\gamma$ and it is seen that, starting with $s(0) = 1 - \epsilon$, $i(0) = \epsilon$, and $r(0) = 0$ for some small $\epsilon > 0$, $i(t)$ is initially increasing if and only if $R_0 > 1$. One difference between this deterministic general epidemic and the stochastic general epidemic is that the deterministic model will surely have an outbreak infecting a substantial community fraction when $R_0 > 1$, whereas in the stochastic setting starting with a small *number* of infectives, a major epidemic *can* happen, but the epidemic may as an alternative still die out infecting only few individuals. So, in the stochastic setting there could be a minor outbreak with a certain probability and a major outbreak with the remaining probability.

In Figure 7.1 we have plotted $\bar{I}_n(t) = I(t)/n$ for a few different n, and its deterministic counterpart $i(t)$, starting with 5 percent infectives, thus assuring a major outbreak also in the stochastic setting. It is seen that the stochastic curve agrees better with the deterministic counterpart the larger n is.

7.2.3   The Reed-Frost epidemic and chain-binomial models

The second choice of infectious period, which has received specific attention is where $I \equiv \iota$, i.e., where the infectious period is non-random and the same for all individuals, a model called the continuous-time Reed-Frost epidemic. This model has received special attention for mathematical rather than for epidemiological reasons. One probabilistic advantage with this model is that when the infectious period is non-random, then the events for an infectious individual to infect different other individuals become *independent*. When the infectious period is random this does not hold: if the infective infects another individual this indicates that most likely the infectious period was long, and this increases the risk to infect another individual. But in the Reed-Frost epidemic these events are independent, so an infective has independent infectious contacts with each other individual, and these contact probabilities all equal $p = 1 - e^{-\beta \iota/n} \approx \beta \iota/n$ (the contact rate to a specific other individual equals β/n).

If individuals are latent for a period prior to the constant infectious period, and assuming the the latent period is long and the infectious period is short, then the new infected people will appear in 'generations', something which can actually even be observed during early stages of outbreaks. This outcome is then called the discrete-time version of the Reed-Frost epidemic. Anyway, then a susceptible individual escapes infection in generation $k + 1$ if the individual avoids getting infected from each of the infected people of the previous generation, so this happens with probability $(1 - p)^{i_k}$, where i_k denotes the number of individuals who got infected in generation k. The probability to get infected is the complimentary

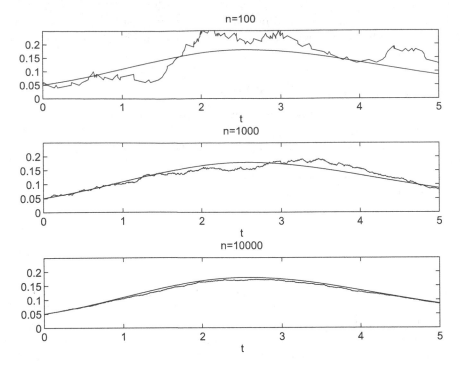

FIGURE 7.1

Time course of proportion infectives in a stochastic model, $\bar{I}_n(t)$ (for $n = 100$, 1,000 and 10,000) and its deterministic limit $i(t)$ against t. Parameters are $\beta = 2$, $\gamma = 1$ (e.g., weeks as time unit and average infectious periods of 1 week), so $R_0 = 2$.

probability $1 - (1 - p)^{i_k}$. This outcome is true for all individuals who were susceptible after generation k and the infection events are independent between different pairs of individuals (due to constant infectious period). As a consequence, if there are i_k individuals getting infected in generation k and s_k remaining susceptible, then it follows that

$$I_{k+1} \sim Bin(s_k,\ 1 - (1 - p)^{i_k}) \text{ and } S_{k+1} = s_k - I_{k+1},$$

where $Bin(n, p)$ denotes the binomial distribution with parameters n and p.

We can use this iteratively over different generations to compute the probability of an entire outbreak in terms of generations. As a small example, suppose that we want to compute the probability that in a community of 10 individuals and starting with 1 infectious and nine susceptibles, we want to compute the probability that first 2 got infected, then 3 followed by 1, and then no more. This computation means that we have $(i_0 = 1, s_0 = 9)$ followed by $(i_1 = 2, s_1 = 7)$, $(i_2 = 3, s_2 = 4)$, $(i_3 = 1, s_1 = 3)$, and $(i_4 = 0, s_4 = 3)$. The probability for this outbreak chain is given by

$$\binom{9}{2}p^2(1 - p)^7 \binom{7}{3}(1 - (1 - p)^2)^3((1 - p)^2)^4 \binom{4}{1}(1 - (1 - p)^3)^1((1 - p)^3)^3 \binom{3}{0}p^0(1 - p)^3.$$

This result should explain why the discrete time version of the Reed-Frost model often is referred to as a *chain binomial model*. It is possible to think of other chain binomial models (e.g., where the infection probabilities are different or there are different types of individuals), but the discrete time Reed-Frost model is by far the most well studied chain binomial model. The final-size probabilities can in principle be determined by summing the different chains given a specified final size, but for more than, for example, five infected people there are too many chains giving such a final size thus making this approach of less practical use.

It is worth pointing out that the time-continuous Reed-Frost model that we started with, in fact, gives the same final outcome probabilities as the discrete time Reed-Frost (having the same p). The order in which individuals get infected, and by whom, differ in the two models, but the same number of individuals will ultimately get infected. For this reason the two models are sometimes used interchangeably.

7.2.4 Asymptotic results

We now present some results for the standard stochastic SIR epidemic valid for large n. All the results can be proven to hold as limit results when $n \to \infty$.

As mentioned earlier, in the beginning of an outbreak in a large community, an infectious individual will have all its infectious contacts with distinct individuals who are susceptible. An infective will hence infect new individuals at constant rate β during the infectious period I, and individuals that the individual infects will do the same and independently. This then satisfies the definition of a continuous-time branching process, where individuals give birth (i.e., infect) at rate β during their life span (infectious period) I.

The mean of the offspring distribution is given by $R_0 = \beta E(I) = \beta \iota$. It is known that if $R_0 \leq 1$, then the branching process (i.e., epidemic) can never take off, and just a small number of individuals will ever get born (be infected). If, however, $R_0 > 1$, then the epidemic may take off infecting large number of individuals. In the beginning of the outbreak, each individual infects a random number X new individuals, and given the duration of the infectious period $I = s$, then the number of infections is Poisson distributed with mean parameter βs (the infection rate multiplied by the duration). Without conditioning on the infectious period, the number of infections is hence what is called a mixed Poission distribution $X \sim MixPoi(\beta I)$, where I is random following the distribution specified by the model. For the continuous time Reed-Frost model $X \sim Poi(\beta \iota)$, since $I \equiv \iota$ is non-random, and for the Markovian SIR where $I \sim Exp(\gamma)$ (having mean $\iota = 1/\gamma$) it is not hard to show that $X \sim Geo(\gamma/(\beta + \gamma))$.

From branching process theory we conclude the following:

(1) An epidemic can take off if and only if $R_0 = \beta E(I) > 1$.

(2) If $R_0 > 1$, the probability π that the epidemic takes off equals the unique strictly positive solution to the equation $1 - \pi = \rho(1 - \pi)$, where $\rho(s) = E(s^X)$ and $X \sim MixPoi(\beta I)$ meaning that X given $I = s$ is $Poi(\beta s)$ and I follows the specified distribution defined in the model. For the Reed-Frost model this equation becomes $1 - \pi = e^{-R_0 \pi}$ and for the Markovian SIR the solution is explicit and equals $\pi = 1 - 1/R_0$.

(3) If the epidemic takes off (hence assuming $R_0 > 1$), then the number of infectives $I(t)$ at time t grows exponentially in t: $I(t) \sim e^{\rho t}$, where ρ is the so-called Malthusian parameter being the unique solution to the equation $\int_0^\infty e^{-\rho t} \beta P(I > t)dt = 1$ (see Figure 7.2 for an illustration).

If the epidemic takes off, the fraction of individuals being susceptible will start decaying so an individual who gets infected will then infect fewer individuals because some of the infectious contacts will be 'wasted' on already infected individuals. This explains why the branching process approximation, which assumes all individuals infect according to the same rules, then breaks down. It is still possible to derive approximately how many individuals will get infected. One way to do this is by analyzing the differential equations

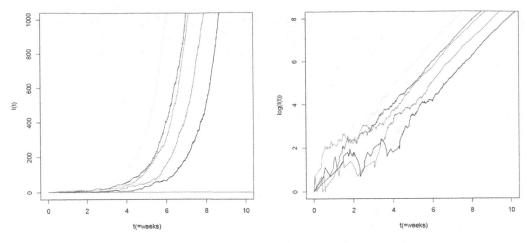

FIGURE 7.2
Time course of number of infectious individuals $I(t)$ during the initial epidemic stage for 10 simulations, original as well as log-scale (for the ones that take off). The population size is $n = 100,000$ so depletion of susceptibles have hardly started when at most 1,000 individuals have been infected. Five of the simulations die out quickly whereas the remaining take off, having different initial delays before taking off. The original scale shows the exponential growth, which is made even more evident on the log-scale where the growth is linear. The model parameters are $\beta = 2$ and $\gamma = 1$ (hence 1 week infectious period and $R_0 = 2$). The model predicts an exponential growth rate of $\rho = \beta - \gamma = 1$, which corresponds to a linear growth with coefficient 1 on the log-scale (agreeing with the slopes of the lines).

defined in Equation (7.1). By manipulating these equations it can be shown that when $t \to \infty$ and the initial fraction infectives is small and the rest are susceptible, then $r(\infty) = 1 - s(\infty)$, and $s(\infty)$, the fraction avoiding infection during the outbreak, is given by the positive solution to $s(\infty) = e^{R_0(1-s(\infty))}$. This equation may equivalently be expressed in terms of $r(\infty) = 1 - s(\infty)$:

$$1 - r(\infty) = e^{R_0 r(\infty)}, \tag{7.2}$$

the so-called final-size equation. In Figure 7.3 we plot the final size $r(\infty)$ as a function of R_0, a solution which has to be obtained numerically.

This result is true irrespective of the distribution of the infectious period I as long as $\beta E(I) = R_0$. From branching process theory (conclusion 2 above), we see that the outbreak probability for the Reed-Frost model is the same as the final-size equation, so for this particular model the probability of a major outbreak (starting with one infective!) equals the final fraction getting infected in case of a major outbreak. As two numerical examples, if $R_0 = 1.5$, then we have $r(\infty) = 0.583$ so approximately 60 percent will get infected if an outbreak takes place in a community without any immunity, and $r(\infty) = 0.98$ if $R_0 = 3$.

For any finite n in the stochastic setting, the ultimate fraction getting infected will, of course, not be exactly identical to $r(\infty)$, there will be some random fluctuations. These, however, will be of order $1/\sqrt{n}$, so close to negligible in large populations (in fact the randomness has been proven to be Gaussian with an explicit standard deviation, which we make use of later).

In the next section we will discuss some extensions of this standard stochastic epidemic model. Here we end by emphasizing that the most important parameter $R_0 = \beta E(I)$

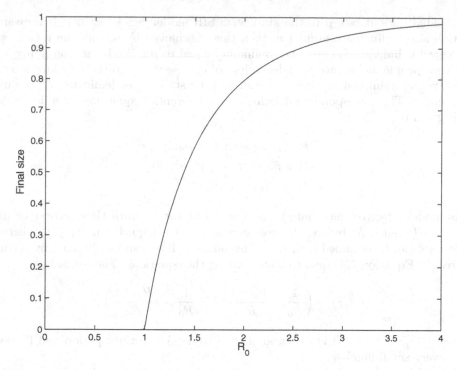

FIGURE 7.3
The final fraction getting infected in case of a major outbreak, $r(\infty)$, as a function of R_0 (for $n \to \infty$).

depends not only on the disease agent but also on the community under study. This connection can be made more explicit by writing $\beta = c \cdot p$, so $R_0 = c \cdot p \cdot E(I)$, where c is the rate at which individuals have close contact with other individuals, p is the transmission probability for such a contact given that one individual is infectious and the other is susceptible, and $E(I)$ is the mean infectious period. Then p and $E(I)$ depend on the disease agent whereas c depends on the community and how frequently people have contact.

7.3 Model Extensions

7.3.1 Including demography giving rise to endemicity

In the model defined in the previous section, it was assumed that the community was fixed and closed. Such an approximation works well if considering a short-term outbreak (e.g., influenza outbreak) taking place over a few months.

If our interest instead concerns diseases staying in the community for longer periods, like with many childhood diseases, then such an approximation is not adequate. Then we should allow for new individuals entering the community and old people leaving the community (e.g., by dying). Such a stochastic model can be achieved by adding a random, but with constant average rate, influx of new susceptible individuals, and assuming that each individual dies at rate μ to the Markovian SIR model defined earlier. If we want the population size to fluctuate around n, then this is achieved by setting the rate at which new susceptible individuals enter the community equal to μn. So, by adding influx at rate μn and that people die at rate μ (independent of disease state) to the standard stochastic epidemic, we get a simplest possible model suitable for studying endemic diseases giving life-long immunity. The corresponding defining set of differential equations for a deterministic model is given by

$$
\begin{aligned}
s'(t) &= \mu - \beta s(t) i(t) - \mu s(t) \\
i'(t) &= \beta s(t) i(t) - \gamma i(t) - \mu i(t) \\
r'(t) &= \gamma i(t) - \mu r(t).
\end{aligned}
\tag{7.3}
$$

For this model infectives have infectious contacts at rate β until they recover or die, so now $R_0 = \beta/(\gamma + \mu)$. As before, the disease will go extinct quickly if $R_0 \leq 1$, whereas an endemic level can be obtained if $R_0 > 1$. This endemic level can be obtained by setting all derivatives in Equation 7.3 equal to 0 and solving the equations. The result is

$$
(\tilde{s}, \tilde{i}, \tilde{r}) = \left(\frac{1}{R_0}, \ \epsilon \frac{R_0 - 1}{R_0}, \ 1 - \frac{1}{R_0} - \epsilon \frac{R_0 - 1}{R_0} \right),
\tag{7.4}
$$

where $\epsilon = \gamma^{-1}/(\mu^{-1} + \gamma^{-1})$ is the ratio of the (average) infectious period and life length; usually a very small number.

It is worth pointing out that the stochastic model, as well as the limiting deterministic model defined by Equation (7.3), assume that the infectious period and also life-length distributions are exponentially distributed. There are extensions to more realistic scenarios, but we omit them here.

7.3.2   Heterogeneities

The stochastic epidemic models defined previously as well as the deterministic counterparts, have all assumed a community consisting of identical individuals that mix uniformly at random with each other. Reality is, of course, more complicated. There are usually different types of individuals who are different in terms of how susceptible they are, how much contact they have with others, and how infectious they become in case of infection. In what follows, we refer to such differences as *individual heterogeneities*. There is also another type of heterogeneity which concerns *whom* individuals have contact with. This latter feature concerns the *social structure* in the community and the fact that usually individual meet more regularly with certain individuals and much less with the remaining majority.

The individual heterogeneities often are dealt with by dividing the population into different *types* of individual and assuming homogeneity within each type, meaning that individuals of the same type have the same susceptibility, total contact rate, and infectivity. A corresponding epidemic is called a multitype epidemic model. Such a *multitype epidemic model* is similar to the original model defined previously, with the difference that now the rate of infecting someone depends on the infector type and the susceptible type. As a consequence, R_0 is now more complicated because the average number of individuals (of different types) an infected individual (of a specified type) infects is now a matrix of numbers. The basic reproduction number R_0 is then the *largest eigenvalue* to this next generation matrix (e.g. [4], Chapter 7).

When it comes to the social structure of a community it depends on what type of disease is considered. For example, when considering influenza or related diseases it is common to consider *household epidemic models* because spreading is usually higher within households than between other individuals. Sometimes also schools or day-care centers are included in the model. If interest is instead on sexually transmitted infections (STIs), then the relevant social structure is the sexual network in the community. Then so-called *network epidemic models* [5] often are used, where the network obeys certain known characteristics of the empirical network but otherwise treated as random, and where an epidemic model is defined on the network.

A different type of heterogeneity is where the contact rates vary with calendar time, often referred to as *seasonality*. The simplest way to include such heterogeneity into a model is to let the infectious contact rate β now depend on calendar time $\beta(t)$. Usually some type of periodic function is assumed, having 1 year as the natural period. Two such choices are $\beta(t) = a + b\sin(\omega + 2\pi t)$ where a is the mean contact rate, b is the amplitude of the seasonality, and ω is the phase shift defining the time location of the yearly peak. A second choice is $\beta(t) = a$ for $t \in k + [t_1, t_2]$ for some integer k and $\beta(t) = b$ otherwise. This $\beta(t)$ is a two step function, often reflecting school terms vs. summer break, the latter having lower overall contact rate.

Finally we mention heterogeneity in terms of the infectivity varying with time since infection. In the presented model, it was assumed that individuals immediately become infectious upon infection and infect others at rate β until the end of the infectious period when infectivity suddenly drops to 0. A more realistic model is to assume that the infectivity depends on the time s since infection $\beta(s)$. For instance, there might be very low infectivity shortly after infection, then the infectivity picks up after a few days and remains high for some time until it starts decaying down to 0. It also could be that $\beta(s)$ is random in the sense that different individuals have different infectivity curves (this is actually the case also for the original model since the end of the infectious period is random). One special case of this more general model is where each individual is a first latent for a random period having no infectivity, followed by an random infectious period I when the individual has infectious contacts at constant rate β, and then the individual recovers, the difference from the original model hence being a latent period prior to infectivity. Such models are called SEIR epidemic models, where 'E' stands for exposed but not yet infectious. In terms of the epidemic, SEIR epidemics will result in the same final size (assuming the same R_0 of course), but the timing and duration of the outbreak will differ. From an inference point of view this means that extending the model in this direction is not important for final size data, but, e.g., when data comes from the beginning of an outbreak time, varying infectivity is often important to take into consideration.

7.3.3 Prior immunity

In the model defined in Section 7.2, it was assumed that initially all individuals were susceptible to the disease except for one or a few index cases. In empirical settings, there is often some natural immunity in the community due to prior history to the disease (see Section 7.5 for immunity due to preventive vaccination).

Suppose as a simple illustration that a fraction s in the community are fully susceptible and the remaining fraction $1 - s$ are completely immune. If the disease is then introduced by a few index cases, then the reproduction number is reduced from R_0 to $R_E = R_0 s$ since, early on in the outbreak, only a fraction s of all contacts will result in infection. An outbreak then is possible only if the effective reproduction number $R_E > 1$. We hence see that an outbreak is only possible if $s > 1/R_0$. How many will get infected in case of an outbreak (as well as the probability for a major outbreak) can be derived analogously to the case without natural immunity. The result is that the fraction of the initially susceptible that ultimately get infected, $r_s(\infty)$, is the solution to the new final-size equation

$$1 - r_s(\infty) = e^{-R_0 s r_s(\infty)}. \tag{7.5}$$

The overall fraction that get infected $r_{overall}$ is hence $r_{overall} = sr_s(\infty)$. As a numerical illustration, suppose $R_0 = 3$ and $s = 50$ percent, so only half of the community are susceptible. Then $r_s(\infty) = 0.583$ so the overall fraction getting infected will be about 29–30 percent. Compare this with the situation where there is no prior immunity (so $s = 100$ percent) when we saw earlier that 98 percent get infected! These differences are also very important when making inference as we shall see later: neglecting prior immunity when estimating R_0 can lead to dramatic *underestimation* of R_0!

7.4   Statistical Inference

In the previous sections we introduced some basic epidemic models and discussed some extensions towards more realistic models. What follows now, which is the main focus of this handbook, concerns how to make inference about model parameters after having observed an outbreak taking place.

Stochastic epidemic modeling is concerned with deriving likely outcomes given some parameter set-up. Epidemic inference goes in the opposite direction: which parameters are best in agreement with an observed outcome? This perspective should explain why knowing some results from stochastic epidemic modeling helps when making inference.

How to make inference depends on two things: what model is considered and what type of data that is available for making inference. In the current section our emphasis is the standard stochastic epidemic model, but we discuss two different types of data: the final size, when we observe how many that were infected at the end of the outbreak, and the situation where we also have some temporal information. We start with the former situation.

7.4.1   Inference based on final size

Consider a community of size n and suppose that prior to the outbreak the fraction s were susceptible to the disease and the rest were immune to the disease. After the outbreak has taken place, we observe that a fraction $\tilde{r}_s$ of the initally susceptibles were infected during the outbreak. This outcome means that we know the population size n and the initial fraction immune $1 - s$, and our observation is the fraction $\tilde{r}_s$ among the susceptibles who got infected. If our data is the overall fraction infected $\tilde{r}_{overall}$, then we get the observed fraction infected among the initially susceptible by the relation $\tilde{r}_s = \tilde{r}_{overall}/s$.

If we only observe the final size, we cannot estimate any rates or durations, so β and $E(I)$ cannot be estimated separately, only their product $R_0 = \beta E(I)$.

From Equation (7.5), we know that $\tilde{r}_s$ should approximately equal the solution of this equation. A very natural estimator is hence to rewrite (7.5) having R_0 on one side and to estimate R_0 by inserting the observed fraction $\tilde{r}_s$ infected. This gives the following estimator:

$$\hat{R}_0 = \frac{-\ln(1 - \tilde{r}_s)}{s\tilde{r}_s} = \frac{-\ln(1 - \tilde{r}_{overall}/s)}{r_{overall}}. \tag{7.6}$$

As mentioned earlier, it has been shown that the final fraction infected is Gaussian having a mean as defined by (7.5) and with an explicit standard deviation of order $1/\sqrt{n}$. This result together with the so-called δ-method (e.g., [6], Ch 4) can be used to obtain a standard error for the estimate $\hat{R}_0$. The result is

$$s.e.(\hat{R}_0) = \frac{1}{\sqrt{ns}} \sqrt{\frac{1 + c_v^2(1 - \tilde{r}_s)\hat{R}_0^2 s^2}{s^2 \tilde{r}_s(1 - \tilde{r}_s)}}, \tag{7.7}$$

where $c_v := \sqrt{V(I)}/E(I)$ denotes the coefficient of variation of the infectious period. For the Reed-Frost epidemic, $c_v = 0$ and for the Markovian SIR, $c_v = 1$ and most often when estimated c_v lies somewhere inbetween these two values. If unknown, a conservative estimate is hence to set $c_v = 1$. Recall that s is the initial fraction susceptible which is assumed to be known. If there is no natural immunity $s = 1$.

This inference assumes that all infected cases are observed, meaning that there is no underreporting. In reality there is, of course, underreporting in that only some fraction π of all cases are reported. However, if all we observe is the fraction of reported cases among the initially susceptible, $r_s^{(rep)}$, it is impossible to deduce how many unreported cases there were. As a consequence, what fraction π of all cases that are reported has to be inferred in some other way. Having done this, we immediately have an estimated of the true fraction infected among the initially susceptible: $\hat{r}_s = r_s^{(rep)}/\hat{\pi}$. This estimate then can be used in the previous expression to obtain an estimate of R_0. The uncertainty of the estimate increases some, how much depends on the uncertainty of the estimate $\hat{\pi}$ – a standard error can be obtained using the δ-method.

7.4.2 Inference based on temporal data

Quite often there is temporal information available from an outbreak, weekly reported number of cases being the most common. The date at which an infected individual is reported is typically when the individual starts showing symptoms, or rather a few days after when a test is taken at a clinic (and later confirmed as positive). It is not always clear how this time relates to the time of infection and time of recovery, and this will depend on the disease in question. A common way to proceed is to assume that the reporting date approximately equals the recovery date (perhaps the individual receives some treatment reducing infectivity and also the illness usually has the effect of reducing social activity). With such an assumption, and neglecting that the recovery time is often truncated to a week, we hence observe $R(t)$ during some time interval $[t_0, t_1]$, often the start and end of the outbreak. There exist inference procedures for this type of data, here we simplify the situation by assuming that we also observe the infection times of individuals, thus saying that we observe $(S(t), I(t), R(t))$ for $t \in [t_1, t_2]$ together with observing the infectious periods $I_1, \ldots, I_k$ for all individuals who also recover during the period. This data is used for inference in this section. The more likely data, observing times of diagnosis rounded to nearest week, is hence less informative but on the other hand more informative as compared to final-size data considered in the previous section.

The parameters we want to make inference about are $R_0 = \beta E(I)$, and possible also the infectious contact rate β and properties of the infectious period separately. In fact, the main advantage from having temporal information lies in the possibility to infer not only R_0 but also the the other parameters separately, and also to be able to check model fit better.

To estimate R_0 from this temporal data can be done by only using the final-size data and using methods of the previous section. This estimate can be improved slightly by inserting the separate estimates obtained below: $\hat{R}_0 = \hat{\beta}\hat{E}(I)$. For standard errors we refer to [4], Section 7.4.2.

To infer parameters of the infectious period is straightforward, since we have i.i.d. observations $I_1, \ldots, I_k$ of the infectious period. So, for example, we can estimate the mean nonparametrically by $\hat{E}(I) = \bar{I}$, the mean length of the infectious periods.

With regard to the transmission parameter β, it should be clear from Equation (7.1) that a sensible estimator for β is obtained by integrating both sides of the top equation of (7.1), and replacing the deterministic fraction with the corresponding observed fractions:

$$\hat{\beta} = \frac{\bar{S}(0) - \bar{S}(t)}{\int_0^t \bar{S}(u)\bar{I}(u)du}. \tag{7.8}$$

In fact, $\bar{S}(0) - \bar{S}(t) - \int_0^t \beta \bar{S}(u) \bar{I}(u) du$ is a so-called *martingale*, which can be used to show that the estimator $\hat{\beta}$ is consistent and asymptotically normally distributed with an explicit standard error. For details we again refer to [4], Section 7.4.2.

As mentioned previously, another advantage with having temporal data is to check model fit. For example, we could plot the deterministic curves of Equation 7.1 with $\hat{\beta}$ and $1/\bar{I}$ replacing β and γ and compare these curves with the corresponding observed curves ($\bar{S}(t)$, $\bar{I}(t)$, and $\bar{R}(t)$). If there is big discrepancy it could be that some heterogeneity has high influence on the observed epidemic, which hence should be investigated further.

Like always, the problem of underreporting is an issue also here. If it is anticipated that underreporting is substantial, then this should be estimated somehow, preferably using other sources of information (there is ongoing research aiming at estimating the underreporting fraction π using only reported data, e.g., [7], the conclusion seems to be that it is problematic).

7.4.3   Inference from emerging outbreaks

In the previous section, the focus was on observing a complete outbreak while also having some temporal information. As mentioned earlier, a complicating factor with inference for infectious diseases are the strong dependencies between infection events clearly manifested in that the rate of having infectious contact is β, but the rate of infecting new people is $\beta \bar{S}(t)$, since only contacts with susceptibles (which happens with probability $\bar{S}(t)$ at time t) result in infection.

During the early stage of an outbreak, for example, before 1 percent of the population has been infected, this dependence is close to negligible; so with good approximation we can assume that individuals infect new individuals independently (remember that we consider a homogeneously mixing community; when spreading is high within households this does not hold true). When individuals infect new individuals independently the epidemic model behaves like a *branching process*, which we will make use of later. In this section, we consider this type of simpler (but still hard!) situation, a suitable approximation when observing an emerging epidemic outbreak (during which typically the number of recovered individuals $R(t)$ grows exponentially with rate ρ say, cf. Section 7.2.4). In Figure 7.4 the reported number of Ebola cases during the beginning of the 2014–15 outbreak are plotted for each of the three countries separately and together (the latter showing a clear exponentially growing behavior).

Suppose that we observe the number of reported cases $R(t)$, also called the reported incidence, from the start $t = 0$ up until some time $t = t_1$. Using previous notation we hence observe $R(t)$, $0 \le t \le t_1$ during the beginning of an outbreak meaning that the overall fraction infected $\bar{R}(t_1)$ is still small (in Figure 7.4 much less than 1 percent have been infected). Questions of interest are: what is R_0, how fast does the epidemic grow, and how many will eventually get infected (with or without some specified preventive measures put in place)?

We start with the easiest question which concerns the exponential growth rate ρ. Since growth is exponential and the depletion of susceptibles is still negligible, taking logarithms of the incidence and performing regression gives a simple and good estimate of ρ.

The remaining questions, what is R_0 and how many will eventually get infected, let's say without preventive measures, is harder. From observing only the initial growth (e.g., Figure 7.4), it is in fact impossible to say anything more than that $R_0 > 1$ and that a substantial fraction will get infected. This outcome should be clear from the following example. Consider two different diseases, both having $R_0 = 1.5$ (and assuming no prior immunity) but one having average an infectious period of 3 days and the other having an average infectious period of 1 week and lower daily infectivity. Since $R_0 = 1.5$ we know from

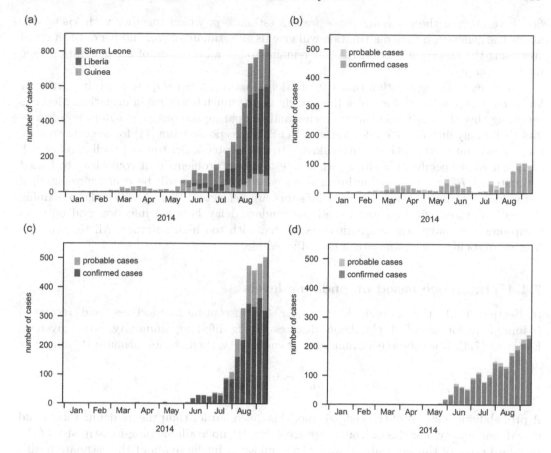

FIGURE 7.4
Reported number of cases during the first 9 months of the Ebola 2014–15 outbreak in West Africa. Data from the patient database as reported by WHO (3 June 2015). (a) West Africa, (b) Guinea, (c) Liberia, and (d) Sierra Leone.

Section 7.2.4 that close to 60 percent will get infected for both diseases. However, from the fact that the first disease has shorter infectious period and hence shorter average generation time, this disease will have a quicker initial growth. So, even though one has quicker growth than the other, they will eventually result in the same final size (approximately, of course).

This example illustrates that some additional information, beside the initial growth rate, is needed in order to infer R_0 and the final fraction getting infected $r(\infty)$. The needed quantity is the so called *generation time distribution* $g(s)$, which quantifies the distribution of the time between getting infected and infecting a new individual (cf. [8] and [9]). Or, equivalently, an individual infects new individuals at average rate $R_0 g(s)$ s time units after infection. For the standard stochastic SIR epidemic $g(s) = P(I > s)/E(I)$ but the generation time distribution can be computed for more realistic models allowing for latent periods and time varying infectivity. Using theory for branching processes (e.g., [10]), it is well-known that, given the generation time distribution $g(s)$, the exponential growth ρ, and the basic reproduction number R_0 are connected to each other through the Lotka equation

$$\int_0^\infty e^{-\rho t} g(t)dt = \frac{1}{R_0},$$

So, if we observe the emerging phase we can estimate ρ, which together with knowledge about the generation time distribution will give us an estimate of R_0, and hence of the final size using the theory of Section 7.2.4. It remains to get an estimate of the generation time distribution $g(\cdot)$.

To estimate the generation time distribution, however, often is quite hard, in particular for an emerging outbreak for which there might not be much historical information. Methods for doing this often rely on contact tracing and comparing the onsets of symptom of cases and their likely infector. We refer to the WHO Ebola response team [11] for a recent treatise on such estimates for the ebola outbreak, and to the chapter 5. Britton and Scalia Tomba [12] highlight some specific difficulties with such estimation problems that could lead to biased estimates of R_0: early in an outbreak short generation times will be over represented, if individuals having multiple potential infectors are neglected, then it will make remaining generation systematically shorter, and the random delay between infection and onset of symptoms can make generation times estimated with too high variance. All three effects lead to R_0 being *underestimated* if not adjusted for.

7.4.4   Inference based on endemic levels

In Section 7.3.1, the endemic levels $(\tilde{s}, \tilde{i}, \tilde{r})$ of susceptibles, infectives, and recovered (=immune), for so-called childhood diseases giving life-long immunity, were given in Equation (7.4). If we observe a community at endemicity, then we can estimate R_0 simply by

$$\hat{R}_0^{(endemic)} = \frac{1}{\tilde{s}}.$$

A probabilistic analysis of the endemic model is much harder than the model in a fixed and closed community. For this reason, there are currently no available plug-in estimates of the standard error of this estimate. However, we can say a bit more about the estimate itself.

At first it might not seem that easy to observe $\tilde{s}$, the fraction susceptible at endemicity. But, since we are considering diseases giving life-long immunity, the length of the susceptible life-period of an individual is identical to the age at which the individual gets infected. Since we are considering a community at equilibrium the fraction of individuals being susceptible will, therefore, equal the average relative part of a life an individual is susceptible, and this is simply the average age of infection a divided by the average life-length ℓ: $\tilde{s} = a/\ell$. Both these numbers are easily obtained: the former from the medical authorities and the latter from national statistics data.

As an illustration, suppose the average life length equals 75 years, and the typical age of infection of some disease not currently vaccinated for, is 5 years, then $\tilde{s} = 5/75 = 1/15$, which hence implies that $\hat{R}_0 = 15$.

7.4.5   Inference for extended models

In Section 7.3.2, several extensions of the standard stochastic SIR epidemics were discussed, bringing in realism in terms of various sorts of heterogeneities. These were, for example, to acknowledge that individuals are of different types, having different susceptibilities and infectivities between different types, for example, due to age, gender, and/or prior history to the disease; models which often are referred to as multitype epidemic models. Another heterogeneity lies in how people mix with each other; if, for example, considering influenza, including household structure into the model makes sense, whereas if considering sexually transmitted infections (STIs), a network mimicking the network of sex-contacts is more relevant. Finally, there might be heterogeneity in infectivity over time, either calendar time because of seasonal differences and/or time since infection where infectivity may first increase, then peak, followed by a slow decay down to 0.

To make inference in such more complicated situations, including also other aspects, is what most of the forthcoming chapters are dealing with. We hence refer to later sections for such statistical analyses except giving a few qualitative statements.

If observing the final outcome of a multitype epidemic the fraction infected in each type is observed, and it is assumed that the community fraction of the different types are known. If there are k types of individuals, then the data vector is hence k-dimensional. However, the number of parameters is greater than k, whether assuming a completely general contact matrix between different types (having dimesion k^2) or assuming separable mixing where the contact rate between two types is the infectivity of the infective type multiplied by the susceptibility of the receiving type (dimension $2k$). As a consequence, it is not possible to estimate all model parameters consistently, and what is worse, it is not even possible to estimate R_0 consistently. A solution might be to include information about the actual contact behavior, see Chapter 6. Without such additional knowledge, all that is possible to do is to give a range of possible values of R_0 (cf. [13]).

When it comes to household models, it is possible to estimate the transmission rates both within and between households whether observing temporal or final-size data. Intuitively, the more cases are clustered in certain households, the more spreading there is within households. From these estimates, it is possible to estimate R_0, or rather another threshold parameter R_* called the household reproduction number (cf. [14]).

Network epidemic models, and inference for such, have received much attention in the literature during the last two decades. From an inference point of view, the statistical methodology differs whether the network is observed globally, locally, or not at all, beside observing infected individuals. If the complete network is observed, then inference is quite straightforward: susceptible individuals are exposed by infectious neighbors, and by observing when infection takes place and how long infectious periods last it is possible to infer disease model parameters. If the network is only observed locally, e.g., the number of neighbors of infected individuals or the more common situation that the underlying network is not observed at all, then except possibly some summary statistics such as mean degree and/or clustering, then inference becomes much harder. Individuals who get infected are usually unrepresentative in having many neighbors thus exposing themselves to higher risk of transmission, and it is not observed which are the underlying links responsible for infection, making estimation of R_0 impossible without additional assumptions.

The final type of heterogeneity regards variation in either calendar time or time since infection. Varying infectivity due to calendar time often is referred to as seasonality and is usually modelled by a sinusoidal curve. It is possible to include such a function and to estimate parameters using, e.g., reported incidence over the year. As for the infectivity function as a function of time since infection, denoted the generation time distribution, often is estimated from contact tracing (see, e.g., [11]). But as mentioned in Section 7.4.3, this often is associated with potential risk for biases.

7.5   Introducing Prevention: Modeling and Inference

One of the main reasons for modeling and making inference for epidemics is to better understand them, and in particular to understand what preventive measures are needed to reduce or preferably completely stop an outbreak. In this section, we focus on the preventive measures which make susceptible individual no longer at risk of infection. This outcome can be acheived in different ways depending on the application: an individual may get vaccinated, isolated, or for STIs stop being sexually active or only having safe sex. In what follows we use the term *vaccination* but bear in mind that this may have alternative meanings.

Suppose that a fraction v of the community is vaccinated prior to the arrival of the outbreak, or, in the endemic setting, suppose that a fraction v of all new-born individuals are vaccinated. Further, assume that the vaccine gives 100 percent protection (there also exist model extensions allowing for partial *vaccine efficacy*). The basic reproduction number is then reduced to $R_v = R_0(1 - v)$, since only the fraction $1 - v$ of the infectious contacts are with non-vaccinated individuals. As a consequence, there will be no outbreak (or the disease will vanish in the endemic setting) if $R_v \leq 1$. But this is equivalent to $v \geq 1 - 1/R_0$. The value giving exact equality is known as the critical vaccination coverage and denoted $v_C = 1 - 1/R_0$, a very important quantity when aiming at preventing an outbreak or making an endemic disease disappear.

Because we have estimates of R_0 from final-size data, an estimate of v_C for the same data is immediate:

$$\hat{v}_C = 1 - \frac{1}{\hat{R}_0} = 1 - \frac{s\tilde{r}_s}{-\ln(1 - \tilde{r}_s)}. \qquad (7.9)$$

Recall that s denotes the initial fraction susceptible in the community in which the outbreak took place, and $\tilde{r}_s$ the observed fraction infected among the initially susceptibles. A standard error for $\hat{v}_C$ can be obtained using similar methods as for $\hat{R}_0$. The result says that

$$s.e.(\hat{v}_C) = \frac{1}{\sqrt{ns}} \sqrt{\frac{1 + c_v^2(1 - \tilde{r}_s)\hat{R}_0^2 s^2}{\hat{R}_0^4 s^2 \tilde{r}_s(1 - \tilde{r}_s)}}, \qquad (7.10)$$

where as before, c_v denotes the coefficient of variation of the infectious period, which can be conservatively estimated to 1 if unknown.

For endemic diseases having a fraction $\tilde{s}$ susceptible, the corresponding estimate of v_C equals

$$\hat{v}_C^{(endemic)} = 1 - \tilde{s}.$$

To obtain a standerd error for this estimate remains an open problem, but the standard error should be of order $1/\sqrt{n}$.

7.6   Discussion

Reality often is complicated, and more realistic models having more complicated inference procedures are many times to be preferred as compared to the simple models discussed in this chapter. However, a recommendation is to complement such analyses with the simpler methods of this chapter. If the estimates from the simpler methods are close to the ones in the more complicated models, this is reassuring, and if not, then it is worth spending some time to understand why this is not the case.

We again stress the importance of acknowledging that not all infected individuals are usually reported, often due to no or minor symptoms (asymptomatic infections).

In this chapter, we did not consider estimation of vaccine efficacy, usually inferred in a clinical trial in which certain individuals are vaccinated and others not. In fact there are several different vaccine efficacies: in terms of susceptibility, symptoms, infectivity if infected, and others. This rather complicated inference problem is investigated in detail in [15] and Chapter 8.

One heterogeneous feature that was not considered in this chapter was spatial aspects, where most likely, the risk of transmitting decreases with the distance between the steady locations of the two individuals (particularly relevant in wildlife and plant populations).

We end by giving a general rule of thumb: various heterogeneities play a bigger role the less transmittable the disease is, so homogeneous mixing models often work satisfactorily for measles and similar childhood diseases, but various heterogeneities need to be included when analyzing, e.g., STI outbreaks.

References

[1] T. Britton. Stochastic epidemic models: A survey. *Math. Biosci.*, 225:24–35, 2010.

[2] T. Britton and F. Giardina. Introduction to statistical inference for infectious diseases. *J. Soc. Franc. Stat.*, 157:53–70, 2016.

[3] N. G. Becker. *Modeling to Inform Infectious Disease Control.* Chapman and Hall/CRC, Boca Raton, FL, 2015.

[4] O. Diekmann, H. Heesterbeek, and T. Britton. *Mathematical Tools for Understanding Infectious Disease Dynamics.* Princeton University Press, Princeton, NJ, 2013.

[5] M. E. J. Newman. The structure and function of complex networks. *SIAM Rev.*, 45(2):167–256 (electronic), 2003.

[6] J. A. Rice. *Mathematical Statistics and Data Analysis.* Brooks/Cole, Pacific Grove, CA, 2006.

[7] G. E. Leventhal, H. F. Günthard, S. Bonhoeffer, and T. Stadler. Using an epidemiological model for phylogenetic inference reveals density dependence in HIV transmission. *Mol. Biol. Evol.*, 31(1):6–17, 2014.

[8] J. Wallinga and M. Lipsitch. How generation intervals shape the relationship between growth rates and reproductive numbers. *Proc. R. Soc. B*, 274(1609):599–604, 2007.

[9] Å Svensson. A note on generation times in epidemic models. *Math. Biosci.*, 208: 300–311, 2007.

[10] P. Jagers. *Branching Processes with Biological Applications.* John Wiley & Sons, New York, 1975.

[11] WHO Ebola Response Team. Ebola virus disease in West Africa–The first 9 months of the epidemic and forward projections. *N. Engl. J. Med.*, 371:1481–1495, 2014.

[12] T. Britton and G Scalia Tomba. Estimation in emerging epidemics: Biases and remedies. *J. Royal Soc. Interface*, 16(150):20180670, 2019. doi:10.1098/rsif.2018.0670.

[13] T. Britton. Estimation in multitype epidemics. *J. Roy. Statist. Soc. B*, 60:663–679, 1998.

[14] F. Ball, D. Mollison, and G. Scalia-Tomba. Epidemics with two levels of mixing. *Ann. Appl. Probab.*, 7:46–89, 1997.

[15] M. E. Halloran, I. M. Longini, and C. J. Struchiner. *Design and Analysis of Vaccine Studies.* Springer, New York, 2010.

8

Analysis of Vaccine Studies and Causal Inference

M. Elizabeth Halloran

CONTENTS

8.1   Introduction

8.1.1   Background

The analysis of vaccine studies enjoys a long history. In 1915, Greenwood and Yule (1915) published an 85-page treatise on "The Statistics of Anti-typhoid and Anti-cholera Inoculations, and the Interpretation of such Statistics in general." In the days before randomization, they stated three conditions for valid inference when estimating protective effects of vaccination (inoculation). "1. The persons must be, *in all material respects*, alike. 2. The effective exposure to the disease must be identical in the case of inoculated and uninoculated persons. 3. The criteria of the fact of inoculation and of the fact of the disease having occurred must be independent." Since the advent of randomized trials, randomization is supposed to ensure the validity of the comparison groups. Greenwood and Yule also discussed heterogeneity in susceptibility and protection and the role of a possible immune threshold level for protection, issues that are still discussed today.

Historically, the focus was on estimating the protective effects of vaccines in vaccinated individuals. In 1916, Sir Ronald Ross (1916) published his general treatise on the Theory of Happenings. He separated different kinds of happenings into two classes, namely "(a) those in which the frequency of the happening is *independent* of the number already affected; and (b) those in which the frequency of the happening depends on this quantity." Infectious diseases belong to the latter. Due to dependent happenings, in infectious diseases, interventions, including vaccination, can have several kinds of effects in populations, not just protective effects in individuals, which require different study designs and methods of analysis for their evaluation.

Halloran and Struchiner (1991, 1995) defined study designs for dependent happenings that allow evaluation of the direct, indirect, total, and overall effects of vaccination, and other infectious disease interventions (Figure 8.1). Consider two clusters, or populations, of individuals. In one of the populations, a certain portion of individuals is vaccinated and the rest remain unvaccinated. In the other population, no one is vaccinated. The *direct effect* of vaccination in the population in which some individuals were vaccinated is defined by comparing the average outcomes in vaccinated individuals with the average outcomes in unvaccinated individuals. The *indirect effects*, also known as *spillover effects*, are defined as a contrast between the average outcomes in unvaccinated individuals in the population

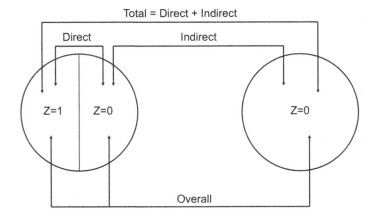

FIGURE 8.1
Study designs for dependent happenings. Two clusters, or populations, are considered under two different scenarios. In the scenario on the left, a certain portion of individuals in the cluster receive vaccination (or other treatment), $Z = 1$, and the other portion of individuals receive control, $Z = 0$. In the scenario on the right, everyone receives control. Control could be current best practice, a placebo, or nothing. The direct, indirect, total, and overall effects of intervention are defined by the indicated contrasts. The figure makes no reference to an assignment mechanism, comparability of possible subgroups within the populations, or inference about the different effects. (Adapted from Halloran, M.E. and Struchiner, C.J. *Epidemiology*, 2, 331–338, 1991; Halloran, M.E. and Struchiner, C.J. *Epidemiology*, 6, 142–151, 1995.)

with vaccination and the average outcomes of unvaccinated individuals in the unvaccinated population. The *total effects* are defined by comparing the average outcomes in the vaccinated individuals in the vaccinated population to the average outcomes in the unvaccinated individuals in the unvaccinated population. The *overall effects* are defined by the contrast in the average outcomes in the entire population where some individuals were vaccinated compared to the average outcomes of the entire population that did not receive vaccine.

8.1.2 Causal inference

In recent decades, causal inference methods have been developed for evaluating some effects of vaccination. Causal inference based on potential outcomes (Rubin, 1980, 1986; Holland, 1986) is a principled framework for carefully defining the causal effects of interventions. A potential outcome is defined as the outcome an individual would have if the individual were to receive a particular intervention. The potential outcomes are generally assumed fixed prior to an individual actually receiving treatment. That is why they are called potential, or counterfactual, outcomes. A common assumption in causal inference is that the treatment assignment in one individual does not affect the potential outcomes in another individual, called the assumption of no interference (Cox, 1958). The Stable Unit Treatment Value Assumption (SUTVA) contains the assumption of no interference, as well as the assumption that all treatments and their potential outcomes are represented (Rubin, 1980). Assuming no interference, if there are only two treatments, such as a vaccine and a control, then an individual has only two potential outcomes.

Causal effects can be defined at the individual level as a contrast of potential outcomes under two different interventions. For example, the individual causal effect of treatment compared to a control is the contrast between the individuals's potential outcome under treatment and the individual's potential outcome under control. Generally only one potential outcome can be observed in an individual, so the individual causal effect cannot be observed. The population average causal effect is defined as the contrast of the average of the difference between outcomes if everyone received treatment and if everyone received control. This measure also is not possible to observe.

Drawing inference about treatment effects requires specification of an assignment mechanism of the treatments to individuals or knowledge of how individuals select their treatment. An assignment mechanism where the treatment assigned is independent of the potential outcomes, such as randomization, is a useful assignment. Under the assumption of no interference between individuals and randomization, we can construct an unbiased estimator of the population average causal effect from the contrast of the observed average outcomes in the two treatment groups. The assumption of randomization to specify estimators of the estimands of interest is our point of departure for estimating effects of interest. Observational studies in which vaccine is not assigned randomly may be subject to biases, but can be viewed as departures from randomized experiments.

Obviously, in interventions for infectious diseases, such as vaccination, the intervention assignment of one individual might affect the potential outcomes of another individual. For example, if an individual is vaccinated, the individual may not become infected or be less infectious if infected, and then not infect another individual that he or she would have infected had he or she not been vaccinated. Thus, the assumption of no interference may be violated, which we consider further herein.

Causal inference methods assuming no interference are useful in understanding vaccine effects on post-infection outcomes (Section 8.2.6) and evaluating surrogates of vaccine-induced protection (Section 8.4). Causal inference where interference may be present is useful in defining estimands and estimators of different population-level effects of vaccination as in Figure 8.1 (Section 8.3.2). Section 8.3.3.1 presents a case study of evaluating and interpreting such estimates. Evaluating the effects of vaccination on infectiousness requires a combination of causal methods (Section 8.2.7).

8.1.3 Focus of this chapter

In this chapter, the focus is on evaluating prophylactic vaccines in populations. However, many of the principles outlined in this chapter could apply to other infectious disease interventions, either prophylactic or treatment, or pharmaceutical or behavioral, or combinations of interventions. The book *Design and Analysis of Vaccine Studies* by Halloran et al. (2010) covers some of the material presented here in much more detail. The book *Cluster Randomised Trials* by Hayes and Moulton (2017, second edition) is an excellent resource for the practical design and analysis of cluster randomized studies, particularly in the infectious disease context. In this chapter, we present some key ideas and recent topics in vaccine studies and causal inference for evaluating vaccination.

8.2 Estimating Different Effects of Vaccination

We present a framework showing the relation among many of the different vaccination effects and the study designs to estimate them. Commonly, vaccine efficacy and effectiveness (VE) are estimated as 1 minus some measure of relative risk, RR:

$$VE = 1 - RR.$$

However, vaccine effects also can be measured on the risk difference scale, the odds ratio scale, and relative risk scale. The vaccine effect of interest determines the choice of comparison groups, the unit of observation, the choice of parameter, and the amount of information about the transmission system required for estimation. The framework draws on the dependent happening relation in infectious diseases. Table 8.1 list several different vaccine effects. Table 8.2 provides a framework for understanding how many of the effects and estimators of different vaccine effects relate to one another.

TABLE 8.1

Some vaccine effects of interest

Symbol	Definition
VE_S	Vaccine efficacy for susceptibility
VE_{SP}	Vaccine efficacy for susceptibility to disease
VE_{col}, VE_{acq}	Vaccine efficacy for colonization (acquisition)
VE_P	Vaccine efficacy for progression or pathogenicity
VE_I	Vaccine efficacy for infectiousness
VE_T	Total vaccine efficacy
$VE_{Indirect}$	Indirect effects of vaccination in those not vaccinated
VE_{Total}	Total effects of vaccination in those vaccinated
$VE_{Overall}$	Overall population-level effects

8.2.1 Protective effects of vaccination, VE$_S$, VE$_{SP}$

VE$_S$, the vaccine efficacy for susceptibility, is a measure of how protective vaccination is against infection. VE$_{SP}$ denotes vaccine efficacy against disease. With most infectious agents, the major interest has been in preventing clinical illness. In studies of vaccines against such infectious agents, including measles, influenza, dengue, and pertussis, ascertainment of the outcome of interest is often on individuals who have symptomatic disease, who then might have a laboratory test done to confirm the infectious agent under study. In this scenario, asymptomatic infections would not be ascertained.

VE$_P$, vaccine efficacy for progression or pathogenicity, measures the efficacy of vaccination in preventing a post-infection outcome. Depending on the situation, the measure of interest can be the effect of prophylactic vaccination on the rate or probability of progressing to disease, conditional on being infected. If ascertainment is on disease, VE$_P$ could be a measure of the effect of vaccination on the probability of severe disease. Although VE$_S$, VE$_{SP}$, and VE$_P$ are all measures of the direct protective effects of vaccination, there is an important difference. Studies to estimate VE$_S$ and VE$_{SP}$ are based on an outcome in participants who are susceptible to infection, whereas studies to estimate VE$_P$ are based on an outcome in participants who are already infected. The denominators in the two different types of studies are different. In randomized studies, as long as the outcome is the first outcome of interest after randomization, whether infection, VE$_S$, or disease, VE$_{SP}$, the validity of the comparison is preserved. This result is not necessarily true with VE$_P$ (Section 8.2.6).

We first consider study designs for estimating the protective effects of vaccination, VE$_S$ (VE$_{SP}$). In the following, we use VE$_S$ to denote both VE$_S$ and VE$_{SP}$, that is, it could be ascertainment on infection or disease, unless there is a need to differentiate the two. In Table 8.2, these are represented in the column labeled "Susceptibility." The estimates of VE$_S$ are obtained from the relative risk of infection or disease in the vaccinated individuals compared to the unvaccinated individuals:

$$\text{VE}_S = 1 - \frac{R(\text{vaccinated people})}{R(\text{unvaccinated people})},$$

where R denotes one of the measures of risk. The measure of risk can be a form of the transmission probability, which conditions on exposure to infection, or the incidence rate, hazard rate, or cumulative incidence (attack rate), which do not condition on exposure to infection. In Table 8.2, the amount of information about the transmission system required for the efficacy estimates decreases from Level I in the top row to Level IV in the bottom row.

The top row of Table 8.2 contains measures of VE that rely on information about exposure to infection and contacts between infectious individuals and susceptible individuals. The first is a measure of VE$_S$ based on the transmission probability, VE$_{S,p}$. Let the *transmission probability*, denoted p_{ij}, be the probability that, conditional upon a contact between an infective source with covariate status i and a susceptible host with covariate status j, successful transfer and establishment of the infectious agent will occur. A related concept is the *secondary attack rate* (SAR$_{ij}$), defined as the proportion of susceptible individuals with covariate status j making contact with an infectious person of covariate status i that becomes infected. The SAR is a special case of the transmission probability.

Let 0 and 1 denote being unvaccinated and vaccinated. Then, for example, p_{01} denotes the transmission probability per contact from an unvaccinated infective person to a vaccinated uninfected person. Let $p_{.0}$ and $p_{.1}$ denote the transmission probability to unvaccinated and vaccinated susceptible individuals, where the dot in the subscript can denote any vaccine status or an average across the population.

TABLE 8.2

Parameters used for measuring various effects of vaccination. The levels form a hierarchy, with higher levels requiring less information about the transmission system, with only level I requiring actual contact information[a]

	Parameter	Comparison Groups and Effect		
		Susceptibility	Infectiousness	Combined Change in Susceptibility and Infectiousness
Level	**Choice**			
I	Conditional on exposure to infection: Transmission probability, p; Secondary attack rate, SAR	$VE_{S,p}^b = 1 - \frac{p_{.0}}{p_{.1}}$	$VE_{I,p} = 1 - \frac{p_{1.}}{p_{0.}}$	$VE_{T,p} = 1 - \frac{p_{11}}{p_{00}}$

		Study Design			
		Direct	Indirect	Total	Overall
II	Unconditional: Incidence rate, IR; Hazard rate, λ	$VE_{S,IR} = 1 - \frac{IR_{A1}}{IR_{A0}}$ $VE_{S,\lambda} = 1 - \frac{\lambda_{A1}}{\lambda_{A0}}$	$VE_{Indirect,IR} = 1 - \frac{IR_{A0}}{IR_{B0}}$ $VE_{Indirect,\lambda} = 1 - \frac{\lambda_{A0}}{\lambda_{B0}}$	$VE_{Total,IR} = 1 - \frac{IR_{A1}}{IR_{B0}}$ $VE_{Total,\lambda} = 1 - \frac{\lambda_{A1}}{\lambda_{B0}}$	$VE_{Overall,IR} = 1 - \frac{IR_{A.}}{IR_{B.}}$ $VE_{Overall,\lambda} = 1 - \frac{\lambda_{A.}}{\lambda_{B.}}$
III	Proportional hazards, PH	$VE_{S,PH} = 1 - e^{\beta_1}$	$VE_{Indirect,PH} = 1 - e^{\beta_{ind}}$	$VE_{Total,PH} = 1 - e^{\beta_{tot}}$	$VE_{Overall,PH} = 1 - e^{\beta_{over}}$
IV	Cumulative incidence, CI; Attack rates, AR	$VE_{S,CI} = 1 - \frac{CI_{A1}}{CI_{A0}}$	$VE_{Indirect,CI} = 1 - \frac{CI_{A0}}{CI_{B0}}$	$VE_{Total,CI} = 1 - \frac{CI_{A1}}{CI_{B0}}$	$VE_{Overall,CI} = 1 - \frac{CI_{A.}}{CI_{B.}}$

[a] Adapted from Halloran et al. (1997). The subscripts 0 and 1 denote unvaccinated and vaccinated people, respectively. Population A contains both vaccinated and unvaccinated people. All people in population B are unvaccinated (Figure 8.1, left = A, right = B). The subscripts S, I, and T denote susceptibility, infectiousness, and combined effects. The Cox proportional hazards estimator is denoted by e^β with the corresponding subscript. Time has been omitted from the table for notational clarity.

[b] Vaccine efficacy/effectiveness

Then $VE_{S,p}$ based on the transmission probability(or secondary attack rate) (Table 8.2, top row) is estimated from

$$VE_{S,p} = 1 - \frac{p_{.1}}{p_{.0}} = 1 - \frac{\frac{\text{vaccinated infections}}{\text{vaccinated contacts}}}{\frac{\text{unvaccinated infections}}{\text{unvaccinated contacts}}} \qquad (8.1)$$

Estimating vaccine efficacy from the transmission probability ratios requires information on who is infectious and when, and whom they contact and how. The concept of a *contact* is very broad and must be defined in each particular study. Often it is defined for individuals within a small transmission unit such as a household or sexual partnership. Analysis of such studies can either assume that the transmission units are independent, such as in the conventional SAR analysis, or that the transmission units are embedded in a community where individuals are exposed to infection within and outside the transmission unit. The latter can be based on final value data or longitudinal data. These topics are handled elsewhere in this book and not considered further here. In the top row of Table 8.2, the vaccine efficacy for infectiousness, $VE_{I,p}$, is the relative reduction in the transmission probability from a vaccinated infected person to a susceptible person compared to the transmission probability from an unvaccinated infected person to a susceptible person. The $VE_{T,p}$ is the relative reduction in the transmission probability if both the infected person and the susceptible person in a contact are vaccinated compared to if both the infected person and the susceptible person in a contact are unvaccinated. VE_I and VE_T are discussed in Section 8.2.7.

Standard parameters for estimating VE_S that do not require exposure to infection information are incidence rates, hazard rates, or cumulative incidence (attack rate). Statistical analysis for estimates of these can be done using standard software, such as the R statistical programming system (R Core Team 2018). Primary vaccine efficacy studies often report $VE_{S,IR}$ based on the relative number of events per person-time,

$$VE_{S,IR} = 1 - \frac{\text{vaccinated events/person-time}}{\text{unvaccinated events/person-time}}. \qquad (8.2)$$

The usual assumption is that the numbers of events follow a Poisson distribution. Similarly, investigators may estimate the hazard rates at time t in the vaccinated and unvaccinated, $\lambda_1(t)$ and $\lambda_0(t)$, using survival analysis methods. Then the VE_S is based on the hazard rate ratio

$$VE_{S,\lambda}(t) = 1 - \frac{\lambda_1(t)}{\lambda_0(t)}. \qquad (8.3)$$

When covariates such as age and gender are added, the analyses are stratified by the covariates or Poisson regression can be used. Under the assumption that the vaccine effect is multiplicative, constant, and homogeneous, the Cox proportional hazards model can be used to estimate $VE_{S,PH}$. In this case, it is not necessary to estimate the hazard rate in the unvaccinated group, but only the relative hazard rate. This situation requires only the ordering of the infection times. Covariates, including time-dependent covariates, can easily be incorporated using standard software, such as the `survival` package in R (Therneau, 2015).

$VE_{S,CI}(T)$ based on the cumulative incidence uses only information about whether persons are infected by the end of the study at time T, that is, final value data:

$$VE_{S,CI}(T) = 1 - \frac{\text{vaccinated infection events/persons--at--risk}}{\text{unvaccinated infection events/persons--at--risk}}$$

$$= 1 - \frac{CI_1(T)}{CI_0(T)}. \qquad (8.4)$$

Using the simple $VE_{S,CI}(T)$ in Equation (8.4) assumes there is no loss to follow-up. However, we also can estimate the cumulative incidence from time-to-event data that allows for censoring. This method may be preferable to using the Poisson model in Equation (8.2) or the Cox regression model because those are both based on parametric assumptions that may fail. Vaccine efficacy at time t based on the cumulative incidence function is

$$VE_{S,CI}(t) = 1 - \frac{CI_1(t)}{CI_0(t)} . \tag{8.5}$$

The estimated vaccine efficacy with simultaneous confidence bands can be plotted as a function of time to visualize the behavior of vaccine efficacy over time.

Neafsey et al. (2015) presented estimates of vaccine efficacy using both 1 minus the ratio (vaccine vs. control) of cumulative incidences and 1 minus the ratio (vaccine vs. control) of hazards, the latter under the assumption that the hazards are proportional over time. The context was to estimate the efficacy of the RTS,S/AS01 malaria vaccine according to genetic diversity of the parasite. The estimates of vaccine efficacy based on the two methods differ significantly in several of the analyses.

If there is no adjustment for covariates, the cumulative incidence function can be estimated by the nonparametric likelihood estimator (Aalen, 1978), implemented in the R `cmprsk` package, based on the Kaplan-Meier estimate of the survival function and the Nelson-Aalen estimates of the cumulative hazard functions. Adjusted analyses that include covariates to estimate the cumulative incidence functions can use targeted maximum likelihood estimation that leverages information in covariates to improve efficiency (Benkeser et al. 2018).

8.2.2 Hierarchy of VE_S parameters

The different VE_S parameters require different levels of information for their estimation and make different demands on study design and data collection (Rhodes et al., 1996) [65]. Levels I through IV in Table 8.2 form a hierarchy, with higher levels requiring less information about the transmission system, and only Level I requiring contact and exposure to infection information. Because of the dependent happening structure of events in infectious diseases, an intrinsic relation exists among the different parameters on which the VE_S estimators are based.

Let p_{ij} be the transmission probability as previously defined. Let c denote the contact rate in a population assuming that people are randomly mixing, and let $P(t)$ denote the prevalence of infectives at time t. Then the hazard rate $\lambda(t)$ (or incidence rate or force of infection) at time t can be expressed as the product of the contact rate, the transmission probability, and the probability that a contact is infectious:

$$\lambda(t) = c p_{ij} P(t). \tag{8.6}$$

So even if the different components of the hazard rate are not measured, we can consider the underlying process that is producing the infections we observe. Similarly, the cumulative incidence, $CI(T)$, at some time T is a function of the hazard rate during the follow-up period, and thus also a function of the transmission probability, contact rate, and prevalence of infection in the contacts.

8.2.3 Vaccine efficacy for colonization and acquisition

Many infectious agents, such as *Streptococcus pneumoniae* (pneumococcus), meningococcus, and *Hemophilus influenzae b* bacteria, colonize the nose and throat passages without causing overt disease. The state of being colonized is also called nasopharyngeal carriage. Colonized individuals generally are asymptomatic, but they play a central role in transmission. They can transmit to other susceptible individuals who in their turn may develop severe disease after being colonized. Individuals can clear the bacteria and then be re-colonized repeatedly. Pneumococcus has over 90 strains. A common pneumococcus vaccine contains antigens to 13 strains, although one is available with even more. VE_{col} measures the efficacy against colonization (Auranen et al., 2000, Käyhty et al., 2006). In particular, the rate of acquisition of pneumococcal carriage also can be used as the outcome measure to estimate vaccine efficacy, VE_{acq} (Rinta-Kokko et al., 2009).

Because carriage is asymptomatic, studies need to do active swabbing of individuals to determine if they are colonized or not. These studies are generally longitudinal, expensive, and invasive, thus interest has developed to estimate VE_{acq} from just one observation of current status data. Auranen et al. (2013) present two examples of vaccine studies estimating vaccine efficacy from just cross-sectional data on nasopharyngeal colonization by pneumococcus. They present a framework for defining and estimating strain-specific and overall vaccine efficacy for susceptibility to acquisition of colonization (VE_{acq}) when there is a large number of strains with mutual interactions and recurrent dynamics of colonization, such as in pneumococcus. They develop estimators based on one observation of the current status per study subject, evaluate their robustness, and re-analyze the two vaccine trials.

Mehtälä et al. (2016) consider the problem of estimating heterogeneous vaccine efficacy against an infection that can be acquired multiple times. Estimation is based on a limited number of repeated measurements of the current status of each individual. They investigate how the choice of time intervals between consecutive samples affects the estimability and efficiency of vaccine efficacy parameters. The authors suggest practical guidelines that allow estimation of all components. For situations in which the estimability of individual components fails, they suggest using summary measures of vaccine efficacy.

8.2.4 Modes of action and time-varying VE_S

Smith et al. (1984) pointed out that the choice of method of analysis may depend on the mode of vaccine protection. They defined Type I and Type II modes of action. In the Type I mechanism, vaccination is assumed to reduce the instantaneous disease rate in all the vaccinated people by a constant proportion. That is, Type I has a multiplicative effect on the baseline hazard. In the Type II mechanism, a certain proportion of the vaccinated individuals are completely protected while the other individuals have no protection, and essentially are at risk like the unvaccinated individuals. Struchiner et al. (1990) used the term "leaky" from the malaria vaccinology literature to replace the term Type I and Halloran et al. (1991) used the term "all-or-none" to replace the term Type II. The assumptions about the mechanism of vaccine protection have implications for the choice of efficacy measures. Assuming the vaccine effect does not wane, in general, estimates of VE_{CI} will be time-invariant under the all-or-none (Type II) mechanism, and estimates of VE_{IR} or VE based on the Cox proportional hazards model will be time-invariant under a leaky (Type I) mechanism. Frailty models can be used for analysis if a combination of leaky and all-or-none is suspected (Halloran et al., 1996).

To estimate waning vaccine efficacy, Durham et al. (1998) used a method based on the smoothed scaled Schoenfeld residuals (Grambsch and Therneau, 1994). Cox models can be fitted using the `survival` package (Therneau, 2015) in the R statistical programming system (R Core Team 2018). Plots of the time trends of vaccine efficacy can be made using the R function VEplot in the `kyotil` package (Fong and Sebestyen, 2018).

The approach in Equation (8.5) to estimate and graph $\text{VE}_{S,CI}(t)$ allows us to visually see how vaccine efficacy changes over time, as in Neafsey et al. (2015). However, if the vaccine has a leaky (Type I) mechanism, the estimate of $\text{VE}_{S,CI}(t)$ based on the cumulative incidence function may change over time even though the vaccine efficacy does not wane.

8.2.5   Observational studies

Much has been written on the use of case-control studies in evaluating vaccine efficacy and effectiveness (Struchiner et al., 1990; Rodrigues and Smith, 1999). We do not cover that here. We highlight two recent developments for observational studies, namely, the test negative design and quasi-experimental designs.

8.2.5.1   Test negative design

The test-negative design to estimate VE_S enrolls cases presenting to a medical facility that have symptoms consistent with the disease of interest. Then a laboratory test is performed to confirm whether the case has the disease of interest or not. Those individuals who test positive are considered the cases and those who test negative are the non-cases. Vaccine efficacy is estimated from the odds ratio comparing the odds of testing positive for the disease among vaccinated individuals with the odds among unvaccinated individuals using logistic regression, adjusting for potential confounders. The method is fairly inexpensive if the tests are being performed anyway. The method has been used extensively for estimating the efficacy of influenza vaccines (Jackson and Nelson, 2013) and, more recently, of rotavirus vaccines in low resource settings (see, for example, Bar-Zeev et al., 2015). A core assumption of the method is that the vaccine does not have an effect on the causes of the symptomatic cases who test negative.

One method of examining how well the test negative design performs has been to use randomized, placebo controlled vaccine trials as a gold standard and compare the estimates that a test negative design would have yielded if it had been performed instead (De Serres et al., 2013). For example, Schwartz et al. (2017) derived test-negative vaccine effectiveness estimates from three large randomized placebo controlled trials of rotavirus vaccines in sub-Saharan Africa and Asia. They found that the test-negative design estimates of vaccine efficacy were nearly equivalent to those from the randomized controlled trials.

Although this result is comforting, it is not a true examination of the validity of the approach. The first use of causal inference to examine the theoretical basis of the test-negative study was by Sullivan et al. (2016). The test-negative design is generally considered to control for care-seeking behavior by using only cases that seek medical care, in contrast to case-control studies that use population-based controls (Jackson and Nelson, 2013). It also is assumed to reduce misclassification of cases by requiring laboratory confirmation of the infectious agent of interest. Using directed acyclic graphs, Sullivan et al. (2016) showed how bias may be reduced in some instances, but may be introduced in others. Directed acyclic graphs are one approach to causal inference. Richardson and Robins (2013) provided a detailed analysis of how causal inference with potential outcomes relates to that using directed acyclic graphs and developed a unified theory of single world intervention graphs (SWIGs) that lies outside the scope of this chapter. Westreich and Hudgens (2016) pointed out further that because the test-negative design is limited to those seeking health care, the study may not be generalizable to the population if vaccine efficacy differs by health-care seeking behavior or associated factors. In addition, the odds ratio is not collapsible in that the conditional causal odds ratio will not in general equal the marginal causal odds ratio (Greenland et al., 1999). Thus further research is left to be done on the use and validity of the test-negative design for evaluating vaccines.

8.2.5.2 Quasi-experimental design

An approach as yet underutilized in public health (Bor et al., 2014; Moscoe et al., 2015) is the quasi-experimental design known as the regression discontinuity design (Thistlewaite and Campbell, 1960). In particular, the design might be useful for evaluating vaccines in some situations when randomized studies are not feasible or ethical. The regression discontinuity design allows for causal inference about the effects of interventions when certain conditions hold. The main idea is that an intervention, such as a vaccine, would be administered to a group based on an arbitrary continuous cut-off, such as age. Then we might assume that those just below the cutoff who do not receive vaccine would be comparable to those just above the cutoff who do receive vaccine. The approach has been used widely in economics studies where randomization is often unfeasible. It seems not yet to have been developed in the context of evaluating vaccines. Aronow et al (2016) consider the regression discontinuity design under interference using a local randomization approach, where the causal estimands are related to those presented in Section 8.3.

8.2.6 Vaccine effects on post-infection outcomes, VE$_P$

Sometimes interest is in the effect of a vaccine on an outcome that occurs after an individual is infected. For example, we might be interested in estimating the probability of developing a symptomatic case in vaccinated infected individuals compared to unvaccinated infected individuals. Then VE$_P$ is defined as 1 minus the ratio of a summary measure of the post-infection outcome in the infected vaccinated individuals and a summary measure of the post-infection outcome in the infected unvaccinated individuals:

$$\text{VE}_P = 1 - \frac{\frac{\text{vaccinated post-infection outcome}}{\text{infected vaccinated people}}}{\frac{\text{unvaccinated post-infection outcome}}{\text{infected unvaccinated people}}}. \tag{8.7}$$

Similarly, if a post-clinical outcome in the clinical cases is of interest, then VE$_P$ is defined as 1 minus the ratio of a summary measure of the post-clinical outcome in the vaccinated cases and a summary measure of the post-clinical outcome in the unvaccinated cases:

$$\text{VE}_P = 1 - \frac{\frac{\text{vaccinated post-clinical outcome}}{\text{vaccinated clinical cases}}}{\frac{\text{unvaccinated post-clinical outcome}}{\text{unvaccinated clinical cases}}}. \tag{8.8}$$

For example, we might be interested to estimate if the severity of disease is lower in vaccinated clinical cases than in unvaccinated clinical cases. Use of Equations (8.7) and (8.8) without further adjustment assumes that those who get infected in the vaccinated and unvaccinated groups are comparable.

However, conditioning on an event, such as infection, that occurs subsequent to receipt of vaccine or control, could result in selection bias, even under randomization. Issues related to interpreting malaria vaccine trials motivated Struchiner et al. (1994) to consider the problem of vaccinated and unvaccinated groups not being comparable after being infected even in randomized trials. With the development of human immunodeficiency virus (HIV) vaccine candidates, and HIV vaccine trials in which infection was actively ascertained, concern grew that the infected individuals in the vaccinated group and infected individuals in the unvaccinated group might not be comparable, leading to biased estimates of the effect of vaccination on post-infection outcomes (Hudgens et al., 2003; Gilbert et al., 2003).

For example, assume that the potential immune response to HIV infection has a distribution in the population before individuals are randomized to vaccine or control. Randomization would assure that in large samples, the potential distribution of the immune response to HIV infection before vaccination would be the same in the vaccine and the control groups. However, vaccination might enhance protection only in individuals who have a stronger immune system, conferring some level of protection against infection if exposed. Then the individuals in the vaccinated group who become infected would be the ones with weaker immune systems, whereas the infected individuals in the unvaccinated group would be those with a weaker immune system as well as those with a stronger immune system. In this situation, if a post-infection outcome in the vaccinated group is compared with that in the unvaccinated group, the vaccine could appear to make things worse, even if vaccination has absolutely no effect on anything after infection.

For example, if individuals with a weaker immune system tend to have a higher viral load after being infected than those with a stronger immune system, then the mean viral load in the infected vaccinated group would be higher than the mean viral load in the infected unvaccinated group. This observation could lead to the false conclusion that the vaccine made the post-infection outcome worse, possibly resulting in rejection of a potentially useful vaccine candidate (Hudgens et al., 2003; Gilbert et al., 2003). However, the vaccine in this case actually does not make anything worse. The problem is that the infected vaccinated group and infected control group are no longer comparable because of selection bias.

Frangakis and Rubin (2002) proposed a method in the causal inference with potential outcomes framework to address this problem. The method, called *principal stratification*, adjusts for post-treatment variables by stratifying on the joint potential post-treatment variables under each of the treatments being considered. A principal stratum is composed of individuals with the same joint post-treatment variable. Causal effects are then defined within the principal strata. In fact, in our situation, the causal effect estimand for VE_P is only defined in the principal stratum in which individuals become infected regardless of being assigned to vaccine or control.

A difficulty in using this approach is that which individuals are in which principal stratum is generally not identifiable without further assumptions. Thus, methods have been developed to do sensitivity analyses and to establish bounds on the degree of selection bias that may be present. Several papers have been published using this approach to assess vaccine effects on post-infection outcomes. In studying HIV vaccines, Hudgens et al. (2003) and Gilbert et al. (2003) adopted the principal stratification approach to assess HIV vaccine effects on the continuous post-infection outcome viral load. Hudgens and Halloran (2006) developed methods for the causal vaccine effects on binary post-infection outcomes with applications to pertussis and rotavirus vaccines.

8.2.7 Vaccine efficacy for infectiousness, VE_I

A vaccinated individual who becomes infected might have a lower probability of transmitting to a susceptible individual during a contact than an unvaccinated individual who becomes infected, either because that individual is less infectious or infectious for a shorter period of time. The vaccine efficacy for infectiousness, VE_I, measures the relative reduction in the ability of a vaccinated infected individual compared to an unvaccinated infected individual to transmit the infectious agent to others. Estimating reduction in infectiousness can be of considerable public health interest, particularly with vaccines that do not protect well against infection.

In Table 8.2, VE_I is a measure that conditions on exposure to infection. When based on the transmission probability it can be estimated as

$$VE_{I,p} = 1 - \frac{p_{1\cdot}}{p_{0\cdot}}. \tag{8.9}$$

The $\cdot$ indicates that the individual being exposed is not stratified by vaccine status. For example, in a study in Niakhar, Senegal, Préziosi and Halloran (2003) estimated the relative reduction in infectiousness to household contacts of a vaccinated case of pertussis compared to an unvaccinated case, VE_I to be 67 percent (95% CI 29, 86). The analysis can be stratified by vaccine status of the exposed individual (Préziosi and Halloran, 2003). The combined effect of having both individuals in a contact being vaccinated compared to neither being vaccinated, denoted VE_T in Table 8.2, also can be estimated.

However, just as with VE_P in Section 8.2.6, VE_I compares the transmission probability only in infected vaccinated and infected unvaccinated individuals. These individuals might not be comparable for the same reasons even if the study is randomized, so estimates of VE_I can be subject to post-randomization selection bias (Hudgens and Halloran, 2006). Using the method described in Equation (8.9) without further adjustment assumes no selection bias. The situation is more complicated than with VE_P, because in estimating the transmission probability, the outcome is dependent on the infection status of another exposed individual.

VanderWeele and Tchetgen Tchetgen (2011), and Halloran and Hudgens (2012a) proposed causal quantities corresponding to the infectiousness effect in the simple situation of households of size two. Halloran and Hudgens (2012a) consider the general case that one or both individuals could be exposed outside the household as well as either, neither or both could be randomized to vaccine. The approach combines causal inference with interference (see Section 8.3.2) with principal stratification (Frangakis and Rubin, 2002). The latter accounts for the fact that the comparison in the groups who become infected may be subject to selection bias. The causal infectiousness effect is not identifiable without further assumptions, but bounds on the selection effects can be set (Halloran and Hudgens, 2012a, 2012b). VanderWeele et al. (2014) presented results for sensitivity analyses for causal infectiousness effects. These approaches assume that interference occurs within households but not across households, known as partial interference (Sobel, 2006). More studies need to be designed and conducted to estimate VE_I for the causal approach to find much application.

8.3 Assessing Indirect, Total, and Overall Effects

8.3.1 Cluster randomized studies

Establishing that vaccination provides population-level effects that go beyond the direct effects in the vaccinated, such as those in Figure 8.1, can have important consequences for public health policy. The overall effect of an intervention program often is the quantity of greatest interest for policy makers, as it summarizes the public health consequences of the choice of intervention strategy if adopted in a population. Establishing that vaccination produces indirect effects in the unvaccinated can make a vaccination strategy more cost-effective. Some vaccines, such as transmission-blocking malaria vaccines, have only indirect effects. The expected magnitude of these population-level effects depends not only on the magnitude of the direct effect, but also factors related to the mixing structure of the population, transmission of the disease in the population, and the distribution of the vaccine.

If evaluating population-level effects of interventions, such as the indirect, total, or overall effects, is of interest, then a cluster-randomized study generally will be the design of choice. There are two main different kinds of cluster randomized designs of interest for evaluating vaccines. In a parallel randomized study, clusters are identified before start of the trial, and assigned to either the vaccine of interest or a control, which could be a different vaccine, standard of care, or a placebo. All clusters stay on their assigned intervention until the end of the study. In a stepped wedge design, the order in which clusters receive vaccination is randomized before the trial (Hussey and Hughes, 2007). The clusters where vaccination has not yet been implemented serve as control clusters until the vaccination is implemented. Thus, eventually all of the clusters receive vaccination by the end of the trial. Such trials are sometimes called phased-implementation trials.

During the 2014–2016, Ebola outbreak in West Africa, a novel form of cluster randomized design was implemented (Ebola ca suffit, 2015; Henao-Restrepo et al., 2015). The novel ring vaccination trial of one of the Ebola vaccine candidates compared outcomes in rings of contacts and contacts of contacts around a detected case and randomized each ring to receive either immediate or delayed vaccination, such as in a stepped wedge design. The idea for the ring vaccination trial was motivated by the ring vaccination strategy around cases that led to the eradication of smallpox, but in the Ebola outbreak as part of a trial design. In the context of the public health emergency and declining incidence, the design took the trial to where the transmission was most intense. The estimated vaccine efficacy was 100 percent (95% CI 79.3, 100.0) (Henao-Restrepo et al., 2015). Although the trial reported its results as efficacy, it is more comparable to total efficacy because the vaccination within a cluster could have reduced transmission in that cluster.

Table 8.2 shows that the indirect, total, and overall effects of vaccination can be estimated using incidence rates, hazard rates, Cox proportional hazards models, or cumulative incidence. This table has been modified from earlier versions where the Cox proportional hazards model was not included for indirect, total, and overall effects with the reasoning that the baseline hazard would not be the same in clusters with different levels of coverage. However, in a cluster-randomized study, before vaccination, the expected value the baseline hazards in the clusters receiving vaccine would equal those in the clusters not receiving vaccine. Thus, its use seems potentially valid. Analysis of cluster randomized studies needs to account for clustering using either a cluster-level random effect or a marginal model such as general estimating equations. Hayes and Moulton (2017) give details on designing and analyzing cluster randomized trials, particularly in the context of infectious disease interventions. Because of the complex effects of vaccination, simulations can be useful for designing and planning the analysis of studies (Halloran et al., 2017).

8.3.2   Causal vaccine effects and two-stage randomization

Most of the research on cluster randomized studies has not been done in the context of causal inference. Here we present some of the progress on evaluating the different effects of vaccination in populations using causal inference based on potential outcomes. Using potential outcomes as described in Section 8.1.2 is more complicated under interference because the potential outcomes of an individual can depend on the treatment assignment in others. If there are two treatments and a binary outcome and no interference, each individual has just two potential outcomes, and the individual causal effect is just the difference in the two. However, if there are N individuals that can potentially interfere with an individual, there are 2^N possible potential outcomes. The notation needs to allow that the potential outcomes for any individual depend on the vector of treatment assignments to other individuals with whom they potentially interfere (Rubin, 1978, 1990; Halloran and Struchiner, 1995). Individual causal estimands can be defined by the difference between the potential outcomes that depend on the treatment assignment vectors of those who interfere with that individual. However, this determination can become quite complex. The key is to define an average individual potential outcome that averages over the potential outcomes under all possible treatment assignments in the population for a particular allocation strategy (Sobel, 2006).

In the following, the population is assumed to be partitioned into groups (clusters) where interference can occur within groups but not across groups, known as partial interference

(Sobel, 2006). The goal is to obtain population-level estimates of the direct, indirect, total, and overall effects defined by comparing different treatment allocation strategies or policies. The question might be how does vaccinating 70 percent of the population with a vaccine of interest compare to vaccinating 30 percent. Hudgens and Halloran (2008) defined group- and population-level causal estimands for direct, indirect, total, and overall causal effects of treatment given two different treatment allocations. As demonstrated herein, we can define similar effects with many different levels of coverage. The potential outcomes are averaged over the individual, the group, and finally the population level. The direct effects are defined as the contrast between the population level average potential outcomes if individuals receive vaccine or control under a given strategy. The indirect effects are the contrast in population level potential outcomes if individuals receive control under one strategy and if they receive control under the other strategy. The total effects are the contrast in the population level potential outcomes if individuals receive vaccine under one strategy and if they receive control under the other strategy. The overall effect is the contrast between the marginal population level potential outcomes under one strategy and the marginal population level potential outcomes under the other strategy.

To obtain unbiased estimators of the group- and population-level causal estimands, Hudgens and Halloran (2008) proposed a two-stage randomization scheme, the first stage of randomization is at the group level, the second stage is at the individual level within groups. There are two approaches to randomization. We can randomize a fixed number of groups to each strategy, then within groups, a fixed number of individuals depending on the strategy assigned to that group. Alternatively, we can randomize each group to a strategy with a certain probability, for example with the flip of a biased coin, then similarly randomize each individual within a group to vaccine or control with a certain probability. Tchetgen Tchetgen and VanderWeele (2012) also developed estimators for the four causal estimands assuming a two-staged randomization scheme. Beyond vaccination, the approach is applicable to other situations with interference in groups of individuals where treatment can be assigned to individuals within groups. Baird et al. (2018) considered the two-stage randomized experimental design in the context of economic experiments to measure indirect/spillover effects.

To do inference about the four effects, variance estimators and confidence intervals are needed. Hudgens and Halloran (2008) made an assumption of stratified inference to develop variance estimators. Stratified inference assumes the effects of an intervention depend on what proportion of individuals in a group receive treatment, but not on exactly which ones. This reduces the complexity of the problem considerably. Tchetgen Tchetgen and VanderWeele (2012) also presented confidence limits for the four causal estimands. Liu and Hudgens (2014) derived the asymptotic distributions of estimators of the causal effects and confidence limits when either the number of individuals per group or the number of groups grows large. Some of these confidence intervals in general are narrower than those in Tchetgen Tchetgen and VanderWeele (2012).

8.3.3 Causal vaccine effects and observational studies

8.3.3.1 Inverse probability weighted estimators

Most studies are not randomized at two stages. In fact, we do not know of any vaccine studies to date that have been randomized at two stages. A study could be randomized at the individual level, at the group (cluster) level, or neither. Then the estimators described herein in general would be biased or inconsistent. For the observational setting where the treatment assignment mechanism is not known and there is no interference, propensity scores are one method to adjust the analysis to resemble results that might be obtained from a randomized trial (Rosenbaum and Rubin, 1983). The propensity score is the probability that an individual receives a treatment assignment based on a function of the observed covariates. The propensity score can be used in different ways to adjust for measured confounders, including weighting by the inverse of the propensity score, called inverse probability weighting (IPW), or stratifying on them (Hong and Raudenbush, 2006).

Tchetgen Tchetgen and VanderWeele (2012) proposed IPW estimators of the direct, indirect, total, and overall causal effects in the presence of partial interference based on group-level propensity scores, and proved the estimators are unbiased when the group-level propensity scores are known. The estimators involve estimating mean potential outcomes by taking weighted averages of the observed responses where the weights include the inverse of group-level propensity scores. These IPW estimators can be viewed as a generalization of the usual IPW estimator of the causal effect of a treatment in the absence of interference. These could theoretically be used for studies that randomize at the group (cluster) level only, the individual level only, or neither.

Perez-Heydrich et al. (2014) used these IPW estimators to estimate the different effects of an individually randomized trial of cholera vaccination. They estimated the propensity scores in the presence of interference. They showed that the estimates were consistent and asymptotically normal, and provided variance estimators. This example provides a case study of how the direct, indirect, total, and overall effects of vaccination can be assessed and interpreted. The vaccine trial was conducted in Matlab, Bangladesh, from 1985–88. All children (2–15 yrs old) and women (>15 yrs old) were randomly assigned with equal probability to either of two killed cholera vaccines or a placebo. Although all women and children were randomized, only a subset participated in the trial. Unvaccinated individuals included eligible non-participants and placebo recipients. Vaccinated individuals included recipients of either vaccine. Of the total eligible population ($N = 121{,}982$), 49,300 women and children received two or more doses of vaccine.

The individuals lived in baris, i.e., clustered patrilineal households. Because this was an individually randomized study, neighborhoods (clusters) were defined from geo-referenced data on the baris using a clustering algorithm. In this study the geographic groups (clusters) were formed post-hoc. Thus, the level of vaccine coverage in each cluster was not randomized. The total number of groups was set to 700 for the main analysis. The analysis was based on the difference of the IPW-adjusted average outcomes in the relevant groups.

The IPW estimates of the direct, indirect, total, and overall effects of vaccination are presented in Figure 8.2. The estimates are given in units of cases of cholera per 1,000 individuals per year. The levels of vaccine coverage are denoted by α and α'. The direct effect estimates (Figure 8.2a) generally decrease with increasing α. The estimates vary from 5.3 (95% CI 2.5, 8.1) at coverage level $\alpha = 0.32$ to 0.6 (95% CI $-1.1, 2.3$) at $\alpha = 0.60$. These two inferences would lead to different conclusions about the vaccine. At the higher coverage, the vaccine does not seem to have a significant effect, illustrating the limitations of analyses that consider only direct effects when interference is present.

The indirect effect estimates are in Figure 8.2b. Here the contrast compares the incidence of cholera among unvaccinated individuals at coverage level α compared to unvaccinated individuals at coverage level α'. On the line along the diagonal where $\alpha = \alpha'$, the indirect effects estimates are zero. This result is because on the diagonal the comparison is between incidence at equal coverage. The indirect effect estimates are symmetric about the diagonal, positive on one side and negative on the other. Considering the positive estimates, the indirect effect estimates tend to increase with the difference between the two coverages. The largest estimate of the indirect effect is 5.3 (95% CI 2.6–8.0) between coverage levels 0.60 and 0.32. That is, we would expect 5.3 fewer cases of cholera per 1,000 person-years in unvaccinated individuals within neighborhoods with 60 percent coverage compared to within neighborhoods with 32 percent coverage.

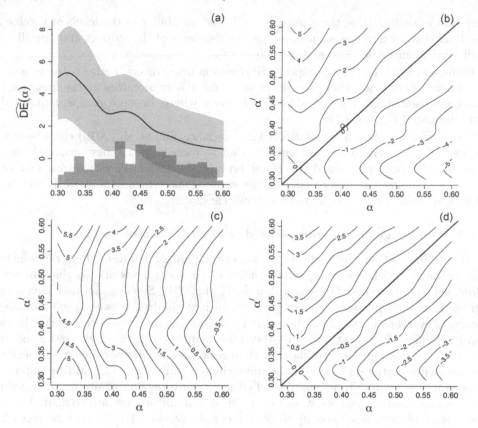

FIGURE 8.2
IPW estimates of (a) direct $\overline{DE}(\alpha)$, (b) indirect $\overline{IE}(\alpha, \alpha')$, (c) total $\overline{TE}(\alpha, \alpha')$, and (d) overall $\overline{OE}(\alpha, \alpha')$ effects based on the cholera vaccine trial data. The estimates are in units of cases per 1,000 individuals per year. In (a) the gray region represents approximate pointwise 95% confidence intervals. The histogram depicts the distribution of observed neighborhood vaccine coverage. (From Perez-Heydrich, C. et al., *Biometrics*, 70, 731–741, 2014.)

The total effect estimates in Figure 8.2c exhibit a different pattern from the indirect estimates. The total effect estimates along the line $\alpha' = \alpha$ equal the direct effects estimates in Figure 8.2a. The total effect contours are roughly vertical, suggesting the estimated risk of cholera when vaccinated tends to be the same regardless of coverage. Of particular interest is the total effect estimate of being vaccinated in a neighborhood with 60 percent coverage compared to being unvaccinated in a neighborhood with coverage 32 percent is 5.9 (95% CI 3.0, 8.8). This result is an order of magnitude greater than the estimated direct effect of 0.6 at 60 percent coverage (Figure 8.2a). Thus, taking the indirect effects into account gives a much different conclusion about the vaccine.

The estimates of overall effects (Figure 8.2d) exhibit a similar pattern to the indirect estimates. They are symmetric about the diagonal.

Details of estimation can be found in Perez-Heydrich et al. (2014). An R package `inference` is available at CRAN that performs these analyses (Saul and Hudgens, 2017). Ali et al. (2005, 2013) found evidence of indirect effects in this cholera vaccine trial using a different, non-causal approach. To be able to estimate the population level effects of vaccination in such studies, there must be sufficient variability in the levels of vaccine coverage. If all clusters have the same coverage, the estimates of the indirect and overall effects will all be 0, as in Figure 8.2b and d where $\alpha' = \alpha$.

Lundin and Karlsson (2014) proposed IPW estimators of direct, indirect, and total causal effects under interference where treatment assignment is randomized at the first stage but not at the second stage. They consider the situation where, in some groups, all individuals remain untreated (Figure 8.1).

IPW estimators often have relatively large variance. Liu et al. (2016) considered other forms of IPW that tend to be less variable, that is, more robust. They proposed unbiased generalized IPW estimators and two Hajek-type (stabilized) IPW estimators. One of the stabilized estimators has substantially smaller variance than the unstabilized IPW estimator proposed by Tchetgen Tchetgen and VanderWeele (2012).

8.3.3.2 One-stage cluster-randomized trial with control vaccine

To estimate indirect and total effects in cluster-randomized studies, where randomization occurs at only the cluster level, some studies use a control vaccine in the clusters not randomized to the vaccine of interest (Moulton et al., 2001). Such studies may have a target subgroup that is eligible to receive the vaccine, such as children between age 6 months and 15 years, or everyone in the population may be the target group. Not everyone in the target group randomized in a cluster to get either vaccine or control will show up, but often the cases are ascertained in the surveillance system regardless of whether they were vaccinated. Thus, estimates of the incidence in the unvaccinated individuals can still be obtained, if vaccine status is known. To estimate total effects, the average outcomes in the individuals in the vaccine clusters who show up to get the vaccine of interest are compared to those in the control clusters who show up to get the control vaccine. To estimate indirect effects, the average outcomes of those who did not get either vaccine are compared. Although these estimates will not necessarily produce the same results as the two-stage randomized design, they produce estimates of total and indirect effects based on populations assumed to be comparable by randomization. Overall effects also can be estimated.

As an example, in a cluster-randomized study of typhoid vaccine in India, Sur et al. (2009) randomized neighborhoods to receive either typhoid vaccine or control (hepatitis A) vaccine. Vaccine effects were estimated by 1 minus the relative incidence of typhoid disease in comparison groups. Total effectiveness in those who had received typhoid vaccine compared to those who had received control (hepatitis A) vaccine was estimated to be 61 percent (95% CI 41, 75). Indirect effectiveness in the unvaccinated individuals in the typhoid vaccine clusters compared to the unvaccinated individuals in the control clusters was 44 percent (95% CI 2, 69). The overall effectiveness in the typhoid clusters compared to the control clusters was 57 percent (95% CI 37, 71). However, incidence of typhoid was higher in the vaccinated individuals than in the unvaccinated individuals in the typhoid vaccine clusters (0.26 versus 0.19 cases per 100,000 person-days), and similarly in the hepatitis A vaccine clusters (0.73 versus 0.35). So if we estimated the direct effect of the typhoid vaccine in this study without any further adjustment, the estimates would be negative. The individuals who showed up to get vaccinated are clearly very different from those who did not show up to get vaccinated, either in their underlying health, health-care seeking behavior, the way they are handled in the health system for diagnosis, or other reason.

More research needs to be done on this design. As illustrated, direct effect estimates are open to extreme bias because the individuals who do not get vaccinated are likely not comparable to those who do get vaccinated, and likely should not be estimated without further consideration. The interpretation of the total and indirect effect estimates is not clear as no clear causal estimands of interest have yet been defined.

8.3.4   Surveillance or other routinely collected data

Cluster-randomized and individually randomized studies can be expensive and/or unfeasible in most situations. Surveillance data on infectious disease occurrence is gathered routinely worldwide. Large administrative databases, such as private insurance and government medical registries, also contain a trove of information on disease outcomes as well as vaccination status of individuals. Routine vaccination also occurs worldwide. It would be useful to use these available data to draw inference about population effects of vaccination (Halloran and Hudgens, 2018). Here we consider two such approaches. Both are based on comparisons of before and after introduction of a vaccination program. The first approach uses medical insurance records to estimate direct, indirect, total, and overall effects of vaccination. The second approach uses surveillance data to estimate the overall effects of introducing a vaccination program. The first approach requires individual level data on both disease outcomes and vaccination status. The second approach requires only incidence data.

Rotavirus vaccine has been available in the USA since 2006, after which the level of rotavirus vaccination in infants increased. Panozzo et al. (2014) estimated direct, indirect, total and overall effectiveness of rotavirus vaccines for the prevention of gastroenteritis hospitalizations in privately insured children in the USA in the years 2007 through 2010. Estimates of the different vaccine effects were based on Cox proportional hazards models to estimate hazard ratios of rotavirus gastroenteritis or acute gastroenteritis hospitalizations. The estimated hazard ratios in infants entering the cohort in 2007, 2008, 2009, and 2010 were used to obtain estimates by calendar year. The direct effect for each calendar year was estimated by comparing outcomes in the vaccinated and unvaccinated infants in each year from 2007 to 2010. To estimate indirect, total, and overall effectiveness during each calendar year, the comparison was made to the unvaccinated infants followed in the pre-vaccine baseline period 2001–2005. In all regression analyses, age served as the underlying time-scale. Children were censored when they experienced their first case of illness. Key to estimating all four effects was having individual-level data on outcomes and vaccination status, and a baseline pre-vaccine comparison group. The estimated direct effectiveness ranged from 87 to 92 percent, with total effectiveness 3–8 percent higher. After 4 years, indirect effectiveness reached over 70 percent and overall effectiveness was over 90 percent.

Interrupted time series analysis is a method for evaluating the overall effectiveness of a vaccination strategy that has been implemented in a population at a defined point in time. It also can be used to look at indirect effects in groups not eligible to receive the vaccine, such as age groups not targeted for vaccination, if the surveillance system has information on such groups. Lopez et al. (2017) provide a tutorial for its use for public health interventions in general. A drawback of inference based on before-and-after comparisons is that temporal trends not related to the vaccination program could reduce incidence of the disease of interest, and bias the estimate of the effectiveness of the program. The interrupted time series analysis adjusts for temporal trends occurring before introduction of the vaccination program.

The basic approach is a segmented regression. Let Y_t be the outcome at time t, X_t be a dummy variable indicating pre-vaccination (X_t set to 0) or post-vaccination period (X_t set to 1), and T is the time since the start of the study. In a simple interrupted time series analysis, the regression model is

$$E[Y_t] = \beta_0 + \beta_1 T + \beta_2 X_t + \beta_3 T X_t, \tag{8.10}$$

where β_0 is the baseline level at $T = 0$, β_1 is the change in outcome associated with time since the begin of the study, so it represents the pre-vaccination trend, β_2 is the level change after the begin of the vaccination program, and β_3 is the slope change following the intervention.

Further complications such as seasonality and other time-varying confounders can be taken into account in more complex models. See Lopez et al. (2017) for further details.

As an example, Ngabo et al. (2016) assessed the effect in Rwanda of introducing rotavirus vaccination in May 2012 into its routine national immunization schedule. Vaccine was administered at 6, 10, and 14 weeks of age. By 2013, coverage reached 99 percent in children under 1 year of age. Compared to the baseline, incidence of hospital admissions specific to rotavirus captured by active surveillance fell by 61-70 percent in the years 2012–2014. The decrease was greater in those age-eligible to be vaccinated, but there was a decrease in nearly all the age groups, suggesting a substantial indirect effect of vaccination for those not age-eligible to receive the vaccine.

8.4   Evaluating Correlates and Surrogates

An important goal of vaccine research is to identify a vaccine-induced immune response that predicts protection from the clinical endpoints of infection and/or disease. If such an immune response were known, it could be used to replace the clinical endpoint in further studies. Thus, if such an immune response were available, it would help avoid large and lengthy new trials and facilitate getting new products and formulations approved. In this section, we consider correlates and surrogates of protection. In a randomized study, the primary clinical endpoint of interest could be clinical disease, infection, or a post-infection outcome. In this section, we assume there is a binary treatment Z, such as vaccine and control, and a binary clinical outcome Y. We assume also that an inexpensive candidate immune surrogate S is measured shortly after randomization.

8.4.1   Terminology

In an important paper, Prentice (1989) defined a surrogate endpoint to be "a response variable for which a test of the null hypothesis of no relationship to the treatment groups under comparison is also a valid test of the corresponding null hypothesis based on the true endpoint." Prentice (1989) also proposed four criteria for a biomarker to be a surrogate endpoint for the clinical outcome of interest. In the context of vaccines (Kohberger et al., 2008), they can be stated as

1. The clinical endpoint is significantly related to the vaccine.

2. The surrogate is significantly related to the vaccine.

3. The surrogate is significantly related to the clinical endpoint.

4. The association of the surrogate with the clinical endpoint is the same in the vaccine and control groups after adjusting for baseline covariates.

For the fourth criterion to be valid, an extra assumption is needed that there are no unmeasured dual correlates of the surrogate and the clinical outcome.

Validation of a Prentice definition surrogate is a challenging task that requires much evidence, and the definition is hard to empirically validate directly (Gilbert et al., 2015). In the fourth criterion, the risk of clinical endpoints is compared in individuals with the observed values of the immunological marker. However, we observe only the immunological value and clinical endpoint that the person has under the actual vaccine assignment. We do not observe the value of the immune marker that the individual would have had under the other assignment. Thus, the fourth criteria can readily fail because of post-randomization selection bias. The Prentice definition is clear and useful, even though the Prentice criteria can be misleading without modification (Gilbert et al., 2015).

Using the framework of potential outcomes in causal inference, Frangakis and Rubin (2002) proposed a definition of a principal surrogate based on the comparison of individuals with the same pair of potential values of the candidate surrogate under two different treatment assignments (see also Sections 8.2.6 and 8.2.7). Following that approach, Gilbert and Hudgens (2008) and Qin et al. (2007), among others, developed a framework delineating different levels of confidence in immunological markers. They particularly distinguish correlates of risk and surrogates of protection. A correlate of risk, the lowest level of confidence, is an immunological measurement that is shown to have an association with the clinical endpoint using some statistical approach. The vaccination status does not necessarily need to be taken into account.

A surrogate of protection is a correlate of risk that also predicts the level of protective vaccine efficacy. Two levels are differentiated: the specific and the general surrogates of protection. The specific surrogates can be applied in the same setting as an efficacy trial used to learn about the surrogate. The general surrogates might be applicable in other settings. Specific surrogates can be further classified as statistical surrogates of protection and principal surrogates of protection. The statistical surrogates of protection are defined in terms of the statistical and observable associations and satisfy the Prentice criteria described above. A principal surrogate is defined by strong modification of vaccine efficacy over immune marker subgroups and by the absence of vaccine efficacy in the subgroup with no vaccine effect on the immune marker.

The vaccinologist Stanley Plotkin had developed a different terminology for correlates of vaccine protection (Plotkin 2010). Plotkin and Glibert (2012) collaborated to propose a new terminology that would supplant the old. In the mapping, a specific correlate of vaccine protection would be equivalent to the specific principal surrogate of protection presented here. A bridging correlate of protection would be equivalent to the general surrogate of protection. Mechanistic and non-mechanistic correlates of protection are also differentiated. However, in the statistical literature, the terminology in Qin et al. (2007) still dominates.

8.4.2   Principal surrogates

The principal surrogates of protection are defined by fixed values of the immune response if assigned vaccine and the immune response if assigned control. The pair of potential immune responses under vaccine and control is assumed fixed before randomization to either vaccine or control, thus the pair is not subject to potential post-randomization selection bias. To begin, consider the simplest case that the potential immune response in the control would be $S(0) = 0$ or some fixed constant c. Let $S(1)$ be the potential response that an unvaccinated subject would have if vaccinated. Let Y denote having the clinical outcome ($Y = 1$) or not ($Y = 0$), and Z be assignment to vaccine ($Z = 1$) or control ($Z = 0$). Assume that the trial is randomized and that there is no interference between the units. For a specific principal surrogate of protection, one needs to estimate

$$\text{VE}(s_1) = 1 - \frac{\Pr[Y = 1 | Z = 1, S(1) = s_1]}{\Pr[Y = 1 | Z = 0, S(1) = s_1]}. \tag{8.11}$$

The definition in expression (8.11) implies that the vaccine efficacy at the immune response level s_1 is one minus the relative reduction in the risk for groups of vaccinees with immune response s_1 compared with their risk if they had not been vaccinated, but if they had been vaccinated, they would have had immune response s_1. A plot of $\text{VE}(s_1)$ by values of s_1 is called the causal effect predictiveness curve (Gilbert and Hudgens, 2008), or simply the vaccine efficacy curve (Huang et al., 2013). A useful principal surrogate is one where $\text{VE}(s_1)$

varies greatly with values of s_1. For vaccine development, it means that increasing the level of that immune marker will increase vaccine efficacy. A good principal surrogate endpoint is relatively easy to measure and, as a strong vaccine efficacy moderator, can be used to reliably predict vaccine effects on clinical endpoints of interest. Gilbert et al. (2015) discuss the relationship of the principal stratification criteria to the Prentice definition. A good principal surrogate is not necessarily a perfect surrogate that would provide exactly the same information as the clinical endpoint, but it could still be valuable.

The problem is that in people in the control group for whom $Z = 0$, the value of s_1, the surrogate value under vaccination, is not observed. That is, s_1 is a missing potential outcome under $Z = 0$. To assess whether an immunological measurement is a specific principal surrogate of protection, knowledge about $S(1)$ is needed. That is, we need to be able to predict the immune response that an unvaccinated participant would have had if vaccinated. Follmann (2006) proposed two augmented vaccine trial designs to address the missing potential outcomes. The first approach, called "baseline immunogenicity predictor" (BIP), needs some variable measured pre-vaccination that predicts the immune response to vaccination. The BIP strategy develops an imputation model for the unobserved baseline immune measure based on the observed relationship between baseline covariates and biomarker values. Follmann (2006) suggested to vaccinate with another vaccine. But that can be hard to implement, and the immune response to two different antigens, the vaccine of interest and the irrelevant vaccine, could be quite different. One option for a good BIP is measurement of the same marker used as the candidate surrogate at baseline.

In the second approach, called "closeout placebo vaccination" (CPV), all or a subset of uninfected participants in the control group are vaccinated with the study vaccine at the end of the trial and their immune responses are recorded. An advantage in using only a subset is that by not entirely depleting the placebo group, the ability to study the durability of vaccine efficacy is retained. Then we assume that the immune response they have at the end of the trial is the response they would have had if vaccinated at the beginning of the trial. By comparing the distribution of immune responses with the full distribution of immune responses in the vaccinated group, because of randomization, we can infer what the distribution of immune responses in the infected participants in the control group would have been. Both of these approaches depend on strong assumptions when used to estimate the $VE(s_1)$ curve.

Huang et al. (2013) proposed an efficient pseudo-score type estimator suitable for the augmented design to assess surrogate endpoint candidates in a two-phase sampling study in which the biomarker is measured in a random subcohort of study participants. Gabriel and Gilbert (2014) extended these methods to evaluating principal surrogate endpoints with time-to-event data and allowing for time-varying vaccine efficacy. The R package `pseval` (Sachs and Gabriel, 2016) on CRAN implements several functions for estimating the VE(s) curve for either a binary or a survival outcome.

8.4.3   General surrogates of protection

Although it is useful to understand the relation of immune responses to protection against infection and disease within a particular setting, the goal of identifying surrogates of vaccine protection is to replace large scale phase III trials using clinical outcomes with immunological measurements in new settings and for new vaccines. A key point is that "general" is with respect to a particular kind of bridge. It is not intended to necessarily be universal for all types of bridges. So a user must define the relevant variation in units in view of a given use of "general" For example, it could be all for one vaccine regimen, but over different pathogen serotypes, or all for one vaccine regimen and one serotype, but over different age groups. It is actually quite difficult without numerous, likely untestable assumptions.

To show that an immunological marker is a general surrogate of protection requires that it predict vaccine effects on risk across different populations, for different strains, and different vaccine products. One possible approach is to use meta-analysis (Gabriel et al., 2016) or other (Gabriel et al., 2017) approaches to combine information from several studies.

Acknowledgments

This work was partially funded by U54 GM111274, R37 AI032042, and R01 AI 085073. The content is solely the responsibility of the author and does not necessarily represent the official views of the NIH. The author is grateful to Peter Gilbert and Erin Gabriel for helpful comments.

References

Aalen O. Nonparametric estimation of partial transition probabilities in multiple decrement models. *Ann Stat*, 6:534–545, 1978.

Ali M, D Sur, YA You et al., Herd protection by a bivalent killed whole-cell oral cholera vaccine in the slums of Kolkata, India. *Clin Inf Dis*, 56:1123–1131, 2013.

Ali M, M Emch, M von Seidlein, M Yunus, DA Sack, M Rao, J Holmgren, and JD Clemens. Herd immunity conferred by killed oral cholera vaccines in Bangladesh: A reanalysis. *Lancet*, 366:44–49, 2005.

Aronow PM, NE Basta, and ME Halloran. The regression discontinuity design under interference: A local randomization approach (invited commentary). *Observational Studies*, 2:129–133, 2016.

Auranen K, E Arjas, T Leino, and AK Takala. Transmission of pneumococcal carriage in families: A latent Markov process model for binary longitudinal data. *J Am Stat Assoc*, 95:1044–1053, 2000.

Auranen K, H Rinta-Kokko, and ME Halloran. Estimating strain-specific and overall efficacy of polyvalent vaccines against pathogens with recurrent dynamics from a cross-sectional study. *Biometrics*, 69:235–44, 2013.

Baird S, JA Bohren, C McIntosh, and B Özler. Optimal design of experiments in the presence of interference. *Review of Economics and Statistics*, 2018. posted Online January 12, 2018, doi:10.1162/REST_a_00716.

Bar-Zeev N, L Kapanda, JE Tate, KC Jere, M Iturriza-Gomara, O Nakagomi et al. Effectiveness of a monovalent rotavirus vaccine in infants in Malawi after programmatic roll-out: An observational and case-control study. *Lancet Infect Dis*, 15:422–428, 2015.

Benkeser D, M Carone, and PB Gilbert. Improved estimation of the cumulative incidence of rare outcomes. *Stat Medicine*, 37:280–293, 2018. doi:10.1002/sim.7337.

Bor J, E Moscoe, P Mutevedzi, M-L Newell, and T Bärnighausen. Regression discontinuity designs in epidemiology: Causal inference without randomized trials. *Epidemiology*, 25(5):729–737, 2014.

R Core Team. *R: A Language and Environment for Statistical Computing*. R Foundation for Statistical Computing, Vienna, Austria, 2018.

Cox DR. *Planning of Experiments*. John Wiley & Sons, New York, 1958.

Durham LK, IM Longini, ME Halloran, JD Clemens, A Nizam, and M Rao. Estimation of vaccine efficacy in the presence of waning: Application to cholera vaccines. *Am J Epidemiol*, 147:948–959, 1998.

Ebola ça suffit ring vaccination trial consortium. The ring vaccination trial: A novel cluster randomised controlled trial design to evaluate vaccine efficacy and effectiveness during outbreaks, with special reference to Ebola. *BMJ*, 351:h3740, 2015.

Follmann D. Augmented designs to assess immune response in vaccine trials. *Biometrics*, 62:1161–1169, 2006.

Fong Y and K Sebestyen. *kyotil: Utility Functions for Statistical Analysis Report Generation and Monte Carlo Studies*, 2018. https://CRAN.R-project.org/package=kyotil.

Frangakis CE and DB Rubin. Principal stratification in causal inference. *Biometrics*, 58:21–29, 2002.

Gabriel EE and PB Gilbert. Evaluating principal surrogate endpoints with time-to-event data accounting for time-varying treatment efficacy. *Biostatistics*, 15:251–265, 2014.

Gabriel EE, MG Sachs, and ME Halloran. Evaluation and comparison of predictive individual-level general surrogates. *Biostatistics*, 2017. doi:10.1093/biostatistics/kxx037.

Gabriel EE, MJ Daniels, and ME Halloran. Comparing biomarkers as trial-level general surrogates. *Biometrics*, 72:1046–1054, 2016. doi:10.1111/biom.12513.

Gilbert PB and MG Hudgens. Evaluating candidate principal surrogate endpoints. *Biometrics*, 64(4):1146–1154, 2008.

Gilbert PB, EE Gabriel, Y Huang, and ISF Chan. Surrogate endpoint evaluation: Principal stratification criteria and the Prentice definition. *J Causal Inf*, 3:157–176, 2015. doi:10.1515/jci-2014-0007.

Gilbert PB, V DeGruttola, MG Hudgens, SG Self, SM Hammer, and L Corey. What constitutes efficacy for a human immunodeficiency virus vaccine that ameliorates viremia: Issues involving surrogate end points in Phase 3 trials. *J Infect Dis*, 188:179–193, 2003.

Grambsch PM and TM Therneau. Proportional hazards test and diagnostics based on weighted residuals. *Biometrika*, 81:515–526, 1994.

Greenland S, JM Robins, and J Pearl. Confounding and collapsibility in causal inference. *Stat Sci*, 14:29–46, 1999.

Greenwood M and UG Yule. The statistics of anti-typhoid and anti-cholera inoculations, and the interpretation of such statistics in general. *Proc R Soc Med*, 8(part 2):113–194, 1915.

Halloran ME and CJ Struchiner. Causal inference for infectious diseases. *Epidemiology*, 6:142–151, 1995.

Halloran ME and CJ Struchiner. Study designs for dependent happenings. *Epidemiology*, 2:331–338, 1991.

Halloran ME and Hudgens MG. Estimating population effects of vaccination using large, routinely collected data. *Stat Med*, 37:294–301, 2018. doi:10.1002/sim.7392.

Halloran ME and MG Hudgens. Causal vaccine effects for infectiousness. *International J Biostat*, 8(2):1–40, 2012a.

Halloran ME and MG Hudgens. Comparing bounds on vaccine effects on infectiousness. *Epidemiology*, 23:931–932, 2012b.

Halloran ME, CJ Struchiner, and IM Longini. Study designs for different efficacy and effectiveness aspects of vaccination. *Am J Epidemiol*, 146:789–803, 1997.

Halloran ME, IM Longini, and CJ Struchiner. *Design and Analysis of Vaccine Studies*. Springer, New York, 2010.

Halloran ME, IM Longini, and CJ Struchiner. Estimability and interpretation of vaccine efficacy using frailty mixing models. *Am J Epidemiol*, 144:83–97, 1996.

Halloran ME, K Auranen, S Baird et al. Simulations for designing and interpreting intervention trials in infectious diseases. *BMC Medicine*, 15(1):223, 2017. doi: 10.1186/s12916-017-0985-3.

Halloran ME, MJ Haber, IM Longini, and CJ Struchiner. Direct and indirect effects in vaccine field efficacy and effectiveness. *Am J Epidemiol*, 133:323–331, 1991.

Hayes RJ and LH Moulton. *Cluster Randomised Trials: A Practical Approach, second edition*. Chapman and Hall/CRC, Boca Raton, FL, 2017.

Henao-Restrepo AM, IM Longini, M Egger et al. Efficacy and effectiveness of an rVSV-vectored vaccine expressing Ebola surface glycoprotein: Interim results from the Guinea ring vaccination cluster-randomised trial. *Lancet*, 386:857–66, 2015.

PW Holland. Statistics and causal inference. *J Am Stat Assoc*, 81:945–960, 1986.

Hong S and G Raudenbush. Evaluating kindergarten retention policy: A case study of causal inference for multilevel observational data. *J Am Stat Assoc*, 101:901–910, 2006.

Huang Y, PB Gilbert, and J Wolfson. Design and estimation for evaluating principal surrogate markers in vaccine trials. *Biometrics*, 69:301–309, 2013.

Hudgens MG and ME Halloran. Causal vaccine effects on binary postinfection outcomes. *J Am Stat Assoc*, 101:51–64, 2006.

Hudgens MG and ME Halloran. Towards causal inference with interference. *J Am Stat Assoc*, 103:832–842, 2008.

Hudgens MG, A Hoering, and SG Self. On the analysis of viral load endpoints in HIV vaccine trials. *Stat Med*, 22:2281–2298, 2003.

Hussey MA and JP Hughes. Design and analysis of stepped wedge cluster randomized trials. *Contemp Clin Trials*, 28:182–191, 2007.

Jackson ML and JC Nelson. The test-negative design for estimating influenza vaccine effectiveness. *Vaccine*, 31(17):2165–2168, 2013.

Käyhty H, K Auranen, H Nohynek, R Dagan, H Mäkelä, and the Pneumococcal Carriage Group. Nasopharyngeal carriage: A target for pneumococcal vaccination. *Expert Rev Vaccines*, 5:651–667, 2006.

Kohberger RC, D Jemiolo, and F Noriega. Prediction of pertussis vaccine efficacy using a correlates of protection model. *Vaccine*, 26:3516–3521, 2008.

Liu L and MG Hudgens. Large sample randomization inference of causal effects in the presence of interference. *J Am Stat Assoc*, 109:288–301, 2014.

Liu L, MG Hudgens, and S Becker-Dreps. On inverse probability weighted estimators in the presence of interference. *Biometrika*, 103:829–842, 2016.

Lopez BJ, S Cummins, and A Gasparrini. Interrupted time series regression for the evaluation of public health interventions: A tutorial. *Int J Epidemiol*, 46:348–355, 2017.

Lundin M and M Karlsson. Estimation of causal effects in observational studies with interference between units. *Stat Methods Appl*, 23:417–433, 2014.

Mehtälä J, R Dagan, and K Auranen. Estimation and interpretation of heterogeneous vaccine efficacy against recurrent infections. *Biometrics*, 72(3):976–985, 2016.

Moscoe E, J Bor, and T Bärnighausen. Regression discontinuity designs are underutilized in medicine, epidemiology and public health: A review of current and best practice. *J Clin Epidemiol*, 68:132–143, 2015.

Moulton LH, KL O'Brien, R Kohberger, I Chang, R Reid, R Weatherholtz, JG Hackell, GR Siber, and M Santosham. Design of a group-randomised *Streptococcus pneumoniae* vaccine trial. *Contr Clin Trials*, 22:438–452, 2001.

Préziosi MP and ME Halloran. Effects of pertussis vaccination on transmission: Vaccine efficacy for infectiousness. *Vaccine*, 21:1853–1861, 2003.

Neafsey DE, M Juraska, T Bedford et al. Genetic diversity and protective efficacy of the RTS, S/AS01 malaria vaccine. *N Engl J Med*, 373(21):2025–2037, 2015.

Ngabo F, JE Tate, M Gatera, C Rugambwa, P Donnen, P Lepage, JM Mwenda, A Binagwaho, and UD Parashar. Effect of pentavalent rotavirus vaccine introduction on hospital admissions for diarrhoea and rotavirus in children in Rwanda: A time-series analysis. *Lancet Glob Health*, 4:e129–36, 2016.

Panozzo CA, S Becker-Dreps, V Pate, DJ Weber, MJ Funk, T Stürmer, and MA Brookhart. Direct, indirect, total, and overall effectiveness of the rotavirus vaccines for the prevention of gastroenteritis hospitalizations in privately insured US children, 2007-2010. *Am J Epidemiol*, 179:895–909, 2014.

Perez-Heydrich C, MG Hudgens, ME Halloran, JD Clemens, M Ali, and ME Emch. Assessing effects of cholera vaccination in the presence of interference. *Biometrics*, 70(3):731–741, 2014.

Plotkin SA and PB Gilbert. Nomenclature for immune correlates of protection after vaccination. *Clin Inf Dis*, 54(11):1615–1617, 2012.

Plotkin SA. Correlates of protection induced by vaccination. *Clin Vaccine Immunol*, 17:1055–65, 2010.

Prentice RL. Surrogate endpoints in clinical trials: Definition and operational criteria. *Stat Med*, 8:431–440, 1989.

Qin L, PB Gilbert, L Corey, MJ McElrath, and SG Self. A framework for assessing immunological correlates of protection in vaccine trials. *J Infect Dis*, 196:1304–1312, 2007.

Rhodes PH, ME Halloran, and IM Longini. Counting process models for differentiating exposure to infection and susceptibility. *J R Stat Soc Series B*, 58:751–762, 1996.

Richardson TS and JM Robins. Single world intervention graphs (SWIGs): A unification of the counterfactual and graphical approaches to causality. Technical Report 128, Center for Statistics and the Social Sciences, University of Washington, Seattle WA, 2013.

Rinta-Kokko H, R Dagan, N Givon-Lavi, and K Auranen. Estimation of vaccine efficacy against acquisition of pneumococcal carriage. *Vaccine*, 27:3831–3837, 2009.

Robins JM. A new approach to causal inference in mortality studies with sustained exposure period—Application to control of the healthy worker survivor effect. *Math Model*, 7:1393–1512, 1986.

Rodrigues L and P Smith. Case-control approach to vaccine evaluation. *Epidemiol Rev*, 21:56–72, 1999.

Rosenbaum PR and DB Rubin. The central role of the propensity score in observational studies. *Biometrika*, 70:41–55, 1983.

Ross R. An application of the theory of probabilities to the study of *a priori* pathometry, Part 1. *Proc R Soc Series A*, 92:204–230, 1916.

Rubin DB. Bayesian inference for causal effects: The role of randomization. *Ann Stat*, 7:34–58, 1978.

Rubin DB. Comment: Neyman (1923) and causal inference in experiments and observational studies. *Stat Sci*, 5:472–480, 1990.

Rubin DB. Discussion of "Randomization analysis of experimental data in the Fisher randomization test" by Basu. *J Am Stat Assoc*, 75:591–593, 1980.

Sachs MC and EE Gabriel. *pseval: Methods for Evaluating Principal Surrogates of Treatment Response*, 2016. R package version 1.3.0. https://cran.r-project.org/web/packages/pseval/vignettes/introduction.html

Saul B and MG Hudgens. A recipe for inferference: Start with causal inference. Add interference. Mix well with R. *J Stat Softw*, 82:1–21, 2017.

Schwartz LM, ME Halloran, A Rowhani-Rahbar, KM Neuzil, and JC Victor. Rotavirus vaccine effectiveness in low-income settings: An evaluation of the test-negative design. *Vaccine*, 35:184–190, 2017.

De Serres C, DM Skowronski, XW Wu, and CS Ambrose. The test-negative design: Validity, accuracy and precision of vaccine efficacy estimates compared to the gold standard of randomised placebo-controlled clinical trials. *Euro Surveill*, 18:1–9, 2013.

Smith PG, LC Rodrigues, and PEM Fine. Assessment of the protective efficacy of vaccines against common diseases using case-control and cohort studies. *Int J Epidemiol*, 13(1):87–93, 1984.

Sobel M. What do randomized studies of housing mobility demonstrate? Causal inference in the face of interference. *J Am Stat Assoc*, 101:1398–1407, 2006.

Struchiner CJ, ME Halloran, JM Robins, and A Spielman. The behavior of common measures of association used to assess a vaccination program under complex disease transmission patterns—A computer simulation study of malaria vaccines. *Int J Epidemiol*, 19:187–196, 1990.

Struchiner CJ, ME Halloran, RC Brunet, JMC Ribeiro, and E Massad. Malaria vaccines: Lessons from field trials. *Cadernos do Saúde Pública*, 10(supplement 2):310–326, 1994.

Sullivan SG, EJ Tchetgen Tchetgen, and BJ Cowling. Theoretical basis of the test-negative study design for assessment of influenza vaccine effectiveness. *Am J Epidemiol*, 184:345–353, 2016.

Sur D, R Ochiai, SK Bhattacharya et al. A cluster-randomized effectiveness trial of Vi typhoid vaccine in India. *N Engl J Med*, 361:335–344, 2009.

VanderWeele TJ, E. Tchetgen Tchetgen, and M.E. Halloran. Interference and sensitivity analysis. *Stat Sci*, 29(4):687–706, 2014.

Tchetgen EJ and TJ VanderWeele. On causal inference in the presence of interference. *Stat Methods Med Res*, 21(1):55–75, 2012.

Therneau TM. *A Package for Survival Analysis in S*, 2015. version 2.38, https://CRAN.R-project.org/package=survival.

Thistlewaite DL and DT Campbell. Regression-discontinuity analysis: An alternative to the ex-post facto experiment. *J Educ Psychol*, 51:309–317, 1960. reprinted with commentaries in Observational Studies 2:119–128, 2016.

VanderWeele TJ and EJ Tchetgen Tchetgen. Effect partitioning under interference in two-stage randomized vaccine trials. *Stat Probabil Lett*, 81:861–869, 2011.

Westreich D and MG Hudgens. Invited commentary: Beware the test-negative design. *Am J Epidemiol*, 184:354–356, 2016.

Part III

Analysis of Outbreak Data

9

Markov Chain Monte Carlo Methods for Outbreak Data

Philip D. O'Neill and Theodore Kypraios

CONTENTS

9.1   Introduction

In this chapter we explain how Markov chain Monte Carlo (MCMC) methods can be employed to analyze data from an outbreak of infectious disease. The basic approach is to (1) formulate a suitable stochastic transmission model, (2) find a way of deriving the likelihood of the observed data under this model, and (3) adopt a Bayesian framework using MCMC methods to make inference about the model parameters. In practice, simply fitting models to data is rarely of scientific interest in itself, but by choosing models and model parameters appropriately it becomes possible to provide quantitative information about the outbreak or the pathogen. This approach might include information on key quantities such as the basic reproduction number, the importance of relative routes of transmission, the length of the infectious period, or other relevant aspects. The epidemic model also could be used for forecasting using the estimated parameters.

Our main focus in this chapter is on the susceptible-infectious-removed (SIR) model, and we describe in detail how to fit this model to outbreak data consisting of removal times for all cases. Although this is a rather specific problem, the methods we use are readily adapted to many other settings, several of which we then discuss. Also, we focus exclusively on stochastic transmission models, although MCMC methods can also be used to fit deterministic epidemic models.

9.2   Bayesian Inference

We start by outlining the key aspects of Bayesian inference that will be relevant to this discussion. This is an enormous topic, and readers who are unfamiliar with it might wish to consult the relevant literature for a deeper understanding (e.g. [1]). However, many of the ideas we now introduce will be illustrated throughout the rest of the chapter.

9.2.1   The Bayesian approach

The Bayesian approach to statistical inference goes as follows. Suppose we have observed data x, and a model for the data $\pi(x|\theta)$, where π is typically a probability mass or density function with parameters denoted by θ. In our context, x might represent data from an outbreak of infectious disease such as the daily number of diagnosed cases, and θ might be parameters of a suitable epidemic model such as infection or recovery rates. Our objective is to learn about θ, in other words to say something about plausible values for the model parameter given the data x.

The Bayesian view is that θ is a random variable, and that attention should therefore focus on the conditional distribution of θ given x, which is known as the *posterior distribution* of θ given x. According to Bayes' Theorem,

$$\pi(\theta|x) = \frac{\pi(x|\theta)\pi(\theta)}{\pi(x)}, \tag{9.1}$$

where $\pi(\theta|x)$ is the *posterior density* (or mass function, if θ is discrete rather than continuous) of θ given x, $\pi(x|\theta)$ is the *likelihood* of the observed data regarded as a function of θ, $\pi(\theta)$ is the *prior* density of θ and $\pi(x)$ is a normalizing constant that ensures that $\pi(\theta|x)$ integrates to 1, so that the posterior distribution is a probability distribution.

Perhaps the most unusual of these quantities for those new to the Bayesian view is the prior density $\pi(\theta)$. One interpretation is that this object represents our initial belief about θ before seeing any data, and hence is something that might be different for different researchers or analysts working with the same data. Although such an apparently subjective approach can seem alien at first, in practice prior distributions often are assigned to be either (1) uninformative or vague: for example, if θ represents a probability, we might assign a uniform distribution on $[0, 1]$ to represent the idea that any value of θ is equally likely in the absence of data, (2) informative, in the sense that in reality we may either know or have good grounds to believe that certain values of θ are more likely than others: for example, if θ represented the mean time that an individual remained infectious, we may be prepared to rule out values greater than some cut-off, and assign $\pi(\theta)$ appropriately, perhaps using results from previous studies in the literature.

9.2.2 Practical challenges

Although at first glance (9.1) looks rather simple, there can be several problems in practice. The first is that the normalizing constant $\pi(x)$ is obtained via the expression

$$\pi(x) = \int_\Theta \pi(x|\theta)\pi(\theta)\,d\theta, \tag{9.2}$$

where Θ is the set of possible values of the model parameter θ. The integral in (9.2) is often analytically intractable, and also may be high dimensional. For instance, if an epidemic model has six parameters, a six-dimensional integral is required.

The second problem is that the likelihood $\pi(x|\theta)$ might also be intractable. A relevant example for this chapter is the situation where we have a standard SIR model, with parameter $\theta = (\beta, \gamma)$ where β is the infection rate and γ is the removal rate, and we observe removal times $x = (r_1, \ldots, r_n)$, say. As described in more detail later, in this case the likelihood $\pi(x|\theta)$ is not analytically available or computationally tractable unless there are very few observed removals.

A third problem is that, even if we have an explicit formula for $\pi(\theta|x)$, this alone might not be all that helpful. In reality, what we really might want to know are quantities such as the mean or variance of θ given the data (these quantities are called the *posterior mean* and *posterior variance* of θ given x, respectively), or other summaries. We also might be interested in quantities derived from the model, such as $R_0 = \beta/\gamma$ for an SIR model. Calculating such quantities from $\pi(\theta|x)$ involves evaluating further integrals; for example the posterior mean is given by

$$E[\theta|x] = \int_\Theta \theta\pi(\theta|x)\,d\theta.$$

MCMC methods provide one way of addressing all three of the problems we have described.

9.3 MCMC Methods

We now give a brief introduction to MCMC methods. As for the material on Bayesian methods, there is a vast amount more that could be said (see, e.g. [2]), so we just explain the key concepts. Readers new to MCMC are strongly encouraged to try implementing it for themselves, since this is undoubtedly the best way to learn the topic.

9.3.1 Overview

MCMC methods are computational techniques for sampling from a non-normalized probability density, often called the *target density*. In other words, if we are able to evaluate a density function $\pi(\theta)$ up to proportionality, where $\theta \in \Theta$ itself might be high-dimensional, MCMC methods provide a way of obtaining a sample $\theta_1, \theta_2, \ldots, \theta_N$ where each θ_i is a sample from the correctly-normalized $\pi(\theta)$. The key idea behind the methods is to construct an ergodic discrete-time Markov chain $\{X_1, X_2, \ldots\}$ with state space Θ which has a unique stationary distribution with density equal to $\pi(\theta)$. If this chain then is simulated, the probability distribution of X_n will converge to the stationary distribution as $n \to \infty$, and thus the X_n values for large values of n are, at least approximately, a sample from $\pi(\theta)$.

Before providing details, we pause to see how MCMC can solve the three implementation problems of Bayesian inference we mentioned. In this setting, the target density is the posterior density $\pi(\theta|x)$. The first problem, namely computation of the normalizing constant in Bayes' Theorem, is avoided since MCMC methods only require us to know the target density up to proportionality. Thus, to use MCMC methods we need to be able to compute $\pi(x|\theta)\pi(\theta)$ for any specific value of θ. The second problem, of an intractable likelihood, can be solved in some cases by introducing additional variables to create a tractable likelihood. For example, for the SIR model it is possible to write down the likelihood of a set of infection and removal times given the initial conditions and the model parameters. The additional variables can be regarded as additional model parameters which can then be estimated as well using MCMC. This approach is often called *data augmentation* since it refers to the idea that we augment the existing data with other quantities that are "missing." The third problem, that of being able to calculate quantities of interest, is addressed because MCMC is a form of so-called *sample-based* inference, meaning that our knowledge of the posterior distribution is represented not by a formula, but rather by a set of samples. These samples then can be used to directly estimate summaries of interest such as means or variances.

9.3.2   Algorithms

The two most commonly used MCMC algorithms are the Metropolis-Hastings algorithm and the Gibbs sampler, described herein. As well as being algorithms in their own right, they can be used as components of more complex algorithms. In general, defining an MCMC algorithm involves specifying how the Markov chain moves at each iteration; i.e., if it is currently at $X_n = \theta$, we need to define how X_{n+1} is generated, doing so in such a way that the Markov chain has the desired stationary distribution $\pi(\theta)$.

Metropolis-Hastings algorithm. This algorithm can be defined iteratively as follows (Algorithm 9.1). In the following, $a \wedge b$ denotes the minimum of a and b, and $x \sim f(x)$ means that x is distributed according to a probability distribution with density f.

Algorithm 9.1 Metropolis-Hastings algorithm

1: Suppose $X_n = \theta$.
2: Propose $\theta^* \sim q(\theta^*|\theta)$.
3: With probability $\alpha = 1 \wedge \frac{\pi(\theta^*)q(\theta|\theta^*)}{\pi(\theta)q(\theta^*|\theta)}$, set $X_{n+1} = \theta^*$;
4: Otherwise, set $X_{n+1} = \theta$.

In this algorithm, $q(\theta^*|\theta)$ denotes the so-called *proposal density*, from which a proposed new value θ^* is proposed. Note that q can and usually does depend on the value of θ; if it does not, then $q(\theta^*|\theta) = q(\theta^*)$ and the resulting algorithm is called an *independence sampler*. The choice of q is essentially arbitrary, subject to ensuring that the resulting Markov chain is ergodic. However, the speed with which the Markov chain can move around the state space Θ is determined by q. In practice, it is sensible to design q such that the chain neither frequently gets stuck in one location (as happens if proposed values are often such that $\pi(\theta^*) \ll \pi(\theta)$, yielding $\alpha \approx 0$) nor needs many steps to properly explore Θ (as can happen if proposed moves have $\pi(\theta^*) \approx \pi(\theta)$, yielding $\alpha \approx 1$).

Gibbs sampler. Suppose now that θ itself has n components, and write $\theta = (\theta_1, \ldots, \theta_n)$. The most common example of this is simply that θ is n-dimensional, and the components are the marginal distributions. The key idea behind Gibbs sampling is to update each of the n components of θ in turn, according to their so-called *full conditional distribution*, i.e. the distribution of that component conditional on the values of the other components. The algorithm is iteratively defined as follows.

Algorithm 9.2 Gibbs sampler

1: Suppose $X_n = \theta = (\theta_1, \ldots, \theta_n)$.
2: Sample $\theta_1^* \sim \pi(\theta_1 | \theta_2, \ldots, \theta_n)$.
3: Sample $\theta_2^* \sim \pi(\theta_2 | \theta_1^*, \theta_3, \ldots, \theta_n)$.

4: $\vdots$
5: Sample $\theta_n^* \sim \pi(\theta_n | \theta_1^*, \ldots, \theta_{n-1}^*)$.
6: Set $X_{n+1} = (\theta_1^*, \ldots, \theta_n^*)$.

Unlike the Metropolis-Hastings algorithm, there is no accept-reject step in the Gibbs sampler. However, the two algorithms are related in the sense that the latter is actually a special case of the former in which the acceptance probability α is guaranteed to equal 1. There is a sense in which Gibbs sampling is preferable to Metropolis-Hastings since it uses additional information about the target density, namely the full conditional distributions. However, it is not always possible to use Gibbs sampling in practice, since full conditional distributions might be non-standard distributions that are hard to sample from.

General MCMC algorithm. Suppose we have a target density $\pi(\theta) = \pi(\theta_1, \ldots, \theta_n)$. A general MCMC algorithm, which simulates the Markov chain for M steps, is as follows.

Algorithm 9.3 General MCMC Algorithm

1: Initialise θ by $\theta = \theta^{(0)} = (\theta_1^{(0)}, \ldots, \theta_n^{(0)})$.
2: **for** $k = 1$ to M **do**
3:    **for** $j = 1$ to n **do**
4:       Update θ_j and store updated value as $\theta_j^{(k)}$.
5:    **end for**
6:    Set $\theta^{(k)} = (\theta_1^{(k)}, \ldots, \theta_n^{(k)})$.
7: **end for**

In essence, all that is required is to update each of the components of θ at each iteration of the algorithm. Here, an update step for θ_j consists of either a Metropolis-Hastings step, in which a new value θ_j^* is proposed and then either accepted or not, or a Gibbs step, in which case θ_j^* is sampled from its conditional distribution with all the other components of θ fixed. Note, therefore, that an update might result in the new value of θ_j being the same as the previous value.

The output of Algorithm 9.3 is a sequence of values $\theta^{(0)}, \ldots, \theta^{(M)}$ that correspond to a single realization of a Markov chain. We usually discard the first m (say) values $\theta^{(0)}, \ldots, \theta^{(m-1)}$, in the so-called *burn-in* period during which the Markov chain is deemed to have not yet reached its equilibrium distribution. In practice, m can be determined by visual inspection of the *trace plots* of the components, i.e., the time series $\theta_j^{(0)}, \ldots, \theta_j^{(M)}$ for $j = 1, \ldots, n$. Examples are provided herein. It is also customary to *thin* the output, meaning that we discard all but every Lth (say) value of the Markov chain. There are two reasons to do this: one is that it reduces the correlation between samples (since in the original output, successive values of the Markov chain are clearly not independent) and the other is that if we only ever record every Lth sample, we reduce the amount of computer memory required. As for the burn-in period, the amount of thinning can be a question of trial and error. However, unlike burn-in, thinning itself is not strictly necessary in order to end up with a sample that can be used for estimation.

Finally, note that the way we partition θ into $\theta_1, \ldots, \theta_n$ is usually problem-specific. The individual components might be univariate or multivariate quantities. We might choose to update certain components together (known as *block updating*) if they are correlated.

9.4 MCMC Methods for the SIR Model Given Removal Data

9.4.1 The problem of interest

In this section we explain how to perform Bayesian inference for the parameters of a stochastic SIR model, given data on the removal process. The reason that this problem is of interest is that, for many diseases, transmission of the pathogen is unobserved, but symptoms are observable. If we make the additional assumption that a symptomatic individual is removed (perhaps by some form of isolation) then there is only one "missing" piece of information for the individual, namely the time of their infection. Clearly, these assumptions do not hold for all diseases, but the methods we develop for this situation can often be adapted to other settings. We start with some notation.

9.4.2 Notation and preliminaries

Consider a stochastic SIR model among a population of N individuals, of whom one is initially infective and the rest susceptible. We denote by $S(t)$ and $I(t)$, respectively, the numbers of susceptible and infective individuals in the population at time t. The infectious period distribution is assumed to be exponential with mean γ^{-1}. Infections are assumed to occur according to an inhomogeneous Poisson process of rate $\beta N^{-1} S(t) I(t)$. We assume that the observed data consist of removal times $r_1, \ldots, r_n$, where n denotes the total number of individuals who are ever infected, including the initial infective. Without loss of generality, we label the infected individuals $1, \ldots, n$, and the other individuals $n+1, \ldots, N$. For convenience we label the n infected individuals in order of removal time, so that $r_1 < r_2 < \ldots < r_n$, although this is not necessary. For $j = 1, \ldots, n$ let i_j denote the infection time of the individual who is removed at time r_j, and for $j = n+1, \ldots, N$ set $i_j = r_j = \infty$. Let κ denote the individual who is the initial infective, so that $i_\kappa < i_j$ for all $j \neq \kappa$. Note that it is not necessarily the case that $\kappa = 1$, since the initial infective need not be the first individual to be removed. Finally, define vectors $\boldsymbol{r} = (r_1, \ldots, r_n)$ and $\boldsymbol{i} = (i_1, \ldots, i_{\kappa-1}, i_{\kappa+1}, \ldots, i_n)$ of all removal times and all infection times other than i_κ, respectively.

9.4.3 Likelihood

Our objective is to perform Bayesian inference for the parameters β and γ, and thus the object of interest is the posterior density $\pi(\beta, \gamma | \boldsymbol{r})$. Unfortunately, in most cases the likelihood $\pi(\boldsymbol{r} | \beta, \gamma)$ is challenging to compute. To see this, consider the slightly simpler problem in which κ and i_κ are known. Then

$$\pi(\boldsymbol{r} | \beta, \gamma, \kappa, i_\kappa) = \int \pi(\boldsymbol{i}, \boldsymbol{r} | \beta, \gamma, \kappa, i_\kappa) \, d\boldsymbol{i},$$

but the range of integration is non-trivial, since we essentially have to consider all possible configurations of infection times that do not result in the epidemic ceasing before time r_n. Although in principle it is possible to do this, the calculations rapidly become prohibitive.

To overcome this problem, we introduce additional variables that enable us to compute an augmented likelihood. Specifically, we introduce the unobserved infection times $\boldsymbol{i}$, along with the initial conditions κ and i_κ. Then

$$\pi(\boldsymbol{i}, \boldsymbol{r} | \beta, \gamma, \kappa, i_\kappa) = \left\{ \prod_{j \neq \kappa} \frac{\beta}{N} I(i_j -) \right\} \exp \left\{ -\frac{\beta}{N} \int_{i_\kappa}^{r_n} S(t) I(t) \, dt \right\}$$

$$\times \gamma^n \exp \left\{ -\gamma \sum_{j=1}^{n} (r_j - i_j) \right\}, \tag{9.3}$$

where $I(i_j -) = \lim_{t \uparrow i_j} I(t)$ denotes the number of infectives just before time i_j. The likelihood at (9.3) contains three parts, which we now briefly explain. The product term accounts for the infections and is obtained by multiplying together the overall Poisson process rate of infection for each infection event. The exponential term accounts for individuals avoiding infection as the epidemic progresses, both those who ever become infected and those who do not. The final part is simply the likelihood of the n infectious periods, each of which is distributed according to an exponential random variable with rate parameter γ. We alternatively might describe this final part as being the likelihood of the removal process.

We now describe how the likelihood at (9.3) is evaluated in practice. The removal process part involves a straightforward sum and poses no difficulties. For the product term, it is necessary to know how many individuals are infected just before each infection time. One way to do this is to observe that an individual k is infective at time t if and only if $i_k \leq t < r_k$, and so $I(i_j -)$ is simply the number of infectives in the population at time i_j other than individual j. Thus

$$I(i_j -) = \sum_{k=1, k \neq j}^{n} \chi_{\{i_k \leq i_j < r_k\}}, \tag{9.4}$$

where χ_A is the indicator function of the event A.

An alternative way to evaluate the product is to (1) put all event times in order (i.e., infections and removals), keeping track of the type of each event and (2) step through the ordered list starting from time i_κ, keeping track of the numbers of susceptibles and infectives present at the time of each event. Note that both $S(t)$ and $I(t)$ are piece-wise constant and can only change at event times. This approach also can be used to evaluate the integral in (9.3), although there is a much easier way. Specifically,

$$\int_{i_\kappa}^{r_n} S(t) I(t) \, dt = \sum_{j=1}^{n} \sum_{k=1}^{N} (r_j \wedge i_k - i_j \wedge i_k). \tag{9.5}$$

One way to see this is to observe that the integral is simply the total time during which susceptibles avoid infection from infectives. For an individual j who becomes infected and an arbitrary individual k, it is not hard to see that the time during which j is infective and k is susceptible is given by $r_j \wedge i_k - i_j \wedge i_k$, and (9.5) follows by summing over j and k. A more formal derivation is to write $S(t)$ and $I(t)$ as sums of indicator functions, e.g., $S(t) = \sum_{k=1}^{N} \chi_{\{t < i_k\}}$, and (9.5) follows after a few lines of algebra.

9.4.4   Bayesian inference and prior distributions

The augmented posterior density of interest is

$$\pi(\beta,\gamma,\kappa,i_\kappa,\boldsymbol{i}|\boldsymbol{r}) \propto \pi(\boldsymbol{i},\boldsymbol{r}|\beta,\gamma,\kappa,i_\kappa)\pi(\beta,\gamma,\kappa,i_\kappa), \qquad (9.6)$$

where the two terms on the right-hand side of (9.6) are the augmented likelihood defined at (9.3) and the joint prior density of β, γ, κ, and i_κ. Although the latter is essentially arbitrary, in practice we usually assign independent vague prior distributions to all four of these parameters. Note that although $\boldsymbol{i}$ is part of our augmentation scheme, (9.6) demonstrates that it does not require a prior distribution.

We will assume the following prior distributions:

- $\beta \sim \Gamma(m_\beta, \lambda_\beta)$,
- $\gamma \sim \Gamma(m_\gamma, \lambda_\gamma)$,
- $P(\kappa = j) = n^{-1}$, $j = 1, \ldots, n$,
- $i_\kappa = r_1 - Y$, where $Y \sim \text{Exp}(\theta)$,

where $X \sim \Gamma(m, \lambda)$ means X has probability density function (p.d.f.) $f_X(x) \propto x^{m-1} \exp(-\lambda x)$, and $X \sim \text{Exp}(\theta)$ means X has p.d.f. $f_X(x) \propto \exp(-\theta x)$. Note that the prior distribution for i_κ has support $(-\infty, r_1)$, which is sensible because the initial infection time must occur before the first removal. The actual choice of the prior parameters (i.e. m_β, λ_β etc.) is arbitrary, although we discuss some common choices later on.

9.4.5   MCMC algorithm

When constructing an MCMC algorithm, it is usually fruitful to start by looking at the full conditional densities of the parameters that need updating. This amounts to writing the target density as a function of the parameter of interest. For example,

$$\pi(\beta|\boldsymbol{i},\boldsymbol{r},\gamma,\kappa,i_\kappa) \propto \pi(\boldsymbol{i},\boldsymbol{r}|\beta,\gamma,\kappa,i_\kappa)\pi(\beta)$$
$$\propto \beta^{n-1+m_\beta-1} \exp\left\{-\beta\left(\frac{1}{N}\int_{i_\kappa}^{r_n} S(t)I(t)\,dt + \lambda_\beta\right)\right\},$$

so in this case we have

$$\beta|\boldsymbol{i},\boldsymbol{r},\gamma,\kappa,i_\kappa \sim \Gamma\left(n+m_\beta-1, \frac{1}{N}\int_{i_\kappa}^{r_n} S(t)I(t)\,dt + \lambda_\beta\right). \qquad (9.7)$$

Since the full conditional distribution for β has a standard form, we could update β using a Gibbs step within an MCMC algorithm. Note that we could equally use a Metropolis-Hastings step instead, but doing so involves more computations (since we need to evaluate the acceptance probability), and fails to take advantage of the information contained in (9.7). Similar calculations for γ yield

$$\gamma|\boldsymbol{i},\boldsymbol{r},\beta,\kappa,i_\kappa \sim \Gamma\left(n+m_\gamma, \sum_{j=1}^{n}(r_j - i_j) + \lambda_\gamma\right). \qquad (9.8)$$

The remaining parameters i, κ and i_κ are less straightforward to deal with. Now,

$$\pi(i, \kappa, i_\kappa | r, \beta, \gamma) \propto \left\{ \prod_{j \neq \kappa} I(i_j -) \right\} \exp\left\{ -\frac{\beta}{N} \int_{i_\kappa}^{r_n} S(t)I(t)\, dt \right\}$$

$$\times \exp\left\{ -\gamma \sum_{j=1}^{n} (r_j - i_j) \right\} \exp\left\{ -(r_1 - i_\kappa)\theta \right\},$$

and note that in addition to the explicit appearance of terms such as i_j and i_κ, in fact the $I(i_j-)$, $S(t)$ and $I(t)$ terms also depend upon the values of i and i_κ. Although it is possible to derive analytic expressions for the full conditional distributions for individual infection times, in practice it is easier to use a Metropolis-Hastings step. This approach requires us to find a way of proposing new values of i, i_κ and κ; there are many ways to do this, one of which is to select an individual i_j at random, and propose their infectious period from a density g. Although g is arbitrary, a sensible choice is to use the actual infectious period distribution, i.e., $\text{Exp}(\gamma)$.

Algorithm 9.4 Updating the infection times

1: Select an individual j uniformly at random from $1, \ldots, n$.
2: Propose a new infection time $i_j^* = r_j - X$, where $X > 0$ has p.d.f. g.
3: Evaluate the acceptance probability

$$\alpha = \min\left\{ 1, \frac{\pi(i^*, i_\kappa^*, \kappa^* | r, \beta, \gamma) g(r_j - i_j)}{\pi(i, i_\kappa, \kappa | r, \beta, \gamma) g(r_j - i_j^*)} \right\}.$$

4: With probability α, accept the proposed new value i_j^*;
5: Otherwise, i_j remains at its current value.

In Algorithm 9.4, note that when i_j^* is proposed, it is possible that new values of i_κ and κ also are proposed by default, since these quantities are, respectively, the minimum of all the infection times, and the identity of the individual with the minimum infection time. So the quantities i_κ^* and κ^* in the Algorithm 9.4 may be the same as i_κ and κ, or may be different. A further consequence of this is that Algorithm 9.4 is sufficient to update all the infection time parameters, and we do not require separate updating steps for i_κ and κ.

Finally, in practice it is sensible to perform the infection time update step several times in each iteration of the MCMC algorithm. This method is to help the chain move around the state space; if we only updated one infection time each iteration, the distributions of β and γ at (9.7) and (9.8) would not change appreciably and it would take longer to obtain suitable samples for these two parameters.

9.4.6   Example: SIR model given removal data

In this section we shall apply the algorithm described in Section 9.4.5 to a simulated data set and illustrate how the algorithm behaves.

Data. We considered a population of size $N = 100$ individuals of whom one is initially infective and the rest susceptible. A realization from an SIR model with $\beta = 2$ and $\gamma = 1$ was simulated and resulted in $n = 78$ individuals becoming infected, including the initial infective. Figure 9.1 shows the cumulative number of removed individuals at time t, $R(t) = N - S(t) - I(t)$.

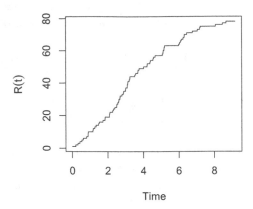

FIGURE 9.1

The cumulative number of removals, $R(t)$, through time for a simulated dataset from the SIR model.

Prior distributions. We assigned independent exponential distributions with rates 10^{-4} to β and γ, i.e., $m_\beta = m_\gamma = 1$ and $\lambda_\beta = \lambda_\gamma = 10^{-4}$. These values correspond to vague prior distributions on the parameters, essentially because these distributions have high variance and their density functions are relatively flat. Equations (9.7) and (9.8) reveal more precisely how these prior choices impact the full conditional distributions of β and γ; from these it is clear that, the larger the values of m_β, λ_β, m_γ and λ_γ, then the larger the impact on the full conditional distributions. It is tempting to conclude that setting all four values to zero would provide a truly uninformative prior distribution, but the problem arises that setting $m_\beta = 0$ or $m_\gamma = 0$ makes the prior distribution sharply peaked at zero, which impacts the resulting inference. Thus, our choice of exponential distribution, in which $m_\beta = m_\gamma = 1$, avoids this problem. Similarly, we assign a prior distribution to the initial infection time i_κ by setting $r_1 - i_\kappa$ to be exponentially distribution with rate 10^{-2}. Finally, a discrete uniform prior distribution on the integers $1, \ldots, 78$ was assigned to represent our ignorance about the identity of the initial infective.

MCMC algorithm. We ran the MCMC algorithm below for $M = 50,000$ iterations. In each iteration the infection time update step, in which we choose an infection time update it, was repeated $n/2 = 78/2 = 39$ times. We illustrate the impact of other choices.

Algorithm 9.5 MCMC Algorithm for the SIR model given removal data

---

1: Choose initial values for β, γ and i.

2: **repeat**

3:     Update β by drawing from $\pi(\beta|i, r, \gamma, k, i_k)$.

4:     Update γ by drawing from $\pi(\gamma|i, r, \beta, k, i_k)$.

5:     **for** $i = 1$ to 39 **do**

6:         Choose j uniformly at random from the set $\{1, 2, \ldots, 78\}$;

7:         update i_j using Algorithm 9.4.

8:     **end for**

9: **until** desired number of iterations is reached.

Trace plots. The panels at the top of Figure 9.2 show the trace plots of the Markov Chain for β and γ obtained from the MCMC algorithm in which the step of updating the infec-

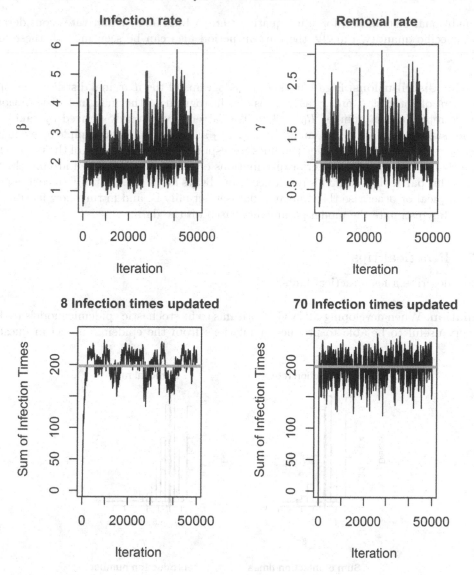

FIGURE 9.2
SIR model: Trace plots of the Markov chain for β and γ (top) and the sum of the infection times when either 8 or 70 infection times are updated in each MCMC iteration (bottom). The grey horizontal lines show the true values.

tion times was repeated 39 times in each iteration. The horizontal lines correspond to the true values of the parameters. Both panels show the initial burn-in phase during which the Markov chain moves towards stationarity. The panels at the bottom are the trace plots of $\sum_{j=1}^{78} i_j$ when either 8 (left) or 70 (right) infection times are updated in each iteration. These graphs illustrate that the more infection times are updated during each iteration, the better the *mixing* of the Markov chain, i.e., the speed with which the chain explores the state space. There are two reasons why we choose to look at the trace plot of the sum of infection times. The first reason is that looking at each of the 78 infection times individually would be highly time consuming, and so considering only the sum provides some kind of summary information. The second reason is that, in this particular example, the sum appears in the full conditional distribution for γ in equation (9.8), which further motivates consideration of this specific quantity. Finally, the burn-in period also can be seen in both these lower panels.

Posterior distributions. Figure 9.3 shows histograms of the marginal distributions of the parameters of interest β and γ as well as the histogram of the marginal distribution of the basic reproduction number $R_0 = \beta/\gamma$. The latter is very easily derived by taking the posterior samples $\beta_1, \beta_2, \ldots, \beta_M$ and $\gamma_1, \gamma_2, \ldots, \gamma_M$ and creating a new sample by evaluating $\beta_1/\gamma_1, \beta_2/\gamma_2, \ldots, \beta_M/\gamma_M$. The vertical lines correspond to the true values of the parameters. We see that both marginal posterior distributions of β and γ are centered around the true values in this particular case. This result need not always happen, essentially since it depends on how typical or otherwise the simulated dataset actually is, and in turn how feasible it is to accurately estimate the model parameters based on the data.

9.4.7 Practical tips

We now describe a few practical hints.

Simulation. When developing MCMC algorithms to fit stochastic epidemic models to data, it is very useful to be able to produce simulations from the epidemic model in question.

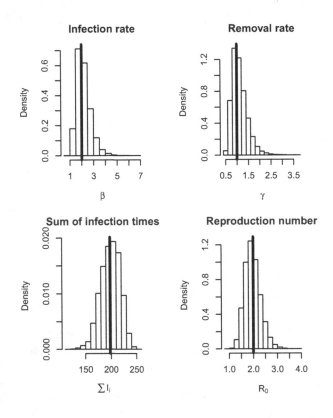

FIGURE 9.3
SIR model: Histograms of the marginal posterior distributions of the infection rate, removal rate, reproduction number, and the sum of the infection times. The bold vertical lines show the true values.

By *simulation* we mean "producing a realization of the model." For the SIR model, this means producing a set of infection and removal times according to the correct distributions inherent in the model. Simulation is useful for four key reasons in this setting. The first is that simulating the model gives some idea how it behaves and whether or not it is capable of producing outcomes that appear realistic. The second is that it can be used to test and validate MCMC code; if we simulate numerous realizations of the epidemic model, with known fixed parameter values, and in each case use an MCMC algorithm to obtain parameter estimates, then we would expect the resulting distribution of these estimates (such as posterior means) to be more or less centered around the true values. If this does not occur then this can indicate an error in the MCMC code, or the inference procedure. The third use of simulation is that it can be used for model assessment. If we estimate model parameter values from a dataset, and then put these estimates back into the epidemic model and simulate it many times, we would hope to see the observed data lying somewhere inside the resulting distribution of outcomes. Conversely, if such simulations consistently look materially different from the observed data, then this suggests that the epidemic model is not adequate. The fourth use of simulation is prediction, meaning that we can use simulations from our model to explore possible what-if scenarios, or make predictions in real-time about the possible future course of an epidemic.

Coding. When writing an MCMC algorithm, it is often very useful to write the different pieces of code separately. For example, to evaluate the likelihood (9.3) it is practically useful to have different a piece of code which computes the integral $\int_{i_k}^{r_n} S(t)I(t)\,dt$ and another piece of code which computes the product term: $\prod_{j \neq \kappa} \frac{\beta}{N} I(i_j-)$. Most MCMC algorithms in this field involve various components, e.g., Gibbs updates, Metropolis-Hastings updates, likelihood evaluations, etc., and it is good practice to carefully check that each component works before proceeding.

Many likelihoods require calculation of products which can in turn lead to numerical instabilities and run-time errors. One way to tackle this issue is to instead work with the log likelihood. The likelihood may involve the calculation of Beta or Gamma functions. For example, R has built-in functions to compute such quantities, i.e. `beta`, `gamma`, but if we are working on the log scale then instead of using `log(gamma(k))`, then we could use the built-in function `lgamma(k)` to improve numerical stability, especially if `k` is large.

9.5 Beyond the SIR Model

The key ideas of using MCMC methods with data augmentation can be applied to numerous other epidemic models and kinds of data. Here we discuss some possible extensions.

9.5.1 General infectious period distributions

In the previous section we assumed that the SIR model of interest had infectious periods distributed according to an exponential distribution. For most infectious diseases such an assumption is not very realistic, and it is preferable to use an alternative distribution such as a Gamma or Weibull distribution. Both of these are two-parameter distributions which enable us to separate the mean and variance of the distribution, unlike the exponential distribution in which the mean determines the variance.

Suppose that the p.d.f. of the infectious period distribution is $f(x|\eta)$, $x \geq 0$, where η is the parameter vector of the distribution. The augmented likelihood corresponding to such a model is given by

$$\pi(\boldsymbol{i}, \boldsymbol{r}|\beta, \eta, \kappa, i_\kappa) = \left\{ \prod_{j \neq \kappa} \frac{\beta}{N} I(i_j-) \right\} \exp\left\{ -\frac{\beta}{N} \int_{i_\kappa}^{r_n} S(t)I(t)\, dt \right\}$$

$$\times \prod_{j=1}^{n} f(r_j - i_j|\eta), \tag{9.9}$$

and it is easy to see that (9.3) is a special case of (9.9). An MCMC algorithm can be constructed in much the same way as before, but instead of an update for γ we now need to update the components of η. Depending on the distribution in question, this may require Metropolis-Hastings steps as opposed to Gibbs steps.

9.5.2   Latent periods

In real life, the ability to transmit an infectious pathogen to other individuals does not usually begin immediately, but after a period of time called the *latent period*. Incorporating this into the SIR model yields the SEIR model (Susceptible-Exposed-Infective-Removed). In this model, susceptible individuals who contact infectives are said to be *exposed*, and after their latent period they become infective as in the SIR model. Thus, the meaning of i_j, the "infection time" of individual j, is now slightly different. Specifically, like the SIR model, i_j is the time that j begins their infectious period, but unlike the SIR model, it is not the time that j was first "infected" with the pathogen.

The corresponding augmented likelihood can be derived as follows. As before, let $\boldsymbol{r}$ denote removal times, but now let $\boldsymbol{i}$ denote *all* infection times $i_1, \ldots, i_n$. Let e_j denote the exposure time of individual j, and as before let κ denote the identity of the first individual to become infective; note that this individual is also the first individual to become exposed. Let $\boldsymbol{e}$ denote all exposure times other than e_κ. Then we have

$$\pi(\boldsymbol{e}, \boldsymbol{i}, \boldsymbol{r}|\beta, \eta, \xi, \kappa, e_\kappa) = \left\{ \prod_{j \neq \kappa} \frac{\beta}{N} I(e_j-) \right\} \exp\left\{ -\frac{\beta}{N} \int_{i_\kappa}^{r_n} S(t)I(t)\, dt \right\}$$

$$\times \prod_{j=1}^{n} f(r_j - i_j|\eta)g(i_j - e_j|\xi), \tag{9.10}$$

where $f(x|\eta)$ and $g(x|\xi)$ denote, respectively, the p.d.f. of the infectious period and latent period distribution. Note that the lower limit of the integral is i_κ; we could equally use e_κ, but since there are no infectives in the population during the time interval $[e_\kappa, i_\kappa)$ then the integrand would be zero on that range.

By following the recipe for the SIR model, we can construct an MCMC algorithm to sample from the joint posterior density $\pi(\beta, \eta, \xi, \boldsymbol{e}, \boldsymbol{i}, \kappa, e_\kappa|\boldsymbol{r})$. However, one issue here is that we are asking rather a lot of the data $\boldsymbol{r}$; specifically, introducing exposure times as well as infection times in our augmentation scheme means that we are essentially trying to estimate two unknown times for each single observation. This approach in turn means that the model is over-parameterized, and within the MCMC scheme we would see strong correlations between parameters. For example, there is nothing in the data to distinguish between scenarios in which (1) latent periods are short, infectious periods are long and the infection rate β is low or (2) latent periods are long, infectious periods are short and β

is high. In practice, it therefore may be necessary to put more informative prior information into the modeling of the latent and/or infectious periods, or even fixing the parameters of one to practically realistic values. One such simple approach is to set latent periods to be of fixed length c, and perform a sensitivity analysis by trying different c values.

9.5.3 General infection rates

In the standard SIR model, there is a single parameter β to govern the infection process. In many real-life settings, the process of transmission between individuals might vary across the population due to many factors such as the status of individuals (e.g., age, vaccination history) or their location (schools, households, workplaces). It can therefore be useful to generalize the SIR model to one in which an infective i makes contact with a susceptible j according to a Poisson process of rate β_{ij}. Define $\boldsymbol{\beta} = \{\beta_{ij} : i, j = 1, \ldots, N\}$. The corresponding augmented likelihood of this model, incorporating a general infectious distribution and using our earlier notation, is

$$
\pi(\boldsymbol{i}, \boldsymbol{r} | \boldsymbol{\beta}, \eta, \kappa, i_\kappa) = \left\{ \prod_{j \neq \kappa} \sum_{k:i_k < i_j < r_k} \beta_{kj} \right\} \exp \left\{ - \sum_{j=1}^{n} \sum_{k=1}^{N} \beta_{jk} (r_j \wedge i_k - i_j \wedge i_k) \right\}
$$
$$
\times \prod_{j=1}^{n} f(r_j - i_j | \eta). \tag{9.11}
$$

In practice, we are not usually interested in such a general model, but one in which β_{ij} has a prescribed form. Examples include household models, in which, e.g., $\beta_{ij} = \beta_H$ if i and j live in the same household and $\beta_{ij} = \beta$ otherwise, spatial models (e.g., for spread of plant or animal diseases) in which β_{ij} is a function of the distance between i and j, and models in which β_{ij} is a function of the ages of i and j (e.g., child-child, adult-child or adult-child combinations). In each case the resulting model has only a few transmission parameters and is therefore amenable to estimation.

9.5.4 Network epidemic models

Another way to improve the realism of the standard SIR model is to relax the underlying assumption of a homogeneously mixing population. One approach is to consider a random graph G in which nodes correspond to individuals and edges correspond to potential contacts between individuals. Given a realization of G, an SIR model then can be propagated on the graph; in the simplest setting, each infective individual has infectious contacts with susceptibles with whom they share an edge according to independent Poisson processes of rate β.

If data on the removal process is available, but we have no information about the realization of G, then an augmented likelihood can be obtained by introducing the realization as an additional (high-dimensional) model parameter. Specifically, if G has parameter vector ψ, the joint posterior density of interest is

$$
\pi(\beta, \eta, \boldsymbol{i}, \kappa, i_\kappa, G, \psi | \boldsymbol{r}) \propto \pi(\boldsymbol{i}, \boldsymbol{r} | \beta, \eta, \kappa, i_\kappa, G) \pi(G | \psi).
$$

To see this, note that the likelihood of a realization of the epidemic, given G, is obtained in a similar manner to (9.11), and we additionally require the likelihood of G given its parameter ψ.

9.6   Example: The 1816 Hagelloch Measles Epidemic

In this section we consider a dataset that describes an historical outbreak of measles in 1861 in the German village of Hagelloch as described in [3]. The outbreak was very severe, as every one of $N = 188$ individuals deemed to be susceptible became infected, these individuals all being children. The data themselves are unusually detailed, consisting for each case of the name, age, sex, date of symptom onset, date of rash onset, class of child in the village school, date of death if this occurred, most likely source of infection, number of days between date of symptom onset in likely infector and infected, complications due to other diseases, location of the child's home, number of cases within the family, maximum temperature, and day of maximum fever.

These data have been considered by a number of authors using different epidemic models of varying complexity. Here, for illustration, we consider the following model taken from [4]. Label the individuals $1, \ldots, N$. Each individual belongs to a household and the community, and either attends school or is of pre-school age. If an individual becomes infected, they undergo a symptom-free infectious period which is assumed to follow a $\Gamma(\omega, \delta)$ distribution, where $\omega = 30$ is fixed and δ is a model parameter. The value $\omega = 30$ is largely chosen for illustration, but such a value means that the coefficient of variation of the symptom-free period is $1/\sqrt{30} \approx 0.18$, meaning that we do not allow much relative variability. As in the previous discussion of latent periods, it would be hard to estimate both ω and δ separately, so fixing one parameter is also pragmatic. At the end of the symptom-free period, the individual displays symptoms and subsequently develops a rash. Both the symptom and rash appearance dates are given by the data and so we do not model the times of these events. Following the rash appearance, the individual is assumed to be recover 3 days later, unless they die first as indicated by the data. An individual is thus removed at either recovery or death, if sooner. The infectious period is assumed to start immediately after initial infection and continue until removal or death.

We assume that, while infectious, individual i makes infectious contacts with susceptible individual j at rate β_{ij} where β_{ij} depends on the relationship of individuals i and j. Any such contact immediately results in the susceptible becoming infected and entering the symptom-free part of the infectious period. The model of [4] assumes that

$$\beta_{ij} = \beta_H \, \chi_{\{\rho(i,j)=0\}} + \beta_C^1 \, \chi_{\{L_i=L_j=1\}} + \beta_C^2 \, \chi_{\{L_i=L_j=2\}} + \beta_G \exp\{-\theta \rho(i,j)\} \qquad (9.12)$$

where $\rho(i,j)$ denotes the Euclidean distance between the households of individuals i and j, L_i denotes the school classroom (either 1 or 2) which individual i belongs to, and $L_i = 0$ if individual i is of pre-school age. The non-negative parameters β_H, β_C^1, and β_C^2 denote the within-household, within-classroom 1, and within-classroom 2 infection rates, respectively. Finally, β_G denotes the global infection rate while θ governs the extent to which distance between individuals reduces the infection rate.

For individual j, denote by i_j, s_j and r_j their infection time, symptom-appearance time, and removal time, respectively. Thus s_j and r_j are fixed according to the data and modeling assumptions, the symptom-free period is $s_j - i_j \sim \Gamma(\omega, \delta)$ and the infectious period is $r_j - i_j$. Let $\boldsymbol{i}$, $\boldsymbol{s}$ and $\boldsymbol{r}$ denote, respectively, the vectors of infection, symptom, and removal times, where as usual $\boldsymbol{i}$ does not include the initial infection time, i_κ, of the initial infective, κ. The likelihood of the observed data is

$$\pi(\boldsymbol{i},\boldsymbol{s},\boldsymbol{r}|\beta_H,\beta_C^1,\beta_C^2,\beta_G,\theta,\delta,\kappa,i_\kappa)$$

$$= \left\{ \prod_{j\neq\kappa} \sum_{k:i_k<i_j<r_k} \beta_{kj} \right\} \exp\left\{ -\sum_{j=1}^{N}\sum_{k=1}^{N} \beta_{jk}(r_j \wedge i_k - i_j \wedge i_k) \right\}$$

$$\times \prod_{j=1}^{N} f(s_j - i_j|\delta), \qquad\qquad (9.13)$$

where f denotes the probability density function of a $\Gamma(30,\delta)$ random variable and β_{kj} is given by (9.12).

Our objective is to perform Bayesian inference for all model parameters, namely β_H, β_C^1, $\beta_C^2, \beta_G, \theta$ and δ. Independent exponential prior distributions with rate 0.1 were assigned to all parameters.

We used an MCMC algorithm similar to the one described in Section 9.4.5. First note that, unlike the SIR model, the full conditional distributions of the infection rate parameters are no longer standard, so instead these were all updated using *Gaussian random walk Metropolis* steps. This approach simply means using a Gaussian proposal distribution centered on the current value. For example, to update β_H, we proposed a new value from $\beta_H^* \sim N(\beta_H, \sigma_H^2)$, where σ_H^2 is the proposal variance, and then accepted or rejected the proposed move according to the Metropolis-Hastings ratio given in Algorithm 9.1. One advantage of using a Gaussian proposal is that, since the density is symmetric about its mean, the q terms in Algorithm 9.1 cancel. The proposal variance σ_H^2 usually requires manual tuning; too small a value leads to frequent acceptances but very small steps, while too large a value leads to infrequent acceptances and the Markov chain remaining in the same state for many iterations. The parameter θ was also updated in this way. Conversely, δ has a standard full conditional distribution, specifically that

$$\delta|\boldsymbol{i},\boldsymbol{s},\boldsymbol{r},\beta_H,\beta_C^1,\beta_C^2,\beta_G,\theta,\kappa,i_\kappa \sim \Gamma\left(\omega N+1, 0.1+\sum_j(s_j-i_j)\right),$$

which follows directly from (9.13) and the prior assumptions, and so δ can be updated using a Gibbs step.

Finally, to update infection times, we used a Metropolis-Hastings step. Specifically we choose an infection time i_j uniformly at random, proposed a new infection time i_j^* by $i_j^* = s_j - X$, where $X \sim \text{Gamma}(30,\delta)$, and then evaluated the acceptance probability as usual. To help the mixing, we updated all infection times during each iteration of the algorithm.

Results for all six model parameters are shown in Figure 9.4. We see, for example, that the transmission rates in households and within classroom 1 are largest which suggests that these two transmission routes were of key importance during the outbreak. Conversely the posterior distributions of β_G and θ suggest that the purely spatial components of the transmission were far less relevant.

In this section we have illustrated that the inference methods described for the SIR model can be readily adapted to a far more complex epidemic model. As for the SIR model, the key practical steps required are to write down a likelihood, derive full conditional distributions, and then design the MCMC algorithm accordingly.

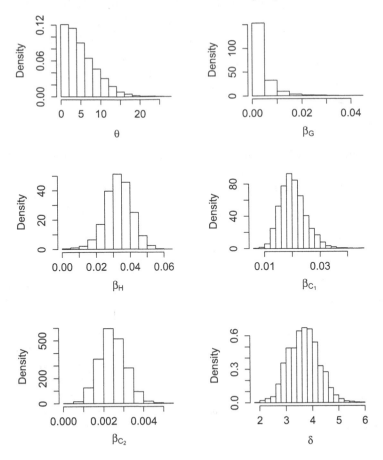

FIGURE 9.4
Hagelloch data: Marginal posterior distributions of the parameters governing the transmission rate β_{ij} and the symptom-free part of the infectious period distribution (δ).

9.7   Concluding Comments

9.7.1   Pros and cons of MCMC methods for outbreak data

Methods of the kind we have described have many positive aspects. First, as illustrated in this chapter the methods are highly flexible and can be adapted to a great many different situations of interest. One particularly notable feature is that the underlying transmission model need not be a Markov process, which is useful in practice since stages of disease (such as latent or infectious periods) are rarely well described by exponential distributions. Second, the methods are relatively straightforward to implement in the sense that they do not usually require extensive algebraic calculations or complicated numerical procedures. Of course, more complex models and datasets may require a lot more bookkeeping within the MCMC code, so the methods can still be rather non-trivial to implement. Third, since the methods are sample-based then it is possible to derive estimates not only of basic model parameters, but associated quantities of interest. Fourth, the methods provide something of a "gold standard" in the sense that they seek to provide samples from the posterior distribution of interest, but without resorting to approximations of any kind within the modelling itself.

There are two main difficulties with MCMC methods, or more particularly with the use of data augmentation within MCMC. The first is that as the amount of data augmentation increases, so the mixing of the Markov chain deteriorates. This result in turn means that it takes far longer to obtain reliable samples from the target distribution. The second difficulty is that the methods require a likelihood, or at least the ability to compute an augmented likelihood. In some situations this is infeasible, either because the amount of data augmentation required is prohibitively large, or because the likelihood itself is intractable. For both of these problems, some of the other methods described in this volume, such as ABC methods or Sequential Monte Carlo methods, can be of use.

9.7.2 Further reading

Our aim in this chapter has been to introduce the key ideas and methods for using MCMC algorithms to analyze data from infectious disease outbreaks within a Bayesian statistical framework. Further introductory material can be found in [5–8] and more advanced techniques for improving MCMC algorithms for epidemic models can be found in [9, 10]. Examples and applications include hospital infections [11], household epidemic models [12, 13], epidemic models on networks [14], spatio-temporal epidemic models [15], smallpox [16] and outbreaks with genomic data [17].

References

[1] Christian P. Robert. *The Bayesian Choice: From Decision-Theoretic Foundations to Computational Implementation, 2nd edition.* Springer, New York, 2007.

[2] Walter R. Gilks, Sylvia Richardson, and David J. Spiegelhalter. *Markov Chain Monte Carlo in Practice.* Chapman & Hall, London, UK, 1996.

[3] Albert Pfeilsticker. *Beiträge zur Pathologie der Masern mit besonderer Berücksichtgung der Statistischen Verhältnisse.* PhD thesis, Eberhard-Karls-Universität, Tübingen, Germany, 1861.

[4] Peter J. Neal and Gareth O. Roberts. Statistical inference and model selection for the 1861 Hagelloch measles epidemic. *Biostatistics*, 5(2):249–261, 2004.

[5] Gavin J. Gibson and Eric Renshaw. Estimating parameters in stochastic compartmental models using Markov chain methods. *Mathematical Medicine and Biology*, 15(1): 19–40, 1998.

[6] Philip D. O'Neill. A tutorial introduction to Bayesian inference for stochastic epidemic models using Markov chain Monte Carlo methods. *Mathematical Biosciences*, 180(1):103–114, 2002.

[7] Philip D. O'Neill. Introduction and snapshot review: Relating infectious disease transmission models to data. *Statistics in Medicine*, 29(20):2069–2077, 2010.

[8] Philip D. O'Neill and Gareth O. Roberts. Bayesian inference for partially observed stochastic epidemics. *Journal of the Royal Statistical Society: Series A (Statistics in Society)*, 162(1):121–129, 1999.

[9] Theodore Kypraios. *Efficient Bayesian inference for partially observed stochastic epidemics and a new class of semi-parametric time series models.* PhD thesis, Lancaster University, Lancaster, UK, 2007.

[10] Peter J. Neal and Gareth O. Roberts. A case study in non-centering for data augmentation: Stochastic epidemics. *Statistics and Computing*, 15(4):315–327, 2005.

[11] Theodore Kypraios, Philip D. O'Neill, Susan S. Huang, Sheryl L. Rifas-Shiman, and Ben S. Cooper. Assessing the role of undetected colonization and isolation precautions in reducing Methicillin-Resistant Staphylococcus aureus transmission in intensive care units. *BMC Infectious Diseases*, 10(29), 2010.

[12] Nikolaos Demiris and Philip D. O'Neill. Bayesian inference for stochastic multitype epidemics in structured populations via random graphs. *Journal of the Royal Statistical Society: Series B (Statistical Methodology)*, 67(5):731–745, 2005.

[13] Edward S. Knock and Philip D. O'Neill. Bayesian model choice for epidemic models with two levels of mixing. *Biostatistics*, 15(1):46–59, 2014.

[14] Tom Britton and Philip D O'Neill. Bayesian inference for stochastic epidemics in populations with random social structure. *Scandinavian Journal of Statistics*, 29(3):375–390, 2002.

[15] Alex Cook, Glenn Marion, Adam Butler, and Gavin Gibson. Bayesian inference for the spatio-temporal invasion of alien species. *Bulletin of Mathematical Biology*, 69(6):2005–2025, 2007.

[16] Jessica E. Stockdale, Philip D. O'Neill, and Theodore Kypraios. Modelling and Bayesian analysis of the Abakaliki smallpox data. *Epidemics*, 19:13–23, 2017.

[17] Colin J. Worby, Philip D. O'Neill, Theodore Kypraios, Julie V. Robotham, Daniela De Angelis, Edward J. P. Cartwright, Sharon J. Peacock, and Ben S. Cooper. Reconstructing transmission trees for communicable diseases using densely sampled genetic data. *The Annals of Applied Statistics*, 10(1):395, 2016.

10

Approximate Bayesian Computation Methods for Epidemic Models

Peter J. Neal

CONTENTS

10.1 Introduction

In this chapter we consider how approximate Bayesian computation (ABC) methods can be used in estimating the (unknown) parameters θ of a parametric model (stochastic process) $\mathcal{M}$, where in our case the parametric model $\mathcal{M}$ will be a stochastic epidemic process. We assume that $\mathcal{M}$ gives rise to realizations $\mathbf{X}$ with the observed data $\mathbf{x}^*$ being one such realization. The foundations for ABC, along with all Bayesian statistics, is Bayes' Theorem which states that

$$\pi(\theta|\mathbf{x}^*) = \frac{\pi(\mathbf{x}^*|\theta)\pi(\theta)}{\pi(\mathbf{x}^*)}, \tag{10.1}$$

where $\pi(\theta|\mathbf{x}^*)$, $\pi(\mathbf{x}^*|\theta)$, $\pi(\theta)$, and $\pi(\mathbf{x}^*)$ denote the posterior density, the likelihood, the prior density, and the marginal likelihood, respectively. We observe that the four components of (10.1) are either probability density or mass functions with the posterior density, the distribution of the parameters θ given the observed data $\mathbf{x}^*$, of primary interest and the focus of this chapter. In Bayesian statistics, we obtain a posterior distribution for the parameters conditional on the data as opposed to obtaining a point estimate for the parameters. From the posterior distribution we can obtain summary statistics such as the (posterior) mean, mode, and variance of the parameters with the latter giving a measure of parameter uncertainty. We also can use the posterior distribution to explore hypotheses concerning the parameters.

The construction of the posterior density is based on the three quantities on the right-hand side of (10.1). The role of the likelihood, $\pi(\mathbf{x}^*|\theta)$, demonstrates that Bayesian statistical inference is a likelihood based method. The prior density $\pi(\theta)$ quantifies knowledge or beliefs about the parameters *prior* to the collection of data. The weight or importance given to our prior beliefs are reflected through our choice of prior density. This choice could reflect substantive knowledge about parameters, for example, from previous epidemic outbreaks, or vague prior information for the parameters for a newly emerging pathogen. The marginal likelihood, also known as the (model) evidence, is given by

$$\pi(\mathbf{x}^*) = \int \pi(\mathbf{x}^*|\boldsymbol{\theta})\pi(\boldsymbol{\theta})\,d\boldsymbol{\theta}. \tag{10.2}$$

Except in a few simple special cases it is not possible to derive an analytical expression for the posterior density $\pi(\boldsymbol{\theta}|\mathbf{x}^*)$ due to complications in computing all the components on the right-hand side of (10.1). The first complication is the marginal likelihood (normalizing constant), $\pi(\mathbf{x}^*)$ through the integral given in (10.2), which is rarely tractable. The second possible complication is computation of the likelihood, $\pi(\mathbf{x}^*|\boldsymbol{\theta})$, which is often not straightforward based upon the available data $\mathbf{x}^*$.

The general solution to not being able to derive the posterior distribution for all but the simplest models is to obtain samples from the posterior distribution using computational methods. The most popular such approach is Markov chain Monte Carlo (MCMC), see [1] and the references therein. MCMC is a serial algorithm for obtaining (dependent) samples $\boldsymbol{\theta}_1, \boldsymbol{\theta}_2, \dots, \boldsymbol{\theta}_N$ from $\pi(\boldsymbol{\theta}|\mathbf{x}^*)$. For $i = 1, 2, \dots, N-1$, given $\boldsymbol{\theta}_i$, a new value for $\boldsymbol{\theta}$ is proposed, $\boldsymbol{\theta}^*$ for example, according to a proposal probability density $q(\cdot|\boldsymbol{\theta}_i)$, which can depend explicitly on $\boldsymbol{\theta}_i$. An acceptance probability

$$A = \min\left\{1, \frac{\pi(\boldsymbol{\theta}^*|\mathbf{x}^*)q(\boldsymbol{\theta}_i|\boldsymbol{\theta}^*)}{\pi(\boldsymbol{\theta}_i|\mathbf{x}^*)q(\boldsymbol{\theta}^*|\boldsymbol{\theta}_i)}\right\}$$

$$= \min\left\{1, \frac{\pi(\mathbf{x}^*|\boldsymbol{\theta}^*)\pi(\boldsymbol{\theta}^*)q(\boldsymbol{\theta}_i|\boldsymbol{\theta}^*)}{\pi(\mathbf{x}^*|\boldsymbol{\theta}_i)\pi(\boldsymbol{\theta}_i)q(\boldsymbol{\theta}^*|\boldsymbol{\theta}_i)}\right\} \tag{10.3}$$

is computed with $\boldsymbol{\theta}_{i+1}$ set equal to $\boldsymbol{\theta}^*$ with probability A and $\boldsymbol{\theta}_{i+1} = \boldsymbol{\theta}_i$ otherwise. The success of MCMC is that, as can be seen in the second line of (10.3), it is not necessary compute $\pi(\mathbf{x}^*)$. However, MCMC requires a tractable likelihood, possibly through the use of data augmentation. That is, we assume that in addition to $\mathbf{X}$, there exists $\mathbf{Y}$, unobserved or unobservable, such that if we observed a realization $\mathbf{y}$ of $\mathbf{Y}$, we could obtain a tractable likelihood $\pi(\mathbf{x}^*, \mathbf{y}|\boldsymbol{\theta})$. We then can adjust the MCMC algorithm to obtain samples from $\pi(\boldsymbol{\theta}, \mathbf{y}|\mathbf{x}^*)$. Large-scale data augmentation can be problematic for MCMC, especially if there is strong correlation between the augmented data, $\mathbf{y}$, and model parameters $\boldsymbol{\theta}$ which can affect performance of the algorithm. Thus, alternatives to MCMC are sought.

For many stochastic epidemic models, as with many stochastic processes, simulation of a realization of an epidemic given a model and parameters is usually straightforward. This approach raises the question, can we use simulation to assist with parameter estimation? Approximate Bayesian computation (ABC) gives us a range of techniques for answering this in the affirmative. Moreover, ABC and simulation based methods more generally have the desirable properties of producing independent samples from the posterior distribution and are trivially parallelizable as opposed to MCMC which produces dependent samples and is inherently serial in its construction.

The aim of this chapter is to give an overview of simulation-based inference for epidemics. This overview starts with the *vanilla* ABC algorithm, a simple rejection algorithm which samples parameters from their prior distribution and decides whether or not to accept the parameter values on the basis of the *closeness* of a simulated data set to the observed data.

We investigate various ways in which simulation-based inference can improve upon the vanilla ABC algorithm by considering the selection of parameters for the simulations, the simulation process to ensure closer agreement between the simulated and observed data and how to determine how closeness is measured. Throughout we demonstrate a trade-off between the simplicity of implementing vanilla ABC and the efficiency gains available from taking a more sophisticated approach to simulation.

The remainder of the chapter is structured as follows. In Section 10.2 we give an overview of ABC with extensions discussed in Section 10.3. In Sections 10.4 and 10.5, we apply the methods to two contrasting datasets to illustrate the wide scope of ABC. In Section 10.4 we consider final outcome data (the total numbers infected) in a measles epidemic in a school estimating the infection rate and the protective effect of vaccination. In Section 10.5 we study a spatial epidemic model for *citrus tristeza virus* (CTV) with the data consisting of two snapshots of the epidemic taken a year apart. The parameters of interest are the rate of infection and the spatial transmission kernel parameters. Finally in Section 10.6 we make some concluding remarks and provide examples of where ABC has been applied to stochastic models in the literature.

10.2 Introduction to Approximate Bayesian Computation

In this section, we introduce the ABC algorithm before discussing extensions to the ABC algorithm in Section 10.3. The starting point is the EBC (exact Bayesian computation) algorithm (Algorithm 10.1), which uses an unbiased estimator of the likelihood $\pi(\mathbf{x}^*|\boldsymbol{\theta})$ to provide *i.i.d.* samples from $\pi(\boldsymbol{\theta}|\mathbf{x}^*)$. The EBC algorithm (Algorithm 10.1) is only appropriate for discrete data, where $\pi(\mathbf{x}^*|\boldsymbol{\theta}) = \mathbb{P}(\mathbf{X} = \mathbf{x}^*|\boldsymbol{\theta})$ is a probability mass function.

Algorithm 10.1 EBC algorithm

For $i = 1, 2, \ldots, N$:

1: Sample $\boldsymbol{\theta}_i$ from $\pi(\cdot)$.
2: Simulate data $\mathbf{x}_i$ from the model $\mathcal{M}$ using parameters $\boldsymbol{\theta}_i$.
3: If $\mathbf{x}_i = \mathbf{x}^*$, set $\chi_i = 1$. Otherwise set $\chi_i = 0$.

The output from the EBC algorithm is $(\boldsymbol{\theta}_1, \chi_1), (\boldsymbol{\theta}_2, \chi_2), \ldots, (\boldsymbol{\theta}_N, \chi_N)$. Throughout we class simulations for which $\chi_i = 1$ as accepted simulations, as it is the parameter values from these simulations that we will use in our analysis.

The first observation with the EBC algorithm is that the $\{(\boldsymbol{\theta}_i, \chi_i)\}$'s are *i.i.d.* by construction. Therefore, we consider $(\boldsymbol{\theta}_1, \chi_1)$ and note that

$$\mathbb{E}[\chi_1|\boldsymbol{\theta}_1] = 1 \times \mathbb{P}(\mathbf{X} = \mathbf{x}^*|\boldsymbol{\theta}_1) + 0 \times \mathbb{P}(\mathbf{X} \neq \mathbf{x}^*|\boldsymbol{\theta}_1)$$

$$= \pi(\mathbf{x}^*|\boldsymbol{\theta}_1). \tag{10.4}$$

By the theorem of total probability

$$\mathbb{E}[\chi_1] = \int \mathbb{E}[\chi_1|\boldsymbol{\theta}_1]\pi(\boldsymbol{\theta}_1)\, d\boldsymbol{\theta}_1$$

$$= \int \pi(\mathbf{x}^*|\boldsymbol{\theta}_1)\pi(\boldsymbol{\theta}_1)\, d\boldsymbol{\theta}_1 = \pi(\mathbf{x}^*). \tag{10.5}$$

Thus, we have that

$$\pi(\boldsymbol{\theta}_1|\chi_1 = 1) = \frac{\mathbb{P}(\chi_1 = 1|\boldsymbol{\theta}_1)\pi(\boldsymbol{\theta}_1)}{\mathbb{P}(\chi_1 = 1)}$$

$$= \frac{\mathbb{E}[\chi_1|\boldsymbol{\theta}_1]\pi(\boldsymbol{\theta}_1)}{\mathbb{E}[\chi_1]}$$

$$= \frac{\pi(\mathbf{x}^*|\boldsymbol{\theta}_1)\pi(\boldsymbol{\theta}_1)}{\pi(\mathbf{x}^*)} = \pi(\boldsymbol{\theta}_1|\mathbf{x}^*). \tag{10.6}$$

Letting $\mathcal{A} = \{i; \chi_i = 1\}$ denote the set of simulations that produce simulated data equal to $\mathbf{x}^*$, we have that $\{\boldsymbol{\theta}_i; i \in \mathcal{A}\}$ are *i.i.d.* samples of size $|\mathcal{A}|$ from $\pi(\boldsymbol{\theta}|\mathbf{x})$. Note that it suffices to keep only $\{\boldsymbol{\theta}_i; i \in \mathcal{A}\}$ as output from Algorithm 10.1 as we do not use in the analysis any realizations where $\chi_i = 0$.

The EBC algorithm is a rejection algorithm with acceptance rate $\mathbb{E}[\chi_1] = \pi(\mathbf{x}^*)$ $(= \mathbb{P}(\mathbf{X} = \mathbf{x}))$ and thus its efficiency, the proportion of simulations accepted $(\chi_i = 1)$ is intrinsically linked with the marginal likelihood. The EBC algorithm as stated previously will generate N simulations, of which a random number $|\mathcal{A}|$ will be accepted. It is trivial to instead run the EBC algorithm until a fixed number of simulations, K, are accepted. This approach will involve a negative binomial distributed number of simulations, B, with parameters K and $p = \mathbb{E}[\chi_1]$ with B having probability mass function

$$\mathbb{P}(B = b) = \binom{b-1}{K-1}p^K(1-p)^{b-K} \quad (b = K, K+1, \ldots). \tag{10.7}$$

Both of these alternatives are used in practice.

The efficiency of the EBC algorithm is linked to the probability that a simulated data set $\mathbf{x}$ exactly matches the observed data $\mathbf{x}^*$. For continuous data, this value will be 0 and hence the EBC algorithm is inappropriate. For discrete data, there is a curse-of-dimensionality with the marginal likelihood becoming exponentially small as the amount of data $\mathbf{x}^*$ grows and although the piecewise approach of [2] offers a partial solution, even for discrete data the probability of accepting a simulation often will be prohibitively small. Thus, the EBC algorithm is often impractical but can be modified to give a practical algorithm at the expense of allowing for approximations.

Let $S(\mathbf{x}^*)$ denote a low dimensional sufficient statistic of the data $\mathbf{x}^*$, then $\pi(\boldsymbol{\theta}|S(\mathbf{x}^*)) = \pi(\boldsymbol{\theta}|\mathbf{x}^*)$. The EBC algorithm still produces *i.i.d.* samples from the posterior distribution if we replace in Step 3 of the algorithm the requirement that $\mathbf{x} = \mathbf{x}^*$ by $S(\mathbf{x}) = S(\mathbf{x}^*)$. This replacement will result in the acceptance probability of the EBC algorithm becoming $\pi(S(\mathbf{x}^*))$, which often will be a significant improvement on $\pi(\mathbf{x}^*)$, especially as the amount of data $\mathbf{x}^*$ increases. However, this approach requires the data to be discrete and a low dimensional sufficient statistic to exist. This requirement is unlikely to be the case in real-life problems where a tractable likelihood is unavailable and we wish to apply the ABC algorithm.

The idea of using sufficient statistics to obtain valid inference, while impractical, is helpful in deriving the ABC algorithm. If we cannot find low-dimensional sufficient statistics can we instead find low-dimensional summary statistics, $T(\mathbf{x}^*)$, that characterize key features of the data and use these in place of sufficient statistics? Also requiring an exact match on any continuous statistic or summary statistic is not feasible, and therefore, what if we accepted simulations that produce summary statistics $T(\mathbf{x}_i)$ that are sufficiently *close* to $T(\mathbf{x}^*)$? This leads us to Algorithm 10.2, the vanilla ABC algorithm, [3].

Algorithm 10.2 The vanilla ABC algorithm

Choose a metric $d(\cdot, \cdot)$ and $\epsilon \geq 0$. For $i = 1, 2, \ldots, N$:

1: Sample $\boldsymbol{\theta}_i$ from $\pi(\cdot)$.
2: Simulate data $\mathbf{x}_i$ from the model $\mathcal{M}$ using parameters $\boldsymbol{\theta}_i$.
3: Compute $T(\mathbf{x}_i)$. If $d(T(\mathbf{x}_i), T(\mathbf{x}^*)) \leq \epsilon$, set $\chi_i = 1$. Otherwise set $\chi_i = 0$.

The output from Algorithm 10.2 is $(\boldsymbol{\theta}_1, \chi_1), (\boldsymbol{\theta}_2, \chi_2), \ldots, (\boldsymbol{\theta}_N, \chi_N)$ and as with Algorithm 10.1 it suffices to keep only $\{\boldsymbol{\theta}_i; i \in \mathcal{A}\}$, where $\mathcal{A} = \{i; \chi_i = 1\}$ is the set of accepted simulations. Note that Algorithm 10.1 (the EBC algorithm) is the special case where $T(\mathbf{x}) = S(\mathbf{x})$ and $\epsilon = 0$.

There are a number of aspects of the ABC algorithm which we will explore further in Section 10.3.

- How should we choose our summary statistics $T(\mathbf{x}^*)$?

- What constitutes a good distance metric?

- How should ϵ be chosen?

- Do our samples $\boldsymbol{\theta}_1, \boldsymbol{\theta}_2, \ldots, \boldsymbol{\theta}_N$ from $\pi_{d,\epsilon}(\boldsymbol{\theta}|T(\mathbf{x}^*))$, the probability density function of accepted values from the ABC algorithm, give us a good approximate sample from $\pi(\boldsymbol{\theta}|\mathbf{x}^*)$?

The most important question and the hardest one to answer is the final one with the others feeding into it. For summary statistics we want to pick out features of the data which are (likely to be) correlated with the parameters or functions of the parameters of interest. In epidemics this choice could be the total number of people infected within the population, or specified sub-populations, which often will be closely associated with R_0, the basic reproduction, the duration of the epidemic that will be linked with the rate parameters of the model, or a measure of spatial correlation in the infectives, such as Moran's I, [4], which will be associated with the parameters of a spatial kernel. Note that to be able to identify p parameters we require at least p summary statistics. In [5], details are given of a semi-automatic procedure for choosing an appropriate subset of summary statistics from a set of candidate summary statistics. This procedure is helpful if there is uncertainty about a suitable set of summary statistics but requires the user to specify the set of candidate summary statistics to be considered.

The distance metric should take into account the importance attached to each summary statistic; for example, in an epidemic data set the total number infected in the epidemic is a key summary. Also, the scale of variability inherent in the summary statistic should be accounted for so that the distance metric can discern between simulated summary statistics that are *close* to the observed summary statistics and those that are not. This requirement leads into the choice of ϵ. Letting $\epsilon \downarrow 0$ ensures that only those simulations that are very close in terms of the distance metric are accepted but typically very few simulations will be accepted. Conversely, letting $\epsilon \to \infty$ ensures the acceptance rate converges to 1 but the sample increasingly resembles the prior distribution. Therefore, there is a trade-off between efficiency and accuracy in the choice of ϵ and it is often chosen pragmatically on a *post-hoc* basis so that the best 100α percentage of simulations are accepted with $\alpha = 0.01$ a common choice, see [6].

10.3   Extensions of the ABC Algorithm

The vanilla ABC algorithm (Algorithm 10.2) offers a substantial practical improvement on the EBC algorithm (Algorithm 10.1) but there is still much room for improvement. There are three components to the ABC algorithm that we will explore further: generating parameter values (simulating from the prior), simulation of data and choice of summary statistics, and closeness. We already have touched upon the choice of summary statistics and the definition of closeness at the end of Section 10.2, although we consider this further in Section 10.3.2. Therefore, we will mainly focus upon the choice of parameter values for the simulations (Section 10.3.1) and the simulation of data (Section 10.3.3).

10.3.1   Parameter choice

For the vanilla ABC algorithm (Algorithm 10.2), the probability that a simulation is accepted is

$$\int \mathbb{P}(d(T(\mathbf{X}), T(\mathbf{x}^*)) \le \epsilon | \boldsymbol{\theta}) \pi(\boldsymbol{\theta}) \, d\boldsymbol{\theta}. \tag{10.8}$$

Suppose that $\boldsymbol{\theta}$ is p-dimensional and let $\Theta \subseteq \mathbb{R}^p$ denote the parameter space. For $0 < \delta \le 1$, let

$$\Gamma_\delta = \{\boldsymbol{\theta} \in \Theta; \mathbb{P}(d(T(\mathbf{X}), T(\mathbf{x}^*)) \le \epsilon | \boldsymbol{\theta}) \ge \delta \sup_{\boldsymbol{\vartheta} \in \Theta} \mathbb{P}(d(T(\mathbf{X}), T(\mathbf{x}^*)) \le \epsilon | \boldsymbol{\vartheta})\}.$$

Then the efficiency of the ABC algorithm is closely related to $\int_{\Gamma_\delta} \pi(\theta) \, d\theta$, the probability that a draw from the prior distribution is from Γ_δ. Thus, the prior distribution has an important impact on the efficiency of the ABC algorithm. In particular, a diffuse, uninformative but proper prior, which might be desirable from a scientific perspective, will lead to a highly inefficient ABC algorithm (where $\int_{\Gamma_\delta} \pi(\theta) \, d\theta$ is small) as most parameter values chosen from the prior will generate a simulation with summary statistics $T(\mathbf{x})$ that are a long way from $T(\mathbf{x}^*)$.

The solution is to use an alternative sampling distribution other than the prior distribution to propose parameter values from. The simplest approach is to use importance sampling by sampling $\boldsymbol{\theta}$ from an alternative probability density $q(\cdot)$, where $q(\cdot)$ is chosen such that $\int_{\Gamma_\delta} q(\theta) \, d\theta > \int_{\Gamma_\delta} \pi(\theta) \, d\theta$, which generates more simulations with parameters in Γ_δ leading to a higher acceptance rate. Then, provided that the ratio $\pi(\boldsymbol{\theta})/q(\boldsymbol{\theta})$ is finite for all $\boldsymbol{\theta}$ for which $\pi(\boldsymbol{\theta}) > 0$, we can apply the ABC importance sampling algorithm (Algorithm 10.3) to obtain weighted samples from $\pi_{d,\epsilon}(\boldsymbol{\theta} | T(\mathbf{x}^*))$.

Algorithm 10.3 ABC Importance sampling algorithm

Choose a metric $d(\cdot, \cdot)$ and $\epsilon \ge 0$. For $i = 1, 2, \ldots, N$:

  1: Sample $\boldsymbol{\theta}_i$ from $q(\cdot)$.
  2: Simulate data $\mathbf{x}_i$ from the model $\mathcal{M}$ using parameters $\boldsymbol{\theta}_i$.
  3: Compute $T(\mathbf{x}_i)$. If $d(T(\mathbf{x}_i), T(\mathbf{x}^*)) \le \epsilon$, set $\chi_i = 1$. Otherwise set $\chi_i = 0$.
  4: Attach weight $\chi_i \pi(\boldsymbol{\theta}_i)/q(\boldsymbol{\theta}_i)$ to sample $\boldsymbol{\theta}_i$.

The output from Algorithm 10.3 is $(\boldsymbol{\theta}_1, \chi_1 \pi(\boldsymbol{\theta}_1)/q(\boldsymbol{\theta}_1)), (\boldsymbol{\theta}_2, \chi_2 \pi(\boldsymbol{\theta}_2)/q(\boldsymbol{\theta}_2)), \ldots, (\boldsymbol{\theta}_N, \chi_N \pi (\boldsymbol{\theta}_N)/q(\boldsymbol{\theta}_N))$ and as with Algorithms 10.1 and 10.2 it suffices to keep only $\{(\boldsymbol{\theta}_i, \pi(\boldsymbol{\theta}_i)/q(\boldsymbol{\theta}_i));$ $i \in \mathcal{A}\}$, where $\mathcal{A} = \{i; \chi_i = 1\}$ is the set of accepted simulations.

Then, for any integrable function $h(\cdot)$,

$$\sum_{i=1}^{N} h(\boldsymbol{\theta}_i)\chi_i\pi(\boldsymbol{\theta}_i)/q(\boldsymbol{\theta}_i) \Bigg/ \sum_{i=1}^{N} \chi_i\pi(\boldsymbol{\theta}_i)/q(\boldsymbol{\theta}_i) \qquad (10.9)$$

is a consistent estimator of

$$\mathbb{E}_{d,\epsilon}[h(\boldsymbol{\theta})] = \int h(\boldsymbol{\theta})\pi_{d,\epsilon}(\boldsymbol{\theta}|\mathbf{x}^*)\,d\boldsymbol{\theta}$$

$$= \frac{\int h(\boldsymbol{\theta})\pi_{d,\epsilon}(\mathbf{x}^*|\boldsymbol{\theta})\{\pi(\boldsymbol{\theta})/q(\boldsymbol{\theta})\}q(\boldsymbol{\theta})\,d\boldsymbol{\theta}}{\int \pi_{d,\epsilon}(\mathbf{x}^*|\boldsymbol{\theta})\{\pi(\boldsymbol{\theta})/q(\boldsymbol{\theta})\}q(\boldsymbol{\theta})\,d\boldsymbol{\theta}}, \qquad (10.10)$$

where $\pi_{d,\epsilon}(\mathbf{x}^*|\boldsymbol{\theta}) = \mathbb{P}(d(T(\mathbf{X}), T(\mathbf{x}^*)) \leq \epsilon|\boldsymbol{\theta})$.

The immediate question which comes to mind is, how do we choose $q(\cdot)$? For $q(\cdot)$ to help the efficiency of the algorithm, we require that $q(\cdot)$ concentrates proposals of $\boldsymbol{\theta}$ values in regions of the parameter space where $\pi_{d,\epsilon}(\mathbf{x}^*|\boldsymbol{\theta})$ is non-negligible and ideally, in such regions we want $\pi(\boldsymbol{\theta})/q(\boldsymbol{\theta})$ close to constant.

A solution to this problem is SMC-ABC (Sequential Monte Carlo approximate Bayesian computation), see [7, 8]. This approach seeks to refine the proposal distribution in a series of L stages to move from an initial proposal $q_1(\cdot) = \pi(\cdot)$ to a final proposal density $q_L(\cdot)$ that better represents the posterior distribution of interest, and thus has a much higher acceptance rate.

Algorithm 10.4 SMC-ABC algorithm

Choose a metric $d(\cdot, \cdot)$, summary statistics $T(\cdot)$ and $\epsilon_1 > \epsilon_2 > \ldots > \epsilon_L \geq 0$.

1: Set $t = 1$.
2: Set $i = 1$ and repeat the following steps until there are N acceptances.
  (a) Sample $\boldsymbol{\theta}'$ from importance density $q_t(\boldsymbol{\theta})$.
  (b) If $\pi(\boldsymbol{\theta}') = 0$ reject and return to (a).
  (c) Simulate data $\mathbf{x}'$ from the model $\mathcal{M}$ using parameters $\boldsymbol{\theta}'$.
  (d) Accept $\boldsymbol{\theta}'$ if $d(T(\mathbf{x}'), T(\mathbf{x}^*)) \leq \epsilon_t$, and otherwise reject.
  (e) If $\boldsymbol{\theta}'$ is accepted, set $\boldsymbol{\theta}_i^t = \boldsymbol{\theta}'$ and increment $i = i + 1$.
3: For $i = 1, 2, \ldots, N$, let $w_i^t = \pi(\boldsymbol{\theta}_i^t)/q_t(\boldsymbol{\theta}_i^t)$.
4: Increment $t = t + 1$ and repeats steps 2 and 3 until $t = L$.

The output of the algorithm is $(\theta_1^L, w_1^L), (\theta_2^L, w_2^L), \ldots, (\theta_N^L, w_N^L)$, the accepted parameters and associated weights from the final iteration L.

In contrast to the ABC algorithms described previously, at each stage we run the algorithm until we obtain N acceptances. In practice, the choice of ϵ_i, and indeed L, often will be determined in a dynamic manner [6]. We typically choose ϵ_i to give a higher acceptance rate than when using the vanilla ABC algorithm (Algorithm 10.2) with an acceptance rate of around 10%, for example. Consequently, for a given precision level ϵ, the SMC-ABC algorithm (Algorithm 10.4) typically requires far fewer simulations than the vanilla ABC algorithm (Algorithm 10.2) and is thus much faster to run.

The key question is, how, for $t > 1$, to choose $q_t(\cdot)$? The solution is to use the sample from iteration $t - 1$ as the basis for the proposal distribution. Specifically, let

$$q_t(\boldsymbol{\theta}) = \sum_{i=1}^{N} w_i^{t-1} K_t(\boldsymbol{\theta}|\theta_i^{t-1}) \Bigg/ \sum_{i=1}^{N} w_i^{t-1}, \qquad (10.11)$$

where $K_t(\cdot|\cdot)$ is a kernel for perturbing samples from iteration $t-1$. The choice of the kernel is arbitrary but [8] shows that a good choice for $K_t(\cdot|\cdot)$ is a multivariate Gaussian distribution with covariance matrix $2\Sigma_{t-1}$, where Σ_{t-1} is the empirical (weighted) covariance matrix of the parameters from iteration $t-1$. This choice works well when the posterior distribution is approximately Gaussian and in Section 10.5 we apply (10.11) to a transformation of the parameter outputs. Note that choosing the perturbation variance that is too small will lead to particle degeneracy (degenerating to point-estimates as t increases with estimation sensitive to the draws of $\boldsymbol{\theta}$ from the prior distribution in stage 1) and under-estimation of parameter variability, while choosing the perturbation variance that is too large will lead to a loss of efficiency in the algorithm.

10.3.2 Kernel weights and regression adjustments

Thus far, we have assumed that equal weight is given to all parameters that result in a summary statistic $T(\mathbf{x}')$ with $d(T(\mathbf{x}'), T(\mathbf{x}^*)) \leq \epsilon$. It is trivial to adjust the previous algorithms to give more weight to those observations with a smaller discrepancy giving weight $w_i = H(d(T(\mathbf{x}_i), T(\mathbf{x}^*))$ to the ith simulation where $H(\cdot)$ is a monotonically decreasing Kernel function with $H(0) = 1$ and $H(x) = 0$ for $x > \epsilon$, see [6]. The special case $H(y) = 1$ for all $y \leq \epsilon$ is the step function used thus far and a common choice of $H(\cdot)$ is the Epanechnikov kernel

$$H(y) = \left\{ \begin{array}{ll} 1 - \left(\frac{y}{\epsilon}\right)^2 & y \leq \epsilon, \\ 0 & \text{otherwise.} \end{array} \right. \tag{10.12}$$

The Epanechnikov kernel is preferable to a Gaussian kernel as it gives zero weight to any simulation with $d(T(\mathbf{x}'), T(\mathbf{x}^*)) > \epsilon$ and thus such simulations can be discarded. By constrast for a Gaussian kernel every simulation has a non-zero weight but those observations with low weight contribute very little to the estimation of the parameters, while slowing down calculations substantially by having to consider many more simulations.

A further innovation introduced in [6] is regression-based adjustment of the parameters to take account of discrepancies between the simulated summary statistics $T(\mathbf{x}')$ and the observed summary statistics $T(\mathbf{x}^*)$. For example, in an epidemic context the total number of infected individuals in an epidemic is correlated with the infection rate. Therefore, for a simulated epidemic with infection rate λ which infects just below (above) the observed number of infected individuals, a small increase (decrease) in the infection rate would have had a reasonable chance of generating a simulated epidemic that infected the correct number of individuals. However, any linear relationship between summary statistics and parameters is only likely to be valid in a small neighborhood of the observed summary statistics, hence the use of local-linear regression. Letting $\mathbf{t}_i = T(\mathbf{x}_i)$ and $\mathbf{t}^* = T(\mathbf{x}')$, this is done by regressing $\boldsymbol{\theta}_i$ on $\boldsymbol{\alpha} + (\mathbf{t}_i - \mathbf{t}^*)^T \boldsymbol{\beta}$ and obtaining the weighted least-squares estimate of $(\boldsymbol{\alpha}, \boldsymbol{\beta})$ by minimizing

$$\sum_{i=1}^{N} \{\boldsymbol{\theta}_i - \boldsymbol{\alpha} - (\mathbf{t}_i - \mathbf{t}^*)^T \boldsymbol{\beta}\}^2 H(d(\mathbf{t}_i, \mathbf{t}^*)). \tag{10.13}$$

The solution is given by

$$(\hat{\boldsymbol{\alpha}}, \hat{\boldsymbol{\beta}}) = (\mathbf{Z}^T W \mathbf{Z})^{-1} \mathbf{Z}^T W \boldsymbol{\theta}, \tag{10.14}$$

where $\boldsymbol{\theta}$ is a column vector of $\{\boldsymbol{\theta}_i\}$ values, W is a diagonal matrix with $W_{ii} = H(d(\mathbf{t}_i, \mathbf{t}^*))$, and

$$\mathbf{Z} = \begin{pmatrix} 1 & t_{11} - t_1^* & \cdots & t_{1q} - t_q^* \\ \vdots & \vdots & \ddots & \vdots \\ 1 & t_{N1} - t_1^* & \cdots & t_{Nq} - t_q^* \end{pmatrix}, \tag{10.15}$$

where q is the total number of summary statistics. Let

$$\tilde{\boldsymbol{\theta}}_i = \boldsymbol{\theta}_i - (\mathbf{t}_i - \mathbf{t}^*)^T \hat{\boldsymbol{\beta}}. \tag{10.16}$$

Then $(\tilde{\boldsymbol{\theta}}_1, \tilde{\boldsymbol{\theta}}_2, \ldots, \tilde{\boldsymbol{\theta}}_N)$ form a regression adjusted sample from the (approximate) posterior distribution and as shown in [6] reduces the root mean square error (RMSE) of the estimates. In Section 10.4, we demonstrate the benefits of using the local-linear regression adjustment and this is computationally inexpensive compared with the simulations required for the ABC algorithm.

10.3.3 Simulation of the data

The final area for consideration is the simulation of data. We assume throughout that this can be done in a simple manner which expedites the use of ABC methods but there are number of considerations with performing simulation. The first observation is that simulation can be viewed as a data augmentation tool and thus there are links to data augmentation MCMC. Specifically we are simulating a realization $\mathbf{y}$ from a stochastic process $\mathbf{Y}$ with parameters $\boldsymbol{\theta}$. We assume that the observed data, $\mathbf{x}^*$, is some function of the realized stochastic process $\mathbf{y}^*$ with either $\mathbf{x}^* = \psi(\mathbf{y}^*)$, a deterministic function of $\mathbf{y}^*$ or that we have $\pi(\mathbf{x}^*|\mathbf{y}^*)$, the probability or density of observing $\mathbf{x}^*$ given $\mathbf{y}^*$. The latter scenario can lead to ABC being used to give exact results if we can use the uncertainty in observing $\mathbf{x}^*$ given $\mathbf{y}^*$. This scenario is closely linked to the observation in [9] that, under the assumption of model error, ABC can be used to obtain exact results. However, such an approach will often be sensitive to the dimension of $\mathbf{x}^*$ and the use of summary statistics may still be preferable.

The simulation of a stochastic process comprises two parts: the parameters underlying the model $\boldsymbol{\theta}$ and the random variables $\mathbf{U}$ used to construct a realization of the process. Typically the random variables $\mathbf{U}$ will depend explicitly upon $\boldsymbol{\theta}$ but there are non-trivial epidemic examples, see [10] and [11], where a non-centered parameterization ([12]) of the stochastic process exists and the random variables $\mathbf{U}$ can be chosen to be independent of $\boldsymbol{\theta}$. In such cases, we can observe a direct link between data augmentation MCMC and ABC, which highlight strengths and weaknesses of both approaches. Suppose that $\mathbf{Y} = \xi(\mathbf{U}, \boldsymbol{\theta})$, where ξ is a function of $\boldsymbol{\theta}$ and $\mathbf{U}$. Then ABC works at each iteration by sampling a new $\boldsymbol{\theta}'$ and a new set of $\mathbf{U}'$ to construct a brand new $\mathbf{Y}'$, which is accepted if the summary statistics of the process $T(\mathbf{x}')$ are sufficiently close to $T(\mathbf{x}^*)$. Data augmentation MCMC will, given a current choice of $\mathbf{u}$ and $\boldsymbol{\theta}$, propose updated values $\mathbf{u}'$ and $\boldsymbol{\theta}'$ based upon the current values. The proposed changes will result in $\mathbf{y}' = \xi(\mathbf{u}', \boldsymbol{\theta}')$ with the proposed move accepted with probability

$$\min\left\{ 1, \frac{\pi(\mathbf{x}^*|\mathbf{y}')\pi(\boldsymbol{\theta}')q(\mathbf{u}', \boldsymbol{\theta}' \to \mathbf{u}, \boldsymbol{\theta})}{\pi(\mathbf{x}^*|\mathbf{y})\pi(\boldsymbol{\theta})q(\mathbf{u}, \boldsymbol{\theta} \to \mathbf{u}', \boldsymbol{\theta}')} \right\}. \tag{10.17}$$

The effectiveness of such an MCMC algorithm is based upon how efficiently the proposal density $q(\cdot \to \cdot)$ can be chosen to explore the joint space of the augmented data and parameters. In [10], Section 4, it is shown that this approach can be effectively done for a model for the evolution of the spread of tuberculosis and applied to tuberculosis data from San Francisco, [13], with the dimension of $\mathbf{U}$ approximately 30,000. In such a case, data augmentation MCMC is preferable to ABC because ABC is wasteful in *throwing away* good simulations (*e.g.*, those which closely match the observed data). What assists the MCMC in [10], Section 4, is that small changes in $(\mathbf{u}, \boldsymbol{\theta})$ result in small changes in $\pi(\mathbf{x}^*|\mathbf{y} = \xi(\mathbf{u}, \boldsymbol{\theta}))$. However, in situations where $\pi(\mathbf{x}^*|\mathbf{y}) = 1_{\{\mathbf{x}^* = \psi(\mathbf{y}^*)\}}$, the MCMC algorithm is likely to get stuck in a local mode and not explore the parameter space (see [11], Section 4 for further discussion). In such circumstances ABC methods come to the fore.

Another consideration is that we ideally want our simulated data to be close to the observed data. However, as observed previously the probability of this happening by chance is usually very small. Therefore, can we *steer* the simulation process such that our simulated data has a greater chance of matching (being close to) the observed data? The answer is yes, but we need to take account of the steering in our analysis.

There are two ways in which we can steer the simulation process. First, given $\boldsymbol{\theta}$, we can simulate $\mathbf{u} = (u_1, u_2, \ldots, u_M)$ such that the simulated data produces $\mathbf{X} = \mathbf{x}^*$. There are two ways in which we can steer the simulation process. First, given $\boldsymbol{\theta}$ we can simulate $\mathbf{u} = (u_1, u_2, \ldots, u_M)$ such that the simulated data produces $\mathbf{X} = \mathbf{x}^*$. In Section 10.4 this is implemented by, for each k, simulating u_k from a set of possible values $\mathcal{S}_k$ dependent on $\boldsymbol{\theta}$ and $\mathbf{u}_{1:k-1}$, to ensure that the simulated epidemic is of the desired size. The simulation is given weight $\prod_{i=1}^M \mathbb{P}(u_k \in \mathcal{S}_k)$, the probability of all the conditioning events imposed on $\mathbf{u}$ occurring by chance. This simulation underpins the pseudo-marginal approach of [14] for fitting the general stochastic epidemic model to temporal data and can be used with an MCMC algorithm. The feasibility of such an approach depends upon how easily the epidemic process can be constructed in a sequential manner under the constraints imposed by the observed data and has been used effectively for simple epidemic models in [14] and [11]. Second, we can generate $\mathbf{u}$ and then find the set of $\boldsymbol{\theta}$ values such that $\psi(\xi(\mathbf{u}, \boldsymbol{\theta})) = \mathbf{x}^*$. This approach underpins the coupled ABC algorithm of [15]. While the coupled ABC algorithm has a far higher acceptance rate than vanilla ABC, it is extremely cumbersome in more than one dimension. Therefore, [16] introduced a partially coupled ABC algorithm which splits $\boldsymbol{\theta}$ into ϕ and λ, which samples ϕ from the prior and generates $\mathbf{u}$ before finding the set of λ values such that $\psi(\xi(\mathbf{u}, (\phi, \lambda))) = \mathbf{x}^*$. In Section 10.5, we show how both of these ideas can be combined to ensure that a simulated dataset matches the observed data.

At first glance the steering of simulations looks to present a perfect solution by guaranteeing simulations match the observed data. However, it relies upon us being able to simulate the conditioned process and compute the weights in a timely manner. Moreover, this approach can lead to the majority of the weight being centered on a small number of simulations, due either to a diffuse prior distribution or large Monte Carlo variability in the simulations, or a combination of the two. Therefore, if w_j is the weight attached to simulation j, it is important to ensure that the effective sample size $(\sum_{j=1}^N w_j)^2 / (\sum_{j=1}^N w_j^2)$ is not too small. In Sections 10.4 and 10.5, we demonstrate how these steered simulation approaches can be applied to final outcome and spatial epidemic data, which allows for comparisons with the simpler to implement ABC algorithms.

10.4   Final Outcome Example: Measles

In this section we apply the ABC methods introduced in Sections 10.2 and 10.3 to final outcome data from a measles outbreak in a Finnish school, [17]. The data have been analyzed previously in [11] using MCMC, which allows us to benchmark the results obtained. We follow [11] in assuming that the school is a homogeneously mixing community and with the exception of the one initial case, all infections are assumed to take place within the school.

The data consist of how many school pupils were infected in a measles outbreak in Honkajoki, a small rural Finnish municipality in 1989, [17]. Pupils belong to one of three types, 0, 1, or 2, where a type k $(k = 0, 1, 2)$ individual has received k doses of measles vaccine. Let x_k^* and n_k denote the total number of infected individuals and the total number of individuals of type k, respectively, with $m = x_0 + x_1 + x_2$ and $N = n_0 + n_1 + n_2$. The data are summarized in Table 10.1.

The final outcome data consist of only three observations: the number infected in each vaccination category. Therefore, there is insufficient data to take account of a vaccine effect in both susceptibility and infectivity of individuals. Thus, we follow [18] and [11] in assuming that the vaccine reduces an individuals susceptibility to the disease but that there is no difference in the infectious behavior of infected individuals irrespective of their vaccine status. Let I denote the infectious period distribution and we assume that during their infectious period individuals make infectious contacts at the points of a homogeneous Poisson point process with rate λ. Without loss of generally we assume that $E[I] = 1$, noting that final outcome data contains no temporal information and therefore the epidemic outcome is invariant to transformations of the timescale. That is, for any $c > 0$, we cannot differentiate between epidemics with parameter sets (I, λ) and $(cI, \lambda/c)$ (see, for example, [19] and [18]).

The model is as follows. There is one initial infective in an otherwise susceptible population. While infectious an individual makes infectious contacts at the points of a homogeneous Poisson point process with rate λ. The person contacted is chosen uniformly at random from the population and if susceptible the individual has probability q_k of becoming infected if they are of type k. We assume that $q_0 = 1$ and $0 < q_1, q_2 < 1$ corresponding to vaccination having a protective effect on individuals.

Let $\boldsymbol{\theta} = (\lambda, q_1, q_2)$ denote the parameters of interest. We assume $U(0,1)$ priors on q_1 and q_2, which allows for the possibility that $q_1 < q_2$, a second dose of the vaccine has a negative effect. For λ we take an Exp(0.1) prior, since λ denotes the basic reproduction number R_0 of the model in an unvaccinated population and the prior mean of 10 is in line with estimates of R_0 for measles (see for example, [20], table 5). Given the parameters, simulation of the epidemic is straightforward. For an infective i, for example, we simulate an infectious period I_i. Then the probability that individual i will make contact with a given susceptible during its infectious period is $1 - \exp(-\lambda I_i/N)$, where N is the total population size. Thus, if there are m_k susceptibles remaining of type k, individual i will infect $\text{Bin}(m_k, q_k\{1 - \exp(-\lambda I_i/N)\})$ of them. Hence, we consider the individuals infected by one infective at a time until there are no infectives remaining in the population with $x_k = n_k - m_k$ individuals of type k ultimately infected in the simulated epidemic. This approach ignores the time course of the epidemic but leaves the final outcome of the epidemic unaffected (see [21]).

We can use an alternative Sellke-type ([22], [11]) construction of the epidemic process to generate simulations conditioned to match the observed data. This construction is based on assigning an infectious threshold to each individual with an individual succumbing to the disease when the total amount of infection they are exposed to exceeds their threshold.

TABLE 10.1

Honkajoki measles data set

Type, k	0	1	2
Total number of infected individuals, x_k^*	18	11	6
Total number of individuals, n_k	79	189	149

The thresholds corresponding to infections at the points of a Poisson point process are exponentially distributed, [22]. We can use properties of the exponential distributions to show that, at a population level, the additional amount of infectious pressure required after the ith infection for the $(i+1)st$ infection to take place is exponentially distributed (see [15] and [11] for further details).

Given parameters $\boldsymbol{\theta} = (\lambda, q_1, q_2)$, we can use the following Sellke-type simulation of the epidemic, which is based upon [11]. We choose a random permutation of the order of infection of the m individuals infected in the epidemic and let $\boldsymbol{\omega} = (\omega_1, \omega_2, \ldots, \omega_m)$ denote the order with $\omega_j = k$ if the jth individual infected is of type k. Let $\mathbf{I} = (I_1, I_2, \ldots, I_m)$ be *i.i.d.* draws from I. For $j = 0, 1, 2$, let $s_{j,i}$ denote the total number of susceptibles of type j after the ith infection with the convention that $s_{j,0} = n_j$, and note that this depends on $\boldsymbol{\omega}$. Moreover, the probability of observing $\boldsymbol{\omega}$ given (q_1, q_2) forms the first part of the conditioning of the epidemic process and is given by

$$\pi(\boldsymbol{\omega}|\mathbf{q}) = \prod_{i=1}^{m} \frac{s_{\omega_i, i-1} q_{\omega_i}}{\sum_{k=0}^{2} s_{k, i-1} q_k}. \tag{10.18}$$

For $i = 1, 2, \ldots$, let $\alpha_i = \sum_{j=0}^{2} s_{j,i} q_j / N$, the probability that following the ith infection, an infectious contact will result in an infection (the contact is with a susceptible and successful). Then, if $L_i \sim \mathrm{Exp}(\alpha_i)$, L_i is the additional amount of infection pressure required after the ith infection for the $(i + 1)st$ infection to take place. Thus, it can be shown (see [11]) that, given $\boldsymbol{\theta}$, $\boldsymbol{\omega}$, $\mathbf{I}$ and $\mathbf{L}$, the epidemic will infect m individuals with x_k infected of type k ($k = 0, 1, 2$), if for all $1 \leq l \leq m - 1$,

$$\sum_{i=1}^{l} L_i \leq \lambda \sum_{i=1}^{l} I_i, \tag{10.19}$$

and

$$\sum_{i=1}^{m} L_i > \lambda \sum_{i=1}^{m} I_i. \tag{10.20}$$

Since the components of $\mathbf{L}$ are independent exponential random variables, it is trivial to simulate these sequentially using inversion of the cumulative distribution function so that (10.19) and (10.20) are satisfied. That is, for $1 \leq l \leq m - 1$, L_l is drawn from $\mathrm{Exp}(\alpha_l)$ conditioned to be less than $V_l = \lambda \sum_{i=1}^{l} I_i - \sum_{i=1}^{l-1} L_i$, which has probability $1 - \exp(-\alpha_l V_l)$ of occurring and L_m is drawn from $\mathrm{Exp}(\alpha_m)$ conditioned to be greater than $V_m = \lambda \sum_{i=1}^{m} I_i - \sum_{i=1}^{m-1} L_i$, which has probability $\exp(-\alpha_m V_m)$ of occurring. Therefore, the conditions imposed on the simulation, the order of infection, given by (10.18) and the conditions on $\mathbf{L}$ give weight

$$w = \left\{ \prod_{i=1}^{m} \frac{s_{\omega_i, i-1} q_{\omega_i}}{\sum_{k=0}^{2} s_{k, i-1} q_k} \right\} \times \left\{ \prod_{l=1}^{m-1} (1 - \exp(-\alpha_l V_l)) \right\} \exp(-\alpha_m V_m). \tag{10.21}$$

We ran the vanilla ABC (Algorithm 10.2), SMC-ABC (Algorithm 10.4), and conditioned simulation (CS) algorithms on the Honkajoki dataset. For the vanilla ABC and SMC-ABC algorithms, we have to specify a distance metric and precision. Specifically, for $k = 0, 1, 2$, let $E_k = |x_k - x_k^*|$ and let $E_T = |\sum_{k=0}^{2} (x_k - x_k^*)|$, the difference between the numbers infected in each group and overall, respectively. Then, for a given $\epsilon \in \mathbb{Z}^+$, we accept a simulation with precision ϵ if

$$\max\{E_0, E_1, E_2, E_T\} \leq \epsilon. \tag{10.22}$$

Note that if $\epsilon = 0$, we obtain from the posterior distribution $\pi(\boldsymbol{\theta}|\mathbf{x}^*)$. For both the vanilla ABC and SMC-ABC algorithms, we applied the local-linear regression corrections (Section 10.3.2 and [6]). Note that for the local-linear regression we regress only (x_0, x_1, x_2) to avoid having a singular matrix as the total number infected is simply $x_0 + x_1 + x_2$.

For the vanilla ABC algorithm we took $\epsilon = 4$ and ran the algorithm until we obtain 1,000 observations from the approximate posterior distribution. This outcome resulted in over 5 million simulations being required. The time taken per simulation varies considerably and is approximately linear in the number of people infected. By observing that any simulation which exceeds $\sum_{k=0}^{2} x_k^* + \epsilon$ infectives will not satisfy (10.22), we can speed the simulation process up considerably by immediately aborting simulations once there are $\sum_{k=0}^{2} x_k^* + \epsilon + 1$ infectives. For the SMC-ABC algorithm, we used the perturbation kernel of [8], (10.11), and we set $L = 3$ for the number of tuning stages with $\epsilon = (10, 7, 4)$. At each step we obtained 1,000 observations from the approximate posterior distribution. This approach resulted in 338,356, 222,571, and 865,451 simulations being required at each of the three stages. The total number of simulations required for the SMC-ABC is less than one-third of the number required for the vanilla ABC algorithm. Note that for stages 2 and 3 approximately 52 and 45 percent of proposed values were not permissible (e.g., q_1 outside the range $(0,1)$), and hence, not used. Given that the time consuming part of the algorithm is the simulations, we report only the number of permissible values generated which led to simulations. Finally, for the CS algorithm we drew $\boldsymbol{\theta}$ from the prior. We ran the algorithm with 1 million sets of parameters, which resulted in an effective sample size of 1,409, which is comparable with the two ABC algorithms (1,000 accepted values).

The posterior estimates of the parameters (means and standard deviations) for all three algorithms are given in Table 10.2 along with estimates obtained using the MCMC algorithm in [11]. The two ABC algorithms show slight biases in the posterior means for the parameters which the local-linear regression corrections (denoted by LL in Table 10.2) assist with correcting in $\mathbf{q}$ at the detriment of λ. The main effect that the local-linear regression correction has is reducing the variance of the parameter estimates to be more in line with those obtained using the CS algorithm or MCMC. The CS and MCMC algorithms give comparable results.

TABLE 10.2
Parameter estimates for the Honkajaki measles outbreak

Algorithm	λ mean	λ sd	q_1 mean	q_1 sd	q_2 mean	q_2 sd	Simulations
ABC	2.851	0.964	0.321	0.156	0.240	0.153	5,141,081
LL ABC	2.966	0.911	0.301	0.132	0.222	0.110	5,141,081
SMC-ABC	2.836	1.006	0.327	0.172	0.246	0.176	1,426,378
LL SMC-ABC	2.974	0.890	0.302	0.140	0.228	0.134	1,426,378
CS	2.785	0.701	0.295	0.115	0.215	0.102	1,000,000
MCMC	2.780	0.691	0.303	0.116	0.220	0.098	100,000

Note: LL denotes local-linear regression corrections.

10.5   Spatial Epidemic Data

In this section we turn to a spatial epidemic example. The model under consideration is a spatial $S \to I$ epidemic model, which is appropriate for a range of agricultural diseases (see, for example [23], [24], [25], [11]). The model is as follows. We assume that there is a closed population of size N and that each member of the population has a spatial location $\mathbf{x} \in \mathcal{S}$, where $\mathcal{S} \subseteq \mathbb{R}^2$. In the examples mentioned previously, the populations are located on a rectangular lattice and, although the model and simulation are not restricted to this scenario, we will work under this assumption. This approach will assist in devising summary statistics for implementing the ABC algorithm. An individual $\mathbf{x}$ is assumed to be infectious immediately on being infected and for each individual $\mathbf{y}$, $\mathbf{x}$ makes infectious contacts with $\mathbf{y}$ at the points of a homogeneous Poisson point process with rate $\lambda F_\alpha(\mathbf{x} - \mathbf{y})$. The function $F_\alpha(\cdot)$ is a spatial transmission kernel and for simplicity usually is taken to be a monotonically decreasing and isotropic function of Euclidean distance but this assumption can be relaxed. If individual $\mathbf{y}$ is susceptible when individual $\mathbf{x}$ makes infectious contact, then individual $\mathbf{y}$ becomes infected. Otherwise, individual $\mathbf{y}$ is already infectious and the contact has no effect. In [23], $\exp(-\alpha|\mathbf{x} - \mathbf{y}|)$ and $|\mathbf{x} - \mathbf{y}|^{-2\alpha}$ are considered for $F_\alpha(\mathbf{x} - \mathbf{y})$, whereas $\exp(-|\mathbf{x}-\mathbf{y}|^2/(2\alpha^2))/(2\pi\alpha^2)$ is used in [25]. The model also may assume a constant background risk of infection rate μ per individual. A key observation is that if $\mathcal{I}$ and $\mathcal{S}$ denote the current sets of infectives and susceptibles, respectively, then the time until the next infection event is exponentially distributed with rate

$$\sum_{\mathbf{y} \in \mathcal{S}} \left\{ \mu + \lambda \sum_{\mathbf{x} \in \mathcal{I}} F_\alpha(\mathbf{x} - \mathbf{y}) \right\}, \tag{10.23}$$

and the probability that individual $\mathbf{z} \in \mathcal{S}$ is the next individual to be infected is

$$\frac{\mu + \lambda \sum_{\mathbf{x} \in \mathcal{I}} F_\alpha(\mathbf{x} - \mathbf{z})}{\sum_{\mathbf{y} \in \mathcal{S}} \left\{ \mu + \lambda \sum_{\mathbf{x} \in \mathcal{I}} F_\alpha(\mathbf{x} - \mathbf{y}) \right\}}. \tag{10.24}$$

We will use CTV as the motivating example for demonstrating ABC algorithms for spatial $S \to I$ epidemics using a dataset obtained by [26] for the spread of CTV in a citrus orchard. This dataset has been analyzed previously using MCMC in [23] and [11]. However, [23], one of the first papers to use MCMC for epidemic models, only infers the spatial parameter α and not the rate parameter λ. Note that in [23] and [11], μ is taken to be 0, an assumption we will maintain here. The more recent work of [11] uses collapsing (see [27]) to integrate out the rate parameter λ, which is later recovered, to obtain a computationally efficient MCMC algorithm. By contrast as we will demonstrate herein, simulation of the epidemic is straightforward and can be used to obtain (approximate) posterior samples from the parameters $\boldsymbol{\theta} = (\lambda, \alpha)$.

The data consists of two snapshots of the epidemic status of the orchard. At the first snapshot in 1981 there are 131 infected trees in an orchard of 1,008 trees situated on a 28×36 rectangular lattice. The rows and columns of the trees are 5.5 meters (m) and 4 m apart, respectively. At the second snapshot taken one year later in 1982, there are an additional 45 infected trees taking the total number of infected trees to 176. We follow [23] and [11] in inferring the parameters based on the 45 infections which occur between the two snapshots by initiating our simulations with the 131 infected trees in 1981. Each simulation then is run for 1 year with the set of new infections compared with the set of 45 new infections in 1982 in the CTV dataset.

As in Section 10.4, we start with the vanilla ABC algorithm (Algorithm 10.2) and build up to sampling from the posterior distribution by conditioning upon which trees gets infected. We will focus on $F_\alpha(\mathbf{x} - \mathbf{y}) = |\mathbf{x} - \mathbf{y}|^{-2\alpha}$. We begin by stipulating our choice of summary statistics because the chances of simulating the epidemic over the course of the year such that it infects exactly the 45 additional infected trees is vanishingly small. In constructing summary statistics for the model we will make explicit use of the lattice structure of the data. In particular, we will take the summary statistics to be the total number of individuals infected, Z, between the two observation time points and the Moran I statistic of the nearest neighbor spatial autocorrelation. Specifically, let p denote the proportion of the population infected at the end of the observation period and let $z_{i,j} = 1 - p$ if individual (i, j) is infected at the end of the observation period and $z_{i,j} = -p$ otherwise. Then we compute

$$I = \frac{N}{2N - n_1 - n_2} \times \frac{\sum_{i=1}^{n_1} \sum_{j=1}^{n_2-1} z_{i,j} z_{i,j+1} + \sum_{i=1}^{n_1-1} \sum_{j=1}^{n_2} z_{i,j} z_{i+1,j}}{\sum_{i=1}^{n_1} \sum_{j=1}^{n_2} z_{i,j}^2},$$

(10.25)

which gives a similarity measure as to the infectious status of nearest neighbors. For the observed data, $(Z^*, I^*) = (45, 0.2015)$ and we require simulated data sets to have similar values of (Z, I). For a given precision $\epsilon = (\epsilon_1, \epsilon_2)$, we accept a simulation that produces summary statistics (Z_S, I_S) if

$$|Z_S - Z^*| \leq \epsilon_1$$

(10.26)

$$|I_S - I^*| \leq \epsilon_2.$$

(10.27)

That is, we specify separate metric and criterion for each summary statistic rather than a joint metric.

Throughout we use $U[0.8, 2.0]$ prior on α based on [23] and $\text{Exp}(0.5)$ prior on λ, which is chosen pragmatically on the basis of the findings of [11]. More generally, the prior on α should reflect the expected spatial decay with distance. For $\alpha = 0.8$ and $\alpha = 2$, a tree is making infectious contacts with its nearest column neighbor 1.66 and 3.57 times more often than with its nearest row neighbor, respectively. Similarly the prior on λ should be such that a moderate number of infections take place between the observation periods.

For the vanilla ABC algorithm, we ran the algorithm until we obtained 1,000 accepted simulations. The acceptance criterion were determined by a pilot run of 1,000 simulations with $\epsilon = (4, 0.01)$. We required 126,343 simulations, which corresponds to accepting approximately 0.79 percent of simulations. As in Section 10.4, the algorithm was speeded up tremendously by aborting all simulations which exceeded $Z^* + 4$ infections as we knew that these simulations would be automatically rejected. The posterior means and standard deviations of the parameters are given in Table 10.3 with the estimates for the other simulation algorithms.

TABLE 10.3

Parameter estimates for the CTV outbreak

Algorithm	λ mean	λ sd	α mean	α sd	Simulations	ϵ
ABC	2.254	1.913	1.237	0.188	126,343	(4, 0.01)
SMC-ABC	2.207	1.860	1.239	0.178	49,255	(4, 0.01)
CS1	2.318	2.002	1.243	0.182	4,504	(0, 0.01)
CS2	2.675	1.533	1.313	0.126	1,000	(0, 0)

For the SMC-ABC algorithm (Algorithm 10.4), we used two stages to estimate the parameters with each stage run until we obtained 1,000 accepted simulations. We used $(9, 0.025)$ and $(4, 0.01)$ for the precisions at stages 1 and 2, respectively. This approach resulted in 25,750 and 23,505 simulations at the two stages, respectively, a significant reduction in the total number of simulations required. It should be noted that the posterior sample for (λ, α) is not approximately normally distributed and therefore we apply the perturbation kernel (10.11) to the transformed parameters $(\log(\lambda), \alpha)$. This method requires us to take account of the Jacobian of the transformation in the weights by multiplying through by λ. The estimated posterior means and standard deviations of the parameters are given in Table 10.3 and show good agreement with the results obtained for the vanilla ABC algorithm.

Given that $\mu = 0$, we can exploit (10.23) to construct simulations which infect exactly 45 individuals between the two observation periods. This approach can be done by simulating the epidemic process with a nominal $\lambda = 1$ until 45 individuals are infected and then determining a value of λ such that these 45 infections only occur within the time interval. The steps are as follow. We sample α from $U[0.8, 2.0]$. Let $\mathcal{I}_t$ and $\mathcal{S}_t$ denote the sets of infectives and susceptibles after the tth infection with $\mathcal{I}_0$ and $\mathcal{S}_0$ denoting the initial sets of infectives and susceptibles, respectively. Let T_t denote the time of the tth infection with $T_0 = 0$. Simulate the epidemic process with the time of the tth infection satisfying

$$T_t = T_{t-1} + \text{Exp}\left(\sum_{\mathbf{y} \in \mathcal{S}_{t-1}} \sum_{\mathbf{x} \in \mathcal{I}_{t-1}} F_\alpha(\mathbf{x} - \mathbf{y}) \right). \qquad (10.28)$$

Then T_{45} and T_{46} represent the time taken until the $45th$ and $46th$ infection, respectively, with λ set equal to 1. We then can exploit the property of the exponential distribution that for any $\varphi, A > 0$, $\text{Exp}(\varphi A)$ is equal in distribution to $\text{Exp}(A)/\varphi$. Therefore, we can speed up time in this simulated epidemic by a factor β to get a realization of the epidemic with $\lambda = \beta$ such that the order of infections are unchanged but the time at which the tth infection occurs is T_t/β. Specifically, if we select λ such that

$$\frac{T_{45}}{\lambda} < 1 < \frac{T_{46}}{\lambda}$$
$$T_{45} < \lambda < T_{46}, \qquad (10.29)$$

we get an epidemic that infects exactly 45 individuals during the course of 1 year. Conditioning upon λ satisfying (10.29) requires us to take account of the probability (from the prior) of this occuring by chance, which is $\exp(-0.5T_{45}) - \exp(-0.5T_{46})$. We then can use inversion of the cumulative distribution function to sample λ from $\text{Exp}(0.5)$ subject to the constraint imposed in (10.29). We term this approach conditioned simulation 1 (CS1). Since the algorithm is guaranteed to generate 45 infections, we can take $\epsilon_1 = 0$ in (10.26). We again use $\epsilon_2 = 0.01$ in (10.27). This algorithm results in a significantly higher acceptance rate for simulations with minimal additional cost per simulation with only 4,504 simulations required to obtain 1,000 accepted simulations, although the effective sample size was reduced by the unequal weights to 341. The posterior summaries of the parameters are presented in Table 10.3 and are similar to those obtained using the ABC algorithms.

Finally, we can implement a conditioned simulation algorithm (CS2) which infects exactly the 45 infected individuals in the interval 1981–1982. To achieve this, we draw $\alpha \in U[0.8, 2.0]$ and choose a random ordering, ω, for the infection of the 45 individuals. The probability of observing the given order of infection with the chosen α then can be determined. The relative times of infection then can be obtained as previously using (10.28) with a nominal $\lambda = 1$. We then can choose λ to satisfy (10.29) and multiply the probability of observing the infection by the corresponding probability of drawing λ from $(T_{45}, T_{46}]$ from the prior distribution.

The CS2 algorithm guarantees an exact match and we ran the algorithm for 1,000 simulations, which gave an effective sample size of 126. The posterior summaries of the parameters complete Table 10.3. The resulting parameter estimates are based on samples from the posterior distribution with $\epsilon = (0, 0)$ and confirm that the ABC algorithms provide a reasonable approximation of the posterior distribution. We note that the cost per simulation varies very little from algorithm to algorithm; therefore, the CS1 and CS2 algorithms offer substantial gains in terms of implementation over the ABC algorithms. More generally, while the vanilla ABC algorithm is often very straightforward to implement, with a bit of thought and work we can make substantial improvements through SMC-ABC and conditioned simulations.

10.6 Conclusions

This chapter introduced the ABC algorithm along with some extensions of the algorithm to make it more efficient. The examples presented in Sections 10.4 and 10.5 are relatively simple models with small datasets that can be analyzed by alternative methods, such as MCMC, but serve to demonstrate the ease and speed with which simulation-based inferential methods can be applied to stochastic epidemic models. Given that ABC methods only require simulation of the epidemic process, they have been successfully applied to model the genotype mutation in a tuberculosis outbreak in San Francisco [5, 28, 29], the spread of HIV-Aids in Cuba, [30], the spread of equine influenza across yards in Newmarket, UK [31], and the spread of bovine tuberculosis, both within cattle in the UK [32] and lions in Kruger National Park, South Africa, [33]. For the San Francisco tuberculosis outbreak, [10] showed how the simulation of the epidemic process could be embedded within an MCMC framework to obtain an effective MCMC algorithm using simulation-based inference. However, there are limitations to ABC especially for large-scale models where simulation can become very time consuming (see [34]). The solution presented in [34] is to combine simulation with a Gaussian process emulator and history matching, where the emulator mimics the behavior of simulations of the stochastic epidemic model but are orders of magnitude faster.

References

[1] P. D. O'Neill and T. Kypraios. Markov chain Monte Carlo methods for outbreak data, this volume.

[2] S.R. White, T. Kypraios, and S.P. Preston. Piecewise approximate Bayesian computation: Fast inference for discretely observed Markov models using a factorised posterior distribution. *Statistics and Computing*, 25:289–301, 2015.

[3] S. Tavaré, D.J. Balding, R.C. Griffiths, and P. Donnelly. Inferring coalescence times from DNA sequence data. *Genetics*, 145:505–518, 1997.

[4] P.A.P. Moran. Notes on continuous stochastic phenomena. *Biometrika*, 37:17–23, 1950.

[5] P. Fearnhead and D. Prangle. Constructing summary statistics for approximate Bayesian computation: Semi-automatic approximate Bayesian computation (with discussion). *Journal of the Royal Statistical Society: Series B*, 74:419–474, 2012.

[6] M.A. Beaumont, W. Zhang, and D.J. Balding. Approximate Bayesian computation in population genetics. *Genetics*, 162:2025–2035, 2002.

[7] S.A. Sisson, Y. Fan, and M.M. Tanaka. Sequential Monte Carlo without likelihoods. *Proceedings of the National Academy of Sciences USA*, 104:1760–1765, 2007.

[8] M.A. Beaumont, J-M. Cornuet, J-M. Marin, and C.P. Robert. Adaptive approximate Bayesian computation. *Biometrika*, 96:983–990, 2009.

[9] R.D. Wilkinson. Approximate Bayesian computation (ABC) gives exact results under the assumption of model error. *Journal Statistical Applications in Genetics and Molecular Biology*, 12:129–141, 2013.

[10] P. Neal and C.L. Huang. Forward simulation MCMC with applications to stochastic epidemic models. *Scandinavian Journal of Statistics*, 42:378–396, 2015.

[11] P. Neal and F. Xiang. Collapsing of non-centered parameterised MCMC algorithms with applications to epidemic models. *Scandinavian Journal of Statistics*, 44:81–96, 2017.

[12] G.O. Roberts, O. Papaspiliopoulos, and M. Sköld. Non-centered parameterisations for hierarchical models and data augmentation. In *Bayesian Statistics 7: Proceedings of the Seventh Valencia International Meeting*, page 307. Oxford University Press, Oxford, UK, 2003.

[13] P.M. Small, P.C. Hopewell, S.P. Singh, A.Paz, J.Parsonnet, D.C. Ruston, G.F. Schecter, C.L. Daley, and G.K. Schoolnik. The epidemiology of tuberculosis in San Francisco. A population-based study using conventional and molecular methods. *New England Journal of Medicine*, 330:1703–1709, 1994.

[14] T.J. McKinley, J.V. Ross, R. Deardon, and A.R. Cook. Simulation-based Bayesian inference for epidemic models. *Computational Statistics and Data Analysis*, 71: 434–447, 2014.

[15] P. Neal. Efficient likelihood-free Bayesian computation for household epidemics. *Statistics and Computing*, 22:1239–1256, 2012.

[16] T. Kypraios, P. Neal, and D. Prangle. A tutorial introduction to Bayesian inference for stochastic epidemic models using approximate Bayesian computation. *Mathematical Biosciences*, 287:42–53, 2017.

[17] M. Paunio, H. Peltola, M. Valle, I. Davidkin, M. Virtanen, and O. Heinonen. Explosive school-based measles outbreak: Intense exposure may have resulted in high risk, even among revaccinees. *American Journal of Epidemiology*, 148:1103–1110, 1998.

[18] M. van Boven, M. Kretzschmar, J. Wallinga, P.D. O'Neill, O. Wichmann, and S. Hahné. Estimation of measles vaccine efficacy and critical vaccination coverage in a highly vaccinated population. *Journal of the Royal Society Interface*, 7:1537–1544, 2010.

[19] F. Ball and P. O'Neill. The distribution of general final state random variables for stochastic epidemic models. *Journal of Applied Probability*, 36:473–491, 1999.

[20] W.J. Edmunds, N.J. Gay, M. Kretzschmar, and R.G. Pebody. The pre-vaccination epidemiology of measles, mumps and rubella in Europe: Implications for modelling studies. *Epidemiology and Infection*, 125:635–650, 2000.

[21] D. Ludwig. Final size distribution for epidemics. *Mathematical Biosciences*, 23:33–46, 1975.

[22] T. Sellke. On the asymptotic distribution of the size of a stochastic epidemic. *Journal of Applied Probability*, 20:390–394, 1983.

[23] G.J. Gibson. Markov chain Monte Carlo methods for fitting spatiotemporal stochastic models in plant epidemiology *Journal of the Royal Statistical Society: Series C*, 46:215–233, 1997.

[24] G.J. Gibson. Investigating mechanisms of spatiotemporal epidemic spread using stochastic models. *American Phytopathological Society*, 87:139–146, 1997.

[25] P.E Brown, F. Chimard, A. Remorov, J.S. Rosenthal, and X. Wang. Statistical inference and computational efficiency for spatial infectious-disease models with plantation data. *Journal of the Royal Statistical Society: Series C*, 63:467–482, 2014.

[26] R. Marcus, F. Svetlana, H. Talpaz, R. Salomon, and M. Bar-Joseph. On the spatial distribution of citrus tristeza virus disease. *Phytoparasitica*, 12:45–52, 1984.

[27] J.S. Liu. The collased Gibbs sampler in Bayesian computations with applications to a gene regulation problem. *Journal of the American Statistical Association*, 89:958–966, 1994.

[28] M.M. Tanaka, A.R. Francis, F. Luciani, and S.A. Sisson. Using approximate Bayesian computation to estimate tuberculosis transmission parameters from genotype data. *Genetics*, 173:1511–1520, 2006.

[29] P. Del Moral, A. Doucet, and A. Jasra. An adaptive sequential Monte Carlo method for approximate Bayesian compuation. *Statistics and Computing*, 22:1009–1020, 2012.

[30] M.G.B. Blum and V.C. Tran. HIV with contact tracing: A case study in approximate Bayesian computation. *Biostatistics*, 11:644–660, 2010.

[31] M. Baguelin, J.R. Newton, N. Demiris, J. Daly, J.A. Mumford, and J.L.N. Wood. Control of equine influenza: Scenario testing using a realistic metapopulation model of spread. *Journal of the Royal Society Interface*, 7:67–79, 2010.

[32] E. Brooks-Pollock, G.O. Roberts, and M.J. Keeling. A dynamic model of bovine tuberculosis spread and control in Great Britain. *Nature*, 511:228–231, 2014.

[33] M. Kosmala, P. Miller, S. Ferreira, P. Funston, D. Keet, and C. Packer. Estimating wildlife disease dynamics in complex systems using an approximate Bayesian computation framework. *Ecological Applications*, 26:295–308, 2016.

[34] I. Andrianakis, I.R. Vernon, N. McCreesh, T.J. McKinley, J.E. Oakley, R.N. Nsubuga, M. Goldstein, and R.G. White. Bayesian history matching of complex infectious disease models using emulation: A tutorial and a case study on HIV in Uganda. *PLoS Computational Biology*, 11:e1003968, 2015.

11

Iterated Filtering Methods for Markov Process Epidemic Models

Theresa Stocks

CONTENTS

11.1 Introduction

In this chapter we describe how iterated filtering methods (Ionides et al., 2006, 2015) can be used to analyze available infectious disease outbreak data in the form of time series. The centerpiece of these methods is the assumption that the outbreak data can be modeled as a noisy and only partially observed realization of a disease transmission process that is assumed to be a Markov process (King et al., 2016). The general inference approach is to (1) formulate a suitable Markovian transmission process, (2) connect the data to the transmission process using some suitable observation process, and (3) use iterated filtering to perform inference for the model parameters. The inference method presented here is likelihood-based. It is designed for models where it is relatively easy to draw samples from the Markov process compared to evaluating its transition probabilities. The iterated filtering algorithm is, among others, implemented in the R package pomp (King et al., 2016), which spans a wide collection of simulation, inference, and model selection methods for partially observed Markov processes (POMP). Other simulation-based inference methods for this model class are simulated moments (Kendall et al., 1999), synthetic likelihood (Wood, 2010), non-linear forecasting (Sugihara and May, 1990) or Bayesian approaches such as approximate Bayesian computations (Toni et al., 2009; Liu and West, 2001), and particle Markov chain Monte Carlo (PMCMC) (Andrieu et al., 2010). However, at present iterated filtering methods are the only currently available, frequentist, full-information, simulation-based inference methods for POMP models (Ionides et al., 2015).

In this chapter we focus on the "simplest" Markovian susceptible-infectious-recovered (SIR) trasmission model and describe in some detail how to fit this model to outbreak data consisting of the number of newly reported cases aggregated over time intervals, e.g. weeks. However, the methods can be easily extended to more complicated settings, several of which will be discussed herein.

The chapter is structured as follows: Section 11.2 gives a short overview about likelihood-based inference and describes some of its general challenges. In Section 11.3, we introduce the model class of partially observed Markov processes and explain how to formulate and evaluate the likelihood of such models with particle filters. In Section 11.4, we present the iterated filtering algorithm and demonstrate its use by a simple example in Section 11.5. In Section 11.6, we discuss possible extensions of this example and, in Section 11.7, illustrate how the method can be applied to a real-world problem which accommodates most of the complications mentioned. Both examples are accompanied by source code and instructions which can be found online at Stocks (2017). We finish the chapter by outlining advantages and disadvantages of the method presented and point the interested reader to further literature in Section 11.8.

11.2   Likelihood-Based Inference

We start by outlining the key aspects of likelihood-based inference that will be relevant to us. This is an extensive topic and for readers new to this area we refer to, e.g., Pawitan (2001) or Held and Sabanés Bové (2013) for a comprehensive overview on likelihood-based inference.

11.2.1   The likelihood approach

The idea behind likelihood-based inference is the following. Suppose we have data in the form of a sequence of N observations $\boldsymbol{y}_{1:N}^*$ at times $t_1, \ldots, t_N$ and a model for the data $f(\boldsymbol{y}_{1:N}; \boldsymbol{\theta})$ where f is typically a probability mass or density function parameterized by a vector of parameters denoted by $\boldsymbol{\theta}$. In our context $\boldsymbol{y}_{1:N}^*$ might, for example, represent the weekly number of newly reported cases over a certain period of time and $\boldsymbol{\theta}$ might contain the parameters of a suitable Markovian epidemic transmission model. To calibrate the model to our observations we would like to find the elements of the parameter vector $\boldsymbol{\theta}$ for which our observations are most likely under the chosen probability model. In other words, we would like to maximize this function f with respect to $\boldsymbol{\theta}$ evaluated at the data $\boldsymbol{y}_{1:N}^*$. This translates to optimizing the function

$$\mathcal{L}(\boldsymbol{\theta}; \boldsymbol{y}_{1:N}^*) = f(\boldsymbol{y}_{1:N}^*; \boldsymbol{\theta}).$$

The function $\mathcal{L}$ is called the *likelihood function* and in the following we will suppress its dependence on the data and simply write $\mathcal{L}(\boldsymbol{\theta})$ for convenience. The parameter vector which maximizes this function is called the *maximum likelihood estimate* (MLE) and is given as

$$\hat{\boldsymbol{\theta}} = \arg\max_{\boldsymbol{\theta}\in\Theta} \mathcal{L}(\boldsymbol{\theta}), \tag{11.1}$$

where Θ is the parameter space containing all possible sets of parameters.

For many applications, it is often more convenient to work with the *log-likelihood function*

$$l(\boldsymbol{\theta}) = \log \mathcal{L}(\boldsymbol{\theta}).$$

This transformation often simplifies optimization, but does not change the location of the MLE since the natural logarithm is a monotonically increasing function.

11.2.2 Practical challenges

In principle, the optimization problem in (11.1) looks rather straightforward; however, there are a number of challenges in practice. First, the evaluation of $\mathcal{L}$ can be difficult because the function might not be available in closed form. Secondly, even if evaluation is possible, it might be very hard to derive the first and higher order derivatives of $\mathcal{L}$ analytically or even numerically that are needed for numerical optimization methods (cf. Nocedal and Wright (1999)). In this case we need derivative-free optimizers. Those optimizers might impose other problems, for example when the likelihood can only be approximated stochastically, e.g., by Monte Carlo methods (Robert and Casella, 2004). In that case standard deterministic derivative-free optimizers fail. All the problems previously mentioned occur for the model class at hand because the likelihood is a complex integral. In the following sections, we will give more rigorous details about the problem and introduce a method which gets around these challenges. The problems mentioned arise in the specific setting of our model formulation. In addition, there are some other general challenges with likelihood-based inference in a statistical context. Usually the point estimate we obtain from maximum likelihood estimation is not very meaningful by itself unless we also quantify the uncertainty of the estimate. One way to solve this problem in a likelihood setting is to construct confidence intervals for the parameters by, e.g., calculating the profile log-likelihood for each parameter of interest and invert the Wilks (1938) likelihood ratio test to get the desired intervals. Another very common challenge is that often there exist multiple local maxima and the optimization algorithm can get stuck in one of these and not return the global maximum. It is, therefore, important to use a wide range of starting values for the numerical algorithm to improve chances that the global maximum is reached. Moreover, it might very well happen that the maximum is not unique because the surface of the likelihood function has ridges. In that case confidence intervals are a good way to quantify the parameter range. In the following, we introduce and formulate the likelihood of partially observed Markov processes and explain how to tackle all of the issues mentioned above.

11.3 Inference for Partially Observed Markov Processes

In the literature partially observed Markov processes are also known as hidden state space models or stochastic dynamical systems. The main assumption is that at discrete points in time we observe some noisy aspect of the true underlying Markov process which is often continuous in time. In the following, we formulate the likelihood of a POMP, give an idea why standard methods to find the MLE do not apply here, and finally describe how iterated filtering methods overcome these problems. In the following, the exposition and notation is adopted from King et al. (2016) and the materials and tutorials in King (2017).

11.3.1 Likelihood of a partially observed Markov process

A POMP consists of two model components: (1) an unobserved Markov process $\{X(t; \theta) : t \geq 0\}$, which can be discrete or continuous in time and (2) an observation model which describes how the data collected at discrete points in time $t_1, \ldots, t_N$, is connected to the transmission model. For notational convenience, we write $X_n = X(t_n; \theta)$ and $X_{0:N} = (X_0, \ldots, X_N)$. In our application, the process $X_{0:N}$ describes the dynamics of the disease spread, e.g., in the case of the simple Markovian SIR model $X_n = (S(t_n), I(t_n), R(t_n))'$ counts the number of susceptible, infectious, and removed individuals at time t_n. Let Y_n denote the random variable counting the observations at time t_n which depend on the state of the transmission process X_n at that time (cf. Figure 11.1). Our data, $y_{1:N}^* = (y_1^*, \ldots, y_N^*)$, are then modeled as a realization of this observation process. Depending on how many aspects of the disease dynamics we observe, $y_{1:N}^*$ can be either a univariate or multivariate time series. Assuming that the observable random variable Y_n is independent of all other variables given the state of the transmission process X_n, the joint density of the states and the observations is defined as the product of the one-step transmission density, $f_{X_n|X_{n-1}}(x_n|x_{n-1}; \theta)$, the observation density, $f_{Y_n|X_n}(y_n|x_n; \theta)$, and the initial density $f_{X_0}(x_0; \theta)$ as

$$
f_{X_{0:N}, Y_{1:N}}(x_{0:N}, y_{1:N}; \theta) = f_{X_0}(x_0; \theta)
$$
$$
\times \prod_{n=1}^{N} f_{X_n|X_{n-1}}(x_n|x_{n-1}; \theta) f_{Y_n|X_n}(y_n|x_n; \theta).
$$

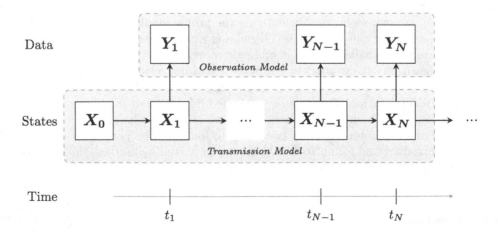

FIGURE 11.1
A partially observed Markov process where $Y_n, n = 1, \ldots, N$, denotes the observations at time t_n, which depend on the state of the transmission process $X_n := X(t_n; \theta)$ at that time.

Hence, the likelihood of the parameter vector can be written as the marginal density for a sequence of observations $\boldsymbol{Y}_{1:N}$ evaluated at the data $\boldsymbol{y}_{1:N}^{*}$ as

$$\mathcal{L}(\boldsymbol{\theta}) = f_{\boldsymbol{Y}_{1:N}}(\boldsymbol{y}_{1:N}^{*}; \boldsymbol{\theta}) = \int f_{\boldsymbol{X}_{0:N}, \boldsymbol{Y}_{1:N}}(\boldsymbol{x}_{0:N}, \boldsymbol{y}_{1:N}^{*}; \boldsymbol{\theta}) d\boldsymbol{x}_{0:N}. \qquad (11.2)$$

The dimension of the integral in (11.2) depends on the number of compartments of the Markov process and the number of observations, so this integral is usually high dimensional and, except for the simplest situations, cannot be solved analytically. The method we will present in the following sections uses the property that it is fairly easy to draw samples from the density $f_{\boldsymbol{X}_n|\boldsymbol{X}_{n-1}}$ rather than evaluating the function. Because the distribution $f_{\boldsymbol{X}_0}$ of the initial state of the Markov process is usually not known, one practical way to deal with this is to fix the initial values of the system at some reasonable values or, treat them as parameters we would like to estimate (see Section 11.6 for further discussion).

11.3.2 Evaluation of the likelihood

Before addressing the question of how to maximize the likelihood in (11.2) in an efficient way, we have to first think about how we actually evaluate $\mathcal{L}$ for a given parameter vector $\boldsymbol{\theta}$. In the special case that the underlying transmission model is deterministic and the initial values are given, $\boldsymbol{X}_n = \boldsymbol{x}_n(\boldsymbol{\theta})$ is a non-random function of $\boldsymbol{\theta}$ for each n, hence $f_{\boldsymbol{X}_n|\boldsymbol{X}_{n-1}}$ and $f_{\boldsymbol{X}_0}$ are point masses. The likelihood equation (11.2) then reduces to

$$\ell(\boldsymbol{\theta}) = \log \mathcal{L}(\boldsymbol{\theta}) = \sum_{n=1}^{N} \log f_{\boldsymbol{Y}_n|\boldsymbol{X}_n}(\boldsymbol{y}_n^{*}; \boldsymbol{x}_n(\boldsymbol{\theta}), \boldsymbol{\theta}). \qquad (11.3)$$

So given that we know the distribution of our observation model, evaluation of the log-likelihood corresponds to summing over the logarithm of the observation density given the states of the deterministic Markov process at each point in time. Maximum likelihood estimation then reduces to a classical numerical optimization problem for a non-linear function of the parameter vector and for optimization we can use a derivative-free optimizer, e.g., the Nelder-Mead (1965). However, in general evaluating (and optimizing) the function $\mathcal{L}$ is unfortunately not as straightforward because the transmission model is not deterministic. Rather, it is a non-trivial problem because of the high dimension of the integral. In the following we describe how to evaluate Equation (11.2) in a general way with particle filters.

11.3.3 Particle filter

One standard approach to solve a high dimensional integral as in Equation (11.2) is to approximate the integral by Monte Carlo methods. However, as it will turn out, for the model class at hand, this approach is highly inefficient in practice. Nevertheless, we will demonstrate this approach first to introduce the reader to the problem. Readers unfamiliar with Monte Carlo methods might want to consult the relevant literature, e.g., Robert and Casella (2004) and Doucet et al. (2001).

The basic idea is that the likelihood in Equation (11.2), which can also be written as the integral

$$\mathcal{L}(\boldsymbol{\theta}) = \int \prod_{n=1}^{N} f_{\boldsymbol{Y}_n|\boldsymbol{X}_n}(\boldsymbol{y}_n|\boldsymbol{x}_n; \boldsymbol{\theta}) f_{\boldsymbol{X}_{0:N}}(\boldsymbol{x}_{0:N}; \boldsymbol{\theta}) d\boldsymbol{x}_{0:N} \qquad (11.4)$$

can be approximated using the Monte Carlo principle as

$$\mathcal{L}(\boldsymbol{\theta}) \approx \frac{1}{J} \sum_{j=1}^{J} \prod_{n=1}^{N} f_{\boldsymbol{Y}_n|\boldsymbol{X}_n}(\boldsymbol{y}_n^*|\boldsymbol{x}_{n,j}; \boldsymbol{\theta}),$$

where $\{\boldsymbol{x}_{0:N,j}, j = 1, \ldots, J\}$ is a sample drawn from $f_{\boldsymbol{X}_{0:N}}(\boldsymbol{x}_{0:N}; \boldsymbol{\theta})$. This result means that if we generate trajectories by simulating from the Markov process, we just have to evaluate the density of the data given the realizations and then average to obtain a Monte Carlo approximation of the likelihood.

It turns out, however, that with this approach the variability in the approximation of the likelihood is very high, because the way of proposing trajectories is entirely unconditional of the data. This result means that in practice this method is very inefficient, because a lot of simulations are necessary in order to obtain an estimate of the likelihood that is precise enough to be useful for parameter estimation or model selection. The longer the time series, the worse the problem gets (King, 2017). As it turns out, a better idea is to parameterize the likelihood in (11.2) as

$$\mathcal{L}(\boldsymbol{\theta}) = \prod_{n=1}^{N} \mathcal{L}_{n|n-1}(\boldsymbol{\theta}), \tag{11.5}$$

where $\mathcal{L}_{n|n-1}(\boldsymbol{\theta})$ is the conditional likelihood, given as

$$\mathcal{L}_{n|n-1}(\boldsymbol{\theta}) = f_{\boldsymbol{Y}_n|\boldsymbol{Y}_{1:n-1}}(\boldsymbol{y}_n^*|\boldsymbol{y}_{1:n-1}^*; \boldsymbol{\theta})$$
$$= \int f_{\boldsymbol{Y}_n|\boldsymbol{X}_n}(\boldsymbol{y}_n^*|\boldsymbol{x}_n; \boldsymbol{\theta}) f_{\boldsymbol{X}_n|\boldsymbol{Y}_{1:n-1}}(\boldsymbol{x}_n|\boldsymbol{y}_{1:n-1}^*; \boldsymbol{\theta}) d\boldsymbol{x}_n, \tag{11.6}$$

with the convention that $f_{\boldsymbol{X}_1|\boldsymbol{Y}_{1:0}} = f_{\boldsymbol{X}_1}$.

In the following we explain how this integral can be efficiently approximated with resampling techniques which are the basis of particle filter methods. Since $\boldsymbol{X}_n$ is a Markov chain it follows from the Chapman Kolmogorov equation that

$$f_{\boldsymbol{X}_n|\boldsymbol{Y}_{1:n-1}}(\boldsymbol{x}_n|\boldsymbol{y}_{1:n-1}^*; \boldsymbol{\theta}) = \tag{11.7}$$
$$\int f_{\boldsymbol{X}_n|\boldsymbol{X}_{n-1}}(\boldsymbol{x}_n|\boldsymbol{x}_{n-1}; \boldsymbol{\theta}) f_{\boldsymbol{X}_{n-1}|\boldsymbol{Y}_{1:n-1}}(\boldsymbol{x}_{n-1}|\boldsymbol{y}_{1:n-1}^*; \boldsymbol{\theta}) d\boldsymbol{x}_{n-1}.$$

From Bayes' theorem it also follows that

$$f_{\boldsymbol{X}_n|\boldsymbol{Y}_{1:n}}(\boldsymbol{x}_n|\boldsymbol{y}_{1:n}^*; \boldsymbol{\theta}) = f_{\boldsymbol{X}_n|\boldsymbol{Y}_n,\boldsymbol{Y}_{1:n-1}}(\boldsymbol{x}_n|\boldsymbol{y}_n^*, \boldsymbol{y}_{1:n-1}^*; \boldsymbol{\theta})$$
$$= \frac{f_{\boldsymbol{Y}_n|\boldsymbol{X}_n}(\boldsymbol{y}_n^*|\boldsymbol{x}_n; \boldsymbol{\theta}) f_{\boldsymbol{X}_n|\boldsymbol{Y}_{1:n-1}}(\boldsymbol{x}_n|\boldsymbol{y}_{1:n-1}^*; \boldsymbol{\theta})}{\int f_{\boldsymbol{Y}_n|\boldsymbol{X}_n}(\boldsymbol{y}_n^*|\boldsymbol{x}_n; \boldsymbol{\theta}) f_{\boldsymbol{X}_n|\boldsymbol{Y}_{1:n-1}}(\boldsymbol{x}_n|\boldsymbol{y}_{1:n-1}^*; \boldsymbol{\theta}) d\boldsymbol{x}_n}, \tag{11.8}$$

where we use the fact that $\boldsymbol{Y}_n$ only depends on $\boldsymbol{X}_n$. The distribution $f_{\boldsymbol{X}_n|\boldsymbol{Y}_{1:n-1}}$ is called the *prediction distribution* and $f_{\boldsymbol{X}_n|\boldsymbol{Y}_{1:n}}$ is called the *filtering distribution* at time t_n. The idea now works as follows. Assume we have a set of J points $\{\boldsymbol{x}_{n-1,j}^F\}_{j=1}^J$, in the following referred to as *particles*, from the filtering distribution at time t_{n-1}. Equation (11.7) then implies that we obtain a sample $\{\boldsymbol{x}_{n,j}^P\}$ from the prediction distribution at time t_n if we just simulate from the Markov model

$$\boldsymbol{x}_{n,j}^P \sim f_{\boldsymbol{X}_n|\boldsymbol{X}_{n-1}}(\cdot|\boldsymbol{x}_{n-1,j}^F; \boldsymbol{\theta}) \quad \text{with} \quad j = 1, \ldots, J. \tag{11.9}$$

Equation (11.8) in turn tells us that resampling from $\{x_{n,j}^P\}$ with weights proportional to

$$\omega_{n,j} = f_{\boldsymbol{Y}_n|\boldsymbol{X}_n}(\boldsymbol{y}_n^*|\boldsymbol{x}_{n,j}^P; \boldsymbol{\theta}) \tag{11.10}$$

gives us a sample from the filtering distribution at time t_n. By the Monte Carlo principle it follows from (11.6) that

$$\mathcal{L}_{n|n-1}(\boldsymbol{\theta}) \approx \frac{1}{J}\sum_{j=1}^{J} f_{\boldsymbol{Y}_n|\boldsymbol{X}_n}(\boldsymbol{y}_n^*|\boldsymbol{x}_{n,j}^P; \boldsymbol{\theta}),$$

where $x_{n,j}^P$ is approximately drawn from $f_{\boldsymbol{X}_n|\boldsymbol{Y}_{1:n-1}}(\boldsymbol{x}_n|\boldsymbol{y}_{1:n-1}^*; \boldsymbol{\theta})$. To obtain the full likelihood, we have to iterate through the data, alternating between simulating (11.9) and resampling (11.10) in every time step, until we reach $n = N$ so that

$$\ell(\boldsymbol{\theta}) = \log \mathcal{L}(\boldsymbol{\theta}) = \sum_{n=1}^{N} \log \mathcal{L}_{n|n-1}(\boldsymbol{\theta}). \tag{11.11}$$

This method to evaluate the likelihood is called a *sequential Monte Carlo* algorithm or *particle filter* (Kitagawa, 1987; Doucet et al., 2001; Arulampalam et al., 2002). The method is implemented as the `pfilter` function in the `pomp` package (King et al., 2016) and returns a stochastic estimate of the likelihood which can be shown to be unbiased (Del Moral, 1996).

It can happen that at some time point a very unlikely particle is suggested. In practice, if the conditional likelihood of this particle is below a certain tolerance value, then that particle is considered to be uninformative. If, at some time point, the conditional likelihood of every particle is below this chosen tolerance a *filtering failure* occurs. When a failure occurs, re-sampling is omitted, the conditional likelihood at that time point is set equal to the tolerance and the iteration through the dataset continues; hence, the time point at which the filtering failure occurred is taken to contain no information. In general, filtering failures are an implication that the model and data might not be consistent (King, 2017).

The variability of the approximation in Equation (11.11) can be reduced by increasing the number J of particles; however, the variability will usually not vanish completely. This result might create problems for standard optimizers, which assume that the likelihood is evaluated deterministically. A better choice in this case is to use stochastic optimizers such as the iterated filtering method that we present in the next section.

11.4 Iterated Filtering Methods

Iterated filtering is a simulation-based method to find the MLE which takes advantage of the structure of POMP models and particle filters. It was first introduced by Ionides et al. (2006) and further improved in Ionides et al. (2015). The iterated filtering method uses the property that it is easy to simulate from $f_{\boldsymbol{X}_n|\boldsymbol{X}_{n-1}}$ while the likelihood is not tractable directly. The basic idea is that a particle filter is applied to a model in which the parameter vector for each particle is following a random walk. As iterations progress, the intensity of the perturbations is successively reduced ("cooling"). It can be shown that the algorithm converges towards the MLE (Ionides et al., 2015). At present this method is the only simulation-based frequentist approach that uses the full information contained in the data. Moreover, iterated filtering methods have been able to solve likelihood-based inference problems for infectious disease related questions which were computationally intractable for available Bayesian methods (Ionides et al., 2015).

11.4.1   Algorithm

In the following we present the pseudocode for iterated filtering as implemented in the `mif2` function in the R package `pomp` and explain how to draw samples from $f_{\boldsymbol{X}_n|\boldsymbol{X}_{n-1}}$.

Pseudocode iterated filtering (`mif2`) cf. Ionides et al. (2015)

Input: Simulators for $f_{\boldsymbol{X}_0}(\boldsymbol{x}_0;\boldsymbol{\theta})$ and $f_{\boldsymbol{X}_n|\boldsymbol{X}_{n-1}}(\boldsymbol{x}_n|\boldsymbol{x}_{n-1};\boldsymbol{\theta})$; evaluator for $f_{\boldsymbol{Y}_n|\boldsymbol{X}_n}(\boldsymbol{y}_n|\boldsymbol{x}_n;\boldsymbol{\theta})$; data $\boldsymbol{y}_{1:N}^*$

Algorithmic parameters: # of iterations M; # of particles J; initial parameter swarm $\{\boldsymbol{\theta}_j^0, j=1,\ldots,J\}$; perturbation density $h_n(\boldsymbol{\theta}|\varphi;\sigma)$; perturbation scale $\sigma_{1:M}$

Procedure:

1:   For m in $1{:}M$

2:     $\boldsymbol{\theta}_{0,j}^{F,m} \sim h_0(\,\cdot\,|\boldsymbol{\theta}_j^{m-1};\sigma_m)$ for j in $1{:}J$

3:     $\boldsymbol{X}_{0,j}^{F,m} \sim f_{\boldsymbol{X}_0}(\,\cdot\,;\boldsymbol{\theta}_{0,j}^{F,m})$ for j in $1{:}J$

4:     For n in $1{:}N$

5:       $\boldsymbol{\theta}_{n,j}^{P,m} \sim h_n(\,\cdot\,|\boldsymbol{\theta}_{n-1,j}^{F,m},\sigma_m)$ for j in $1{:}J$

6:       $\boldsymbol{X}_{n,j}^{P,m} \sim f_{\boldsymbol{X}_n|\boldsymbol{X}_{n-1}}(\,\cdot\,|\boldsymbol{X}_{n-1,j}^{F,m};\boldsymbol{\theta}_{n,j}^{P,m})$ for j in $1{:}J$

7:       $w_{n,j}^m = f_{\boldsymbol{Y}_n|\boldsymbol{X}_n}(\boldsymbol{y}_n^*|\boldsymbol{X}_{n,j}^{P,m};\boldsymbol{\theta}_{n,j}^{P,m})$ for j in $1{:}J$

8:       Draw $k_{1:J}$ with $P(k_j=i)=w_{n,i}^m\big/\sum_{u=1}^J w_{n,u}^m$

9:       $\boldsymbol{\theta}_{n,j}^{F,m}=\boldsymbol{\theta}_{n,k_j}^{P,m}$ and $\boldsymbol{X}_{n,j}^{F,m}=\boldsymbol{X}_{n,k_j}^{P,m}$ for j in $1{:}J$

10:    End For

11:    Set $\boldsymbol{\theta}_j^m=\boldsymbol{\theta}_{N,j}^{F,m}$ for j in $1{:}J$

12:   End For

Output: Final parameter swarm, $\{\boldsymbol{\theta}_j^M, j=1,\ldots,J\}$

In the algorithm the initial parameter values are perturbed (line 2) by a perturbation density where its standard deviation σ_m is a decreasing function of m. The Markov process is initialized (line 3) as a draw from the initial density dependent on the proposed parameter vector. What follows in lines 4–10 is a particle filter as described in the section above with the only difference being that the parameter vector is stochastically perturbed in every iteration through the data. The M loop repeats the particle filter with decreasing perturbations and throughout the algorithm the superscripts F and P denote filtering and prediction distribution, respectively. The algorithm returns the best guess of the parameter swarm after M iterations. In the R package `pomp` the point estimate that the function `mif2` returns is the mean of the parameter swarm.

To generate realizations from $f_{\boldsymbol{X}_n|\boldsymbol{X}_{n-1}}$ we can use the Gillespie (1977) algorithm. Given the current state of the system, the algorithm simulates the waiting time of the next event and updates the number of individuals in each compartment and the overall time is incremented accordingly. The whole procedure is repeated until a pre-defined stopping time is reached. In the case of constant per capita transition rates, the simulation of every individual event gives us a complete and detailed history of the process; however, it is usually a very time-consuming task for systems with large population and state space, because of the enormous number of events that can take place. As a way to speed up such simulations an approximate simulation method can be used, the so called τ-*leap algorithm* which is based on the Gillespie (2001) algorithm. The τ-leap algorithm holds all rates constant in a small time interval τ and simulates the numbers of events that will occur in this interval, then updates all state variables, computes the transition rates again and the procedure is repeated until the stopping time is reached (Erhard et al., 2010; King, 2017). Given the total number of jumps, the number of individuals leaving any of the states by any available route during a time interval τ is then multinomially distributed. Note that the simulation time step is not identical with the timescale the observation process evolves on. Both simulation algorithms are conveniently implemented in the `pomp` package as the functions `gillespie.sim` and `euler.sim`.

11.5 Iterated Filtering for SIR Model Given Incidence Data

11.5.1 The problem of interest

Typical infectious disease data collected by public health authorities often consists of reported incidences in given time periods. Other important characteristics of an epidemic such as recovery times of the individual or contact network are not observed. The method presented is a useful tool to analyze routinely collected surveillance data because it gives insights into the mechanism of disease spread which is crucial if one wants to assess the risk of emerging pathogens or evaluate the impact of control measures such as vaccination.

In this section we describe how to carry out inference for the parameters of a POMP where the underlying disease transmission model is assumed to be a simple Markovian SIR model, given that we observe the number of newly reported cases aggregated by week. We use the algorithm presented in Section 11.4 for a simulated data set and illustrate how the algorithm performs.

To keep things simple, in the specific example of this section, we assume that the time of reporting coincides with the time of infection. Of course, this assumption does not hold for all diseases but the method presented here can be easily adopted to other settings, e.g., when the time of reporting coincides with the time of removal.

The implementation of the following example is made available by Stocks (2017).

11.5.2 Formulation of a POMP model

We will first formulate a Markov transmission model and in a second step relate the data to the transmission model via some observation model which then gives us $f_{Y_n|X_n}$.

Transmission model. As transmission model we choose a stochastic SIR model among a closed population of $\mathcal{N}$ individuals where $\boldsymbol{X}(t) = (S(t), I(t), R(t))$ denotes the number of susceptible, infectious and recovered individuals at time t. Individuals are mixing homogeneously and β is the average number of infectious contacts an infectious individual has per time unit. Furthermore, we assume that the time an individual is infectious is exponentially distributed with mean γ^{-1}. We will now formulate this in a way which makes understanding of the code in Stocks (2017) easier. So let $\{N_{AB}(t) : t \geq 0\}$ denote a stochastic process which counts the number of individuals which have transitioned from compartment A to compartment B during the time interval $[0, t)$ with $A, B \in \mathcal{X}$, where $\mathcal{X} = \{S, I, R\}$ contains all model compartments. The infinitesimal increment probabilities of a jump between compartments fully specify the continuous-time Markov process describing the transmission dynamics. With this notation, $\Delta N_{AB}(t) = N_{AB}(t+\tau) - N_{AB}(t)$ counts the number of individuals changing compartment in an infinitesimal time interval $\tau > 0$. Thus,

$$\mathbb{P}[\Delta N_{SI}(t) = 1|\boldsymbol{X}(t)] = \beta I(t)S(t)\mathcal{N}^{-1}\tau + o(\tau)$$

$$\mathbb{P}[\Delta N_{IR}(t) = 1|\boldsymbol{X}(t)] = \gamma I(t)\tau + o(\tau). \tag{11.12}$$

Moreover, the state variables and the transition probabilities (11.12) are related in the following way:

$$\Delta S(t) = -\Delta N_{SI}(t)$$

$$\Delta I(t) = \Delta N_{SI}(t) - \Delta N_{IR}(t) \tag{11.13}$$

$$\Delta R(t) = \Delta N_{IR}(t).$$

Observation model. We now relate the transmission model to our observations of the weekly number of newly reported cases. With the notation above the true number of newly infected individuals accumulated in each observation time period $(t_{n-1}, t_n], n \in \{1, 2, \ldots, N\}$ is given as

$$H(t_n) = N_{SI}(t_n) - N_{SI}(t_{n-1}). \tag{11.14}$$

To incorporate the count nature of the observations a natural assumption is to model the actual reported cases as realizations of a Poisson-distributed random variable with a given time-dependent mean. The number of recorded cases Y_n within a given reporting interval $(t_{n-1}, t_n]$, is then

$$Y_n \sim \text{Pois}\left(H(t_n)\right). \tag{11.15}$$

This distribution then corresponds to $f_{\boldsymbol{Y}_n|\boldsymbol{X}_n}$ which is easy to evaluate. One interpretation of this choice of observation noise is to account for uncertainty in classification of cases, including false positives.

11.5.3   Inference

In the following we perform inference for the two epidemiological parameters β and γ on a set of simulated data from the model where we apply the iterated filtering algorithm presented in Section 11.4.

Data. We consider a closed population with $\mathcal{N} = 10{,}000$ individuals of whom one is initially infectious and the rest are susceptible. A realization from the model presented previously with $\beta = 1$ and $\gamma = 0.5$ for $N = 50$ weeks where $t_n = n$ for $n = 1, \ldots, N$ was simulated. Figure 11.2 shows the number of weekly reported cases where it is assumed that all cases are reported.

Implementation details. We use the iterated filtering algorithm as implemented in the function `mif2` in the R package `pomp` to infer the epidemic parameters β and γ assuming the initial values and total population size were known. We run the algorithm for $M = 100$ iterations and $J = 500$ particles. As starting values for the fitting algorithm, we use 10 parameter constellations drawn uniformly from a hypercube which contains biologically meaningful parameter values for β and γ. With this procedure, we address the potential problem of local maxima in the optimization. In general, if all searches converge to the

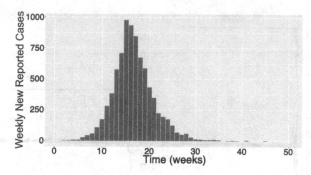

FIGURE 11.2

Weekly number of newly reported cases over time, for a simulated set from the POMP model with an underlying Markovian SIR transmission model as defined in Equations (11.13) and (11.15).

same MLE for starting values drawn at random from a hypercube, then this increases the chances that a global maximum has been found (King, 2017). For the perturbation of the parameters, we choose a random walk with an initial standard derivation of 0.02 for both parameters. As a cooling scheme, we use geometric cooling which means that on the n-th `mif2` iteration, the relative perturbation intensity is $k^{n/50}$, where we chose $k = 0.05$. That is, after 50 iterations the perturbation is only half of the intensity compared to the first iteration. In each iteration the variance of the random walk is successively reduced so the log-likelihood of the perturbed model gradually approaches the log-likelihood of the model we are interested in. However, after a finite number of iteration steps, the log-likelihoods of the two models, the one with and the one without perturbed parameters, are not identical. To get around this issue, a particle filter evaluation of the `mif2` model output using Equation (11.11) is necessary. Hence, for each of the 10 `mif2` outputs we obtain, we run 10 particle filters, each with 1,000 particles. From the multiple particle filter evaluation we then can calculate the average log-likelihood and the standard error of the Monte Carlo approximation for every parameter set. Consequently, we choose the parameter constellation of the 10 possible with the highest average log-likelihood as the MLE. To quantify the associated uncertainties of the parameter estimates based on our observations we calculate the 95% confidence intervals for each parameter. For this, we construct the profile likelihood of each parameter and apply the Monte Carlo adjusted profile (MCAP) algorithm (Ionides et al., 2017). This recently developed methodology accounts for the presence of Monte Carlo error in the likelihood evaluation and adjusts the width of the confidence interval accordingly. This procedure might seem overly complicated at first sight because, intuitively, the parameter swarm we obtain as an output from the iterated filtering algorithm should contain some measure of uncertainty. However, due to particle depletion, which is the situation when only very few different particles have significant weight (Doucet and Johansen, 2011), the information about the local shape of the likelihood surface contained in the particles is not very reliable. The profile likelihood is much more robust in this case since it relies on multiple independent `mif2` searches (King, 2017).

Results. The inference results are visualized in Figures 11.3 and 11.4. As shown in Figure 11.3, the randomly drawn starting values for both parameters are converging towards the true values at the same time as the likelihood increases and the number of filtering failures disappears. Both 95% confidence intervals constructed from the profile log-likelihoods cover the true parameters as shown in Figure 11.4.

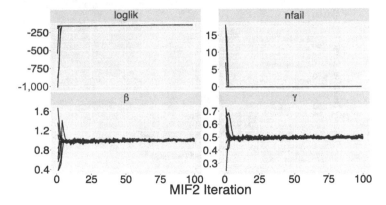

FIGURE 11.3
Diagnostic plot of the iterated filtering algorithm for 100 iterations for simulated incidence data. Shown is the evolution of the log-likelihood (loglik), the number of filtering failures in each `mif2` iteration (nfail), and parameter estimates for parameters β and γ per iteration for 10 trajectories with random starting values drawn from a hypercube.

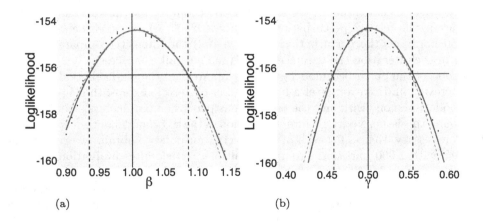

FIGURE 11.4
The smoothed profile likelihoods (solid curves) for both parameters of interest where the solid vertical lines show the true values and the dashed vertical lines contain the corresponding MCAP 95% confidence interval. The quadratic approximation in a neighborhood of the maximum is shown as the dashed curves. (a) Profile log-likelihood for β and (b) Profile log-likelihood for γ.

11.5.4   Practical advice

In the R package pomp a partially observed Markov process together with observations in the form of a uni- or multivariate time series can be represented through a so-called pomp object. The whole package's functionality such as simulation and inference is centered around this object. Depending on which functions used, the model can be implemented by specifying some or all model components. To help identify possible error sources that can occur while applying the algorithm, we now describe a few practical hints.

The first step after constructing the `pomp` object is to simulate realizations from the model to check that the code is working and the model gives the expected output. A good idea at this stage also is to construct the corresponding deterministic skeleton of the stochastic Markov transmission model to have a simplified version of the model and also to generate trajectories and compare if the mean of the stochastic model corresponds to the deterministic version. Another benefit of simulating from the model in general is that it helps to identify a range of likely parameters which generate realizations that resemble the data. Before the data comes into play and the actual fitting starts, we find it very helpful to first test the algorithm with simulated data. For this, a realization of the model is generated, then the known set of parameters which was used to generate the realization is evaluated with the particle filter. This way we make sure that the core function in the iterated filtering method is working. Then the algorithm can be applied to the simulated set and it should give back the values used for simulation. This procedure also helps understanding how the parameter estimators are correlated and if they are identifiable.

Now, let us move to the data. As a last step before applying the iterated filtering algorithm to our observations, we recommend to fit the data first to the simpler, deterministic model to get a feeling for how the parameters behave and identify possible problems with the likelihood surface, etc. Then, when the `mif2` is finally used, it makes sense to choose likely values as starting values for the parameters we want to estimate first. However, in a last step a global search should be carried out, which means that random starting values are chosen and, ideally, then all searches converge to the same MLE regardless of their starting values. In practice, the likelihood is often ridged so some searches can get stuck in local maxima. That is why it is important to use many initial values from many different starting values. Another common problem in practice is that parameter values are suggested that are very unlikely, which in turn leads to filtering failures. In that case it can be useful to add stochasticity to the model, which accounts for model misspecifications or unmodeled disease characteristics.

Working with the `mif2` algorithm can be a time consuming task because the method is simulation based. This is the price we pay for not needing to be able to evaluate the density function of the Markov model directly. That is why we also want to give some hints of how to speed up the procedure to some extent. The first idea is to parallelize the code so that multiple searches can be carried out at the same time. This, in turn, poses some challenges in preventing repetition of expensive computations and trying to ensure reproducibility and we present one way of doing this in the manual by Stocks (2017); more can be found in the tutorials at King (2017). To ensure that the information about the likelihood surface is continually improved, it is useful to keep a record of all parameter vectors estimated with the `mif2` function, together with the computed likelihood for each parameter set, e.g., by saving the obtained results in a CSV file (King, 2017). Moreover, it is sometimes worth accepting approximation errors by choosing the simulation time step in the τ leaping algorithm to be not too small, which can lead to significant gains in computational speed; for a short discussion on numerical solutions based on discretizations in the context of POMP models see Bretó et al. (2009).

11.6 Extensions

In the previous section we used a simple model to explain the concept of iterated filtering to facilitate understanding. However, reality is often way more complicated than this toy example. In the following, we discuss some important complications of infectious disease data and how they can be included in POMP models.

Underreporting. Underreporting is a common problem appearing in surveillance data and is usually the more pronounced the less severe the disease is. It arises for different reasons, e.g., it can result from asymptomatic cases, cases where individuals do not consult the doctor, cases that are not identified as such (misdiagnosis), or cases that just get lost in the reporting system (Gibbons et al., 2014). One way to include underreporting in a POMP model is to change the observation model to

$$Y_n \sim \text{Pois}\left(\kappa \cdot H(t_n)\right).$$

where $\kappa \in (0,1]$ is the reporting rate which then also can be estimated.

Seasonality. For many diseases such as childhood diseases or vector borne diseases the transmission rate β is not constant but varies through time. This might be due to social aggregations of the host such as in daycare institutions and schools which are closed during summer, changes in environment that influence the biology of vector populations or changes in weather such as temperature or precipitation. One way to introduce this complexity into our models is through seasonal forcing of the transmission rate so that the number of infectious contacts changes through time as $\beta(t)$. Following Keeling and Rohani (2008), one possible choice is

$$\beta(t) = \beta\left(1 + \rho\cos\left(\frac{2\pi}{w}t + \phi\right)\right),\tag{11.16}$$

where $\rho \in [0,1]$ is the amplitude of the forcing, $2\pi/w \in \mathbb{R}^+$ is the period of the forcing and $\phi \in [0,2\pi]$ is the phase shift parameter. With this choice of forcing function the parameter β can be interpreted as the average transmission rate of an individual which varies between $(1-\rho)\beta$ and $(1+\rho)\beta$ during the forcing period.

A more flexible way to choose the forcing function is through splines. If $s_i(t)$, $i = 1,\ldots,k$ is a periodic B-spline basis, then we can for example define

$$\beta(t) = \sum_{i=1}^{k} b_i s_i(t).$$

Variation of the coefficients b_i then gives a wide variety of shapes for $\beta(t)$. For the reader new to the theory of splines we recommend Stoer and Bulirsch (2002). A comprehensive overview of the problems of seasonal forcing can be found in Keeling and Rohani (2008).

Overdispersion. A common phenomenon in calibration of models from data is the presence of greater variability in the set of observations than would be expected under the assumed model (cf. e.g., McCullagh and Nelder (1989); Bretó et al. (2009)). Reasons for this include heterogeneities in the population, model misspecifications or unmodeled processes which we either cannot quantify or they are very hard to measure in any way. This phenomenon is called overdispersion and we can account for it in two different ways. On the one hand, we can introduce overdispersion into the observation model by changing the observation distribution from the Poisson distribution to a distribution where the variance can be adjusted separately from the mean. In the case of count data, a natural distribution would be the negative binomial distribution, so

$$Y_n \sim \text{NegBin}\left(H(t_n), \frac{1}{\psi}\right),\tag{11.17}$$

with $H(t_n)$ being the true number of accumulated incidences per time unit $(t_{n-1}, t_n]$ and NegBin$(\mu, 1/\psi)$ with $\psi > 0$ denotes the negative binomial distribution with mean μ and variance $\mu + \psi\mu^2$. Another choice could be the truncated normal distribution where the results are rounded to integers.

However, in outbreak data, we often see fluctuations which clearly are not only due to variation in data collection, but due to phenomena not captured by the model. In the toy example in Section 11.5, we have accounted for stochasticity in the underlying system by assuming that individuals move between classes at random times. However, for large population sizes the stochastic system approaches the deterministic system and, hence, the role of randomness decreases as the population size increases (for details cf. e.g., Fuchs (2013)). One way to account for overdispersion in the transmission model is to stochastically perturb the transmission rate by multiplying a continuous-time white noise process $\xi(t)$, which fluctuates around the value 1 with the transmission rate. In Bretó et al. (2009), it is shown that by choosing the corresponding integrated noise process $\Gamma(t)$ in a way such that its increments are independent, stationary, non-negative, and unbiased the Markov property is retained. One suitable example for such a process is a Lévy process with

$$\xi(t) = \frac{d}{dt}\Gamma(t), \quad \text{where marginally} \quad \Gamma(t+\tau) - \Gamma(t) \sim \text{Gamma}\left(\frac{\tau}{\sigma^2}, \sigma^2\right),$$

and where τ/σ^2 denotes the shape and σ^2 the scale parameter with corresponding mean τ and variance $\tau\sigma^2$. The parameter σ^2 is called the *infinitesimal variance* parameter (Karlin and Taylor, 1981). We can include this into the model by letting the transmission rate be

$$\beta(t) = \beta \cdot \xi(t). \tag{11.18}$$

More details about this kind of overdispersion can be found in Bretó et al. (2009) and Bretó and Ionides (2011).

Structured populations. To make mathematical models for disease spread more realistic different kinds of host heterogeneities can be introduced (Keeling and Rohani, 2008). For example, age structure, spatial heterogeneity, or varying risk structures of the individuals might play an important role in disease transmission and can be easily accommodated in a POMP.

Covariates. It can be interesting to investigate what impact a vector-valued covariate process $\{Z(t) : t \geq 0\}$ has on the disease dynamics. That might be environmental covariates such as temperature, precipitation, or demographic information such as numbers of births and deaths over time. Inclusion of such a covariate vector is unproblematic in a POMP setting because the densities $f_{\boldsymbol{X}_0}$, $f_{\boldsymbol{X}_n|\boldsymbol{X}_{n-1}}$ and $f_{\boldsymbol{Y}_n|\boldsymbol{X}_n}$ can depend on the observed process $\{Z(t) : t \geq 0\}$ (King et al., 2016). If we are interested in investigating the influence of a specific covariate on the transmission rate we could check the model's capability to fit the data with and without this covariate and compare the results.

Initial values. In our toy example of Section 11.5, we assumed that the distribution of the initial values of the Markov process, $f_{\boldsymbol{X}_0}$, is known. Besides some special cases that could arise in some experimental situations, this distribution is, however, not known or observable. If the disease we observe is endemic in the population and does not vary significant over time, it might make sense to assume that the initial values originate from the stationary distribution of the system. If this is not the case, we can treat the value of $\boldsymbol{X}_0$ as a parameter to be estimated. In this case, $f_{\boldsymbol{X}_0}$ is a point mass, the concentration of which depends on $\boldsymbol{\theta}$ (King et al., 2016).

Missing data. Missing values in outbreak data are a common complication. When using the R package `pomp`, the `pomp` object can handle missing values if the observation model probability density function is implemented so as to deal with them appropriately. One way is to construct the observation density so it returns a log-likelihood of 0 for the missing data entries; for implementational details see the FAQ in King (2017).

11.7   Rotavirus Example

After presenting a simple toy example as a proof of concept, we now give a short illustration of a real-world problem which accommodates some of the complications presented in the previous section and was analyzed with iterated filtering. A detailed description of the model and inference results can be found in Stocks et al. (2018).

The data which were analyzed in that paper are the weekly reported number of new laboratory-confirmed rotavirus cases among children, adults, and elderly from 2001 until 2008 in Germany, scaled up by an underreporting rate (see Section 11.6) as inferred and described in more detail in Weidemann et al. (2013). Surveillance of rotavirus infection is relevant to public health authorities because it is the primary cause for severe gastroenteritis in infants and young children and causes significant morbidity, mortality, and financial burdens worldwide (Atkins et al., 2012). Individuals can get the disease more than once but the highest reported incidence is observed in children under the age of 5 and rises again later in life. Parameter estimation from surveillance data is crucial if we want to assess the effect of vaccination campaigns or other public health control measures.

In Stocks et al. (2018), the disease transmission was modeled as an age-stratified SIRS Markov process with overdispersion in the observation (cf. Equation (11.17)) as well as in the transmission model (cf. Equation (11.18)). As rotavirus in Germany varies seasonally peaking around March, a forcing function (cf. Equation (11.7)) was used.

Here, we will present a simplified version of the model which ignores age-structure and perform inference for one realization of this model; the simulated case report data (black line) is shown in Figure 11.5. The initial values were fixed at the stationary distribution

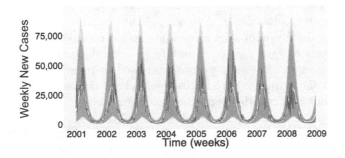

FIGURE 11.5
The 95 percent prediction interval (light shading) for 1,000 realizations of the model for rotavirus evaluated at the MLE for the simulated case report data (solid back line) and the median (solid white line). Furthermore, the 95 percent prediction interval of these 1,000 realizations for only the transmission model is shown (darker shading).

of the system and the waning of immunity rate, $\omega > 0$, also was assumed to be fixed and known. With the notation as in Section 11.5, this translates mathematically into

$$\mathbb{P}[\Delta N._S(t) = 1 | \boldsymbol{X}(t)] = \mu \mathcal{N} \tau + o(\tau)$$

$$\mathbb{P}[\Delta N_{SI}(t) = 1 | \boldsymbol{X}(t)] = \beta(t) I(t) S(t) \mathcal{N}^{-1} \tau + o(\tau)$$

$$\mathbb{P}[\Delta N_{IR}(t) = 1 | \boldsymbol{X}(t)] = \gamma I(t) \tau + o(\tau) \tag{11.19}$$

$$\mathbb{P}[\Delta N_{RS}(t) = 1 | \boldsymbol{X}(t)] = \omega R(t) \tau + o(\tau)$$

$$\mathbb{P}[\Delta N_A.(t) = 1 | \boldsymbol{X}(t)] = \mu A(t) \tau + o(\tau) \quad \text{with } A \in \{S, I, R\}$$

where $\mu > 0$ denotes the birth and death rate which was assumed to be constant and known. Moreover, $N._A(t)$ counts the number of births and $N_A.(t)$ counts the number of deaths with $A \in \mathcal{X}$ in the respective compartment up until time t. The seasonal-forced transmission rate was defined as

$$\beta(t) = \beta \left(1 + \rho \cos \left(\frac{2\pi}{w} t + \phi \right) \right) \xi(t),$$

where $\xi(t)$ is defined as in Equation (11.18). The transition probabilities from (11.19) are related to the state variables in the following way:

$$\Delta S(t) = \Delta N._S(t) - \Delta N_{SI}(t) + \Delta N_{RS}(t) - \Delta N_S.(t)$$

$$\Delta I(t) = \Delta N_{SI}(t) - \Delta N_{IR}(t) - \Delta N_I.(t)$$

$$\Delta R(t) = \Delta N_{IR}(t) - \Delta N_{RS}(t) - \Delta N_R.(t).$$

With this notation the true number of newly infected individuals accumulated in each observation time period $(t_{n-1}, t_n]$, $n \in \{1, 2, \dots, N\}$ is given as

$$H(t_n) = N_{SI}(t_n) - N_{SI}(t_{n-1}).$$

The number of recorded cases Y_n within this time period was modeled as

$$Y_n \sim \text{NegBin} \left(H(t_n), \frac{1}{\psi} \right),$$

compare Equation (11.17). In this example we inferred the susceptibility parameter β, the seasonal forcing parameters ρ and ϕ and the overdispersion parameters σ and ψ, hence $\boldsymbol{\theta} = (\beta, \rho, \phi, \sigma, \psi)'$. A diagnostic plot similar to the one in Figure 11.3 (available online) shows that the iterated filtering algorithm performs well as the parameter estimates converge towards the parameters used for simulation. Figure 11.5 shows the model evaluated at the MLE obtained from the iterated filtering. Further implementational details for this example are available at Stocks (2017).

The aim of the analysis in Stocks et al. (2018) was to compare the impact of different kinds of variabilities in the transmission as well as the observation model. The paper concluded that a model which accounts for overdispersion in both model components (dark and light shading in Figure 11.5) is best suited to explain the analyzed data. The strength of using iterated filtering in this context was that the method allowed for efficient MLE for a POMP where the underlying transmission model was stochastic. Hence, it facilitated model comparison with respect to different choices of variability in both model components.

11.8   Concluding Comments

11.8.1   Pros and cons of iterated filtering methods for outbreak data

The method we have described has many positive aspects. First of all, as illustrated in this chapter, the method is highly flexible and can be easily adapted to many different situations of interest. The great strength of the method is that it is necessary only to simulate from the transmission model if the complete likelihood is not directly tractable. Facilitated by the R package `pomp` the method is very straightforward to implement and can be easily adapted for a wide range of settings. The package is optimized for computational efficiency, in particular the simulation functions (such as `euler.sim` or `gillespie.sim`) facilitate implementation considerably and give rise to substantial gains in speed by accessing C code. Secondly, the method facilitates dealing with unobserved variables and has no problem with the fact that transmission is continuous in time, while observations are made at discrete points in time. Furthermore, it is easy to combine transmission noise and observation noise as long as the Markov property is retained. The method also allows the inclusion of covariates in mechanistically reasonable ways. As mentioned earlier, to date this is the only simulation-based frequentist approach for POMP models that does not rely on summary statistics and can perform efficient inference for POMP models in situations where available Bayesian methods cannot (Ionides et al., 2015).

However, there is one main difficulty with the method. Since it is purely simulation-based, it comes at the cost of being computationally very expensive in particular when the time series becomes long and the state space increases. In Section 11.5.4, we gave some practical hints of how to mitigate the problem. Moreover, the method requires the transmission model to be Markovian, which can be problematic because in practice the stages of diseases are rarely well described by exponential distributions. An easy way to mitigate the problem is by subdividing the respective compartments so that the waiting times individuals stay in each compartment change from being exponentially distributed to gamma distributed, i.e., having a more pronounced mode. Sometimes it is also possible to formulate non-Markovian processes as alternate Markov processes with additional state variables (e.g., if X_n depends on both X_{n-1} and X_{n-2}, i.e., is not Markov, it would be possible to define a new, bivariate Markov process $Z_n = (X_n, X_{n-1})$). However, these strategies increase the dimension of the unobserved state space of the transmission model which can result in an increase of Monte Carlo noise in the particle filter. Hence, those strategies are only effective up to the point where it becomes computationally too expensive to handle this increase of noise.

11.8.2   Further reading

For the reader interested in more details about the theoretical background of iterated filtering methods, we recommend Ionides et al. (2006) and Ionides et al. (2015) for further reading. For the reader interested in learning how to work with the R package `pomp`, we recommend the study of King et al. (2016) and to follow some of the very comprehensive online tutorials available through King (2017). The package already has been applied to answer many different epidemiological questions for different infectious diseases, e.g., for cholera (King et al., 2008), measles (He et al., 2010), malaria (Bhadra et al., 2011), polio (Martinez-Bakker et al., 2015), ebola (King et al., 2015), and rotavirus (Martinez et al., 2016; Stocks et al., 2018). Finally, iterated filtering has facilitated the development and analysis of many mechanistic models; a recent and comprehensive review of which can be found in Bretó (2018).

Acknowledgments

I would like to thank Aaron A. King for making the tutorials and, especially, the codes in King (2017) available. Furthermore, I would like to thank Carles Bretó and Philip O'Neill for their constructive comments and suggestions. TS was supported by the Swedish research council, grant number 2015_05182_VR.

References

Andrieu, C., Doucet, A., and Holenstein, R. (2010). Particle Markov chain Monte Carlo methods. *Journal of the Royal Statistical Society: Series B*, 72(3):269–342.

Arulampalam, M. S., Maskell, S., Gordon, N., and Clapp, T. (2002). A tutorial on particle filters for online nonlinear, non-Gaussian Bayesian tracking. *IEEE Transactions on Signal Processing*, 50(2):174188.

Atkins, K. E., Shim, E., Pitzer, V. E., and Galvani, A. P. (2012). Impact of rotavirus vaccination on epidemiological dynamics in England and Wales. *Vaccine*, 30(3):552–564.

Bhadra, A., Ionides, E. L., Laneri, K., Pascual, M., Bouma, M., and Dhiman, R. (2011). Malaria in northwest India: Data analysis via partially observed stochastic differential equation models driven by Lévy noise. *Journal of the American Statistical Association*, 106(494):440–451.

Bretó, C. (2018). Modeling and inference for infectious disease dynamics: A likelihood-based approach. *Statistical Science*, 33(1):57–69.

Bretó, C., He, D., Ionides, E. L., and King, A. A. (2009). Time series analysis via mechanistic models. *The Annals of Applied Statistics*, 3(1):319–348.

Bretó, C. and Ionides, E. L. (2011). Compound Markov counting processes and their applications to modeling infinitesimally over-dispersed systems. *Stochastic Processes and Their Applications*, 121(11):2571–2591.

Del Moral, P. (1996). Non linear filtering: Interacting particle solution. *Markov Processes and Related Fields*, 2(4):555–580.

Doucet, A., de Freitas, N., and Gordon, N. (2001). *Sequential Monte Carlo Methods in Practice*. Springer-Verlag, New York.

Doucet, A. and Johansen, A. M. (2011) A tutorial on particle filtering and smoothing: Fifteen years later. *The Oxford Handbook of Nonlinear Filtering*. Oxford University Press, Oxford.

Erhard, F., Friedel, C. C., and Zimmer, R. (2010). FERN- stochastic simulation and evaluation of reaction networks. *Systems Biology for Signaling Networks*. Systems Biology. Springer, New York.

Fuchs, C. (2013). *Inference for Diffusion Processes: With Applications in Life Sciences*. Springer-Verlag, Berlin, Germany.

Gibbons, C. L., Mangen, M. J., Plass, D., Havelaar, A. H., Brooke, R. J., Kramarz, P., Peterson, K. L. et al. (2014). Measuring underreporting and under-ascertainment in infectious disease datasets: A comparison of methods. *BMC Public Health*, 14(147).

Gillespie, D. T. (1977). Exact stochastic simulation of coupled chemical reactions. *The Journal of Physical Chemistry*, 81(25):2340–2361.

Gillespie, D. T. (2001). Approximate accelerated stochastic simulation of chemically reacting systems. *Journal of Chemical Physics*, 115(4):1716–1733.

He, D., Ionides, E. L., and King, A. A. (2010). Plug-and-play inference for disease dynamics: Measles in large and small populations as a case study. *Journal of the Royal Society Interface*, 7(43):271283.

Held, L. and Sabanés Bové, D. (2013). *Applied Statistical Inference*. Springer, Berlin, Germany.

Ionides, E. L., Bretó, C., and King, A. A. (2006). Inference for nonlinear dynamical systems. *PNAS*, 103(49):18438–18443.

Ionides, E. L., Bretó, C., Park, J., Smith, R. A., and King, A. A. (2017). Monte Carlo profile confidence intervals for dynamic systems. *Journal of The Royal Society Interface*, 14(132).

Ionides, E. L., Nguyen, D., Atchadé, Y., Stoev, S., and King, A. (2015). Inference for dynamic and latent variable models via iterated, perturbed Bayes maps. *PNAS*, 112(3): 719–724.

Karlin, S. and Taylor, H. M. (1981). *A Second Course in Stochastic Processes*. Academic Press, San Diego, CA.

Keeling, M. J. and Rohani, P. (2008). *Modeling Infectious Diseases in Humans and Animals*. Princeton University Press, Princeton, NJ.

Kendall, B. E., Briggs, C. J., Murdoch, W. W., Turchin, P., Ellner , S. P., McCauley, E., Nisbet, R. M., and Wood, S. N. (1999). Why do populations cycle? A synthesis of statistical and mechanistic modeling approaches. *Ecology*, 80(6):1789–1805.

King, A. A. (2017). Project pomp on github. http://kingaa.github.io/pomp/, [Accessed September 15, 2017].

King, A. A., Domenech de Cells, M., Magpantay, F. M. G., and Rohani, P. (2015). Avoidable errors in the modelling of outbreaks of emerging pathogens, with special reference to Ebola. *Proceedings of the Royal Society of London B*, 282:20150347.

King, A. A., Ionides, E. L., Pascual, M., and Bouma, M. J. (2008). Inapparent infections and cholera dynamics. *Nature*, 454:877–888.

King, A. A., Nguyen, D., and Ionides, E. L. (2016). Statistical inference for partially observed Markov processes via the R package pomp. *Journal of Statistical Software*, 69(12):1–43.

Kitagawa, G. (1987). Non-gaussian state-space modeling of nonstationary time series. *Journal of the American Statistical Association*, 82(400):10321041.

Liu, J. and West, M. (2001). Combinig parameter and state estimation in simulation-based filtering. *Sequential Monte Carlo Methods in Practice*, pages 197–223. Springer, New York.

Martinez, P. P., King, A. A., Yunusd, M., Faruqued, A. S. G., and Pascual, M. (2016). Differential and enhanced response to climate forcing in diarrheal disease due to rotavirus across a megacity of the developing world. *PNAS*, 113(15):4092–4097.

Martinez-Bakker, M., King, A. A., and Rohani, P. (2015). Unraveling the transmission ecology of polio. *PLoS Biology*, 13(6):e1002172.

McCullagh, R. and Nelder, J. (1989). *Generalized Linear Models*. 2nd ed. Chapman & Hall, London, UK.

Nelder, J. A. and Mead, R. (1965). A simplex method for function minimization. *The Computer Journal*, 7(4):308–313.

Nocedal, J. and Wright, S. J., Eds. (1999). *Numerical Optimization*. Springer Series in Operations Research and Financial Engineering. Springer, New York.

Pawitan, Y. (2001). *In All Likelihood: Statistical Modelling and Inference Using Likelihood*. Oxford University Press, Oxford, UK.

Robert, C. P. and Casella, G. (2004). *Monte Carlo Statistical Methods*. Springer-Verlag, New York.

Stocks, T. (2017). Chapter on iterated filtering methods on github. https://github.com/theresasophia/chapter_IFmethods, [Accessed September 10, 2017].

Stocks, T., Britton, T., and Höhle, M. (2018). Model selection and parameter estimation for dynamic epidemic models via iterated filtering: Application to rotavirus in Germany. *Biostatistics*. doi:10.1093/biostatistics/kxy057.

Stoer, J. and Bulirsch, R. (2002). *Introduction to Numerical Analysis*. Springer, New York.

Sugihara, G. and May, R. M. (1990). Nonlinear forecasting as a way of distinguishing chaos from measurement error in time series. *Nature*, 344(6268):734–741.

Toni, T., Welch, D., Strelkowa, N., Ipsen, A., and Stumpf, M. P. (2009). Approximate Bayesian computation scheme for parameter inference and model selection in dynamical systems. *Journal of the Royal Society Interface*, 6(31).

Weidemann, F., Dehnert, M., Koch, J., Wichmann, O., and Höhle, M. (2013). Bayesian parameter inference for dynamic infectious disease modeling: Rotavirus in Germany. *Statistics in Medicine*, 33(9):1580–1599.

Wilks, S. S. (1938). The large-sample distribution of the likelihood ratio for testing composite hypotheses. *The Annals of Mathematical Statistics*, 1(9):60–62.

Wood, S. N. (2010). Statistical inference for noisy nonlinear ecological dynamic systems. *Nature*, 466(7310):1102–1104.

12

Pairwise Survival Analysis of Infectious Disease Transmission Data

Eben Kenah

CONTENTS

12.1 Introduction

The statistical analysis of infectious disease data is complicated by the fact that infections in different individuals are not independent, especially when disease is transmitted directly from person to person (Andersson and Britton, 2000; Becker, 1989). This problem was recognized long ago; Sir Ronald Ross called it "dependent happenings" (Ross, 1916). In this chapter, we show how dependent happenings can be handled using methods adapted from survival analysis. Instead of considering failure times in individuals, we consider failure times in ordered pairs ij that consist of an infectious individual i and a susceptible individual j who is at risk of infection from i. We call this approach *pairwise survival analysis*, and these methods are being implemented in the `transtat` package for R (available at `github.com/ekenah/transtat`).

12.1.1   Contact intervals

Pairwise survival analysis is based on *contact intervals*. The contact interval τ_{ij} in the ordered pair ij is the time from the onset of infectiousness in i to infectious contact from i to j, where we define infectious contact to be a contact sufficient to infect j if j is susceptible (Kenah, 2011; Kenah et al., 2008). If individual i is infected at time t_i and becomes infectious immediately, then infectious contact from i to j will happen at time $t_{ij} = t_i + \tau_{ij}$. If i is infectious and j is susceptible at time t_{ij}, then i infects j. Otherwise, j escapes infection from i. The contact interval distribution determines several important epidemiological properties of disease transmission.

If i has an infectious period ι, the probability of infectious contact from i to j is $1 - S_{ij}(\iota)$ where

$$S_{ij}(\tau) = \Pr(\tau_{ij} > \tau), \tag{12.1}$$

is the survival function of the contact interval distribution. If i and j are members of a household, this is called the *household secondary attack rate*. Secondary attack rates (SAR) can also be defined in hospital wards or other settings with a clearly defined population at risk of infection.

The contact interval distribution also determines how the infectiousness of i varies over time. We call the time τ since the onset of infectiousness in i the *infectious age* of i. The cumulative hazard function of the contact interval from i to j is $H_{ij}(\tau) = -\ln S_{ij}(\tau)$, and the hazard function is

$$h_{ij}(\tau) = H'_{ij}(\tau) = -\frac{S'_{ij}(\tau)}{S_{ij}(\tau)}. \tag{12.2}$$

If j is susceptible at time $t_i + \tau$ and $d\tau$ is small, then j is infected by i in the time interval $(t_i + \tau, t_i + \tau + d\tau]$ with probability approximately equal to

$$h_{ij}(\tau)d\tau. \tag{12.3}$$

Thus, the hazard function $h_{ij}(\tau)$ gives the instantaneous infectiousness of i to j as a function of the infectious age of i. A scaled version of this function is sometimes called the *infectiousness profile* or *infectivity curve*.

In a mass-action model, the hazard of infection from i to j is inversely proportional to the population size. Let

$$h_{ij}^{(n)}(\tau) = \frac{h_{ij}(\tau)}{n-1} \tag{12.4}$$

be the hazard of infection from i to j at infectious age τ of i in a population of size n. Suppose that i is infectious and all other individuals in the population are identical to j. When n is large, the total number of infectious contacts made by i at or before infectious age τ is approximately

$$\int_0^\tau (n-1)h_{ij}^{(n)}(u)du = \int_0^\tau h_{ij}(u)du = H_{ij}(\tau). \tag{12.5}$$

If i is identical to all other individuals, the basic reproductive number is

$$R_0 = \mathbb{E}[H_{ij}(\iota)] \tag{12.6}$$

where the expectation is taken over the distribution of infectious periods ι.

Contact interval distributions are used implicitly in many standard epidemic models. A good example is the stochastic Kermack-McKendrick model, which is a mass-action model. In this model,

$$S'(t) = -\beta S(t)I(t) \tag{12.7}$$

where $S(t)$ and $I(t)$ are the susceptible and infectious proportions of the population, respectively, at time t. Multiplying both sides by the population size n, we get

$$nS'(t) = \frac{\beta}{n}n^2 S(t)I(t). \tag{12.8}$$

The left-hand side is the derivative of the number of susceptible individuals. On the right-hand side, $n^2 S(t)I(t)$ is the total number of infectious-susceptible pairs and $n^{-1}\beta$ is the hazard of infectious contact in each pair. (For large n, we can ignore the difference between n and $n-1$.) The corresponding contact interval distribution has the hazard function $h(\tau) = \beta$ and cumulative hazard function $H(\tau) = \beta\tau$. The total number of infectious contacts for an individual with infectious period ι is $H(\iota) = \beta\iota$. The basic reproductive number is $R_0 = \beta\mathbb{E}[\iota]$. In the standard Kermack-McKendrick model, the infectious period ι has an exponential distribution with rate γ, so $\mathbb{E}[\iota] = \gamma^{-1}$ and

$$R_0 = \frac{\beta}{\gamma}. \tag{12.9}$$

In the Kermack-McKendrick model, infectious individuals have constant infectiousness, which is reflected in the contact interval hazard function $h(\tau) = \beta$.

12.1.2 Contact intervals and generation intervals

If i is infected at time t_i and i infects j at time t_j, the *generation interval* is $t_j - t_i$. The *serial interval* is the time between the onset of symptoms in i and the onset of symptoms in j. Although generation and serial interval distributions are often thought to be stable biological properties of an infectious disease (Fine, 2003), these distributions change systematically over the course of an epidemic (Kenah et al., 2008; Svensson, 2007). Given that i infected j, i must have infected j before anyone else. As the prevalence of infection increases, generation and serial intervals contract because of this competition to infect susceptibles.

If there is no latent period (between infection and the onset of infectiousness), then the generation interval $t_j - t_i$ is equal to the contact interval τ_{ij}. However, the generation interval is defined only if transmission occurs. When j is not exposed to any other source of infection, the survival function of the generation interval distribution is

$$S_{ij}^{\text{gen}}(\tau) = \frac{S_{ij}(\tau) - S_{ij}(\iota)}{1 - S_{ij}(\iota)} \tag{12.10}$$

where ι is the infectious period of i. Because $S_{ij}^{\text{gen}}(\iota) = 0$, the cumulative hazard $H_{ij}^{\text{gen}}(\tau) = -\ln S_{ij}^{\text{gen}}(\tau)$ is unbounded in the interval $(0, \iota]$. Regardless of the underlying hazard of infectious contact, the hazard function $h_{ij}^{\text{gen}}(\tau) = \left(H_{ij}^{\text{gen}}\right)'(\tau)$ is also unbounded in $(0, \iota]$.

For simplicity, we have considered generation intervals when there is a fixed infectious period. The situation does not improve if we consider variation in the infectious period or if we use serial intervals. The contact interval distribution is a more practical and general foundation for the statistical analysis of infectious disease transmission data.

12.1.3   General stochastic S(E)IR model

To describe how the contact interval distribution leads to pairwise survival analysis, we first give a more formal description of its role in the general stochastic Susceptible-(Exposed)-Infectious-Removed or S(E)IR model.

At any time, each individual $i \in \{1, \ldots, n\}$ is in one of four states: susceptible (S), exposed (E), infectious (I), or removed (R). Person i moves from S to E at his or her *infection time* t_i, with $t_i = \infty$ if i is never infected. After infection, i has a *latent period* of length ε_i during which he or she is infected but not infectious. At time $t_i + \varepsilon_i$, i moves from E to I, beginning an *infectious period* of length ι_i. At time $t_i + \varepsilon_i + \iota_i$, i moves from I to R, where he or she can no longer infect others or be infected. The latent period ε_i is a nonnegative random variable, and the infectious period ι_i is a strictly positive random variable. Both have finite mean and variance.

After becoming infectious at time $t_i + \varepsilon_i$, person i makes infectious contact with $j \neq i$ at the *infectious contact time* $t_{ij} = t_i + \varepsilon_i + \tau_{ij}^*$. The *infectious contact interval* τ_{ij}^* is a strictly positive random variable with $\tau_{ij}^* = \infty$ if infectious contact never occurs. Since infectious contact can only occur when i is infectious, $\tau_{ij}^* \in (0, \iota_i]$ or $\tau_{ij}^* = \infty$. Because we define infectious contact to be sufficient to cause infection in a susceptible individual, $t_j \leq t_{ij}$.

For each ordered pair ij, let C_{ij} indicate whether infectious contact from i to j would be possible if i were infectious. We assume the infectious contact interval τ_{ij}^* is generated as follows: A contact interval τ_{ij} is drawn from a distribution with hazard function $h_{ij}(\tau)$. If $\tau_{ij} \leq \iota_i$ and $C_{ij} = 1$, then $\tau_{ij}^* = \tau_{ij}$. Otherwise, $\tau_{ij}^* = \infty$.

12.1.4   Exposure sets, infector sets, and transmission trees

An *external* infection occurs when an individual is infected from a source outside the observed population. External infections can be caused by community, zoonotic, or environmental sources. An *internal* infection occurs when infection is transmitted from one individual to another within the observed population. Let $\mathcal{I}_{\text{ext}}$ denote the set of individuals infected externally, let $\mathcal{I}_{\text{int}}$ denote the set of individuals infected internally, and let $\mathcal{I}$ denote the set of all infected individuals. If $j \in \mathcal{I}_{\text{ext}}$, let $v_j = 0$. If $j \in \mathcal{I}_{\text{int}}$, let v_j denote the index of his or her infector. If $j \notin \mathcal{I}$, let $v_j = \infty$.

For each j, the *exposure set* is the set of all individuals from whom j was at risk of infectious contact:

$$W_j = \{i : t_i + \varepsilon_i < t_j \text{ and } C_{ij} = 1\} \tag{12.11}$$

If j is not infected, $t_j = \infty$ so W_j consists of all infected i such that $C_{ij} = 1$. For each $j \in \mathcal{I}_{\text{int}}$, the *infector set* V_j is the set of possible infectors of j:

$$V_j = \{i : C_{ij} = 1 \text{ and } t_j \in (t_i + \varepsilon_i, t_i + \varepsilon_i + \iota_i]\} \tag{12.12}$$

For all $j \in \mathcal{I}_{\text{int}}$, $v_j \in V_j$ and $V_j \subseteq W_j$. For $j \in \mathcal{I}_{\text{ext}}$, $V_j = \{0\}$. For $j \notin \mathcal{I}$, $V_j = \varnothing$ (the empty set). For each $i \in V_j$, the *infector probability* p_{ij} is the probability that i infected j. For $i \notin V_j$, let $p_{ij} = 0$.

The *transmission tree* is a directed network with an edge from v_j to j for each $j \in \mathcal{I}$. It is a directed tree rooted at node 0, which represents external sources of infection.

Following Wallinga and Teunis (2004), it can be represented by a vector $\mathbf{v} = (v_1, \ldots, v_n)$. Let $\mathcal{V}$ denote the set of all possible $\mathbf{v}$ consistent with the observed data. A transmission tree $\mathbf{v} \in \mathcal{V}$ can be generated by choosing a $v_j \in V_j$ for each $j \in \mathcal{I}_{int}$.

12.1.5   Observation, censoring, and asymptotics

Our population has size n, and there are $m < n$ internal infections. We observe the times of all S $\to$ E (infection), E $\to$ I (onset of infectiousness), and I $\to$ R (removal) transitions in the population between time 0 and time T. We also observe C_{ij} for all ordered pairs ij such that i is infected. We assume that $\mathcal{I}_{ext}$ is known and that all other individuals have no risk of external infection. We first consider the case where who-infects-whom (equivalently, the transmission tree) is observed and then consider the more realistic case where it is not.

Throughout this chapter, we assume that τ_{ij} can be observed only if j is infected by i at time $t_{ij} = t_i + \varepsilon_i + \tau_{ij}$. This can happen only if $C_{ij} = 1$. We also have right-censoring of τ_{ij}:

1. Infectious contact can occur only while i is infectious, so τ_{ij} can be right-censored by the end of infectiousness in i. Let $I_i(t) = \mathbf{1}_{t-t_i-\varepsilon_i \in (0, \iota_i]}$ indicate whether i remains infectious at time t.

2. Infectious contact from i infects j only if j is susceptible, so τ_{ij} can be right-censored by infection in j. Let $S_j(t) = \mathbf{1}_{t \leq t_j}$ indicate whether j remains susceptible at time t.

3. Finally, τ_{ij} can be right-censored by the end of observation. Let $\mathcal{Y}(t) = \mathbf{1}_{t \leq T}$ indicate whether observation is ongoing at time t.

Because $I_i(t)$, $S_j(t)$, and $\mathcal{Y}(t)$ are left-continuous,

$$Y_{ij}(t) = C_{ij} I_i(t) S_j(t) \mathcal{Y}(t) \tag{12.13}$$

is a left-continuous process that indicates the risk of an observed infectious contact from i to j at time t. The assumptions made in the stochastic S(E)IR model ensure that $I_i(t)$ and $S_j(t)$ independently censor τ_{ij}. We also require that T is a stopping time with respect to the observed data so that $\mathcal{Y}(t)$ independently censors τ_{ij} for all ij. The possible censoring mechanisms are illustrated in Figure 12.1.

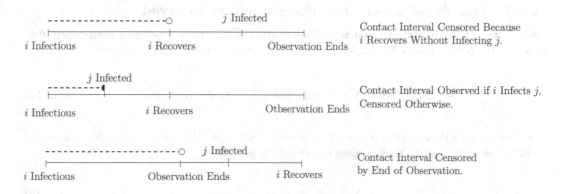

FIGURE 12.1
Right censoring of the contact interval τ_{ij}. At the top, τ_{ij} is censored because $I_i(t_{ij}) = 0$. In the middle, τ_{ij} is observed if $S_j(t_{ij}) = 1$ and censored otherwise. At the bottom, τ_{ij} is censored because $\mathcal{Y}(t_{ij}) = 0$.

For consistency and asymptotic normality of parametric and nonparametric estimates of the contact interval distribution, the number of susceptibles at risk of infection should grow at least as fast as the number of pairs at risk of transmission (Kenah, 2015). More formally, the hazard of infection in the susceptible member of a randomly chosen pair should be bounded as the number of pairs at risk of transmission heads toward infinity. This would be violated if, for example, the number of pairs at risk grew without limit but the number of susceptibles was fixed—each being exposed to more and more infectious individuals. In practice, both the number of pairs at risk of transmission and the number of susceptibles at risk of infection should be large. As in standard survival analysis, statistical power is determined primarily by the number of events (transmissions of infection) that are observed (Aalen et al., 2009; Kalbfleisch and Prentice, 2002).

12.2   Parametric Pairwise Survival Analysis

In parametric pairwise survival analysis (Kenah, 2011), we assume that all contact intervals are independent and identically distributed (IID) with an absolutely continuous distribution such that $h_{ij}(\tau) = h(\tau, \theta_0)$ for all ij. Our goal is to estimate θ_0. For regularity of maximum likelihood estimation (MLE), we assume that θ_0 is unique and that $h(\tau, \theta)$ is strictly positive with continuous second derivatives with respect to θ in an open neighborhood of θ_0. Our derivations use counting processes and martingales, which are reviewed in Aalen et al. (2009) and Kalbfleisch and Prentice (2002).

The contact interval distribution in these models can be any parametric failure time distribution. Many standard stochastic S(E)IR models assume an exponential distribution, which can be parametrized by the rate parameter λ. The Weibull distribution is a generalization of the exponential distribution that is parameterized by $\theta = (\lambda, \gamma)$ where λ is the rate parameter and γ is the shape parameter. It has the cumulative hazard function $H(t, \theta) = (\lambda t)^{\gamma}$. The log-logistic distribution is a two-parameter distribution that allows non-monotonic hazards. It has the cumulative hazard $H(\tau, \theta) = \ln[1 + (\lambda t)^{\gamma}]$ where λ is the rate parameter and γ is the shape parameter.

12.2.1   Likelihood when who-infects-whom is observed

Let $\mathcal{N}_{ij}(t) = \mathbf{1}_{t \geq t_{ij}}$ count the first infectious contact from i to j. Assume j is susceptible at time $t = 0$, so $\mathcal{N}_{ij}(0) = 0$. Then $\mathcal{M}_{ij}(t, \theta_0)$ is a mean-zero martingale,[1] where

$$\mathcal{M}_{ij}(t, \theta) = \mathcal{N}_{ij}(t) - \int_0^t h(u - t_i - \varepsilon_i, \theta) C_{ij} I_i(u) \mathrm{d}u. \qquad (12.14)$$

We observe infectious contacts from i to j only while j is still susceptible and ij is under observation, which gives us the observed counting process

$$N_{ij}(t) = \int_0^t Y_{ij}(u) \mathrm{d}\mathcal{N}_{ij}(u). \qquad (12.15)$$

---

[1] Technically, $M_{ij}(t, \theta_0)$ is a random variable and $\{M_{ij}(t, \theta_0) : t \geq 0\}$ is a martingale with respect to a natural filtration.

Similarly, let

$$M_{ij}(t, \theta) = \int_0^t Y_{ij}(u) \mathrm{d} \mathcal{M}_{ij}(u, \theta). \tag{12.16}$$

Then $M_{ij}(t, \theta_0)$ is a mean-zero martingale because it is the integral of a predictable process with respect to $\mathcal{M}_{ij}(t, \theta_0)$.

When we observe infectious contacts from i to j between time 0 and time T, we get the log likelihood

$$\ell_{ij}(\theta) = \int_0^T \ln h(u - t_i - \varepsilon_i, \theta) \mathrm{d} N_{ij}(u) - \int_0^T h(u - t_i - \varepsilon_i, \theta) Y_{ij}(u) \mathrm{d} u. \tag{12.17}$$

This is a standard survival likelihood: The first term is $\ln h(t_j - t_i - \varepsilon_i, \theta)$ if $v_j = i$ and zero otherwise. The second term is negative cumulative hazard of infectious contact while $Y_{ij}(t) = 1$. The score process of $\ell_{ij}(\theta)$ is

$$U_{ij}(t, \theta) = \int_0^t \left[\frac{\partial}{\partial \theta} \ln h(u - t_i - \varepsilon_i, \theta) \right] \mathrm{d} M_{ij}(u, \theta), \tag{12.18}$$

which is a mean-zero martingale when $\theta = \theta_0$.

Now fix j. If we observe all pairs ij from time 0 until time T, the log likelihood is

$$\ell_{\cdot j}(\theta, v_j) = \sum_{i \in W_j} \ell_{ij}(\theta) \tag{12.19}$$

with score process

$$U_{\cdot j}(t, \theta, v_j) = \sum_{i \in W_j} U_{ij}(t, \theta). \tag{12.20}$$

Because it is a sum of independent mean-zero martingales, $U_{\cdot j}(t, \theta_0, v_j)$ is also a mean-zero martingale.

When we observe who-infects-whom, the complete-data log likelihood is

$$\ell(\theta, \mathbf{v}) = \sum_{j=1}^n \ell_{\cdot j}(\theta, v_j) \tag{12.21}$$

and its score process is

$$U(t, \theta, \mathbf{v}) = \sum_{j=1}^n U_{\cdot j}(t, \theta, v_j). \tag{12.22}$$

Because it is a sum of independent mean-zero martingales, $U(t, \theta_0, \mathbf{v})$ is also a mean-zero martingale. Differentiating $\ell(\theta, \mathbf{v})$, evaluating at θ_0, and taking expectations yields

$$E\left[-\frac{\partial^2}{\partial \theta^2} \ell(\theta_0, \mathbf{v}) \right] = E\left[\langle U(\theta_0, \mathbf{v}) \rangle(T) \right], \tag{12.23}$$

where $\langle U(\theta_0, \mathbf{v}) \rangle(\tau)$ is the predictable variation process of $U(\tau, \theta_0, \mathbf{v})$. Under our regularity assumptions for $h(\tau, \theta)$, this establishes the consistency and asymptotic normality of the maximum likelihood estimate $\hat{\theta}$ as the number of observed infections $m \to \infty$ (Kenah, 2011).

12.2.2   Likelihood when who-infects-whom is not observed

Now suppose we do not observe v_j if j is infected. Instead of seeing each $N_{ij}(t)$, we see only $N_{\cdot j}(t) = \sum_{i \in W_j} N_{ij}(t)$. The total hazard of infectious contact with j at time t is $h_{\cdot j}(t, \theta_0)$ where

$$h_{\cdot j}(t, \theta) = \sum_{i \in W_j} h(t - t_i - \varepsilon_i, \theta) C_{ij} I_i(t). \tag{12.24}$$

The corresponding counting process martingale is $M_{\cdot j}(t, \theta_0)$ where

$$M_{\cdot j}(t, \theta) = \sum_{i \in W_j} M_{ij}(t, \theta) = N_{\cdot j}(t) - \int_0^t h_{\cdot j}(u, \theta) S_j(u) \mathcal{Y}(t) du. \tag{12.25}$$

When j is observed from time 0 to time T, the log likelihood is

$$\ell_{\cdot j}(\theta) = \int_0^T \ln h_{\cdot j}(u, \theta) dN_{\cdot j}(u) - \int_0^T h_{\cdot j}(u, \theta) S_j(u) du, \tag{12.26}$$

and its score process is

$$U_{\cdot j}(t, \theta) = \int_0^t \left[\frac{\partial}{\partial \theta} \ln h_{\cdot j}(u, \theta) \right] dM_{\cdot j}(u, \theta). \tag{12.27}$$

Because it is the integral of a predictable process with respect to a mean-zero martingale, $U_{\cdot j}(t, \theta_0)$ is a mean-zero martingale.

The complete-data log likelihood when we do not observe who-infected-whom is

$$\ell(\theta) = \sum_{j=1}^n \ell_{\cdot j}(\theta), \tag{12.28}$$

and its score process is

$$U(t, \theta) = \sum_{j=1}^n U_{\cdot j}(t, \theta). \tag{12.29}$$

Because it is a sum of independent mean-zero martingales, $U(t, \theta_0)$ is a mean-zero martingale. Differentiating $\ell(\theta)$, evaluating at θ_0, and taking expectations yields

$$E\left[-\frac{\partial^2}{\partial \theta^2} \ell(\theta_0) \right] = E\left[\langle U(\theta_0) \rangle(T) \right], \tag{12.30}$$

where $\langle U(\theta_0) \rangle(\tau)$ is the predictable variation process of $U(\tau, \theta_0)$. Under our regularity assumptions for $h(\tau, \theta)$, this establishes the consistency and asymptotic normality of the maximum likelihood estimate $\hat{\theta}$ as the number of observed infections $m \to \infty$ (Kenah, 2011).

12.2.2.1   Relationship between the likelihoods

When who-infected-whom is unknown, the contact interval hazard function induces a probability distribution over V_j for each internally infected j (Kenah et al., 2008). For each ij such that $j \in \mathcal{I}_{\text{int}}$ and $i \in V_j$, let

$$p_{ij}(\theta) = \frac{h(t_j - t_i - \varepsilon_i, \theta)}{h_{\cdot j}(t_j, \theta)}. \tag{12.31}$$

Then the probability that i infected j is $p_{ij}(\theta_0)$.

A transmission tree $\mathbf{v} \in \mathcal{V}$ can be generated by choosing an $i \in V_j$ for each $j \in \mathcal{I}_{\text{int}}$. These choices are conditionally independent given the observed data (Kenah et al., 2008), so the probability of $\mathbf{v}$ given θ is

$$\Pr(\mathbf{v}|\theta) = \prod_{j \in \mathcal{I}_{\text{int}}} p_{v_j j}(\theta). \tag{12.32}$$

Let $L(\theta, \mathbf{v})$ be the likelihood that we would calculate if we observed the transmission tree $\mathbf{v}$, and let $L(\theta)$ be the likelihood when who-infects-whom is not observed. Then

$$L(\theta, \mathbf{v}) = \prod_{j=1}^{n} h(t_j - t_{v_j} - \varepsilon_{v_j})^{\mathbf{1}_{j \in \mathcal{I}_{\text{int}}}} \exp\left(-\int_0^T h_{\cdot j}(u, \theta) S_j(u) \mathrm{d}u\right) \tag{12.33}$$

$$= \Pr(\mathbf{v}|\theta) L(\theta). \tag{12.34}$$

Because $\sum_{\mathbf{v} \in \mathcal{V}} \Pr(\mathbf{v}|\theta) = 1$ for all θ, it follows that

$$L(\theta) = \sum_{\mathbf{v} \in \mathcal{V}} \Pr(\mathbf{v}|\theta) L(\theta) = \sum_{\mathbf{v} \in \mathcal{V}} L(\theta, \mathbf{v}). \tag{12.35}$$

Thus, the likelihood when who-infects-whom is not observed is the sum of the likelihood contributions of all possible transmission trees.

12.2.3 Accelerated failure time regression models

Many important questions in infectious disease epidemiology involve the effects of covariates on the risk of transmission. For transmission from an individual i to an individual j, there are three types of covariates. Covariates for i could affect infectiousness, covariates for j could affect susceptibility, and pairwise covariates (e.g., membership in the same household) could affect the risk of transmission independently of the infectiousness of i or susceptibility of j. Estimation of these effects can help design public health responses to emerging infections and evaluate vaccine efficacy (Halloran et al., 1997, 2010).

The same derivations used previously can be adapted to develop regression models for infectious disease transmission. For a given failure time distribution, the shape parameter γ (if it exists) is assumed to be the same for all ij, but each pair ij has a rate parameter λ_{ij} determined by its covariates:

$$\ln \lambda_{ij} = \beta_0^\top X_{ij}, \tag{12.36}$$

where β_0 is an unknown coefficient vector and X_{ij} is a vector of covariates for the pair ij. The first component of X_{ij} equals one for all ij, and the first component of β_0 is an intercept term that equals the log rate for a pair in which all other components of X_{ij} are zero. Except for the intercept, each coefficient can be interpreted as the log rate ratio for a one-unit increase in the corresponding covariate when all other covariates are held constant.

In these regression models, $\theta_0 = \beta_0$ for the exponential distribution or $\theta_0 = (\beta_0, \gamma_0)$ for the Weibull or log-logistic distributions. If we replace $h(\tau, \theta)$ with $h(\tau, \theta, X_{ij})$ and make corresponding changes to the cumulative hazard and survival functions, the previous arguments show that we will get consistent and asymptotically normal MLEs of θ_0.

These models are similar to accelerated failure time (AFT) models from standard survival analysis. However, AFT models are typically defined using the scale parameter $\sigma = \lambda^{-1}$, and a ratio of scale parameters is called an *acceleration factor*. The two parameterizations lead to identical models; we prefer rate ratios because they are used more often in epidemiologic research.

12.3   Nonparametric Pairwise Survival Analysis

In nonparametric pairwise survival analysis (Kenah, 2013), we assume only that the contact interval distribution is continuous with the hazard function $h_0(\tau)$ and cumulative hazard

$$H_0(\tau) = \int_0^\tau h_0(u)\mathrm{d}u. \tag{12.37}$$

When who-infects-whom is observed, the Nelson-Aalen estimator (Aalen, 1978; Nelson, 1972) generates an unbiased estimate $\hat{H}(\tau, \mathbf{v})$ of $H_0(\tau)$. When who-infects-whom is not observed, we cannot calculate the Nelson-Aalen estimate because we do not know which contact intervals end in infectious contact and which are censored. We still can obtain an unbiased estimate of $H_0(\tau)$ because

$$H_0(\tau) = \mathbb{E}\big[\hat{H}(\tau, \mathbf{v})\big] = \mathbb{E}\Big[\mathbb{E}\big[\hat{H}(\tau, \mathbf{v})\big|\text{observed data}\big]\Big] \tag{12.38}$$

by the law of iterated expectation. Because the probability of each $\mathbf{v} \in \mathcal{V}$ is unknown, we use an Expectation-Maximization (EM) algorithm (Dempster et al., 1977) to iteratively reweight each possible $\mathbf{v}$, obtaining a sequence of estimates that converges to a nonparametric maximum likelihood estimate of $H_0(\tau)$. This method adapts easily to a situation where the infectors any subset of $\mathcal{I}_{\text{int}}$ are observed; the EM algorithm operates only on j with unknown v_j.

Parametric estimators of the contact interval distribution were derived using counting processes and martingales defined in absolute time. To derive nonparametric estimators, we use counting processes and martingales defined in infectious age. This change of timescale is allowed because the distribution of the contact interval τ_{ij} does not depend on the infection time t_i of i. Throughout the rest of this section, let $Y_{ij}(\tau)$ indicate whether there is a risk of transmission from i to j at infectious age τ of i. More formally,

$$Y_{ij}(\tau) = C_{ij} I_i(t_i + \varepsilon_i + \tau) S_j(t_i + \varepsilon_i + \tau) \mathcal{Y}(t_i + \varepsilon_i + \tau) \tag{12.39}$$

where C_{ij} indicates whether infectious contact from i to j is possible, $I_i(t)$ indicates infectiousness of i at time t, $S_j(t)$ indicates susceptibility of j at time t, and $\mathcal{Y}(t)$ indicates whether observation is ongoing at time t. Whereas absolute-time processes are defined for all ordered pairs ij, infectious-age processes are defined only for those ij in which $i \in W_j$.

To estimate $H_0(\tau)$ nonparametrically in an interval $(0, \mathcal{T}]$, the infectious period should be greater than $\mathcal{T}$ with positive probability (Kenah, 2015). The price of nonparametric estimation is that we cannot extrapolate outside the range of the observed data.

12.3.1   Estimation when who-infects-whom is observed

First, suppose there is no censoring, so we observe the contact interval in each ordered pair ij such that $i \in W_j$. Then $\mathcal{N}_{ij}(\tau) = \mathbf{1}_{\tau \geq t_j - t_i - \varepsilon_i}$ and

$$\mathcal{M}_{ij}(\tau) = \mathcal{N}_{ij}(\tau) - \int_0^\tau h_0(u)\mathrm{d}u \tag{12.40}$$

is a mean-zero martingale. In the presence of censoring, we have the observed counting process

$$N_{ij}(\tau) = \int_0^\tau Y_{ij}(u)\mathrm{d}\mathcal{N}_{ij}(u) \tag{12.41}$$

and the mean-zero martingale

$$M_{ij}(\tau) = \int_0^\tau Y_{ij}(u) \mathrm{d}\mathcal{M}_{ij}(u). \tag{12.42}$$

For a fixed j, the combined observations of all ij give us the counting process

$$N_{.j}(\tau) = \sum_{i \in W_j} N_{ij}(\tau), \tag{12.43}$$

which has a jump of size one at $\tau = t_j - t_{v_j} - \varepsilon_{v_j}$ if $j \in \mathcal{I}_{\text{int}}$. Because it is a sum of mean-zero martingales,

$$M_{.j}(\tau) = \sum_{i \in W_j} M_{ij}(\tau) = N_{.j}(\tau) - \int_0^\tau h_0(u) Y_{.j}(u) \mathrm{d}u \tag{12.44}$$

is a mean-zero martingale, where

$$Y_{.j}(\tau) = \sum_{i \in W_j} Y_{ij}(u) \tag{12.45}$$

is the number of infectives who could have made an observed infectious contact with j at infectious age τ. The combined observations of all j give us the counting process

$$N(\tau) = \sum_{j=1}^n N_{.j}(\tau), \tag{12.46}$$

which counts the number of observed infectious contacts occurring at infectious age $\leq \tau$. Since it is a sum of mean-zero martingales,

$$M(\tau) = \sum_{j=1}^n M_{.j}(\tau) = N(\tau) - \int_0^\tau h_0(u) Y(u) \mathrm{d}u \tag{12.47}$$

is a mean-zero martingale, where

$$Y(\tau) = \sum_{j=1}^n Y_{.j}(\tau) \tag{12.48}$$

is the total number of contact intervals of length greater than or equal to τ that were observed.

The Nelson-Aalen estimate of $H_0(\tau)$ is

$$\hat{H}(\tau, \mathbf{v}) = \int_0^\tau \frac{\mathbf{1}_{Y(u)>0}}{Y(u)} \mathrm{d}N(u) \tag{12.49}$$

Let $\mathcal{T} = \max\{\tau : Y(\tau) > 0\}$ and $\tau \wedge \mathcal{T} = \min(\tau, \mathcal{T})$. Then

$$\hat{H}(\tau, \mathbf{v}) - H_0(\tau \wedge \mathcal{T}) = \int_0^\tau \frac{\mathbf{1}_{Y(u)>0}}{Y(u)} \mathrm{d}M(u), \tag{12.50}$$

is a mean-zero martingale. Therefore, $\hat{H}(\tau, \mathbf{v})$ is an unbiased estimate of $H_0(\tau)$ for each $\tau \in (0, \mathcal{T}]$. It maximizes the log likelihood

$$\ell(H) = \sum_{j:t_j \leq T_j} \ln \mathrm{d}H(t_j - t_{v_j} - \varepsilon_{v_j}) - \int_0^\infty Y(u) \mathrm{d}H(u) \tag{12.51}$$

over all step functions $H(\tau)$, and it is asymptotically efficient (Van der Vaart, 1998). An unbiased estimate of $\mathrm{Var}(\hat{H}(\tau, \mathbf{v}))$ is

$$\hat{\sigma}^2(\tau, \mathbf{v}) = \int_0^\tau \frac{\mathbf{1}_{Y(u)>0}}{Y(u)^2} \mathrm{d}N(u), \tag{12.52}$$

which is the optional variation process of (12.50). Using the martingale central limit theorem and a log transformation, we get the large-sample pointwise $1 - \alpha$ confidence limits

$$\hat{H}(\tau, \mathbf{v}) \exp\left(\pm \frac{\hat{\sigma}(\tau, \mathbf{v})}{\hat{H}(\tau, \mathbf{v})} \Phi^{-1}\left(1 - \frac{\alpha}{2}\right) \right), \tag{12.53}$$

where Φ is the standard normal cumulative distribution function.

12.3.2   Estimation when who-infects-whom is not observed

If we do not observe who-infects-whom, the conditional probability that j was infected by $i \in V_j$ given the observed data is

$$p_{ij} = \frac{h_0(t_j - t_i - \varepsilon_i)}{\sum_{k \in V_j} h_0(t_j - t_k - \varepsilon_k)}. \tag{12.54}$$

Given the observed data, the conditional probability of each $\mathbf{v} \in \mathcal{V}$ is

$$\Pr(\mathbf{v}) = \prod_{j \in \mathcal{I}_{\mathrm{int}}} p_{v_j j}. \tag{12.55}$$

Equations (12.54) and (12.55) are identical to equations (12.31) and (12.32), respectively, except for the specification of the hazard function.

Given the observed data, the conditional expectation of the counting process $N_{ij}(\tau)$ from equation (12.41) for each $i \in V_j$ is

$$\mathbb{E}_c N_{ij}(\tau) = p_{ij} \mathbf{1}_{\tau \geq t_j - t_i - \varepsilon_i}, \tag{12.56}$$

which is a cadlag function with a jump of size p_{ij} at $\tau = t_j - t_i - \varepsilon_i$. The conditional expectation of $N_{\cdot j}(\tau)$ from equation (12.43) is

$$\mathbb{E}_c N_{\cdot j}(\tau) = \sum_{i \in V_j} \mathbb{E}_c N_{ij}(\tau), \tag{12.57}$$

and the conditional expectation of $N(\tau)$ from equation (12.46) is

$$\mathbb{E}_c N(\tau) = \sum_{j=1}^n \mathbb{E}_c N_{\cdot j}(\tau). \tag{12.58}$$

Let $\mathbf{V}$ denote the random graph of which each $\mathbf{v} \in \mathcal{V}$ is a possible realization. The conditional expectation of $\hat{H}(\tau, \mathbf{V})$ is

$$\mathbb{E}_c \hat{H}(\tau, \mathbf{V}) = \sum_{\mathbf{v} \in \mathcal{V}} \Pr(\mathbf{v}) \hat{H}(\tau, \mathbf{v}) = \int_0^\tau \frac{\mathbf{1}_{Y(u)>0}}{Y(u)} \mathrm{d}\mathbb{E}_c N(u), \qquad (12.59)$$

where the second equality holds because $Y(\tau)$ does not depend on $\mathbf{v}$. By the law of iterated expectation,

$$\mathbb{E}\left[\mathbb{E}_c \hat{H}(\tau, \mathbf{V})\right] = H_0(\tau) \qquad (12.60)$$

so $\mathbb{E}_c \hat{H}(\tau, \mathbf{V})$ is an unbiased estimate of $H_0(\tau)$ for each $\tau \in (0, \mathcal{T}]$.

When $h_0(\tau)$ is unknown, we cannot calculate $\mathbb{E}_c \hat{H}(\tau, \mathbf{V})$ exactly. However, suppose we have an estimate $\hat{h}(\tau)$ of $h_0(\tau)$. Then the estimated infector probability of $i \in V_j$ is

$$\hat{p}_{ij} = \frac{\hat{h}(t_j - t_i - \varepsilon_i)}{\sum_{k \in V_j} \hat{h}(t_j - t_k - \varepsilon_k)}. \qquad (12.61)$$

The corresponding estimate of $\mathbb{E}_c N_{ij}(\tau)$ is

$$\hat{N}_{ij}(\tau) = \hat{p}_{ij} \mathbf{1}_{\tau \geq t_j - t_i - \varepsilon_i}, \qquad (12.62)$$

and the estimated $\mathbb{E}_c N(\tau)$ is

$$\hat{N}(\tau) = \sum_{j=1}^n \sum_{i \in V_j} \hat{N}_{ij}(\tau). \qquad (12.63)$$

Let $\hat{\Pr}(\mathbf{v})$ be the estimated probability of $\mathbf{v}$ where we replace p_{ij} with $\hat{p}_{ij}$ in equation (12.55). The *marginal Nelson-Aalen estimate* (Kenah, 2013) is

$$\hat{H}(\tau) = \sum_{\mathbf{v} \in \mathcal{V}} \hat{\Pr}(\mathbf{v}) \hat{H}(\tau, \mathbf{v}) = \int_0^\tau \frac{\mathbf{1}_{Y(u)>0}}{Y(u)} \mathrm{d}\hat{N}(u). \qquad (12.64)$$

Smoothing $\hat{H}(\tau)$ and differentiating gives us a new estimate of $h_0(\tau)$. This new estimate can be used to recalculate $\hat{H}(\tau)$, and so on. This is an EM algorithm (Kenah, 2013), so the estimates of $H_0(\tau)$ converge. The entire process is summarized in Algorithm 12.1.

Algorithm 12.1 EM algorithm for nonparametric estimation of $H_0(\tau)$

1: Start with an initial $\hat{h}^{(0)}(\tau)$
2: $k \leftarrow 0$
3: **while** convergence criterion not met **do**
4:    *E-step:* Calculate the infector probabilities $\hat{p}_{ij}^{(k)}$.
5:    *M-step:* Calculate the marginal Nelson-Aalen estimate $\hat{H}^{(k+1)}(\tau)$.
6:    *Smoothing step:* Smooth $\hat{H}^{(k+1)}(\tau)$ and differentiate to get $\hat{h}^{(k+1)}(\tau)$.
7:    $k \leftarrow k + 1$
8: **end while**

The variance $\hat{\sigma}^2(\tau)$ of $\hat{H}_0(\tau)$ can be estimated using the conditional variance formula. Conditioning on $\mathbf{V}$, we get

$$\hat{\sigma}^2(\tau) = \mathbb{E}\left[\hat{\sigma}^2(\tau, \mathbf{V})\right] + \text{Var}\left[\hat{H}(\tau, \mathbf{V})\right]. \tag{12.65}$$

Let $\hat{h}(\tau)$ denote the estimated hazard function corresponding to $\hat{H}(\tau)$. Let $\hat{N}_{.j}(\tau)$ and $\hat{N}(\tau)$ denote the estimates of $\mathbb{E}_c N_{.j}(\tau)$ and $\mathbb{E}_c N(\tau)$. The first term of equation (12.65) reduces to

$$\mathbb{E}\left[\hat{\sigma}^2(\tau, \mathbf{V})\right] = \int_0^\tau \frac{\mathbf{1}_{Y(u)>0}}{Y(u)^2} d\hat{N}(u). \tag{12.66}$$

Kenah (2013) shows that the second term reduces to

$$\text{Var}\left[\hat{H}(\tau, \mathbf{V})\right] = \int_0^\tau \frac{\mathbf{1}_{Y(u)>0}}{Y(u)^2} d\hat{N}(u) - \sum_{j \in \mathcal{I}_{\text{int}}} \left(\int_0^\tau \frac{\mathbf{1}_{Y(u)>0}}{Y(u)} d\hat{N}_{.j}(u)\right)^2. \tag{12.67}$$

Therefore,

$$\hat{\sigma}^2(\tau) = 2 \int_0^\tau \frac{\mathbf{1}_{Y(u)>0}}{Y(u)^2} d\hat{N}(u) - \sum_{j \in \mathcal{I}_{\text{int}}} \left(\int_0^\tau \frac{\mathbf{1}_{Y(u)>0}}{Y(u)} d\hat{N}_{.j}(u)\right)^2. \tag{12.68}$$

Using the martingale central limit theorem and a log transformation, we get the large-sample pointwise $1 - \alpha$ confidence limits

$$\hat{H}(\tau) \exp\left(\pm \frac{\hat{\sigma}(\tau)}{\hat{H}(\tau)} \Phi^{-1}\left(1 - \frac{\alpha}{2}\right)\right). \tag{12.69}$$

12.3.2.1 Estimating the hazard function

Obtaining $\hat{h}^{(k)}(\tau)$ from $\hat{H}^{(k)}(\tau)$ in the smoothing step of Algorithm 12.1 is nontrivial. The increments of $\hat{H}^{(k)}(\tau)$ cannot be used directly. To see why, consider an infected person j. For each $i \in V_j$, $\hat{p}_{ij}^{(k)}$ is the estimated probability that i infected j after the kth iteration of the EM algorithm, and $p_{ij}^{(0)}$ is the initial estimate. If $\hat{h}^{(k)}(\tau)$ equaled the increment of $\hat{H}^{(k)}(\tau)$ at $\tau = t_j - t_i - \varepsilon_i$, we would have

$$p_{ij}^{(k)} \propto \frac{p_{ij}^{(0)}}{Y(t_j - t_i - \varepsilon_i)^k}. \tag{12.70}$$

after k iterations. Because $Y(\tau)$ is usually decreasing in τ, Algorithm 12.1 would converge to a Nelson-Aalen estimate that assigns infector probability one to the $i \in V_j$ with the largest value of $t_j - t_i - \varepsilon_i$. The lengths of the intervals between the increments of $\hat{H}^{(k)}(\tau)$ contain information about $h_0(\tau)$ that is ignored if the increments are used directly. Therefore, some form of smoothing is required to estimate $\hat{h}^{(k)}(\tau)$ from $\hat{H}^{(k)}(\tau)$. Algorithm 12.1 is not sensitive to the smoothing method used. In practice, cubic smoothing splines and kernel smoothers produce nearly identical results.

12.3.2.2   Partially observed transmission trees

Suppose we observe the infectors of a subset of $\mathcal{I}_{\text{int}}$. For each j with a known v_j, let $\hat{N}_{\cdot j}(\tau) = N_{v_j j}(\tau)$, which has a jump of size one at $\tau = t_j - t_{v_j} - \varepsilon_{v_j}$. Taking $V_j = \{v_j\}$ for each such j, equations (12.61) through (12.64) define a marginal Nelson-Aalen estimator that uses the partially observed transmission tree, and equations (12.68) and (12.69) can be used to get confidence intervals.

12.4   Semiparametric Pairwise Relative-risk Regression

Kenah (2015) showed that nonparametric estimates in Section 12.3 can be generalized to get a semiparametric relative-risk regression model similar to that of Prentice and Self (1983). In this model, the hazard of infectious contact from i to j at infectious age τ of i is

$$h_{ij}(\tau) = r\big(\beta_0^{\top} X_{ij}(\tau)\big) h_0(\tau), \tag{12.71}$$

where $h_0(\tau)$ is an unspecified baseline hazard function, $r : \mathbb{R} \to (0, \infty)$ is a relative risk function, β_0 is an unknown coefficient vector, and $X_{ij}(\tau)$ is a predictable covariate process taking values in a set $\mathcal{X}$. We assume that r has a continuous second derivative, $r(0) = 1$, and $\ln r(\beta^{\top} X)$ is bounded on $\mathcal{X}$. The relative risk function $r(x) = \exp(x)$ gives us a model similar to that of Cox (1972). As in the AFT models of Section 12.2.3, the covariates $X_{ij}(\tau)$ can include individual-level covariates predicting the infectiousness of i and the susceptibility of j as well as pairwise covariates that predict the hazard of infectious contact from i to j.

12.4.1   Model fitting when who-infects-whom is observed

Given β, the Breslow (1972) estimator of $H_0(\tau)$ is

$$\hat{H}(\beta, \tau, \mathbf{v}) = \int_0^{\tau} \frac{1}{Y(\beta, u)} dN(u), \tag{12.72}$$

where

$$Y(\beta, u) = \sum_{j=1}^{n} \sum_{i \in W_j} r\big(\beta^{\top} X_{ij}(u)\big) Y_{ij}(u). \tag{12.73}$$

The Breslow estimator has two desirable properties. First, $\hat{H}(\beta_0, \tau, \mathbf{v})$ is an unbiased estimator of $H_0(\tau)$. Second, $\hat{H}(\beta, \tau, \mathbf{v})$ maximizes the log likelihood

$$\ell(\beta, H) = \sum_{j : t_j < T} \ln \Big[r\big(\beta^{\top} X_{v_j j}(t_j - t_{v_j} - \varepsilon_{v_j})\big) dH(t_j - t_{v_j} - \varepsilon_{v_j}) \Big]$$
$$- \int_0^{\infty} Y(\beta, u) dH(u) \tag{12.74}$$

over all step functions $H(\tau)$. Substituting $\hat{H}(\beta, \tau, \mathbf{v})$ into $\ell(\beta, H)$, we get the log profile likelihood

$$\ell_p(\beta, \mathbf{v}) = \sum_{j \in \mathcal{I}_{\text{int}}} \ln \frac{r\big(\beta^{\top} X_{v_j j}(\tau_{v_j j})\big)}{Y(\beta, \tau_{v_j j})}. \tag{12.75}$$

This derivation of the partial likelihood as a profile likelihood follows that of Johansen (1983). When $\beta = 0$, the Breslow estimator in equation (12.72) reduces to the Nelson-Aalen estimator in equation (12.49), and the likelihood in equation (12.74) reduces to that of equation (12.51).

Let $\hat{\beta}$ denote the value of β that maximizes $\ell_p(\beta, \mathbf{v})$, and let $\hat{H}(\hat{\beta}, \tau, \mathbf{v})$ be the corresponding Breslow estimate of the baseline cumulative hazard. When both the number of pairs at risk and the number of susceptibles is large, hypothesis tests and confidence intervals for β_0 can be obtained using Wald, score, or likelihood ratio statistics. The variance of $\hat{H}(\hat{\beta}, \tau, \mathbf{v})$ is estimated consistently

$$\hat{\sigma}^2(\beta, \tau, \mathbf{v}) = \left(\frac{\partial}{\partial \beta} \hat{H}(\beta, \tau, \mathbf{v}) \right)^{\top} I_p(\beta)^{-1} \left(\frac{\partial}{\partial \beta} \hat{H}(\beta, \tau, \mathbf{v}) \right) + \int_0^{\tau} \frac{1}{Y(\beta, u)^2} dN(u), \quad (12.76)$$

where $I_p(\beta)$ is the observed information function.

Using the martingale central limit theorem and a log transformation, we get the large-sample pointwise $1 - \alpha$ confidence limits

$$\hat{H}(\hat{\beta}, \tau, \mathbf{v}) \exp\left(\pm \frac{\hat{\sigma}(\hat{\beta}, \tau, \mathbf{v})}{\hat{H}(\hat{\beta}, \tau, \mathbf{v})} \Phi^{-1}\left(1 - \frac{\alpha}{2}\right) \right). \quad (12.77)$$

12.4.2   Model fitting when who-infects-whom is not observed

Given the observed data, the probability that j was infected by $i \in V_j$ is

$$p_{ij} = \frac{h_{ij}(t_j - t_i - \varepsilon_i)}{\sum_{k \in V_j} h_{kj}(t_j - t_i - \varepsilon_i)} \quad (12.78)$$

where $h_{ij}(\tau)$ is given by equation (12.71). This is identical to equation (12.54) except for the relative risk function. The probability of each $\mathbf{v} \in \mathcal{V}$ is given by equation (12.55).

The conditional expectation of $\ell_p(\beta, \mathbf{V})$ is

$$\ell_p(\beta) = \sum_{\mathbf{v} \in \mathcal{V}} \Pr(\mathbf{v}) \ell_p(\beta, \mathbf{v}) = \sum_{j=1}^{n} \sum_{i \in W_j} \int_0^{\infty} \ln \frac{r\left(\beta^{\top} X_{ij}(u)\right)}{Y(\beta, u)} d\mathbb{E}_c N_{ij}(u) \quad (12.79)$$

where $\mathbb{E}_c N_{ij}(\tau)$ is defined in equation (12.56). Similarly, the conditional expectation of $\hat{H}(\beta_0, \tau, \mathbf{V})$ is

$$\mathbb{E}_c H(\beta_0, \tau, \mathbf{V}) = \sum_{\mathbf{v} \in \mathcal{V}} \Pr(\mathbf{v}) \hat{H}_0^*(\beta_0, \tau, \mathbf{v}) = \int_0^{\tau} \frac{1}{Y(\beta, u)} d\mathbb{E}_c N(u) \quad (12.80)$$

where $\mathbb{E}_c N(\tau)$ is defined in equation (12.58). By the law of iterated expectation,

$$\mathbb{E}\left[\mathbb{E}_c \hat{H}(\beta_0, \tau, \mathbf{V})\right] = H_0(\tau), \quad (12.81)$$

so $\mathbb{E}_c \hat{H}(\beta_0, \tau, \mathbf{V})$ is an unbiased estimate of $H_0(\tau)$ for each $\tau \in (0, \mathcal{T}]$.

Without knowing β_0 and $h_0(\tau)$, we cannot calculate $\mathbb{E}_c \hat{H}(\beta_0, \tau, \mathbf{V})$. If we have estimates $\hat{\beta}$ and $\hat{h}(\tau)$, the corresponding estimate of p_{ij} is

$$\hat{p}_{ij} = \frac{\hat{h}_{ij}(t_j - t_i - \varepsilon_i)}{\sum_{k \in V_j} \hat{h}_{kj}(t_j - t_i - \varepsilon_i)} \quad (12.82)$$

where $\hat{h}_{ij}(\tau) = r(\hat{\beta}^{\top} X_{ij}(\tau))\hat{h}(\tau)$. The estimated $\ell_p(\beta)$ is

$$\hat{\ell}_p(\beta) = \sum_{\mathbf{v} \in \mathcal{V}} \hat{\Pr}(\mathbf{v})\ell_p(\beta, \mathbf{v}) = \sum_{j=1}^{n} \sum_{i \in W_j} \int_0^{\infty} \ln \frac{r(\beta^{\top} X_{ij}(u))}{Y(\beta, u)} d\hat{N}_{ij}(u) \qquad (12.83)$$

where $\hat{N}_{ij}(\tau)$ is defined in equation (12.62). The *marginal Breslow estimate* (Kenah, 2015) is

$$\hat{H}_0(\hat{\beta}, \tau) = \sum_{\mathbf{v} \in \mathcal{V}} \hat{\Pr}(\mathbf{v})\hat{H}(\hat{\beta}, \tau, \mathbf{v}) = \int_0^{\tau} \frac{1}{Y(\hat{\beta}, u)} d\hat{N}(u) \qquad (12.84)$$

where $\hat{N}(\tau)$ is defined in equation (12.63). As in Algorithm 12.1, $\hat{H}_0(\hat{\beta}, \tau)$ can be smoothed and differentiated with respect to τ to get a new estimate of $h_0(\tau)$, and so on. The estimates of $H_0(\tau)$ converge (Kenah, 2015) because this is an Expectation-Conditional Maximization (ECM) algorithm (Meng and Rubin, 1993), which generalizes the EM algorithm by splitting the M-step into a series of conditional maximizations. The entire process is summarized in Algorithm 12.2.

Algorithm 12.2 ECM algorithm for semiparametric regression

1: Start with an initial $\hat{\beta}^{(0)}$ and $\hat{h}^{(0)}(\tau)$
2: $k \leftarrow 0$
3: **while** convergence criterion not met **do**
4:    *E-step:* Calculate the infector probabilities $\hat{p}_{ij}^{(k)}$.
5:    *CM1-step:* Find $\hat{\beta}^{(k+1)} = \arg\max_{\beta} \hat{\ell}_p(\beta)$.
6:    *CM2-step:* Calculate the marginal Breslow estimate $\hat{H}^{(k+1)}(\hat{\beta}^{(k+1)}, \tau)$.
7:    *Smoothing step:* Smooth $\hat{H}^{(k+1)}(\hat{\beta}^{(k+1)}, \tau)$ and take the first derivative with respect to τ to get $\hat{h}^{(k+1)}(\tau)$.
8:    $k \leftarrow k + 1$
9: **end while**

If it is known that $\beta_0 = 0$, then Algorithm 12.2 reduces to Algorithm 12.1 and the marginal Breslow estimate reduces to the marginal Nelson-Aalen estimate. Therefore, convergence of both $\hat{\beta}^{(k)}$ and $\hat{H}^{(k)}(\hat{\beta}^{(k)}, \tau)$ should be monitored.

Let $\hat{\beta}$ denote the estimate of β_0 to which Algorithm 12.2 converges. The observed information (Louis, 1982) is

$$\hat{I}_p(\beta) = \sum_{\mathbf{v} \in \mathcal{V}} \hat{\Pr}(\mathbf{v})I_p(\beta, \mathbf{v}) - \sum_{\mathbf{v} \in \mathcal{V}} \hat{\Pr}(\mathbf{v})U_p(\beta, \infty, \mathbf{v})^{\otimes 2} \qquad (12.85)$$

where $U_p(\beta, \infty, \mathbf{v})$ is the score function that we would obtain if we observed the transmission tree $\mathbf{v}$.

The first term in equation (12.85) is

$$\sum_{\mathbf{v} \in \mathcal{V}} \hat{\Pr}(\mathbf{v})I_p(\beta, \mathbf{v}) = -\sum_{j=1}^{n} \sum_{i \in W_j} \int_0^{\infty} \frac{\partial^2}{\partial \beta^2} \ln \frac{r(\hat{\beta}^{\top} X_{ij}(u))}{Y(\hat{\beta}, u)} d\hat{N}_{ij}(u). \qquad (12.86)$$

This is the observed information matrix in a weighted Cox regression model (Therneau and Grambsch, 2000) with two copies of each pair ij such that $i \in V_j$: an uncensored copy with weight $\hat{p}_{ij}$ and a censored copy with weight $1 - \hat{p}_{ij}$. If $i \in W_j \setminus V_j$, then there is only a censored copy of ij. To evaluate the second term in equation (12.85), let

$$\hat{U}_{\cdot j}(\beta, \tau) = \sum_{i \in W_j} \int_0^\tau \frac{\partial}{\partial \beta} \ln \frac{r(\hat{\beta}^\top X_{ij}(u))}{Y(\hat{\beta}, u)} \mathrm{d}\hat{N}_{ij}(u) \tag{12.87}$$

be the contribution to the score of $\hat{\ell}_p(\beta)$ from all pairs in which j is susceptible. Because $\sum_j \hat{U}_{\cdot j}(\hat{\beta}, \infty) = 0$, each $j \in \mathcal{I}_{\text{int}}$ has only one infector, and the infectors of different individuals can be chosen independently given the observed data, the second term in equation (12.85) equals

$$\sum_{j=1}^n \sum_{i \in V_j} \int_0^\infty \left(\frac{\partial}{\partial \beta} \ln \frac{r(\hat{\beta}^\top X_{ij}(u))}{Y(\hat{\beta}, u)} \mathrm{d}\hat{N}_{ij}(u) \right)^{\otimes 2} \mathrm{d}\hat{N}_{ij}(u) - \sum_{j=1}^n \hat{U}_{\cdot j}(\hat{\beta}, \infty)^{\otimes 2}.$$

Using this variance estimate, hypothesis tests and confidence intervals for β_0 can be obtained using Wald, score, or likelihood ratio tests.

Let $\hat{H}(\hat{\beta}, \tau)$ be the marginal Breslow estimate of $H_0(\tau)$ to which Algorithm 12.2 converges. Kenah (2015) derives the variance estimate $\hat{\sigma}^2(\hat{\beta}, \tau)$ where

$$\hat{\sigma}^2(\beta, \tau) = \left(\frac{\mathrm{d}}{\mathrm{d}\beta} \hat{H}(\beta, \tau) \right)^\top \hat{I}_p(\beta)^{-1} \left(\frac{\mathrm{d}}{\mathrm{d}\beta} \hat{H}(\beta, \tau) \right)$$

$$+ 2 \int_0^\tau \frac{1}{Y(\beta, u)^2} \mathrm{d}\hat{N}(u) - \sum_{j=1}^n \left(\int_0^\tau \frac{1}{Y(\beta, u)} \mathrm{d}\hat{N}_{\cdot j} \right)^2 \tag{12.88}$$

The martingale central limit theorem and a log transformation give us the large-sample pointwise $1 - \alpha$ confidence limits

$$\hat{H}(\hat{\beta}, \tau) \exp\left(\pm \frac{\hat{\sigma}(\hat{\beta}, \tau)}{\hat{H}(\hat{\beta}, \tau)} \Phi^{-1}\left(1 - \frac{\alpha}{2}\right) \right). \tag{12.89}$$

12.5   Limitations, Extensions, and Implications

The methods described in this chapter offer important theoretical and practical advantages over existing methods for the analysis of infectious disease transmission data, but there are several limitations that must be addressed.

12.5.1   Missing data

As explained in Section 12.1.5, we have assumed that infection times, latent periods, and infectious periods are observed for each infected individual. In practice, these variables usually must be imputed from the observed clinical course of infection. The problem of missing data is ubiquitous in infectious disease epidemiology, and data-augmented Markov chain Monte Carlo (MCMC) methods (Gibson and Renshaw, 1998; O'Neill, Philip D. and Roberts, 1999) are a general and practical solution to this problem. In this approach, a Metropolis-Hastings algorithm is used to integrate over missing data on infection times, latent periods, and infectious periods. These methods apply directly to the parametric estimators in Section 12.2.

The partial likelihood in Section 12.4 is a profile likelihood where the baseline hazard $h_0(\tau)$ is treated as a nuisance parameter. Strictly speaking, a profile likelihood does not fit within standard Bayesian statistical inference. However, a profile likelihood can incorporated into a data-augmented MCMC algorithm using a profile sampler (Lee et al., 2005). Based on the results of Cheng and Kosorok (2008), we expect the mean and credible sets of the posterior profile likelihood to produce accurate point and interval estimates of β_0 and $H_0(\tau)$ in semiparametric regression models. Similarly, we expect a profile sampler to produce accurate point and interval estimates of $H_0(\tau)$ in the nonparametric estimators of Section 12.3.

12.5.2   External sources of infection

Another limitation from Section 12.1.5 is the assumption that the set $\mathcal{I}_{\text{ext}}$ of external infections is known. This assumption was made so that we could focus on the estimation of the contact interval distribution. In practice, the set of external infections is usually unknown. The chain binomial model for household transmission handles exogenous infections by including a per-time-unit probability of infection from outside the household (Rampey et al., 1992). Similarly, pairwise survival models need to include a hazard of infection from external sources. These external infection models are based on individuals rather than infectious-susceptible pairs, and the hazard functions are defined on an absolute time scale rather than an infectious age time scale. Let C_{0j} indicate whether individual j is at risk of infection from an external source, and let V_j include zero when $C_{0j} = 1$.

The AFT models of Section 12.2.3 can be extended by letting individual j have an external rate parameter

$$\mu_j = \alpha_0^\top X_j, \tag{12.90}$$

where α_0 is an unknown coefficient vector and X_j is a vector of individual-level covariates for j. The coefficient vector α_0 could overlap the coefficient vector β_0 for the internal hazard of infection. For example, the rate ratio for the effect of vaccination on susceptibility to infection could be the same for both internal and external infection. There also could be covariates associated with different rate ratios in the two models, or covariates included in only one of the models. For example, infectiousness or pairwise covariates in the internal hazard model would not be included in the external hazard model. The failure time distribution in the internal and external models need not be the same. For example, we might assume a constant hazard of infection from the outside but a log-logistic hazard of infection between individuals. Let θ include all coefficients from both models as well as the shape parameter(s). Then external likelihood contribution from j in the time interval $(0, T]$ is

$$\ell_{0j}(\theta) = \int_0^T \ln h_*(u, \theta) \mathrm{d}N_{0j}(u) - \int_0^T h_*(h, \theta) Y_{0j}(u) \mathrm{d}u \tag{12.91}$$

where $h_*(t, \theta)$ is the external hazard of infection at time t, $N_{0j}(t)$ counts external infectious contacts with j, and $Y_{0j}(t) = C_{0j} S_j(u) \mathcal{Y}(u)$ indicates the risk of an observed external infection in j. The total likelihood contribution from person j is

$$\ell_{\cdot j}(\theta) = \ell_{0j}(\theta) + \sum_{i \in W_j} \ell_{ij}(\theta), \tag{12.92}$$

and the overall likelihood is given by equation (12.21). If who-infects-whom is not observed, the likelihood contribution of person j is given by equation (12.26) where

$$h_{\cdot j}(t, \theta) = h_*(t, \theta) C_{0j} + \sum_{i \in W_j} h(t - t_i - \varepsilon_i, \theta) C_{ij} I_i(t), \tag{12.93}$$

and the overall likelihood is given by equation (12.28). These models are being developed in Sharker and Kenah (2019).

The semiparametric regression models of Section 12.4 can be extended by allowing individual j to have an external hazard of infection

$$h_{0j}(t) = r_*\big(\alpha_0^\top X_j(t)\big) h_*(t) \tag{12.94}$$

where $r_* : \mathbb{R} \to (0, \infty)$ is a relative risk function, α_0 is an unknown coefficient vector, $X_j(t)$ is a covariate process for person j, and $h_*(t)$ is an unspecified baseline hazard function. If individual j is infected at time t_j, he or she is an external infection with probability

$$p_{0j} = \frac{h_{0j}(t_j)}{h_{0j}(t_j) + \sum_{i \in V_j \setminus \{0\}} h_{ij}(t_j - t_i - \varepsilon_i)}. \tag{12.95}$$

As in the extended AFT models, the coefficient vector α_0 can have overlap with β_0 and have its own coefficients. Algorithm 12.2, can be extended to update this probability iteratively along with the p_{ij} for $i \in V_j \setminus \{0\}$. This will allow simultaneous semiparametric estimation of α_0, β_0, $H_0(\tau)$, and $H_*(t) = \int_0^t h_*(u)\mathrm{d}u$. This model is being developed in Kenah (2019).

12.5.3 Contact intervals and infectious periods

A more fundamental limitation from Section 12.1.5 is that the infectious period of i is assumed to independently censor the contact intervals τ_{ij} in all ij such that $i \in W_j$. The independent censoring assumption allowed us to deal with the contact interval distribution alone—a mathematical convenience rather than a reasonable scientific approximation. For some diseases, it may be reasonable to assume a constant infectious period, which implies independent censoring by infectious periods. For other diseases, contact intervals and variation in the infectious period may be determined by the same underlying biology. Relaxing the assumption of independent censoring requires simultaneous estimation of the contact interval distribution and the infectious period distribution, leading us into the domain of multivariate survival analysis. The extensions required are likely to be pathogen-specific, depending on within-host dynamics and immunology.

12.5.4 Incorporation of pathogen phylogenies

The increasing availability of whole-genome sequence data has renewed interest in combining pathogen genetic sequence data with epidemiologic data to reconstruct transmission trees. The transmission tree from one outbreak does not generalize to future outbreaks, but a phylogenetic tree linking pathogens sampled from infected individuals provides partial information about who-infected-whom. In pairwise survival analysis, estimates of the contact interval distribution are based on sums or averages over the set of possible transmission trees. By reducing the number of possible transmission trees, pathogen phylogenies can improve the precision of all of the estimators described above.

A pathogen phylogeny can be consistent with many different transmission trees and vice versa. Branching events in a phylogeny do not necessarily correspond to transmissions, and the topology of the phylogenetic tree need not be the same as the topology of the transmission tree (Pybus and Rambaut, 2009; Romero-Severson et al., 2014; Ypma et al., 2013). These differences are especially important for diseases with significant within-host pathogen diversity and long latent or infectious periods (Didelot et al., 2014; Romero-Severson et al., 2014). Kenah et al. (2016) developed a recursive algorithm to enumerate the set of all transmission trees consistent with a pathogen phylogeny. The relationship between phylogenies and transmission trees enforced by the algorithm is similar to the pioneering work of Cottam et al. (2008) and logically equivalent to the more recent approaches of Ypma et al. (2013), Didelot et al. (2014), and Hall and Rambaut (2015).

Let Φ be a pathogen phylogeny, and let $\mathcal{V}_\Phi$ be the set of transmission trees consistent with Φ. Let θ be a parameter vector for the contact interval distribution, and η be a parameter vector for a model of within-host pathogen evolution. Then the likelihood is

$$L(\theta, \eta) = \sum_{\mathbf{v} \in \mathcal{V}_\Phi} \Pr(\Phi, \mathbf{v} | \theta, \eta) = \sum_{\mathbf{v} \in \mathcal{V}_\Phi} \Pr(\Phi | \eta, \mathbf{v}) \ell(\theta, \mathbf{v}), \tag{12.96}$$

where $\Pr(\cdot)$ denotes probabilities or probability densities as necessary. The second equality follows from the fact that the phylogeny contributes no more information to estimation of the contact interval distribution if $\mathbf{v}$ and all infection times, latent periods, and infectious periods are observed. The factor $\Pr(\Phi | \eta, \mathbf{v})$ depends on within-host pathogen evolution and could incorporate genetic distances and branching times, allowing the joint estimation of parameters for within-host evolution and between-host transmission.

Likelihood calculation with a phylogeny is more computationally intensive than that in Section 12.2.2. Given Φ, the infectors of different $j \in \mathcal{I}_{int}$ are not conditionally independent. Monte Carlo methods will be needed to handle estimation of the contact interval inference with a phylogeny. Nonetheless, simulation studies indicate that, for a given number of observed infections, the inclusion of a phylogeny leads to greater precision in coefficient estimates for infectiousness and pairwise covariates (Kenah et al., 2016).

12.5.5 Data on individuals who escape infection

Data on individuals who were exposed to infection but not infected play a crucial role in pairwise survival analysis. Many studies of emerging infections are based on epidemic curves or other population-level data that includes only infected individuals. Because there are no pathogen genetic sequences to collect from uninfected individuals, the introduction of methods from phylogenetics has reinforced this tendency. Under strong assumptions, it is possible to derive estimators for mass-action models that depend only on data about infected individuals (Kenah, 2011, 2013). However, simulation studies (Kenah, 2011; Kenah et al., 2016) show that the failure to include data on individuals who escape infection can lead to severely biased point and interval estimates even when the pathogen phylogeny is known. The exclusion of individuals who escape infection should be justified from first principles under clearly stated assumptions, and greater emphasis should be given to studies of disease transmission in settings with a clearly defined population at risk.

Acknowledgements

This research was supported by National Institute of General Medical Sciences (NIGMS) grant F32 GM085945 and National Institue of Allergy and Infectious Diseases (NIAID) grants K99/R00 AI095302 and R01 AI116770. The content is solely the responsibility of the author and does not necessarily represent the official views of NIGMS, NIAID, or the National Institutes of Health.

References

Aalen, O. Nonparametric inference for a family of counting processes. *Annals of Statistics*, 6:701–726, 1978.

Aalen, O., Ørnulf Borgan, and Hakon Gjessing. *Survival and Event History Analysis: A Process Point of View*. Statistics for Biology and Health. Springer-Verlag, New York, 2009.

Andersson, H. and Tom Britton. *Stochastic Epidemic Models and Their Statistical Analysis*. Lecture Notes in Statistics. Springer, New York, 2000.

Becker, Niels G. *Analysis of Infectious Disease Data*. Monographs on Statistics and Applied Probability. Chapman & Hall/CRC Press, Boca Raton, FL, 1989.

Breslow, N. Contribution to discussion of paper by D. R. Cox. *Journal of the Royal Statistical Society B*, 34:216–217, 1972.

Cheng, Guang and Michael R. Kosorok. General frequentist properties of the posterior profile distribution. *Annals of Statistics*, 36:1819–1853, 2008.

Cottam, Eleanor M. Gaël Thébaud, Jemma Wadsworth, John Gloster, Leonard Mansley, David J. Paton, Donald P. King, and Daniel T. Haydon. Integrating genetic and epidemiological data to determine transmission pathways of foot-and-mouth disease virus. *Proceedings of the Royal Society B*, 275:887–895, 2008.

Cox, David R. Regression models and life-tables. *Journal of the Royal Statistical Society, Series B*, 34:187–220, 1972.

Dempster, Arthur. P., N. M. Laird, and D. B. Rubin. Maximum likelihood from incomplete data via the EM algorithm. *Journal of the Royal Statistical Society, Series B*, 39:1–38, 1977.

Didelot, Xavier, Jennifer Gardy, and Caroline Colijn. Bayesian inference of infectious disease transmission from whole-genome sequence data. *Molecular Biology and Evolution*, 31: 1869–1879, 2014.

Fine, Paul E. M. The interval between successive cases of an infectious disease. *American Journal of Epidemiology*, 158:1039–1047, 2003.

Gibson, Gavin J. and Eric Renshaw. Estimating parameters in stochastic compartmental models using Markov chain methods. *IMA Journal of Mathematics Applied in Medicine & Biology*, 15:19–40, 1998.

Hall, Matthew. and Andrew Rambaut. Epidemic reconstruction in a phylogenetics framework: Transmission trees as partitions of the node set. *PLoS Computational Biology*, 11: e1004613, 2015.

Elizabeth Halloran, M. Claudio Struchiner, and Ira M. Longini, Jr. Study designs for evaluating different efficacy and effectiveness aspects of vaccines. *American Journal of Epidemiology*, 146:789–803, 1997.

Elizabeth Halloran, M. Ira M. Longini, Jr., and Claudio Struchiner. *Design and Analysis of Vaccine Studies*. Statistics for Biology and Health. Springer-Verlag, New York, 2010.

Johansen, Soren An extension of Cox's regression model. *International Statistical Review*, 51:165–174, 1983.

Kalbeisch, John D. and Ross L. Prentice. *The Statistical Analysis of Failure Time Data*. Wiley Series in Probability and Statistics. John Wiley & Sons, Hoboken, NJ, second edition, 2002.

Kenah, Eben Contact intervals, survival analysis of epidemic data, and estimation of R_0. *Biostatistics*, 12:548–566, 2011.

Kenah, Eben Nonparametric survival analysis of epidemic data. *Journal of the Royal Statistical Society, Series B*, 75:277–303, 2013.

Kenah, Eben Semiparametric relative-risk regression for infectious disease transmission data. *Journal of the American Statistical Association*, 110:313–325, 2015.

Kenah, Eben Semiparametric relative-risk models for infectious disease transmission within and between households. 2019. In preparation.

Kenah, Eben, Marc Lipsitch, and James M. Robins. Generation interval contraction and epidemic data analysis. *Mathematical Biosciences*, 213:71–79, 2008.

Kenah, Eben, Tom Britton, M. Elizabeth Halloran, and Jr Longini, Ira M. Molecular infectious disease epidemiology: Survival analysis and algorithms linking phylogenies to transmission trees. *PLoS Computational Biology*, 12:e1004869, 2016.

Lee, Bee Leng, Michael R. Kosorok, and Jason P. Fine. The profile sampler. *Journal of the American Statistical Association*, 100:960–969, 2005.

Louis, Thomas A. Finding the observed information matrix when using the EM algorithm. *Journal of the Royal Statistical Society, Series B*, 44:226–233, 1982.

Meng, Xiao-Li. and Donald Rubin. Maximum likelihood estimation via the ECM algorithm: A general framework. *Biometrika*, 80:267–278, 1993.

Nelson, Wayne Theory and applications of hazard plotting for censored failure data. *Technometrics*, 14:945–966, 1972.

Philip D. O'Neill and Gareth O. Roberts. Bayesian inference for partially observed stochastic epidemics. *Journal of the Royal Statistical Society, Series A*, 162:121–129, 1999.

Prentice, Ross L. and Steven G. Self. Asymptotic distribution theory for Cox-type regression models with general relative risk form. *Annals of Statistics*, 11:804–813, 1983.

Pybus, Oliver G. and Andrew Rambaut. Evolutionary analysis of the dynamics of viral infectious disease. *Nature Reviews Genetics*, 10:540–550, 2009.

Rampey, Alvin H., Jr, Ira M. Longini, Jr, Michael Haber, and Arnold S. Monto. A discrete-time model for the statistical analysis of infectious disease incidence data. *Biometrics*, 48:117–128, 1992.

Romero-Severson, Ethan, Helena Skar, Ingo Bulla, Jan Albert, and Thomas Leitner. Timing and order of transmission events is not directly reflected in a pathogen phylogeny. *Molecular Biology and Evolution*, 31:2472–2482, 2014.

Ross, Ronald An application of the theory of probabilities to the study of *a priori* pathometry: Part I. *Proceedings of the Royal Society of London, Series A*, 92:204–230, 1916.

Sharker, Yushuf and Eben Kenah. Pairwise accelerated failure time models for infectious disease transmission within and between households. 2019. In preparation. arXiv: https://arxiv.org/abs/1901.04916

Svensson, Ake A note on generation times in epidemic models. *Mathematical Biosciences*, 208:300–311, 2007.

Therneau, Terry M. and Patricia M. Grambsch. *Modeling Survival Data: Extending the Cox Model*. Statistics for Biology and Health. Springer-Verlag, New York, 2000.

Van der Vaart, A W. *Asymptotic Statistics*. Cambridge University Press, Cambridge, UK, 1998.

Wallinga, Jacco and Peter Teunis. Different epidemic curves for severe acute respiratory syndrome reveal similar impacts of control measures. *American Journal of Epidemiology*, 160:509–516, 2004.

Ypma, Rolf J. F., W. Marijn van Ballegooijen, and Jacco Wallinga. Relating phylogenetic trees to transmission trees of infectious disease outbreaks. *Genetics*, 195:1055–1062, 2013.

13

Methods for Outbreaks Using Genomic Data

Don Klinkenberg, Caroline Colijn, and Xavier Didelot

CONTENTS

13.1 Introduction

In most methods described in other chapters, outbreaks were analysed using host data such as day of symptom onset, age, sex, or profession, and environmental data such as daily temperature or presence of particular control measures. These data were used to infer individual-level parameters such as incubation periods and risk factors for infection, and population-level parameters such as the basic reproduction ratio and the reduction in transmission due to control. A third type of data can greatly contribute to these analyses: genomic data from the pathogen. Molecular typing data from viruses or bacteria isolated from infected individuals can contain additional information on the likely links in the contact network that have led to transmission. Higher genetic similarity between isolates is likely indicative of a closer link in the transmission chain.

The general idea of the use of molecular data is as follows. Viruses contain RNA or DNA, and bacteria contain DNA, in the form of one or several long molecules called chromosomes. These chromosomes are chains of nucleotides, with four different nucleotides in a specific order. These nucleotides are adenine, cytosine, guanine, and thymine (uracil in RNA), or in short, A, C, G, or T (U). When the pathogens reproduce during infection of a host, the DNA or RNA is replicated, but this replication process is not completely without errors and gives rise to mutations. A mutation could be a deletion or insertion of one or more nucleotides, but more frequently it is a replacement of a nucleotide by another one. This type of mutation produces a Single Nucleotide Polymorphism (SNP). Once a mutation occurs, the changed DNA is further copied to the pathogen's offspring. In the course of a transmission chain, mutations slowly accumulate, so two isolates from patients that are closely linked in the transmission chain are likely to have more similar genomes than two isolates further apart. Conversely, from an inference point of view, data on the molecular differences between patient isolates can be used to infer the likely transmission history.

The most complete data includes all mutations and requires sequencing of the complete genome (whole genome sequencing, WGS). This process involves not only molecular sequencing machines, but also bioinformatics to process the output of these machines. The machines cut the long sequence molecules into shorter fragments, read these fragments, and return the sequences of these fragments as output (next generation sequencing, NGS). However, the output does not give the genomic location of each fragment, and the reads contain many mistakes. Bioinformatic algorithms are needed to transform the NGS data to a complete genome. There are basically two strategies to do this: aligning the reads to a complete reference genome or performing *de novo* assembly, in which partially overlapping reads are used to construct longer concatenated sequences. Sequencing ambiguities are found if different reads of the same sequence have a different nucleotide at a particular position. Although WGS is becoming more and more the standard, it is also possible to use sequences of only a subset of genes. For more detail, see, e.g., [1].

13.1.1   An example dataset

In the context of this section on outbreak analysis, we concentrate on methods for densely sampled outbreaks, i.e., outbreaks with most or all cases notified and sampled. We will use an example dataset to illustrate some of the methods. This is a dataset from a small foot-and-mouth disease (FMD) outbreak in Surrey, UK, which took place in 2007 [2]. The dataset consists of 11 whole genome sequences (8,176 nucleotides) from 10 infected premises. Figure 13.1 shows the 27 SNPs in this FMD dataset and Table 13.1 shows the corresponding genetic distance matrix with pairwise SNP differences.

13.2   Sparse Sampling

Most epidemiological analyses based on pathogen sequence data use sequences from only a limited subset of all cases in an outbreak or endemic situation, which results in a sparse sampling situation. This can be because not all notified cases have been sampled and sequenced, because not all cases have been observed and notified, or in most cases a combination of both. For many research questions, it is not necessary to have all cases sampled. Before turning to methods to analyze densely sampled outbreaks, we first briefly present some methods for sparsely sampled epidemics—methods that have been under development for longer and which have been the starting point for the more recently developed methods for densely sampled outbreaks.

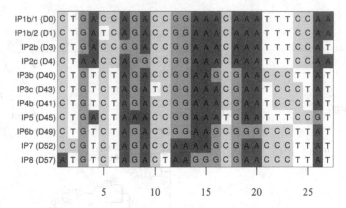

FIGURE 13.1
Single Nucleotide Polymorphisms (SNPs) in the foot-and-mouth disease (FMD) dataset. Each row indicates the infected premise (IP) and sampling day since first sample (D), followed by the nucleotides on all 27 loci with a SNP. The first two samples are from the same IP.

TABLE 13.1
Distance matrix of the foot-and-mouth disease dataset, indicating for each pair of samples the number of loci on which they differ (Figure 13.1)

	IP1b/1	IP1b/2	IP2b	IP2c	IP3b	IP3c	IP4b	IP5	IP6b	IP7	IP8
IP1b/1	0	1	2	2	10	8	7	6	12	13	16
IP1b/2	1	0	3	3	11	9	8	7	13	14	17
IP2b	2	3	0	4	10	8	7	6	12	13	16
IP2c	2	3	4	0	12	10	9	8	14	15	18
IP3b	10	11	10	12	0	4	3	10	2	3	6
IP3c	8	9	8	10	4	0	1	8	6	7	10
IP4b	7	8	7	9	3	1	0	7	5	6	9
IP5	6	7	6	8	10	8	7	0	12	13	16
IP6b	12	13	12	14	2	6	5	12	0	5	8
IP7	13	14	13	15	3	7	6	13	5	0	5
IP8	16	17	16	18	6	10	9	16	8	5	0

13.2.1   Methods based on genetic distance

Two of the most frequently used methods to visualize and analyze sequence data are the Minimum Spanning Tree (MST) and the Neighbor Joining (NJ) algorithm. Both methods build a tree from the distance matrix rather than from the complete sequences. The main difference in the result is that MST makes a tree in which every node represents one or more samples, whereas the NJ algorithm returns a phylogenetic tree, in which the samples are only located on the tip nodes, and the internal nodes represent putative ancestors.

A MST is a tree which connects all samples in such a way that the sum of the distances along all edges is minimized. There are several algorithms to build an MST, implemented in R, which give the tree in Figure 13.2a for the FMD outbreak data. Because all nodes represent a sample, it is possible to interpret the tree in Figure 13.2a as a transmission tree if you would know which was the index case. However, that is not possible with identical samples (which are concentrated on one node), or in sparsely sampled outbreaks.

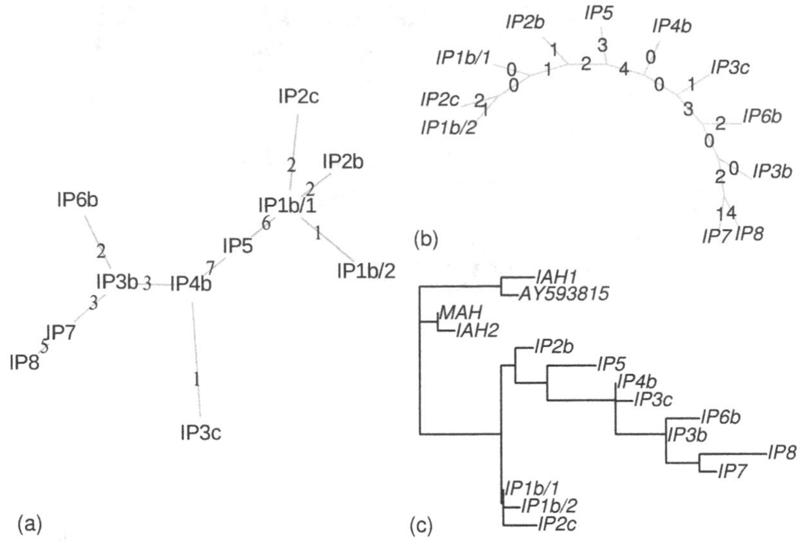

FIGURE 13.2
Distance-based trees of FMD data. (a) MST with distances on the edges; (b) unrooted NJ
tree with distances on the edges; (c) rooted NJ tree with four outgroup genomes.

A NJ tree is a binary tree built with the NJ algorithm, which iteratively connects
clusters (which are single samples or groups of samples connected in previous steps) by
selecting the pair of least distant clusters, until all samples are connected. If possible, this
algorithm returns the tree where all distances between pairs of leaves are equal to the
distances in the distance matrix, which is the case with the FMD outbreak data (Figures
13.2b and c). NJ trees are unrooted, but they can be used as the basis to make (rooted)
phylogenies, where the direction of evolution is known for each branch, and the internal
nodes represent ancestors. The root can be defined as the midpoint of the tree, but more
often it is defined by including samples known to be well separated from the sequences under
study, called outgroups. Figure 13.2c shows such a tree for the FMD outbreak, where four
reference genomes that are not part of the outbreak were used to root the tree. NJ trees
are examples of phylogenetic trees which describe the inferred evolutionary relationships
between the samples (or taxa). There are many more approaches to infer phylogenetic trees,
for example UPGMA, maximum parsimony, maximum likelihood, and various Bayesian
approaches [1, 3].

13.2.2   Model-based inference

Distance-based methods are useful to show genetic relations, but genetic data contains
much more information about the history of pathogen dynamics, which can only be
revealed by using model-based inference. The widely used BEAST software (Bayesian
Evolutionary Analysis through Sampling of Trees) provides an environment to carry out
such analyses, and new model theory with new add-ons are continuously developed and
used within BEAST[1] [4, 5]. Here we briefly introduce the models in BEAST, so that it

---

[1] There are two BEAST versions, where BEAST2 is a modular version of the original BEAST. The basic
   model as described here is identical, but add-ons related to transmission models may vary.

becomes clear what the relation is between the data (sequences and sampling days) and the epidemiological results.

Although BEAST fits its models simultaneously using a Markov Chain Monte-Carlo (MCMC) algorithm, it is easier to understand it by thinking of it as a sequence of models from data to result.

The first model is the substitution model, which links the sequences to the phylogenetic tree [6]. The substitution model describes the rates by which specific nucleotide changes occur. In the simplest substitution model (Jukes-Cantor, JC), all substitutions are equally likely. More complicated models assume different rates by correcting for nucleotide baseline frequencies (adding three parameters), or different (reversible) transition rates per nucleotide pair (adding five parameters). It is also possible to let the substitution rate depend on position within a codon (a triplet of nucleotides coding for an amino acid).

The second model is the clock model [7], which considers the nodes of the tree on the time axis. The tips of the tree are placed according to their sampling time, and the internal nodes are placed backwards in time. This model leans on the molecular clock assumption, which states that substitutions occur at a constant rate over a long period of time, so that the number of substitutions along an edge of the tree is proportional to the time interval between the nodes. This rate parameter, i.e., the mean substitution rate throughout the entire tree, may be estimated from the data if the sampling times are sufficiently spread over time; otherwise, an informative prior distribution is needed. BEAST also allows the use of "relaxed" substitution rate models where the rate is allowed to vary between lineages.

The third model is the phylodynamic model [8], which reconstructs the history of the population size from the time-stamped phylogenetic tree. Because it is a tree for the pathogen, the population history is about the pathogen, not the host. However, by assuming that the size of the pathogen population is proportional to the number of infected hosts over time—which seems reasonable if cases are sparsely sampled—it also reflects prevalence. The phylodynamic model typically connects the tree to the population size through the Kingman coalescent, which is the continuous-time version of ancestries in a Wright-Fisher population [9].

Ancestries in the Wright-Fisher model are described by a stochastic process starting at the tips and going backwards in time, generation by generation. The model assumes that each lineage in generation g has a random parent in generation $g - 1$, independent of the parents of other lineages. As a consequence, if the population size in each generation is equal to N, two lineages in generation g have the same parent in generation $g - 1$ with probability $1/N$, so the distribution of the number of generations back in time until two lineages share a most recent common ancestor (that the two lineages coalesce), is a geometric distribution with mean N. To translate the number of generations to real time, the mean should be multiplied by the generation interval T_g, resulting in the effective population size $N_e = N \cdot T_g$.

The Kingman coalescent is the continuous-time equivalent, with an exponential distribution instead of a geometric distribution. The likelihood of a tip i at time t_i coalescing with an existing tree at time t_{c_i} is equal to $\exp(-A_i/N_e)$, where A_i is the sum of all branch lengths on the existing tree between t_{c_i} and t_i. By ordering the tips from young to old (starting with the most recent leaf), the likelihood of the complete tree can be calculated by considering the probability of adding these tips one by one to the growing tree:

$$\ell(N_e) = \prod_i \exp(-A_i/N_e) \tag{13.1}$$

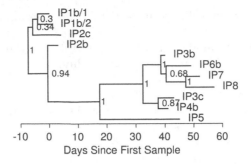

FIGURE 13.3
Phylogenetic tree of the FMD data, obtained with BEAST with posterior clade probabilities
indicated at the internal nodes.

More complicated population models can also be used by including a parametric function
$N_e(t)$, e.g. exponential growth, in which case A_i/N_e is replaced by a sum of areas under
the curve of $1/N_e(t)$. BEAST also allows for a piecewise constant population size, called
the Bayesian Skyline model [10].

Applying a constant population size model in BEAST to analyse the FMD data results
in the tree in Figure 13.3. It is topologically identical to the NJ tree, but the nodes are
now placed on a time axis and annotated with the posterior credibility of each clade (how
frequently that clade was sampled in the MCMC).

13.3   Dense Sampling

Now we come to the central topic of this chapter, which is the analysis of densely sampled
outbreaks with sequence data. With these datasets, epidemiological questions are addressed
through inference of who infected whom during the outbreak, even though the exact
transmission tree may not be the main object of interest in itself. Combining transmission
models and evolutionary models in outbreak analysis can help in addressing questions
such as: was the outbreak the result of a single or multiple introductions, how often did
transmission occur between two sub-populations in the dataset (e.g., two geographical
areas), what was the contribution of particular individuals to the outbreak (e.g., health
care workers in a hospital)?

It is sometimes possible to address these questions in the analysis, or sometimes the
analysis will consist of outbreak reconstruction first, followed by interpretation of the results.
Methods for densely sampled outbreaks combine epidemiological and evolutionary models
(similarly to the combination of phylodynamic and evolutionary models described above
in BEAST), so that a Bayesian approach based on MCMC sampling is well suited. In
this chapter we describe a subset of published methods which were selected because the
underlying models are relatively simple, so they are useful to illustrate the basic concepts,
and also because they are freely available in the form of R packages.

Here the focus is on the models, not the MCMC sampling algorithms or the analysis of
the MCMC output, i.e., checking the convergence and mixing of the chain, and summarizing

the output. A key output summary is a consensus transmission tree, for which several methods are available. All described R packages have functions to obtain consensus trees.

13.3.1 Notation

All methods are for an outbreak with N observed cases, each identified by index $i = 1, \ldots, N$, infected at unknown times $\mathbf{I} = \{I_1, \ldots, I_N\}$, and sampled at known times $\mathbf{S} = \{S_1, \ldots, S_N\}$. The infectors are indicated by the vector $\mathbf{M} = \{M_1 \ldots M_N\}$, with $M_i = 0$ if case i has been infected from an external source. The genetic data are sequences $\mathbf{G} = \{G_1, \ldots, G_N\}$.

The models include a sampling interval distribution $d_S(\Delta t)$, which is the distribution of the time interval between infection and sampling of a case, and a generation interval distribution $d_I(\Delta t)$, which is the distribution of the time interval between infection and transmission to other hosts. The means of these distributions are m_S and m_I. Furthermore, the models contain a substitution rate μ, which is the expected number of substitutions per site (nucleotide position) per unit of time.

13.3.2 No within-host evolution or diversity

By assuming that pathogens do not evolve within the host and substitutions take place at transmission, it is possible to reconstruct outbreaks by using the sampling times and the distance matrix, rather than the complete sequences. This process is done in the R package OUTBREAKER, developed by Jombart et al. [11]. The reconstructed transmission tree has nodes (hosts) placed on a time axis to indicate when they were infected and to show the order of transmission events. An illustration of such a tree is shown in Figure 13.4a. Since the model allows for unsampled cases, the edges on the tree indicate for each host i the most recent ancestor case in the dataset $\tilde{M}_i$, separated from host i by $K_i - 1$ unsampled intermediate transmission links. The probability that a case was sampled is denoted by π. The complete outbreak graph in Figure 13.4a is thus described by the variables:

$$\mathbf{I} = \begin{pmatrix} 0 \\ 1 \\ 3 \\ 4 \end{pmatrix}; \mathbf{S} = \begin{pmatrix} 1 \\ 3 \\ 4 \\ 6 \end{pmatrix}; \mathbf{M} = \begin{pmatrix} 0 \\ 1 \\ 2 \\ 2 \end{pmatrix}; \mathbf{K} = \begin{pmatrix} 0 \\ 1 \\ 2 \\ 2 \end{pmatrix} \qquad (13.2)$$

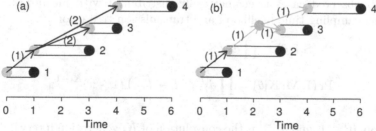

FIGURE 13.4

Outbreak of four observed cases. Each pod is a case with the grey dot at the time of infection and the black dot at the time of sampling; arrows indicate the direction of transmission, with (a) between brackets the numbers of generations between cases (as in OUTBREAKER), or (b) one possible placement of an unsampled case in the same outbreak.

The sampling time vector $\mathbf{S}$ is known, whereas $\mathbf{I}$, $\mathbf{M}$ and $\mathbf{K}$ are unobserved and sampled in the MCMC algorithm.

13.3.2.1   The posterior distribution and likelihood

The OUTBREAKER algorithm samples transmission trees and infection times as well as the the parameter vector $\theta = (\tilde{\mu}, \pi)$. The target posterior probability can be decomposed using Bayes' rule as follows:

$$\Pr\left(\mathbf{I}, \mathbf{M}, \mathbf{K}, \theta | \mathbf{G}, \mathbf{S}\right) \propto \Pr\left(\mathbf{G}, \mathbf{S} | \mathbf{I}, \mathbf{M}, \mathbf{K}, \theta\right) \cdot \Pr\left(\mathbf{I}, \mathbf{M}, \mathbf{K}, \theta\right)$$
$$= \Pr\left(\mathbf{G} | \mathbf{M}, \mathbf{K}, \tilde{\mu}\right) \cdot \Pr\left(\mathbf{S} | \mathbf{I}, \pi\right) \cdot \Pr\left(\mathbf{I}, \mathbf{M}, \mathbf{K} | \theta\right) \cdot \Pr\left(\tilde{\mu}, \pi\right) \tag{13.3}$$

The first two terms on the second line are the genetic and sampling time likelihoods, the third term is the transmission tree prior, and the final term is the prior on the parameters. The substitution rate $\tilde{\mu}$ is the number of substitutions per site per transmission event, not per unit of time, but since both are generally very low they are approximately related through the mean generation interval: $\tilde{\mu} \approx \mu \cdot m_I$.

To make the likelihood calculation easier and faster, all links in the transmission tree are assumed to be independent, even though in fact there could be an unobserved host between an ancestor and two secondary cases (Figure 13.4b). Both likelihoods are thus approximated by pseudo-likelihoods, which are expressed as products of likelihood terms for each host-ancestor combination $\left\{ \tilde{M}_i, i \right\}$.

In the genetic model it is assumed that each host harbors a single genetic sequence, which is sampled and transmitted to secondary cases. Mutations take place during the transmission event so that the next host in the transmission chain may carry a slightly different sequence. Each nucleotide changes with probability $\tilde{\mu}$ at each transmission event. Thus, the genetic likelihood is a product of terms for each edge in the transmission tree:

$$\Pr\left(\mathbf{G} | \mathbf{M}, \mathbf{K}, \tilde{\mu}\right) = \prod_i \tilde{\mu}^{d\left(G_i, G_{\tilde{M}_i}\right)} \left(1 - \tilde{\mu}\right)^{K_i l\left(G_i, G_{\tilde{M}_i}\right) - d\left(G_i, G_{\tilde{M}_i}\right)}, \tag{13.4}$$

in which $d\left(G_i, G_j\right)$ is the genetic distance between hosts i and j, and $l\left(G_i, G_j\right)$ is the total shared sequence length of hosts i and j.

The epidemiological model assumes knowledge of the generation interval distribution $d_I\left(\Delta t\right)$, and of the sampling interval distribution $d_S\left(\Delta t\right)$. The number of generations separating two observed cases is geometrically distributed with mean $1/\pi$. This results in the following sampling time likelihood and transmission tree prior:

$$\Pr\left(\mathbf{S} | \mathbf{I}, \theta\right) = \prod_i d_S\left(S_i - I_i\right)$$
$$\Pr\left(\mathbf{I}, \mathbf{M}, \mathbf{K} | \theta\right) = \prod_i d_I^{(K_i)}\left(I_i - I_{\tilde{M}_i}\right) \left(1 - \pi\right)^{K_i - 1} \pi \tag{13.5}$$

In this equation, $0^0 \equiv 1$, and $d_I^{(K_i)}$ is the convolution of K_i generation interval distributions.

13.3.2.2   Results for the FMD dataset

Applying OUTBREAKER to the FMD dataset requires setting the sampling and generation interval distributions, which we estimated based on the original publication [2]. We also assumed complete observation of cases ($\pi = 1$). The resulting consensus transmission tree is shown in Figure 13.5, with darkness of the arrows indicating the level of support. Only three transmission links (to IP1b/2, IP5, and IP3b) have support $< 100\%$.

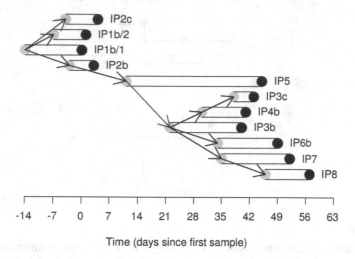

FIGURE 13.5
Consensus FMD transmission tree according to OUTBREAKER. The darkness of the arrows indicates posterior support of the transmission links.

13.3.3 Within-host evolution without diversity

OUTBREAKER reconstructs the transmission tree under the assumption that pathogen sequences do not change while they are in the host, but that after transmission a slightly different variant of the pathogen establishes infection in the next host. By contrast, in the following models substitutions accumulate in continuous time within the host. Consequently, these models not only describe the relationship between the sampled hosts in a transmission tree, and but also the evolutionary relationship between the sampled pathogens in a phylogenetic tree.

The simplest way to combine a transmission model with a continuous-time substitution model is to assume no instantaneous within-host variation but a single strain infecting each host that may slowly change during the course of the infection. Figure 13.6 shows an outbreak with four cases, displaying both the transmission tree and phylogenetic tree. In both graphs, the thick horizontal lines indicate lineages along which substitutions may have taken place. The assumption of a single lineage in each host and no within-host variation implies that there is a one-to-one translation from the transmission tree to the phylogenetic tree, with each internal node of the phylogenetic tree corresponding to transmission or sampling (indicated in Figure 13.6). The variables of the outbreak in Figure 13.6 are

$$\mathbf{I} = \begin{pmatrix} 0 \\ 0.8 \\ 2.5 \\ 4 \end{pmatrix}; \mathbf{S} = \begin{pmatrix} 1.2 \\ 3 \\ 4 \\ 6 \end{pmatrix}; \mathbf{M} = \begin{pmatrix} 0 \\ 1 \\ 2 \\ 2 \end{pmatrix} \tag{13.6}$$

As in OUTBREAKER, the vector $\mathbf{S}$ is known whereas the other vectors are sampled in the MCMC algorithm.

13.3.3.1 The posterior distribution and likelihood

This model is implemented in the R package PHYBREAK [12]. The evolutionary model with one dominant strain was used by Morelli et al. [13], to analyze the same FMD dataset we use in this chapter. However, they used a much more complex epidemiological model,

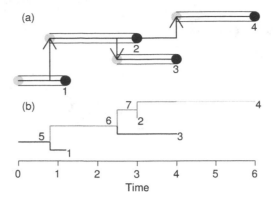

FIGURE 13.6

Outbreak of four cases with one dominant lineage in each host. (a) transmission tree where each pod is a case with the grey dot at the time of infection and the black dot at the time of sampling; arrows indicate the direction of transmission; numbers indicate the host. (b) phylogenetic tree with "colored" branches to distinguish the hosts; numbers indicate the node.

including spatial data (the locations of the farms) affecting the transmission likelihood, a more mechanistic transmission model including farms that did not get infected, and observations on symptom onset and culling dates to put constraints on times of transmission events. The PHYBREAK method samples from the posterior distribution

$$\Pr\left(\mathbf{I}, \mathbf{M}, \theta | \mathbf{G}, \mathbf{S}\right) \propto \Pr\left(\mathbf{G}, \mathbf{S} | \mathbf{I}, \mathbf{M}, \theta\right) \cdot \Pr\left(\mathbf{I}, \mathbf{M}, \theta\right)$$
$$= \Pr\left(\mathbf{G} | \mathbf{I}, \mathbf{M}, \mu\right) \cdot \Pr\left(\mathbf{S} | \mathbf{I}, \theta\right) \cdot \Pr\left(\mathbf{I}, \mathbf{M} | \theta\right) \cdot \Pr\left(\theta\right) \tag{13.7}$$

The first term is the genetic likelihood, depending on the substitution rate μ; the second term the sampling likelihood, depending on the distribution for the sampling interval; the third term is the epidemiological prior, depending on the distribution for the generation interval; and the final term is the prior distribution of all parameters involved. In PHYBREAK the sampling and generation intervals are gamma distributed, and it is possible to estimate the means of these distributions, but not their shape parameters.

The genetic model assumes a constant substitution rate and Jukes-Cantor substitution model, so that substitution probabilities are identical for each site and for each nucleotide change. The substitution process can be described by a set of differential equations for the probability of a site carrying nucleotide $g \in \{A, C, G, T\}$ at time t:

$$\frac{dp_g\left(t\right)}{dt} = \frac{1}{4}\mu\left(1 - p_g\left(t\right)\right) - \frac{3}{4}\mu p_g\left(t\right) = \frac{1}{4}\mu - \mu p_g\left(t\right), \tag{13.8}$$

which has as solution

$$p_g^-\left(t\right) = \tfrac{1}{4} + \tfrac{3}{4}\exp\left(-\mu t\right) \text{ if } \ p_g\left(0\right) = 1 \text{ (without substitution)}$$
$$p_g^+\left(t\right) = \tfrac{1}{4} - \tfrac{1}{4}\exp\left(-\mu t\right) \text{ if } \ p_g\left(0\right) = 0 \text{ (with substitution)} \tag{13.9}$$

The sites are independent, so the likelihood can be written as a product of likelihood contributions per site.

We now derive the likelihood for a single site, using a procedure known as Felsenstein pruning. We number all tips and internal nodes in the tree (as in Figure 13.6), and define for all internal nodes i their child nodes $c_1(i)$ and $c_2(i)$. For example, in Figure 13.6, $c_1(6) = 7$ and $c_2(6) = 3$. Further, we define $L_i^{(l)}(g)$ as the likelihood for site l on the tree with node i as root node, with node i carrying nucleotide g on site l. If node i is a tip node, $L_i^{(l)}(g)$ is 0 or 1, as given by the data. If node i is an internal node, $L_i^{(l)}(g)$ can be written as a function of the likelihoods of the two child trees:

$$L_i^{(l)}(g) = \prod_{j \in \{c_1(i), c_2(i)\}} \left(L_j^{(l)}(g)\, p_g^-(t_j - t_i) + \sum_{g' \neq g} L_j^{(l)}(g')\, p_g^+(t_j - t_i) \right), \qquad (13.10)$$

Thus, $L_r^{(l)}(g)$ can be calculated for the root node r of the complete tree, from which the likelihood $L^{(l)}$ for site l on the complete tree is calculated as

$$L^{(l)} = \sum_{g \in \{A,C,G,T\}} \tfrac{1}{4} L_r^{(l)}(g) \qquad (13.11)$$

Finally, the complete genetic likelihood for all sites is

$$\Pr(\mathbf{G}|\mathbf{I}, \mathbf{M}, \theta) = \prod_l L^{(l)} = \prod_l \sum_g \tfrac{1}{4} L_r^{(l)}(g) \qquad (13.12)$$

By assuming that all cases have been observed, the epidemiological model is simpler than in OUTBREAKER with the following sampling likelihood and transmission tree prior:

$$\Pr(\mathbf{S}|\mathbf{I}, \theta) = \prod_i d_S(S_i - I_i)$$

$$\Pr(\mathbf{I}, \mathbf{M}|\theta) = \prod_{i|M_i \neq 0} d_I(I_i - I_{M_i}) \qquad (13.13)$$

13.3.3.2 Results for the FMD dataset

We applied PHYBREAK with the dominant strain model to the FMD data with the same sampling interval and generation interval distributions as used with OUTBREAKER. The transmission tree is shown in Figure 13.7, as well as a corresponding phylogenetic tree with colour transitions indicating transmission. In comparison with the OUTBREAKER output, the posterior probabilities of specific transmission events are generally much lower. Although this result may seem disappointing at first, it correctly reflects the increase in uncertainty that happens when within-host evolution is accounted for.

13.3.4 Within-host evolution and diversity

The next step in generalizing models for sequence evolution during infectious disease outbreaks is to relax the assumption of a single dominant lineage in each host. In fact, when a host is sampled and sequenced, only a small number of bacteria or virus particles in that host is sequenced. This sequence may contain SNPs recently developed within that host, and if the host infects another host the next day, the transmitted pathogen may not contain these same recent SNPs. From the perspective of the observer, it may seem as if new SNPs in an early case of an outbreak are "lost" in the subsequent cases, but in reality these SNPs were never transmitted as a result of a large and diverse pathogen population within each host. In the following methods, this diversity is explicitly modelled, though still under the assumption of a complete transmission bottleneck, which means that at transmission only a single variant is passed on to the next host.

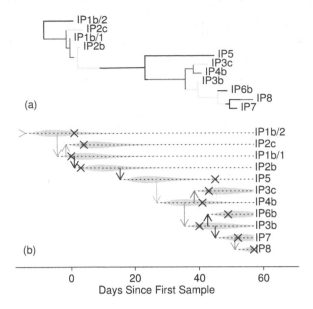

FIGURE 13.7

Consensus FMD transmission tree with the dominant strain model. (a) phylogenetic tree taken from the MCMC chain (consensus topology but not infection times) with change in "color" indicating transmission or (b) transmission tree with darkness of the arrows indicating posterior support of the transmission links, placed at median posterior infection times; crosses indicate sampling times.

In the model with the single dominant strain, there was a single possible translation from the transmission tree to the phylogenetic tree, as in Figure 13.6. Thus, the transmission tree (variables **I**, **S**, **M**) also described the phylogenetic tree, and these variables were sufficient to calculate the complete likelihood. Note that the reverse translation was not absolute, as at each bifurcation at transmission, either branch could be transmitted or stay in the infector. For example, in node 6 in Figure 13.6, host 3 could have transmitted to host 2, or vice versa. Now that we relax the assumption of a single dominant strain, bifurcations in the phylogenetic tree are not linked to transmission or sampling anymore, so each transmission tree can correspond to many phylogenetic trees.

To solve this ambiguity, Didelot et al. [14] proposed to color the branches on phylogenetic trees, to indicate in which host each branch resided. In the bottom panel of Figure 13.6 this is shown for the dominant strain model, in which color changes always happen at bifurcation points. However, this idea can also be used in a model with within-host diversity, in which case color changes can happen anywhere on phylogenetic branches. Figure 13.8 shows how a single transmission tree can correspond to multiple colored phylogenetic trees. Conversely, Didelot et al proved that by coloring the branches on a phylogenetic tree, there exists only a single possible translation to a transmission tree. Thus, a colored phylogenetic tree is a complete description of both the transmission and phylogenetic trees, and is sufficient to calculate the full likelihood. They used this principle to sample possible transmission trees, i.e., color schemes, for a given phylogenetic tree. That method is available in the R package TRANSPHYLO [14].

A description of such a tree requires additional variables for the phylogenetic tree: we number the nodes $j = 1, \ldots, n$ and define their times $\mathbf{t} = \{t_1, \ldots, t_n\}$, and their parent

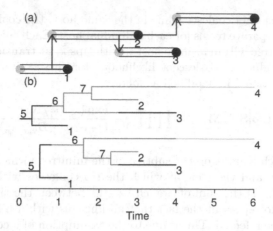

FIGURE 13.8

Outbreak of four cases with within-host diversity. (a) Transmission tree where each pod is a case with the grey dot at the time of infection and black dot at the time of sampling; arrows indicate the direction of transmission; numbers indicate the host. (b) Two possible matching phylogenetic trees with "colored" branches to distinguish the hosts; numbers indicate the node.

nodes $\mathbf{p} = \{p_1, \ldots, p_n\}$ with $p_j = 0$ if j is the root node. Then, the bottom colored tree in Figure 13.8 is completely described by

$$
\mathbf{I} = \begin{pmatrix} 0 \\ 0.8 \\ 2.5 \\ 4 \end{pmatrix} ; \mathbf{S} = \begin{pmatrix} 1.2 \\ 3 \\ 4 \\ 6 \end{pmatrix} ; \mathbf{M} = \begin{pmatrix} 0 \\ 1 \\ 2 \\ 2 \end{pmatrix} ; \mathbf{t} = \begin{pmatrix} 1.2 \\ 3 \\ 4 \\ 6 \\ 0.5 \\ 1.6 \\ 2.3 \end{pmatrix} ; \mathbf{p} = \begin{pmatrix} 5 \\ 7 \\ 7 \\ 6 \\ 0 \\ 5 \\ 6 \end{pmatrix} . \tag{13.14}
$$

TRANSPHYLO uses $\mathbf{S}$, $\mathbf{t}$, and $\mathbf{p}$ as input data, where $\mathbf{t}$ and $\mathbf{p}$ can be the output of a BEAST analysis for example.

13.3.4.1 The posterior distribution and likelihood

The TRANSPHYLO package samples transmission trees and infection times from the posterior distribution

$$
\begin{aligned}
\Pr(\mathbf{I}, \mathbf{M}, \theta | \mathbf{t}, \mathbf{p}, \mathbf{S}) &\propto \Pr(\mathbf{t}, \mathbf{p}, \mathbf{S} | \mathbf{I}, \mathbf{M}, \theta) \cdot \Pr(\mathbf{I}, \mathbf{M}, \theta) \\
&= \Pr(\mathbf{t}, \mathbf{p} | \mathbf{S}, \mathbf{I}, \mathbf{M}, \theta) \cdot \Pr(\mathbf{S} | \mathbf{I}, \theta) \cdot \Pr(\mathbf{I}, \mathbf{M} | \theta) \cdot \Pr(\theta)
\end{aligned} \tag{13.15}
$$

The first term is the phylodynamic likelihood, for the coalescent processes in each host; the second term is the sampling likelihood; the third term is the transmission tree prior; and the final term is the prior for all parameters. Note that there is no genetic likelihood in this posterior, because the phylogenetic tree is fixed. The coalescent model depends on the pathogen population in each individual host. In the Kingman coalescent as described in Equation 13.1, all extant lineages at time t are at risk of coalescing in the next time interval dt. In the context of an outbreak, however, lineages that are in different hosts cannot coalesce until they come together in the same host through transmission. The coalescent model goes backward in time, so that the process ends when all lineages come together in the index case.

Because lineages can only coalesce while in the same host, the coalescent likelihood can be deconstructed into separate terms for each individual host. Each color in the phylogenetic tree demarcates a minitree within a single host i, with tips k_i at transmission and sampling. The likelihood is a product of coalescent likelihoods for these minitrees, each calculated using a version of Equation 13.1 modified as follows:

$$\Pr(\mathbf{t}, \mathbf{p} | \mathbf{S}, \mathbf{I}, \mathbf{M}, \theta) = \prod_i \prod_{k_i} \frac{\exp(-A_{k_i}/N_e)}{N_e(1 - \exp(-B_{k_i}/N_e))}. \tag{13.16}$$

A_{k_i} is the sum of branch lengths on the subtree of the minitree formed by all younger tips, between the time of k_i and the time at which the tip coalesces with that subtree (as in Equation 13.1); and B_{k_i} is the sum of branch lengths between the time of k_i and I_i. The latter term is needed to represent the fact that all lineages within a host need to coalesce before that host became infected. This is due to the assumption of a complete bottleneck at transmission, such that only a single variant from the infector is transmitted to the newly infected host.

The sampling likelihood and transmission tree prior are the same as in PHYBREAK:

$$\Pr(\mathbf{S}|\mathbf{I}, \theta) = \prod_i d_S(S_i - I_i)$$

$$\Pr(\mathbf{I}, \mathbf{M}|\theta) = \prod_{i|M_i \neq 0} d_I(I_i - I_{M_i}) \tag{13.17}$$

13.3.4.2 Results for the FMD dataset

We applied TRANSPHYLO to the FMD phylogenetic tree reconstructed by BEAST (Figure 13.3) with the same sampling interval and generation interval distributions as used with OUTBREAKER. The consensus transmission tree is shown in Figure 13.9.

13.3.5 Simultaneous inference of transmission and phylogenetic trees

Finally, we consider how to infer the transmission tree by taking within-host diversity into account, plus the uncertainty regarding the phylogenetic relation between the samples.

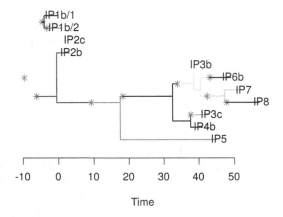

FIGURE 13.9
Consensus FMD transmission and phylogenetic tree obtained with TRANSPHYLO.

This is done in the R package PHYBREAK [12]. The correspondence between phylogenetic and transmission trees are as in Figure 13.8, described by the vectors in Equation 13.14. However, in TRANSPHYLO **t** and **p** are input data, whereas in PHYBREAK these are also sampled in the MCMC algorithm, informed by the sequence data and sampling times.

Because in PHYBREAK there is no single phylogenetic tree on which transmission trees are sampled in the MCMC algorithm, the model description in terms of "coloring the branches" of a phylogenetic tree is less straightforward. Instead, PHYBREAK is best described as a transmission tree with each host harboring a phylogenetic "minitree," as already introduced for the coalescent likelihood computation in TRANSPHYLO. These minitrees are linked through the transmission events to form a single phylogenetic tree that explains the evolutionary history of all isolates (Figure 13.10).

13.3.5.1 The posterior distribution and likelihood

The PHYBREAK package samples transmission trees, infection times, and phylogenetic minitrees from the posterior distribution

$$
\begin{aligned}
\Pr\left(\mathbf{I}, \mathbf{M}, \mathbf{t}, \mathbf{p}, \theta | \mathbf{G}, \mathbf{S}\right) &\propto \Pr\left(\mathbf{G}, \mathbf{S} | \mathbf{I}, \mathbf{M}, \mathbf{t}, \mathbf{p}, \theta\right) \cdot \Pr\left(\mathbf{I}, \mathbf{M}, \mathbf{t}, \mathbf{p}, \theta\right) \\
&= \Pr\left(\mathbf{G} | \mathbf{t}, \mathbf{p}, \theta\right) \cdot \Pr\left(\mathbf{t}, \mathbf{p} | \mathbf{S}, \mathbf{I}, \mathbf{M}, \theta\right) \cdot \Pr\left(\mathbf{S} | \mathbf{I}, \theta\right) \cdot \Pr\left(\mathbf{I}, \mathbf{M} | \theta\right) \cdot \Pr\left(\theta\right)
\end{aligned}
\tag{13.18}
$$

In fact, this model with within-host diversity is an extension of the PHYBREAK model with one single dominant lineage (Section 13.3.3), so the posterior distribution is the same with one additional term: the likelihood for the coalescent processes in all hosts (the minitrees), $\Pr\left(\mathbf{t}, \mathbf{p} | \mathbf{S}, \mathbf{I}, \mathbf{M}, \theta\right)$. In PHYBREAK, the within-host pathogen population size is modeled with linear growth, $w\left(\tau\right) = r\tau$, so that the coalescent rate $1/w\left(\tau\right)$ approaches infinity at infection. This forces all lineages to coalesce within the host, resulting in a complete bottleneck. As a consequence, the coalescent likelihood in PHYBREAK is different from the one in TRANSPHYLO: the denominator in Equation 13.16 to condition on a complete bottleneck is not needed, but the coalescent rate is not constant anymore, so the likelihood cannot be written in terms of sums of branch lengths. Instead, for each minitree i a function $L_i\left(\tau\right)$ is defined that describes the number of lineages at time τ since infection, from which the likelihood is formulated as

$$
\Pr\left(\mathbf{t}, \mathbf{p} | \mathbf{S}, \mathbf{I}, \mathbf{M}, \theta\right) = \prod_i \exp\left(-\int_0^\infty \binom{L_i\left(\tau\right)}{2} \frac{1}{w\left(\tau\right)} d\tau\right) \prod_{c_i} \frac{1}{w\left(\tau_{c_i}\right)}
\tag{13.19}
$$

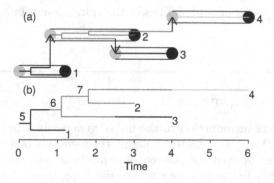

FIGURE 13.10

Outbreak of four cases with within-host diversity, displayed as (a) transmission tree with phylogenetic minitrees or (b) phylogenetic tree with "colored" branches.

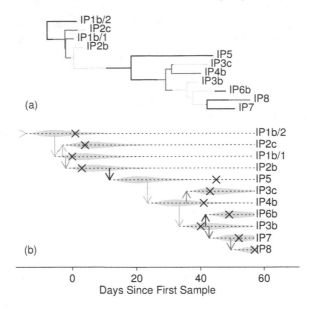

(a)

(b)

0   20   40   60
Days Since First Sample

FIGURE 13.11
Consensus FMD transmission tree with PHYBREAK within-host diversity model. (a) phylogenetic tree taken from the MCMC chain (consensus topology but not infection times); (b) transmission tree with darkness of the arrows indicating posterior support of the transmission links, placed at median posterior infection times; crosses indicate sampling times.

Here, the integral is the area under the curve of coalescent rates needed (by exponentiation) for the probability to not have coalescence in the intervals between the coalescent, sampling, and transmission events. The last term is the product of coalescent rates at the coalescent times.

13.3.5.2 Results for the FMD dataset

We applied PHYBREAK with within-host diversity to the dataset, resulting in the consensus tree in Figure 13.11. Because PHYBREAK takes more uncertainty into account than all previous methods, the posterior probabilities of the transmission links are the lowest.

13.4 Further Developments

This chapter gave a brief introduction to the use of genetic data in outbreak analysis. To present the underlying theory and models in detail, the focus was on single baseline scenario: outbreaks with all cases observed and one sequence available per host. The chapter also was based on easy availability in the form of ready-to-use R packages. All methods are already capable of dealing with more complex scenarios, and as this text is written, new theory is being developed, and methods are further extended or newly developed. We finish this chapter with a non-exhaustive list of some of these developments, within the R packages already described, and in other implementations:

1. BEASTLIER [15]: an extension in BEAST to infer transmission trees at the same time as the timed phylogeny. Apart from specific choices of the submodels, e.g. for the within-host pathogen population or mutation, BEASTLIER's model is similar to TRANSPHYLO and PHYBREAK.

2. SCOTTI (Structural Coalescent Transmission Tree Inference) [16]: an extension in BEAST2 to infer transmission trees. SCOTTI treats hosts as demes and models transmission of pathogens as migration events between demes. This makes it easier to include multiple samples per host and multiple infections (which could have resulted from a wide bottleneck), and it is also possible to include unsampled hosts. However, inference requires input of exposure intervals for each host to indicate when they were most likely part of the outbreak, and infection times are not inferred.

3. BITRUGS (Bayesian inference of transmission routes using genome sequences) [17]: an R package to infer transmission trees. The BITRUGS method allows for multiple samples per patient and the use of epidemiological data, for example admission and discharge data in a hospital setting. The method also infers whether the observed cases are a result of multiple introductions from the general community. The genetic likelihood makes use of genetic distance data (not the sequences), but unlike OUTBREAKER includes the genetic distances between all pairs of sequences, with different geometric distributions for samples within a host, in the same transmission tree depending on the number of links separating the samples, or in a different tree in the case of multiple introductions.

4. TRANSPHYLO [14, 18]. In TRANSPHYLO it is also possible to infer unobserved cases as part of the phylogenetic tree that is used as input data. In that case, the likely presence of intermediate unobserved links in the transmission tree is informed by the sampling times and generation interval distribution, but the unobserved hosts are given a specific place in the transmission tree as informed by the genetic data (unlike OUTBREAKER, where they are only counted between observed hosts). By explicitly modelling the observation process with a sampling probability, TRANSPHYLO also estimates the number of unobserved hosts that are not part of the phylogenetic tree, i.e., which have not led to further transmission themselves. Finally, the observation model is used to allow inference in ongoing outbreaks by including the possibility of hosts that have not yet been observed by the time that sampling ended.

5. PHYBREAK [12]. In PHYBREAK it is possible to use multiple sequences per host, which are modelled as additional tips in the within-host minitrees. The method has also been adapted to relax the assumption of a complete bottleneck. That is done by using a different model for the within-host pathogen population (starting at a positive population size), so that the coalescent process in a host can end with more than one lineage at the time of infection.

6. BADTRIP (Bayesian epidemiological transmission inference from polymorphisms) [19]: an extension in BEAST2 to reconstruct transmission trees with Next Generation Sequencing (NGS) data. BADTRIP makes use of the raw sequence data instead of consensus sequences. The genetic model treats each site on the genome independently: monomorphic sites (with only A, C, G, or T) may mutate to become polymorphic (two nucleotides present), whereas polymorphic sites display neutral drift which changes the relative frequencies of those nucleotides. That approach treats the whole within-host population size at once so that the relation between the phylogenetic and transmission trees is as with the dominant

strain model described in Section 13.3.3. Furthermore, BADTRIP includes a wide bottleneck by resampling the polymorphic site distributions at transmission. It is possible to include multiple samples per host in the analysis.

7. PHYLOSCANNER [20]: identifying transmission events from multiple phylogenies obtained with NGS data. PHYLOSCANNER consists of two parts. The first part, written in Python, is a tool to make phylogenies from NGS data: it partitions the genome in small segments and makes phylogenies for each segment. The second part is an R package that uses these phylogenies to infer likely transmission events. As a part of the analysis, the tool cleans the raw NGS sequence data, quantifies within-host diversity, and identifies multiple infections and recombination events. It does not explicitly estimate times of infection.

As molecular sequencing techniques become cheaper, faster, and more accurate, methods to analyse these data will continue to be developed. There seem to be two directions where progress will be made in the near future. The first one is with the focus on the complexity of molecular data, i.e., how to make most use of all information hidden in the (raw) sequence data. The BEAST implementations and PHYLOSCANNER seem best prepared for that direction as they have their focus on explicitly modelling the evolutionary process. The second direction is with the focus on the complementary use of epidemiological data, where sequence data are just one of the sources of information. The R packages may be the more natural environments to move into that direction.

References

[1] P. Lemey, M. Salemi, and A.-M. Vandamme. *The Phylogenetic Handbook.* Cambridge University Press, Cambridge, 2009.

[2] E. M. Cottam, J. Wadsworth, A. E. Shaw, R. J. Rowlands, L. Goatley, S. Maan et al. Transmission pathways of foot-and-mouth disease virus in the United Kingdom in 2007. *PLoS Pathog.*, 4(4):e1000050, 2008.

[3] Z. Yang and B. Rannala. Molecular phylogenetics: Principles and practice. *Nat. Rev. Genet.*, 13(5):303–14, 2012.

[4] A. J. Drummond, M. A. Suchard, D. Xie, and A. Rambaut. Bayesian phylogenetics with BEAUti and the BEAST 1.7. *Mol. Biol. Evol.*, 29(8):1969–1973, 2012.

[5] R. Bouckaert, J. Heled, D. Kuhnert, T. Vaughan, C. H. Wu, D. Xie, M. A. Suchard, A. Rambaut, and A. J. Drummond. BEAST 2: A software platform for Bayesian evolutionary analysis. *PLoS Comput. Biol.*, 10(4):e1003537, 2014.

[6] P. Liò and N. Goldman. Models of molecular evolution and phylogeny. *Genome Res.*, 8(12):1233–1244, 1998.

[7] L.D. Bromham, S. Duchene, X. Hua, A.M. Ritchie, D.A. Duchene, and S.Y.W. Ho. Bayesian molecular dating: Opening up the black box. *Biol. Rev.*, 93(3):1165–1191, 2018.

[8] E. M. Volz, K. Koelle, and T. Bedford. Viral phylodynamics. *PLoS Comput. Biol.*, 9(3):e1002947, 2013.

[9] N. A. Rosenberg and M. Nordborg. Genealogical trees, coalescent theory and the analysis of genetic polymorphisms. *Nat. Rev. Genet.*, 3(5):380–90, 2002.

[10] A. J. Drummond, A. Rambaut, B. Shapiro, and O. G. Pybus. Bayesian coalescent inference of past population dynamics from molecular sequences. *Mol. Biol. Evol.*, 22(5):1185–1192, 2005.

[11] T. Jombart, A. Cori, X. Didelot, S. Cauchemez, C. Fraser, and N. Ferguson. Bayesian reconstruction of disease outbreaks by combining epidemiologic and genomic data. *PLoS Comput. Biol.*, 10(1):e1003457, 2014.

[12] D. Klinkenberg, J. A. Backer, X. Didelot, C. Colijn, and J. Wallinga. Simultaneous inference of phylogenetic and transmission trees in infectious disease outbreaks. *PLoS Comput. Biol.*, 13(5):e1005495, 2017.

[13] M. J. Morelli, G. Thebaud, J. Chadceuf, D. P. King, D. T. Haydon, and S. Soubeyrand. A Bayesian inference framework to reconstruct transmission trees using epidemiological and genetic data. *PLoS Comput. Biol.*, 8(11):e1002768, 2012.

[14] X. Didelot, J. Gardy, and C. Colijn. Bayesian inference of infectious disease transmission from whole-genome sequence data. *Mol. Biol. Evol.*, 31(7):1869–1879, 2014.

[15] M. Hall, M. Woolhouse, and A. Rambaut. Epidemic reconstruction in a phylogenetics framework: Transmission trees as partitions of the node set. *PLoS Comput. Biol.*, 11(12):e1004613, 2015.

[16] N. De Maio, C. H. Wu, and D. J. Wilson. SCOTTI: Efficient reconstruction of transmission within outbreaks with the structured coalescent. *PLoS Comput. Biol.*, 12(9):e1005130, 2016.

[17] C. J. Worby, P. D. O'Neill, T. Kypraios, J. V. Robotham, D. De Angelis, E. J. Cartwright, S. J. Peacock, and B. S. Cooper. Reconstructing transmission trees for communicable diseases using densely sampled genetic data. *Ann. Appl. Stat.*, 10(1):395–417, 2016.

[18] X. Didelot, C. Fraser, J. Gardy, and C. Colijn. Genomic infectious disease epidemiology in partially sampled and ongoing outbreaks. *Mol. Biol. Evol.*, 34(4):997–1007, 2017.

[19] N. De Maio, C. J. Worby, D. J. Wilson, and N. Stoesser. Bayesian reconstruction of transmission within outbreaks using genomic variants. *PLoS Comput. Biol.*, 14(4):e1006117, 2018.

[20] C. Wymant, M. Hall, O. Ratmann, D. Bonsall, T. Golubchik, M. de Cesare, A. Gall, M. Cornelissen, and C. Fraser. PHYLOSCANNER: Inferring transmission from within- and between-host pathogen genetic diversity. *Mol. Biol. Evol.*, 35(3):719–733, 2018.

Part IV

Analysis of Seroprevalence Data

14

Persistence of Passive Immunity, Natural Immunity (and Vaccination)

Amy K. Winter and C. Jessica E. Metcalf

CONTENTS

14.1   Immunity in Context

Infection with many pathogens leaves hosts protected from subsequent infection by the same pathogen. This protection is rooted in a response of the adaptive immune system, and may last from a few years (for antigenically variable pathogens, like influenza) to lifelong protection, also called sterilizing immunity (for many childhood infections such as measles). Understanding the dynamics of immunity, and thus susceptibility, is essential because infection can spread only if there is contact between an infected individual and a susceptible individual. Knowledge of susceptibility thus defines outbreak risk, but also can identify timing and targets for vaccination, a source of immunity.

Here, we introduce mathematical and statistical methods developed to define and characterize the landscape of immunity. We focus our overview on directly transmitted immunizing infections, such as measles or rubella. For these pathogens, the life-cycle is relatively straightforward: individuals are typically born immune to infection as a result of antibodies transferred from their mothers; this passive maternal immunity wanes and individuals become susceptible; they then are at risk of acquiring the infection. Infection is followed by recovery, after which individuals are completely protected from re-infection by immunity. A vaccine that confers lifelong immunity is often available, which can transfer individuals directly from the susceptible to the immune category. The life-cycle can be schematically described as shown in Figure 14.1a.

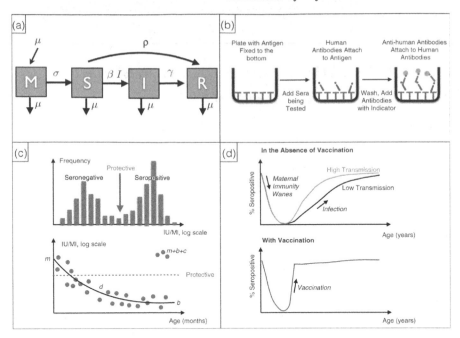

FIGURE 14.1

The landscape of immunity of directly transmitted immunizing infections: (a) Simplified life cycle: Individuals are born (at rate μ) into the maternally immune class (M); following waning of maternal immunity (at rate σ) and if they avoid mortality (at rate μ), they become susceptible (S); they then may die (at rate μ), be vaccinated (at rate ρ), or enter the infected class (I) at rate βI, where β is the rate of contact and successful transmission between S and I individuals; once infected, again, they may die or enter the recovered class (R) at rate γ. For immunizing infections, this stage is never left and is also the endpoint for vaccinated individuals; (b) Enzyme-immunoassays: Sera sampled from a focal individual are added to a well whose surface is coated with antigens. After washing away the unbound material, the amount of antibody that remains bound to the surface provides a measure of antibody concentration of that individual, and is calibrated by a third step in which anti-antibodies labeled with a detectable marker are added and washed away; and optical density of the well is measured. The process is repeated across a range of dilutions to obtain the titer of each sample. (c) Titers measured across a population often are distributed bimodally (top panel). Individuals to the left of a threshold (vertical grey arrow, here denoted "protective") are typically seronegative (i.e., susceptible, thus in the S class); individuals to the right, are typically seropositive (i.e., immune, in the M, I, or R class). Methods exist to identify the cutoff between "seronegative" (left) and "seropositive" (right) individuals that minimizes misclassification. Changes in titers for example during loss of maternal antibodies (bottom panel) can be framed parametrically (see text—m is the starting log titer of newborn individuals, d is the rate at which this decays over age, b is the baseline level of log titers, and c is the excess titer in individuals who have seroconverted (by vaccination or infection)); (d) Seropositivity often is plotted as a proportion across age. Very young individuals have a high proportion of seropositivity as a result of maternal antibodies. This proportion declines as maternal antibodies wane and more individuals fall below the protective threshold (e.g., previous panel, grey horizontal dashed line), and then increases as individuals either acquire infection (top panel) at a rate determined by the magnitude of transmission, or are vaccinated (bottom panel). Acquisition of seropositivity can reflect a mixture of infection and vaccination.

Since immunity following infection or vaccination is often life-long, the only source of new susceptible individuals is by birth (following waning of maternal passive immunity), or immigration of susceptible individuals. This simplicity means that it is theoretically possible to reconstruct the profile of susceptibility through time by combining incidence data with the underlying birth rates and vaccination coverage data, an approach called "susceptible reconstruction" [1]. Taking as a time-step the serial interval of the infection (e.g., approximately 2 weeks for measles), and ignoring migration and delays associated with maternal immunity for simplicity, the number of susceptible individuals at $t+1$, S_{t+1}, is defined by the recursion

$$S_{t+1} = S_t + B_t - I_{t+1} + u_t, \tag{14.1}$$

where I_{t+1} is the number of infected individuals, B_t is the number of births, and u_t is additive noise such that $\mathbb{E}[u_t] = 0$. In endemic settings, the number of susceptible individuals will fluctuate around a mean proportion seronegative, $\bar{S}$, given a population size, N, such that $S_t = \bar{S}N + Z_t$, where Z_t is the deviation around mean number of susceptibles at time t. Reframing the equation through successive iterations around a starting condition, Z_0, and a reporting rate, ρ, we obtain

$$\sum_{k=0}^{t-1} B_k = -Z_0 + 1/\rho \sum_{k=0}^{t-1} I_k^{(r)} + Z_t + u_t, \tag{14.2}$$

implying that, where u_t is small, Z_t can be estimated from the deviations of a locally varying regression of the cumulative number of births, B, on the cumulative number of infected individuals reported, $I^{(r)}$.

This approach has been successively deployed to characterize fluctuations in susceptibility, and from this, to disentangle transmission dynamics for a number of childhood infections [1–4]. However, data on incidence is often under-reported [5], reporting norms may change through time [6], and data on vaccination coverage is often imprecise for a variety of reasons [7]. These issues may bias estimates of susceptibility, and particularly estimates of the age profile of susceptibility [8], an important variable to the design of control strategies. Key programmatic decisions that knowing the age profile of susceptibility can inform include the age of routine immunization (9 or 12 months [9]), or the age range targeted by each vaccination campaign (also known as Supplementary Immunization Activities; e.g., up to 5, 10 or 15 years old, or even higher).

To address questions related to age-specific susceptibility, where age incidence data is available, it is possible to infer age profiles of susceptibility. For example, assuming a fully susceptible birth cohort (again ignoring maternal immunity for simplicity), the number of susceptibles of each age, a, can be calculated recursively via

$$S_a = \frac{S_{a-1} - I_{a-1}}{N_{a-1}} N_a, \tag{14.3}$$

where I_a is the number of infected individuals of age a, and N_a is the population size of individuals age a [10]. However, this data is also subject to uncertainties previously described, further amplified if there is any variability in reporting across age.

The most direct source of data on susceptibility over age is serology, the study of, and testing for circulating antibodies against a pathogen using sera. With enzyme immunoassays (Figure 14.1b, one of many possible approaches for testing sera), sera can be tested for Immunoglobulin M (IgM), an antibody whose titers rise immediately after infection, but then quickly fall, thus making this antibody a good marker of recent infection; and Immunoglobulin G (IgG), an antibody whose titers rise, and then stay high for decades, after either infection or vaccination. Measles virus-specific, and rubella virus-specific IgG antibodies above a known threshold are recognized correlates of immunity [11, 12] whether resulting from the transfer of maternal antibodies, natural infection, or vaccination (Figure 14.1c). Age-specific IgG serology thus can inform directly patterns of immunity (and in turn susceptibility) over age, and their complex fluctuations. In this chapter, we focus on IgG serology, and consider approaches for interpreting serological profiles over age commonly available from cross-sectional studies. We first broadly introduce the age profile of immunity for immunizing infections, and its determinants and discuss the basic tool-set for inference around this type of data, introducing methods for both continuous and binary response variables, indicating how this can reveal the underlying dynamical drivers. We conclude with a case study on use of IgG serology for rubella across the spectrum from endemic to elimination settings and outline some directions for further statistical and methodological innovation.

14.2   Expectations for Serological Age Profiles

The proportion of individuals seropositive over age for measles and rubella has a broadly consistent shape, with high early seropositivity that falls, and then rises again, eventually plateauing (Figure 14.1d). Several biological drivers underpin this pattern. First, seropositivity for measles and rubella in young infants is a consequence of the transplacental transfer of maternal IgG antibodies to the fetus. Maternal antibody titers subsequently decay as the infant ages, and eventually fall below the threshold for immunity, such that children become seronegative (Figure 14.1c, bottom panel). After this age, the proportion of seropositive children rises at a rate determined by the rate at which children either acquire infection or are immunized through vaccination (Figure 14.1d). In the absence of vaccination, settings with higher rates of transmission will show a faster increase in seropositivity over age, as children acquire the infection earlier, a pattern immediately indicating the role that serology can play in interpreting historical dynamics of transmission. The footprint of vaccination on age profiles of seropositivity can be abrupt; that is if all children are vaccinated around 12 months of age with high coverage, then seropositivity will take a sudden jump at this age. In some circumstances, the footprint of past vaccination campaigns can be observed on profiles of age-specific seropositivity. For example, 3 years after a campaign targeting 1 to 5 year olds had occurred in Zambia, one might expect a sharp increase in the proportion seropositive for children aged approximately 4 years old, indicating the footprint of the campaign-; these 4-year- old children would have been just older than the lower age margin of the campaign [13]. Indeed, both vaccination campaigns and historical fluctuations in the magnitude of transmission will tend to disrupt the smooth monotonic increases in seropositivity after loss of maternal immunity both expected and most tractable by the simplest statistical and mathematical approaches to such data.

14.3   Methods for Analysis of IgG Titers

The binary classification for individuals as seronegative or seropositive, used for much analysis of serology, emerges from classifying the antibody concentration or titer in sera relative to a threshold considered protective [11, 12, 14]. Patterns of titers across populations are often bimodal (Figure 14.1c, top panel). In the simplest case, this might indicate directly the existence of individuals who are seronegative and therefore susceptible, and thus have been neither infected nor vaccinated (low titer); and individuals who are seropositive or immune, and thus have either been infected or vaccinated (high titer). Identifying the appropriate threshold that indicates protection associated with this distribution is a classic epidemiological challenge (see Chapter 19), and one complicated by the fact that mechanisms of immune protection are likely to be diverse and redundant, with cellular immunity playing a role as well as antibodies. For example, the absence of antibodies does not necessarily indicate absence of protection, and protection can be of various possible degrees, for example against infection, or against disease, or against clinical disease, etc. [14]. Focusing on protection against infection, if there is overlap in the distribution of titers for immune and non-immune individuals, placing the threshold (arrow in Figure 14.1c) too far to the right will increase the number of false negatives (individuals with a titer below the chosen threshold, and yet in fact immune), while reducing the number of false positives (individuals with a titer above the threshold who are not immune); and *vice versa*. Analyses designed to characterize the appropriate threshold may be rooted in slightly more biologically relevant approaches to measuring antibody titers than Enzyme Immunoassays (depicted in Figure 14.1b), such as Plaque Reduction Neutralization assays, where the antibodies' ability to interfere with viral spread cell to cell *in vivo* is directly measured [15]. Positive and negative controls also provide a powerful source of information with which to strengthen inference as to the mapping between titers and protection, available, for example, through outbreaks in schools where blood drives had recently occurred [15]. For less well-described pathogens, where few controls are available, or in situations where overlap between the two distributions is marked, one option is to apply mixture models to the distribution of titers [16, 17]; individuals then can be characterized as probabilistically belonging to one or the other distribution, and this information can be used in further analyses (e.g., to establish the force of infection [18], see Chapter 19).

Interest in the absolute magnitude of titers is not restricted to defining the protective threshold, but also in characterizing the dynamics of titers as individuals age. A classic question concerns the rate of loss of passively acquired maternal antibodies in infants (Figure 14.1c, lower panel), since this affects both the vulnerability of children at young ages, but also the age at which vaccine can be delivered, since maternal antibodies interfere with vaccination. Cohort studies provide a direct window to characterizing how loss of maternal immunity occurs [19, 20]. Where detailed individual follow-up is not possible, cross-sectional studies also can be leveraged by defining a functional form describing loss of antibodies over age. For example, following [21], $w(a_i)$, the expected log titer level of individual i at age a can be defined by:

$$w(a_i) = p_i \log(me^{-da_i} + b) + (1 - p_i) \log(m + b + c), \qquad (14.4)$$

where p_i is the probability that individual i has not seroconverted yet through infection or vaccination (set to 1 for individuals aged < 6 months, since they are known not to seroconvert), m is the average level of maternal antibodies at birth, d is the rate at which maternal antibodies decay over age, b is the baseline antibody titer, and c is the excess titer in individuals who have seroconverted (by vaccination or infection); the resulting patterns will resemble those depicted in Figure 14.1c. Since titer levels tend to be approximately normally distributed on a log scale, this model can be fit to data using maximum likelihood approaches, and further hypotheses such as the difference in baseline levels, or rates of decay of children from naturally immune and vaccinated mothers [19] or other covariates [22] can be evaluated.

Another stage at which the dynamics of antibodies is of policy relevance is in waning of antibodies at late ages (see Chapter 15); a concern for mumps control given evidence of outbreaks among vaccinated individuals [23], and to a lesser degree a concern for measles and rubella. Longitudinal [24, 25] and cross-sectional [26] serological surveys have been used to characterize these patterns of decay, and in turn to help predict future outbreak risk [27]. There is also opportunity to expand statistical and mathematical approaches to analyzing quantitative levels of IgG (and potentially other antibodies) to deepen our understanding of basic natural history features of infection. For example, understanding the degree to which boosting of immunity through exposure to wild-type virus plays a role in maintaining immunity is an increasingly important question for these types of infections, as vaccine-derived immunity becomes increasingly prevalent. Seasonal cycles of boosting of rubella immunity suggest that this may be important in maintaining population immunity [28], but further investigation across broader population contexts would be necessary to disentangle this. Finally, there may be innovations in using nuances in the magnitude of antibodies (perhaps combining IgM and IgG) to characterize timing of infection [29]; see Chapter 15.

14.4   Methods for Analysis of Seropositivity

We now consider analysis of a binary classification of IgG serological status, rather than underlying titers, distinguishing seropositive individuals (defined as $Y_i = 1$, where i indexes individual observations, corresponding to individuals to the right of the threshold shown on Figure 14.1c) from seronegative individuals ($Y_i = 0$, to the left of the threshold on Figure 14.1c). For subsequent analyses, individuals whose seropositivity might be the result of passively transferred maternal antibodies are dropped (e.g., individuals aged less than 6 or 9 months, depending on the pathogen and data permitting), because disentangling maternal immunity from other sources of immunity is inferentially challenging. With this assumption in place, interpreting seropositivity requires considering the dynamical context of infection or vaccination, because we do not know exactly when individuals were infected (or vaccinated), only that if they are seropositive, they were infected (or vaccinated) at some age younger than their current age.

14.4.1   Fitting to data

We denote $\pi(a)$ as the probability of being infected before age a. We assume that $\pi(a)$ equates to being seropositive by age a. Since infection is immunizing, for an individual to be infected at a particular age requires that they first avoid infection up to that age, and then become infected at that age (initially assuming that vaccination is not occurring). The data now takes a binary form, so in subsequent analyses, model fitting is based around generalized linear models using binomial likelihoods. The log likelihood for the most basic framing for N observations is defined by

$$\ell = \sum_{t=1}^{N} Y_i \log[\pi(a_i)] + (1 - Y_i) \log[1 - \pi(a_i)], \tag{14.5}$$

and defining $\eta(a)$ as the linear predictor (linear function of coefficients used to predict the dependent variable) and g as a link function (function defining the relationship between the linear predictor and the mean of the distribution function), we have [18]:

$$g(P(Y = 1|a)) = g(\pi(a)) = \eta(a). \tag{14.6}$$

Here, we focus mostly on inference based around the logit link, the popularly used link function for binary responses, defined as $\log[\pi/(1 - \pi)]$.

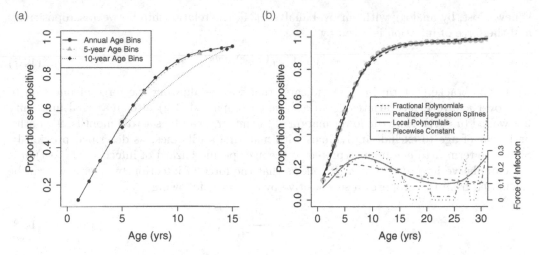

FIGURE 14.2

Analysis of seropositivity illustrated with simulated data: (a) Estimates of age-specific seropositivity at the mid-age of each age bin (yearly, 5-year, and 10-year age bins) as points (black dots, grey triangles, and black diamonds) and fitted lines using a smooth spline (solid black, dashed grey, dotted black), illustrating increasing bias as the width of age classes increases. (b) Estimates of age-specific seropositivity and force of infection. Grey points represent the data. Fractional polynomials, local polynomial estimators, penalized regression splines, and piecewise constants were used to fit age-specific seroprevalence curves to the data. Age-specific force of infection was inferred based on equation 14.8. Note that the default option was used whenever choices needed to be made for other parameters such as the degrees of freedom or the spline basis functions and number of knots. While all our methods produce qualitatively similar results, there are also clear differences with, for example, large increases at late ages emerging for the local polynomials as a result of fluctuations in the underlying spline. See Supplementary Code for details on fitting seroprevalence curves and estimation of force of infection.

While the framing so far assumes a continuous measure of age ("*a*" in the previous equations), in reality, proportion seropositive is often reported by age group. Chosen age bins may vary considerably (e.g., [30–32]) and groups can encompass up to 10 years of age, often reflecting constraints imposed by data collection circumstances. This variance is an important consideration in evaluating the use of serological surveys in public health settings, as age binning may bias estimates of age-specific seropositivity. Binning ages where age-specific seroprevalence curve tends to follow a concave function will underestimate seroprevalence [33], such that for measles and rubella bias will be exaggerated when binning children of ages 5–15 (Figure 14.2a) who experience high levels of contact and seroconversion. Further, in populations where the history of natural infection or vaccination has resulted in profiles where proportion seropositive does not always increase with age, age binning could distort the complexities in these profiles.

14.4.2   Estimating the force of infection

To move from modeling the probability of being infected over age to considering the dynamical underpinnings of this pattern, we focus on settings with no vaccination. The force of infection, λ, is defined as the rate at which susceptible individuals become infected. Because $\pi(a)$ indicates the probability of being infected before age a, and immune status is never lost, by analogy with survival analysis [34], the relationship between seropositivity and the force of infection is given by

$$\pi(a) = 1 - e^{\left(-\int_A^a \lambda(u)du\right)}, \tag{14.7}$$

where the bracketed term in $\lambda(u)$ indicates that we are allowing the force of infection to vary over age (other covariates could also be encompassed [18]) after maternal immunity has waned ($a \leq A$). Here the lower margin of the integral can be set to 6 months, 9 months, or 1 year of age to exclude individuals with maternal antibodies, as described previously. Since the term $\lambda(u)$ can be interpreted as the age specific hazard of infection, $\int_A^a \lambda(u)du$ is the cumulative hazard by age a. It follows that the force of infection by age, $\lambda(a)$, can be calculated from the proportion seropositive by age, $\pi(a)$ following

$$\lambda(a) = \frac{\pi'(a)}{(1 - \pi(a))}, \tag{14.8}$$

where the acute marker indicates the first derivative. For cases where $\pi(a)$ is fitted using a logit function, we can express the estimated force of infection as

$$\lambda(a) = \eta'(a)\frac{e^{\eta(a)}}{1 + e^{\eta(a)}}, \tag{14.9}$$

see [18] for other link functions. Importantly, this does not necessarily constrain estimates of $\lambda(a)$ to be positive [18], and this must be considered carefully in the analysis. Various additional approaches to constrain estimates of the force of infection to be positive exist, and are further detailed in [18], illustrated in the Supplement.

Given this basic framework, the core question is how to frame the linear predictor, $\eta(a)$. A variety of options are possible. The simplest possible framing is to assume that the force of infection is constant over age. In this setting, a simple catalytic model [35], modeled with a log link, indicates that in the absence of vaccination the proportion of seropositive individuals by age a corresponds directly to the cumulative proportion of infected individuals, and is defined by

$$\pi(a) = 1 - e^{(-\lambda a)}. \tag{14.10}$$

The force of infection is easily estimated (excluding individuals less than age 1), by identifying the value of λ that maximizes the binomial likelihood of seropositive individuals by age a given the probability $\pi(a)$ in Equation 14.1. However, age-related changes in the force of infection are well established for communicable infections, generally attributed to changes in the pattern of contact over age [8, 36–38]. A first approach to formally accounting for this is to assume piecewise constant variation in the force of infection over age [18]. The proportion seropositive is then defined by

$$\pi(a) = 1 - e^{\left(-\sum_{i=1}^n \lambda_i \Delta_i(a)\right)}. \tag{14.11}$$

where $\Delta_i(a)$ is the number of years spent in age category i for individuals of age a, and λ_i is the force of infection for each age category i. As previously given, estimates of λ_i for each age category i can be obtained by maximizing the binomial likelihood of the probability of being seropositive. Where fine-scale age data is available, this method has the benefit of allowing monotonicity in seropositivity over age to be enforced by choosing age groups for which this is the case. However, this *ad hoc* approach to enforcing monotonicity highlights the need for more objective approaches to characterizing age variation in the force of infection.

A range of approaches can be used to address the issue of fitting continuous curved shapes to the force of infection over age. Parametric, non-parametric, and semi-parametric approaches have been developed since the introduction of the catalytic model, providing different degrees of flexibility [39]. A comprehensive overview can be found in [18], including in depth discussions of the strength and limitations of each method. In Figure 14.2b we demonstrate an example of a subset of approaches highlighted by [18] see Supplement for Code.

14.4.3 Inference into age profile of infection

For pathogens like rubella and parvovirus B19, whose burden manifests in an age-specific manner, one key question is establishing the age-specific profile of infection [32, 40], or probability of being infected at any age, $i(a)$. To be infected at any age requires that individuals avoid infection up to that age, and then become infected. This requires knowing the force of infection over age, and harnessing the estimates it provides of both the probabilities of escaping infection, and becoming infected, which can be expressed as

$$i(a) = [1 - \pi(a)][1 - e^{-\lambda(a)}], \tag{14.12}$$

with indexing suitably modified if discrete age classes are being used. The probability of being infected at any age differs from the force of infection by directly identifying the most at risk age groups, and as such is an important measure for pathogens with age heterogenous disease severity. These estimates assume time homogenous age-specific force of infection such that the risk of infection at each age is identical across birth cohorts, an issue further discussed in this chapter.

14.5 Case Study—Use of Serological Data for Rubella

In the last decades, vaccination programs for measles and rubella have expanded globally. The Pan-American Health Organization has successfully eliminated both pathogens, measles elimination goals are in place in all other World Health Organization (WHO) member states, and three WHO regions have set rubella control or elimination goals [41]. Since the measles and rubella vaccines are easily combined into the Measles-Rubella (MR) vaccine, policies for rubella are generally framed and assessed within the context of existing measles vaccination programs. While the benefit of increasing measles vaccination coverage is straightforward, given the potentially high case fatality rate of this infection [42], the situation for rubella is more complex [43]. Rubella is a mild infection in children, and the main burden is associated with infection of women during pregnancy. The outcome may be birth of a child with congenital rubella syndrome (CRS), associated with blindness, deafness, and an array of other issues [44]. The resulting age specificity of the burden associated with rubella raises an important challenge for vaccination policy: childhood vaccination short of the threshold of elimination has the potential to increase the average age of infection. As a result, although total incidence may decline, the number of cases occurring in the one group of individuals we are most concerned about, i.e., women of childbearing age, may increase [45]. Serology has played an important role in development of policy for rubella, from establishing the burden of CRS to considering the impact of vaccination coverage [32]. As we move towards rubella elimination, serology has the potential to further contribute to informing public health [46]: elimination implies avoiding outbreaks, and successfully closing important immunity gaps by vaccination. Importantly, because of the feedback loops inherent in the life cycle of infections like rubella (Figure 14.1a) in the face of heterogenous vaccination, immunity gaps over age will fluctuate in non-linear ways over the time course from endemicity to elimination. Serology provides the most direct approach to estimate the current state of immunity in the population and, given the assumption of time homogeneity, to estimate key epidemiological parameters (moving away from assumptions of time-homogeneity is discussed next). In this case study, we illustrate use of serology to estimate the age-profile of immunity and by inferring transmission parameters to estimate the burden of CRS, as well to evaluate whether the vaccine should be introduced.

14.5.1 Using serology to estimate the burden of CRS

Characterizing the burden of CRS requires knowing the distribution of age of infection within the population, the age profile of fertility, and the risk that an infected woman will give birth to a child with CRS. We illustrate this using three examples of pre-vaccination rubella seropositivity surveys from the literature, featuring Côte d'Ivoire in 1987 [47], Tehran, Iran, in 1996 [48] and Bangladesh in 2008 [49]; Figure 14.3. Setting aside for the moment the issue of adequacy of laboratory techniques and consistency of testing across settings, these three examples illustrate the diversity of possible patterns of seropositivity for rubella pre-vaccination, as well as the footprint of sampling procedures (only Iran has samples of young enough individuals to reveal the impact of maternal immunity). We can fit local polynomials to these seropositivity curves (see Supplement), excluding samples from children aged less than 6 months or 1 year of age (depending on data availability), to avoid issues linked to maternal immunity, see previous discussion. Côte d'Ivoire shows

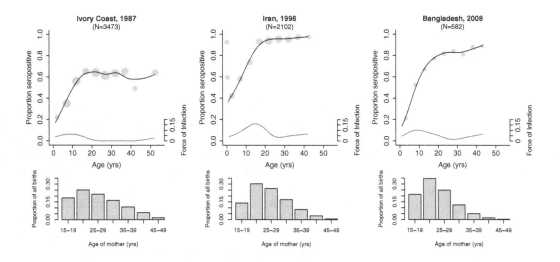

FIGURE 14.3

Age-specific serology and policy decisions for rubella: Top panel shows three example serological surveys from the literature (Côte d'Ivoire in 1987 [47], Tehran, Iran, in 1996 [48] and Bangladesh in 2008 [49]), grey points represent the age-specific seroprevalence data and the size of each point indicates the number of individuals within each age bin, black lines show fitted seropositivity curve using non-parametric local polynomial estimators, and dashed black lines show the inferred force of infection over age. The bottom panel shows the distribution of births across reproductive ages for each respective country and year based on [51]. See Supplementary Code for details on fitting and estimation of public health key indicators such as CRS incidence and R_0, also described in the text.

an increase in seropositivity to a plateau, followed by a decline in seropositivity at late ages, Tehran goes rapidly up to near 100 percent seropositivity, and Bangladesh increases initially fast and then more slowly after age 20 years. The late age decline in Côte d'Ivoire could indicate either waning of immunity (although evidence in the literature to support this scale of decline is slight for rubella), or, alternatively low transmission about 30 to 40 years prior to the sample being taken, and a cohort that subsequently aged through avoiding exposure to infection, a pattern that requires non-equilibrium dynamics, and strong structuring of patterns of contact over age. Without rubella incidence data, it is hard to robustly infer which explanation is appropriate. The plateau in Côte d'Ivoire could indicate a subpopulation that for some reason avoided mixing and thus exposure to rubella infection (which could be formally fitted, as an extra parameter [18]).

Assuming that this pattern of seropositivity nevertheless supplies reasonable inference into the broad pattern of the force of infection over age (obtained by taking the derivative as described previously, and shown as black dashed lines in Figure 14.3, top panel), we can estimate the burden of CRS from these age profiles of seropositivity. This method requires estimating the probability that individuals remain susceptible up until the age at which they become pregnant, then become infected during the first trimester of pregnancy, and that this results in birth of a child with CRS. Previous work suggests that 65 percent of babies born to mothers infected during the first 16 weeks of pregnancy have CRS [50]. Using the expression of seropositivity and the force of infection defined previously, we can first estimate CRS incidence per 100,000 live births per each reproductive age, a (15–49 years old), as

$$\hat{I}_{CRS}(a) = (1 - \hat{\pi}(a)) \times (1 - e^{-16\hat{\lambda}(a)/52}) \times 0.65 \times 100,000. \tag{14.13}$$

Extending this across ages requires accounting for age-specific fertility rates. The population CRS incidence per 100,000 live births at time t, $\hat{I}_{CRS}(t)$, is the weighted mean of CRS incidence per 100,000 live births for each reproductive age a, $\hat{I}_{CRS}(a)$, by births to women of reproductive age a at time t, $B_{a,t}$ (Figure 14.3, bottom panel), defined as

$$\hat{I}_{CRS}(t) = \frac{\sum_{a=15}^{49} \hat{I}_{CRS}(a) B_{a,t}}{\sum_{a=15}^{49} B_{a,t}}, \tag{14.14}$$

The highest resolution of age classes for numbers of live births in any given year is generally 5-year reproductive age classes between 15 and 49 years of age (i.e., 15–19, 20–24, 25–29, 30–34, 35–39, 40–44, and 45–49) [51]). Therefore, $B_{a,t}$ is equal to the number of births in each 5 year reproductive age class associated with reproductive age a and time t divided by 5 [51]. As defined here, $\hat{I}_{CRS}(t)$ yields estimates of 24, 88, and 148 CRS incidence per 100,000 live births, for Côte d'Ivoire in 1987, Iran in 1996, and Bangladesh in 2008, respectively. These estimates are within the broader range across pre-vaccination countries found in other studies [32]. The degree to which these magnitudes reflect an important health burden will be dependent on other health burdens within these countries at the time; but whatever the magnitude, an important consideration is that CRS is entirely preventable giving sufficient deployment of the relatively inexpensive vaccine.

14.5.2 Using serology to determine whether vaccine should be introduced

Mathematical models have been used to show that the magnitude of transmission of rubella in endemic settings is a key variable in the outcome of vaccine introduction [52], that is settings with lower rates of rubella transmission are more likely to successfully reduce the burden of CRS with the introduction of rubella vaccination [52]. The magnitude of transmission is generally framed in terms of R_0, the number of new infections per infectious individual in a completely susceptible population. Theory reveals that R_0 is related to the average age of infection, A, by the relationship $R_0 = G/A$ where G is the inverse of the crude birth rate [53]. Through this effect, R_0 thus defines the burden of CRS in the absence of vaccination through its effect on average age of infection, such that a higher average age of infection is associated with a lower R_0 and a larger burden of CRS [52]. The average age of infection also modulates the minimum vaccination coverage required to reduce the burden of CRS relative to vaccination free settings, with settings with higher levels of R_0 requiring greater coverage because it is harder to sufficiently reduce incidence to reduce the CRS burden [54].

Based on this theory, we can estimate R_0 in Côte d'Ivoire, Iran, and Bangladesh using serology data. The average age of infection is estimated from age-specific proportion seropositive in the absence of vaccination, given by $A = \int_0^u (1 - \pi(a)) da$ ignoring maternal immunity [55]. We estimated the average age of infection in Côte d'Ivoire, Iran, and Bangladesh was 13, 9, and 11 years old, respectively (setting the upper age limit to $u = 30$ years as irregularities in the proportion seropositive beyond this age suggest non-linear past dynamics that will disrupt estimation of the current average age) (Figure 14.3). Using data on country specific crude birth rates made available by the World Bank for the appropriate years to obtain G, we can then estimate the associated R_0 as 2, 5, and 4 for Côte d'Ivoire, Iran, and Bangladesh, respectively. These R_0 estimates are within the range estimated for rubella [52, 56], suggesting all countries would benefit from RCV introduction given a higher average age of infection, and the minimum required vaccination coverage for introduction of rubella-containing-vaccine of 80 percent is sufficient to reduce the burden of CRS [52]. Since rubella vaccination is generally introduced by adding it into existing measles programs, the required level of coverage could have been mapped to contemporary estimates of current measles vaccination coverage to evaluate the benefits of introducing the vaccine.

More nuanced approaches to estimating R_0 from age-serology are also available [57], but these often require some knowledge of the age structure of transmission, and frequently require assuming time-homogeneity. We do not further illustrated these methods here.

14.5.3   Using serology to determine core areas for vaccine introduction

Even in the absence of vaccination, in settings where incidence is sufficiently low, dynamics may be dominated by demographic stochasticity, and rubella may go locally extinct. As extinction can allow buildup of susceptible individuals, identifying such areas may be useful for targeting earlier vaccine introduction: locations where extinction has persisted the longest will provide time for individuals to age while remaining susceptible, thus potentially contributing to an increased burden of CRS once the pathogen is reintroduced. A combination of age-specific incidence, metrics of remoteness, and models of the expected transmission dynamics have been used to identify areas of low immunity resulting from extinction [58, 59]. However, uncertainties in data streams (discussed previously), especially problematic in the case of rubella by asymptomatic infection [44], make identifying areas where extinction has occurred challenging [60]. Spatial seroprevalence data is thus a potentially powerful extension for identifying at risk populations [27], particularly if regularly administered (i.e., sero surveillance). Since nationally representative serological surveys are likely to be beyond the scope of most public health programs, either nesting such efforts with other household survey efforts (e.g., Demographic Health Surveys) or informing deployment of serological surveys using predictions from dynamic models (e.g., using vaccination data to highlight at risk areas [61]) are potentially powerful ways of adding spatial targeting to the age-based targeting that age-serological surveys most naturally lend themselves to. However, given the costs inherent in deploying serological surveys, the potential gain in inference should be considered with care before such surveys are deployed.

14.6 Challenges and Next Directions

A core assumption of the methods presented above for estimation of the force of infection and its variability over age is that of time-homogeneity or steady state dynamics. In reality, this is rarely likely to be the case. For example, seasonality in transmission, driven by features ranging from aggregation of children during school term times [1] to climatic drivers [62], is a feature of many human infections. While regular epidemics driven by seasonality can be encompassed in analysis of age-serology (particularly given age contact assumptions) [63], more complex outcomes such as multi-annual [1] or chaotic dynamics [64, 65] are likely to pose a greater challenge resulting in inferential biases [66]. Further, aspects from demography [6] to vaccination coverage [67] are rapidly changing over time. By altering patterns of susceptible replenishment [68], this will modulate the history of infection and thus the force of infection across populations.

Assuming equilibria allows the assumption that $\lambda(a)$ of years in the past is equal to $\lambda(a)$ at the time of the cross-sectional survey. Stepping away from this assumption implies that the probability of being seropositive at age a depends on potentially varying forces of infection for every age and time-step preceding the current one. In other words, where the force of infection is both age specific and changing through time, seropositivity at every age will reflect its own unique history (Figure 14.4). One way to reduce the dimensionality of this challenge is to assume that the rate at which susceptibles become infected depends only on overall prevalence of infection [6], and is independent of the age incidence profile. This is equivalent to assuming that the shape of the force of infection over age remains the same, but its magnitude increases or decreases in response to overall prevalence of infection. As a result, fluctuations in $\lambda(a)$ through time can be inferred if data on prevalence is available. Another approach is to assume that the pattern of contact over age (i.e., Who-Acquires-Infection-From-Whom matrix, WAIFW) is known, for example from diary studies during the course of which individuals are asked to record numbers and aspects of who they interact with [38]. Various metrics of contacts recorded within diary studies such conversation, touch, etc., have been compared to identify those with greatest power to predict seropositivity [69], indicating that more intimate contacts have greatest predictive power across a range of settings. Another approach took diary contacts as a foundation and layered proportional scaling of transmission onto this to predict seropositivity [70].

A key element of the inferential challenge in disentangling seropositivity profiles in the vaccine era is that there is currently no straightforward way to distinguish between seropositivity that arises from natural infection or from vaccine-induced immunity. Yet, knowledge of the magnitude of vaccination coverage is of considerable public health relevance, and often poorly defined by the "supply side" statistics that emerge from dose delivery. In particular, repeated vaccination of the same individuals can result in large discrepancies between so-called "administrative coverage" (the ratio between number of doses deployed and the target population size) and the actual proportion of individuals immunized by vaccination [71]. Statistical approaches can be developed to infer vaccination coverage from age profiles of serology [6, 72], potentially leveraging simultaneous delivery of multiple antigens such as measles, mumps, and rubella by the MMR vaccine [70, 73]. These

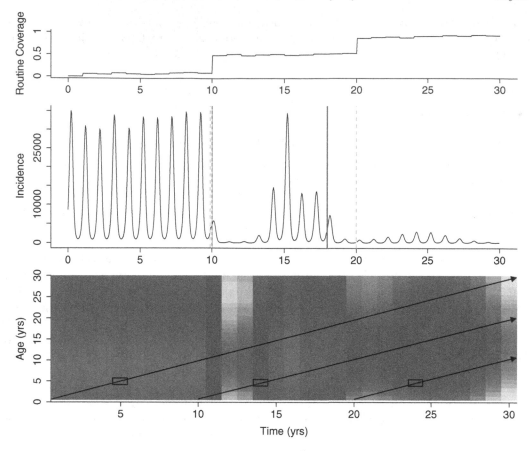

FIGURE 14.4

Seroprofile variation through time and age. Many vaccine preventable diseases in contemporary populations will have experienced fluctuations in incidence (middle panel) as
a result of introduction of routine vaccination (simulated here as occurring at the first
vertical grey dashed line on the middle panel, level of coverage achieves in the routine
program is illustrated in the top panel), occurrence of vaccination campaigns (black vertical
lines, middle panel, in both cases targeting individuals aged 9 months to 5 years) and
strengthening of routine vaccination (second vertical grey dashed line, see also top panel).
The result will be fluctuations in the force of infection over age (lower panel, shading
indicates the magnitude of force of infection, defined as I × WAIFW used in the simulation),
as opposed to the usual assumption of constant pattern over age (see text). As a result, in
this example, for a serological profile obtained in the 30th year of the simulation, for example,
individuals aged 30 years old will have experienced a much higher force of infection as 5
year olds (shown by the first box, lower panel) than individuals aged 20 years old when they
were 5 (second small box, lower panel), yet these may, in fact, have experienced a similar
magnitude when 5 years old as current 10 year olds (final small box, lower panel).

approaches generally require additional data, which might encompass information ranging
from demographic rates (births and potentially mortality) to the timing and magnitude of
vaccination efforts, to incidence data. With this in hand, dynamic models can be calibrated
to age serology [72], (see also Chapter 17). Repeated (e.g., annual) serology would strengthen
the inferential power of such approaches (see also Chapter 16).

14.7 Conclusions

The interpretation of serological surveys can be framed in the context of a rich body of theory on the dynamics of immunizing infections, opening the way to inference into a diversity of variables of public health relevance. Yet, the complex and changing reality of both human demography and vaccination policies also require extending analysis to integrate a diversity of data sources, from diary studies on human contacts to estimates of vaccination coverage. Increasingly statistical and inferential tools are being developed to meet this challenge. Further developments in the laboratory techniques associated with serological assays, provided potentially more nuanced windows into aspects such as time since infection, etc, are likely to further increase the potential insights generated from this important public health tool.

Acknowledgments

We thank Daniel Navarrete who digitized published rubella serological data used in the case study.

References

[1] O.N. Bjornstad, B. Finkenstadt, and B.T. Grenfell. Endemic and epidemic dynamics of measles: Estimating epidemiological scaling with a time series SIR model. *Ecological Monographs*, 72:169–184, 2002.

[2] C.J.E. Metcalf, O.N. Bjornstad, B.T. Grenfell, and V. Andreasen. Seasonality and comparative dynamics of six childhood infections in pre-vaccination Copenhagen. *Proceedings of the Royal Society of London, Series B*, 276:4111–4118, 2009.

[3] S. Takahashi, Q. Liao, T.P. Van Boeckel, W. Xing, J. Sun, V.Y. Hsiao, C.J.E. Metcalf, Z. Chang, F. Liu, and J. Zhang. Hand, foot, and mouth disease in China: Modeling epidemic dynamics of enterovirus serotypes and implications for vaccination. *PLoS Medicine*, 13(2):e1001958, 2016.

[4] A. Mahmud, C. Metcalf, and B. Grenfell. Comparative dynamics, seasonality in transmission, and predictability of childhood infections in Mexico. *Epidemiology and Infection*, 145(3):607–625, 2017.

[5] S. Tanihara, E. Okamoto, T. Imatoh, Y. Momose, A. Kaetsu, M. Miyazaki, and H. Une. Evaluating measles surveillance: Comparison of sentinel surveillance, mandatory notification, and data from health insurance claims. *Epidemiology and Infection*, 139(04):516–523, 2011.

[6] S. Li, C. Ma, L. Hao, Q. Su, Z. An, F. Ma, S. Xie et al. Demographic transition and the dynamics of measles in six provinces in China: A modeling study. *PLoS Medicine*, 14(4):e1002255, 2017.

[7] V. Mitchell, V.J. Dietz, J.M. Okwo-Bele, and F.T. Cutts. *Immunization in Developing Countries.*, chapter 70, pages 1369–1394. Elsevier Saunders, Philadelphia, PA, 6th edition, 2013.

[8] B.T. Grenfell and R.M. Anderson. The estimation of age-related rates of infection from case notifications and serological data. *Journal of Hygiene of Cambridge*, 95:419–436, 1985.

[9] C.J.E. Metcalf, P. Klepac, M. Ferrari, R.F. Grais, A. Djibo, and B.T. Grenfell. Modeling the first dose of measles vaccination: The role of maternal immunity, demographic factors, and delivery systems. *Epidemiology and Infection*, 139:265–274, 2010.

[10] N. Hens, M. Aerts, Z. Shkedy, P.K. Kimani, M. Kojouhorova, P. Van Damme, and P. Beutels. Estimating the impact of vaccination using age-time-dependent incidence rates of hepatitis b. *Epidemiology and Infection*, 136(3):341–351, 2008.

[11] J.M. Best and S. Reef. *Immunological Basis for Immunization: Module 11: Rubella.* World Health Organization, Geneva, 2008.

[12] W.J. Moss and S. Scott. *The Immunological Basis for Immunization Series : Module 7: Measles—Update 2009.* World Health Organisation, 2009.

[13] J. Lessler, W.J. Moss, S.A. Lowther, and D.A. Cummings. Maintaining high rates of measles immunization in Africa. *Epidemiology and Infection*, 139(7):1039–1049, 2011.

[14] S. A. Plotkin. Correlates of protection induced by vaccination. *Clinical and Vaccine Immunology*, 17(7):1055–1065, 2010.

[15] R.T. Chen, L.E. Markowitz, P. Albrecht, J.A. Stewart, L.M. Mofenson, S.R. Preblud, and W.A. Orenstein. Measles antibody: Reevaluation of protective titers. *Journal of Infectious Diseases*, 162(5):1036–1042, 1990.

[16] A.J. Vyse, N.J. Gay, L.M. Hesketh, R. Pebody, P. Morgan-Capner, and E. Miller. Interpreting serological surveys using mixture models: The seroepidemiology of measles, mumps and rubella in England and Wales at the beginning of the 21st century. *Epidemiology and Infection*, 134(6):1303–1312, 2006.

[17] A.J. Peel, T.J. McKinley, K.S. Baker, J.A. Barr, G. Crameri, D.T. Hayman, Y.-R. Feng, C.C. Broder, L.-F. Wang, and A.A. Cunningham. Use of cross-reactive serological assays for detecting novel pathogens in wildlife: Assessing an appropriate cutoff for henipavirus assays in African bats. *Journal of Virological Methods*, 193(2):295–303, 2013.

[18] N. Hens, Z. Shkedy, M. Aerts, C. Faes, P. Van Damme, and P. Beutels. *Modeling Infectious Disease Parameters Based on Serological and Social Contact Data: A Modern Statistical Perspective.* Statistics for biology and health. Springer, New York, 2012.

[19] E. Leuridan, N. Hens, V. Hutse, M. Ieven, M. Aerts, and P. Van Damme. Early waning of maternal measles antibodies in era of measles elimination: Longitudinal study. *BMJ*, 340:c1626, 2010.

[20] E. Leuridan, N. Hens, V. Hutse, M. Aerts, and P. Van Damme. Kinetics of maternal antibodies against rubella and varicella in infants. *Vaccine*, 29(11):2222–2226, 2011.

[21] S. Waaijenborg, S.J. Hahn, L. Mollema, G.P. Smits, G.A. Berbers, F.R. van der Klis, H.E. de Melker, and J. Wallinga. Waning of maternal antibodies against measles, mumps, rubella, and varicella in communities with contrasting vaccination coverage. *Journal of Infectious Diseases*, 208(1):10–16, 2013.

[22] V.M. Cceres, P.M. Strebel, and R.W. Sutter. Factors determining prevalence of maternal antibody to measles virus throughout infancy: A review. *Clinical Infectious Diseases*, 31(1):110–119, 2000.

[23] J. Eriksen, I. Davidkin, G. Kafatos, N. Andrews, C. Barbara, D. Cohen, A. Duks et al. Seroepidemiology of mumps in Europe (1996–2008): Why do outbreaks occur in highly vaccinated populations? *Epidemiology and Infection*, 141(3):651–666, 2013.

[24] J.R. Kremer, F. Schneider, and C.P. Muller. Waning antibodies in measles and rubella vaccinees—a longitudinal study. *Vaccine*, 24(14):2594–2601, 2006.

[25] I. Davidkin, S. Jokinen, M. Broman, P. Leinikki, and H. Peltola. Persistence of measles, mumps, and rubella antibodies in an mmr-vaccinated cohort: A 20-year follow-up. *Journal of Infectious Diseases*, 197(7):950–956, 2008.

[26] C. Poethko-Muller and A. Mankertz. Seroprevalence of measles-, mumps- and rubella-specific igg antibodies in German children and adolescents and predictors for seronegativity. *PLoS One*, 7(8), 2012.

[27] S. Abrams, P. Beutels, and N. Hens. Assessing mumps outbreak risk in highly vaccinated populations using spatial seroprevalence data. *American Journal of Epidemiology*, 179(8):1006–1017, 2014.

[28] L.S. Rosenblatt, M. Shifrine, N.W. Hetherington, T. Paglierioni, and M.R. MacKenzie. A circannual rhythm in rubella antibody titers. *Biological Rhythm Research*, 13(1): 81–88, 1982.

[29] K.M. Pepin, S.L. Kay, B.D. Golas, S.S. Shriner, A.T. Gilbert, R.S. Miller, A.L. Graham, S. Riley, P.C. Cross, and M.D. Samuel. Inferring infection hazard in wildlife populations by linking data across individual and population scales. *Ecology Letters*, 20(3):275–292, 2017.

[30] J.L. Goodson, B.G. Maresha, A. Dosseh, C. Byabamazima, D. Nshimirimana, S.L. Cochi, and S. Reef. Rubella epidemiology in Africa in the prevaccine era, 2002–2009. *Journal of Infectious Diseases*, 204:S215–S225, 2011.

[31] K.M. Thompson and C.L. Odahowski. Systematic review of measles and rubella serology studies. *Risk Analysis*, 36:1459–1486, 2015.

[32] E. Vynnycky, E.J. Adams, F.T. Cutts, S.E. Reef, A.M. Navar, E. Simons, L.-M. Yoshida, D.W. Brown, C. Jackson, and P.M. Strebel. Using seroprevalence and immunisation coverage data to estimate the global burden of congenital rubella syndrome, 1996–2010: A systematic review. *PLoS One*, 11(3):e0149160, 2016.

[33] J.L.W.V. Jensen. Sur les fonctions convexes et les inégalités entre les valeurs moyennes. *Acta Mathematica*, 30(1):175–193, 1906.

[34] D.A. Griffiths. A catalytic model of infection from measles. *Applied Statistics*, 23: 330–339, 1974.

[35] H. Muench. *Catalytic Models in Epidemiology.* Harvard University Press Cambridge, MA, 1959.

[36] R.M. Anderson and R.M. May. Vaccination against rubella and measles: Qualitative investigations of different policies. *Journal of Hygiene of Cambridge,* 90:259–325, 1983.

[37] R.M. Anderson and R.M. May. Age related changes in the rate of disease transmission: Implications for the design of vaccination programmes. *Journal of Hygiene of Cambridge,* 94:365–436, 1985.

[38] J. Mossong, N. Hens, M. Jit, P. Beutels, K. Aranen, R. Mikolajczyk, M. Massari et al. Social contacts and mixing patterns relevant to the spread of infectious diseases. *PLoS Medicine,* 5:e74, 2008.

[39] N. Hens, M. Aerts, C. Faes, Z. Shkedy, O. Lejeune, P. van Damme, and P. Beutels. Seventy-five years of estimating the force of infection from current status data. *Epidemiology and Infection,* 138(6):802–812, 2010.

[40] J. Mossong, N. Hens, V. Friederichs, I. Davidkin, M. Broman, B. Litwinska, J. Siennicka et al. Parvovirus b19 infection in five European countries: Seroepidemiology, force of infection and maternal risk of infection. *Epidemiology and Infection,* 136(8):1059–1068, 2008.

[41] World Health Organization. *Global Measles and Rubella Strategic Plan, 2012–2020.* Naturaprint, Metz-Tessy, 2012.

[42] L.J. Wolfson, R.F. Grais, F.J. Luquero, M.E. Birmingham, and P.M. Strebel. Estimates of measles case fatality ratios: A comprehensive review of community-based studies. *International Journal of Epidemiology,* 38:195–205, 2009.

[43] F. Cutts, C. Metcalf, J. Lessler, and B. Grenfell. Rubella vaccination: Must not be business as usual. *The Lancet,* 380(9838):217–218, 2012.

[44] L.Z. Cooper. The history and medical consequences of rubella. *Reviews of Infectious Diseases,* 7:S2–S10, 1985.

[45] E.G. Knox. Strategy for rubella vaccination. *International Journal of Epidemiology,* 9:13–23, 1980.

[46] F.T. Cutts and M. Hanson. Seroepidemiology: An underused tool for designing and monitoring vaccination programmes in lowand middleincome countries. *Tropical Medicine and International Health,* 21(9):1086–1098, 2016.

[47] S. Ouattara, J. Brettes, R. Kodjo, K. Penali, G. Gershy-Damet, A. Sangare, Y. Aron, and V. Akran. Seroepidemiology of rubella in the Ivory Coast. Geographic distribution. *Bulletin de la Societe de pathologie exotique et de ses filiales,* 80(4):655–664, 1986.

[48] S. Modarres, S. Modarres, and N.N. Oskoii. Immunity of children and adult females to rubella virus infection in tehran. *Iranian Journal of Medical Sciences,* 21:69–73, 1996.

[49] A. Nessa, M. Islam, S. Tabassum, S. Munshi, M. Ahmed, and R. Karim. Seroprevalence of rubella among urban and rural bangladeshi women emphasises the need for rubella vaccination of pre-pubertal girls. *Indian Journal of Medical Microbiology,* 26(1):94, 2008.

[50] F.T. Cutts and E. Vynnycky. Modelling the incidence of congenital rubella syndrome in developing countries. *International Journal of Epidemiology,* 28:1176–1184, 1999.

[51] United Nations. World population prospects: The 2015 revision, dvd edition, United Nations, New York, 2015.

[52] J. Lessler and C.J.E. Metcalf. Balancing evidence and uncertainty when considering rubella vaccine introduction. *PLoS One*, 8:e67639, 2013.

[53] A.R. McLean and R.M. Anderson. Measles in developing countries. Part I: Epidemiological parameters and patterns. *Epidemiology and Infection*, 100:111–133, 1988.

[54] C.J.E. Metcalf, J. Lessler, P. Klepac, F.T. Cutts, and B.T. Grenfell. Impact of birth rate, seasonality and transmission rate on minimum levels of coverage needed for rubella vaccination. *Epidemiology and Infection*, 16:1–12, 2012.

[55] C.P. Farrington. Modelling forces of infection for measles, mumps and rubella. *Statistics in Medcine*, 9:953–967, 1990.

[56] R.M. Anderson and R.M. May. *Infectious Diseases of Humans*. Oxford University Press, Oxford, UK, 1991.

[57] C.P. Farrington, M.N. Kanaan, and N.J. Gay. Estimation of the basic reproduction number for infectious diseases from age-stratified serological survey data. *Applied Statistics*, 50:251–292, 2001.

[58] C.J.E. Metcalf, C.V. Munayco, G. Chowell, B.T. Grenfell, and O.N. Bjornstad. Rubella meta-population dynamics and importance of spatial coupling to the risk of congenital rubella syndrome in peru. *Journal of the Royal Society Interface*, 8:369–376, 2011.

[59] A. Wesolowski, K. Mensah, C.A. Brook, M. Andrianjafimasy, A. Winter, C.O. Buckee, R. Razafindratsimandresy, A.J. Tatem, J.-M. Heraud, and C.J.E. Metcalf. Introduction of rubella-containing-vaccine to madagascar: Implications for roll-out across low-income countries. *Journal of the Royal Society Interface*, 13:117, 2016.

[60] C.E. Gunning and H.J. Wearing. Probabilistic measures of persistence and extinction in measles (meta) populations. *Ecology Letters*, 16(8):985–994, 2013.

[61] S. Takahashi, C.J.E. Metcalf, M.J. Ferrari, A.J. Tatem, and J. Lessler. The geography of measles vaccination in the African Great Lakes region. *Nature Communications*, 8:15585, 2017.

[62] V.E. Pitzer, C. Viboud, W.J. Alonso, T. Wilcox, C.J. Metcalf, C.A. Steiner, A.K. Haynes, and B.T. Grenfell. Environmental drivers of the spatiotemporal dynamics of respiratory syncytial virus in the United States. *PLoS Pathogens*, 11(1):e1004591, 2015.

[63] H.J. Whitaker and C.P. Farrington. Estimation of infectious disease parameters from serological survey data: The impact of regular epidemics. *Statistics in Medcine*, 23:2429–2443, 2004.

[64] M.J. Ferrari, R.F. Grais, N. Bharti, A.J.K. Conlan, O.N. Bjornstad, L.J. Wolfson, P.J. Guerin, A. Djibo, and B.T. Grenfell. The dynamics of measles in sub-Saharan Africa. *Nature*, 451:679–684, 2008.

[65] B.D. Dalziel, O.N. Bjornstad, W.G. van Panhuis, D.S. Burke, C.J.E. Metcalf, and B.T. Grenfell. Persistent chaos of measles epidemics in the prevaccination United States caused by a small change in seasonal transmission patterns. *PLoS Computational Biology*, 12(2), 2016.

[66] M.J. Ferrari, A. Djibo, R.F. Grais, B.T. Grenfell, and O.N. Bjornstad. Episodic outbreaks bias estimates of age specific force of infection: A corrected method using measles in Niamey, Niger as an example. *Epidemiology and Infection*, 138:108–116, 2010.

[67] M.J. Ferrari, B.T. Grenfell, and P. Strebel. Think globally, act locally: The role of local demographics and vaccination coverage in the dynamic response of measles infection to control. *Philosophical Transactions of the Royal Society*, 368:2012014, 2013.

[68] D.J.D. Earn, P. Rohani, B.M. Bolker, and B.T. Grenfell. A simple model for complex dynamical transitions in epidemics. *Nature*, 287:667–670, 2000.

[69] A. Melegaro, M. Jit, N. Gay, E. Zagheni, and W.J. Edmunds. What types of contacts are important for the spread of infections? Using contact survey data to explore European mixing patterns. *Epidemics*, 3(3):143–151, 2011.

[70] N. Goeyvaerts, N. Hens, B. Ogunjimi, M. Aerts, Z. Shkedy, P.V. Damme, and P. Beutels. Estimating infectious disease parameters from data on social contacts and serological status. *Journal of the Royal Statistical Society: Series C (Applied Statistics)*, 59(2):255–277, 2010.

[71] J. Lessler, C.J.E. Metcalf, R.F. Grais, F.J. Luquero, D.A.T. Cummings, and B.T. Grenfell. Measuring the performance of vaccination programs using cross-sectional surveys. *PLoS Medicine*, 8:e1001110, 2011.

[72] F. Trentini, P. Poletti, S. Merler, and A. Melegaro. Measles immunity gaps and the progress towards elimination: A multi-country modelling analysis. *Lancet Infectious Diseases*, 17(10):1089–1097, 2017.

[73] J.G. Wood, N. Goeyvaerts, C.R. MacIntyre, R.I. Menzies, P.B. McIntyre, and N. Hens. Estimating vaccine coverage from serial trivariate serologic data in the presence of waning immunity. *Epidemiology*, 26(3):381–389, May 2015.

15

Inferring the Time of Infection from Serological Data

Maciej F. Boni, Kåre Mølbak, and Karen A. Krogfelt

CONTENTS

15.1 Introduction

15.1.1 Characterizing past epidemiology with serological data

Seroepidemiology aims to cover two main individual-level questions, whether antibody levels in the blood are indicative of past infection and protective against future infection. The answers, if available, are readily translatable to populations. A seroepidemiological study focused on past infection will aim to describe the historical force of infection or historical incidence of a particular pathogen. A seroepidemiological study focused on protection will aim to determine whether a population has enough herd immunity to prevent an epidemic from occurring. In this chapter, we will address questions on past infection. Specifically, we will investigate the informativeness of an individual antibody measurement on inferring the time of past infection (for an individual) and we will discuss whether estimates of time of past infection can be used to reconstruct historical incidence.

Population-level inference on past infection, or past force of infection (FOI), typically makes one of two assumptions: either that the FOI is constant in time (i.e., that we are looking at an endemic disease at a constant level of circulation) or that the FOI acts equally on all age groups (see also Chapter 14). If both of these conditions are met, the annual FOI can be inferred easily from an age-seroprevalence curve constructed from a single population cross-section. All we need to be sure of is which individuals are seropositive and which individuals are seronegative, and a curve of the form $1 - e^{-\phi a}$ will fit these data, with a representing age and ϕ the annual FOI. See the top row of Figure 15.1.

If the FOI is constant in time but varying with age, a similar calculation can be made by allowing ϕ_a, $\phi_{a'}, \phi_{a''}$, etc. to represent the FOI on different age groups. In the second row

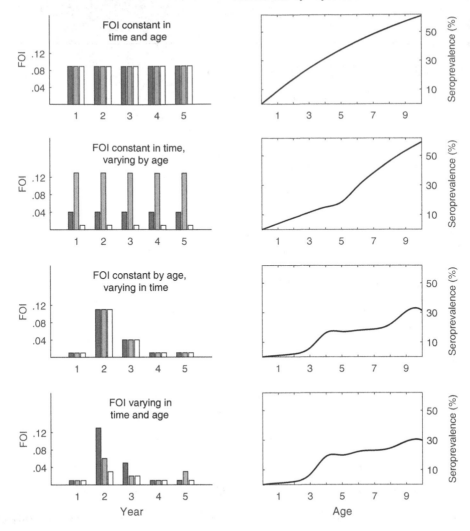

FIGURE 15.1

Effects of time-dependence and age-dependence on the force of infection (FOI). The dark gray bars represent the FOI on the 0–5 age group. The light gray bars represent the FOI on the 5–15 age group. The white bars represent the FOI on the >15 age group. We assume that the FOI has been cycling periodically in the past, with the previous 5 years looking exactly like the current 5 years shown in the left-hand column. Each age-seroprevalence curve on the right corresponds to its FOI diagram on the left. The age-seroprevalence curve was constructed from a cross-sectional study conducted at the end of year 5.

of Figure 15.1, the age-seroprevalence curve turns upwards at age 5 because 5–15 year-olds experience a higher FOI than young children (<5), and thus seropositivity in the 5–15 age range will increase more quickly than it did in the 0–5 age range. If the FOI varies in time but is constant across age groups, an age-seroprevalence curve from a population cross-section allows us to infer a varying FOI from year to year. Again in Figure 15.1, the third row shows a time-varying age-constant FOI and a corresponding age-seroprevalence curve. The curve turns sharply upward at age 4, because of a large epidemic that occurred 4 years ago, causing a large portion of the population (which is the current "over-4" population) to be seropositive. The curve also turns up sharply at age 9, because in this example we have assumed that the FOI cycle repeats every 5 years in the pattern shown.

In the case that the FOI varies both in time and age, an age-seroprevalence curve alone is not sufficient for inferring the past age-specific dynamics of the FOI (see Chapter 16). Notice that in the bottom row of Figure 15.1 the age-seroprevalence curve turns upwards at age 4 because of the high FOI experienced 4 years ago by the 0–5 age group. This result is consistent with our expectation. However, this age-seroprevalence behavior has an alternative explanation: that the FOI is simply higher for children over the age of 4. The only way to differentiate these two scenarios is to add information on recency of infection. If the 4-year-olds in the current cross section appear to have recently acquired antibodies, then the scenario is more likely explained by an age-varying FOI with the ≥4 age group having higher exposure. If the 4-year-olds in the current cross section appear to have older or non-recent antibodies, then it is more likely that they acquired them 4 years ago and the scenario is more plausibly explained by a time-varying FOI that peaked 4 years ago. This is the key rationale for understanding antibody recency and antibody waning in seroepidemiology. These measures allow us to reconstruct past FOI that is both time-dependent and age-dependent. Estimating time of infection from a serological data point is the essential statistical inference that makes this possible, as it allows us to reconstruct a historical infection process that varied with time and age.

15.1.2 Estimating the antibody waning rate

To estimate time of past infection, the process of antibody waning must be characterized. To do this accurately, patients with a confirmed infection should be recruited into a basic clinical observational study shortly after onset of symptoms. A follow-up visit should be scheduled about 1 month after symptoms onset so that antibody levels (antibody titers) can be measured. After the initial visit, follow-up visits should be scheduled every month or every several months as is convenient for the patients, allowed for in the study setting, and appropriate for the pathogen in question. The more follow-up visits, the better the estimates of the antibody waning rate will be. Two or three follow-up visits will typically not be enough to obtain an accurate estimate of the waning rate. Four or more follow-up visits over a 6–18 month period following infection is a good starting point for an observational study aiming to estimate an antibody waning rate. For some infections, antibodies will wane more slowly and a follow-up period of several years may be required.

Antibody waning rates post-infection are useful for assessing the duration of immune protection conferred by an episode of disease. Despite this apparent utility, studies with statistical estimates of the waning rate are not common. A few diseases for which we do have sufficient long-term follow-up with antibody measurements are whooping cough (*Bordetella pertussis*) [1–5], salmonella (non-typhoidal *Salmonella* spp.) [6–10], and campylobacter [11,12], for which these research groups have carried out multi-year follow-up on hundreds of individuals post-infection, with follow-up typically including four or more time points. Smaller numbers of patients have been enrolled in influenza studies [13–18] and have enabled us to approximate the rate of antibody waning after an acute infection with influenza virus. Multiple sequential follow-ups are common in vaccine studies [19–24] but in this chapter we will focus on antibody waning post-infection only.

15.1.3 Details of the waning process

The decay of antibody concentrations acts like a clock that allows measurement of when an infection took place. However, some important caveats and details about the antibody waning process need to be known when using it to estimate when an infection occurred.

First, post-infection antibody levels are commonly described using a variety of terms like life-long, long-lived, short-lived, persistent, and transient. These terms need to be understood so that an appropriate statistical model can be formulated to capture the relevant features of antibody dynamics. When immunity levels are described as "life-long", this usually refers to protection from a second infection and does not necessarily mean that antibody levels stay constant throughout life; rather, it means that antibody levels stay protective throughout life. This is of course a simplification. Immune protection is not adequately described by an antibody concentration alone as cellular and non-antibody components of the immune system are associated with protection from pathogens. However, because most assays measure antibody levels (they are easier to measure than the cellular components of the immune system), antibody concentrations are inevitably translated into quantities that are associated with individuals' protection from infection. In the case of long-lived immune protection, an antibody assay may indicate seropositivity many years after an infection; again, seropositivity does not mean that antibodies have not waned during this period, but that antibody levels have remained above a predefined threshold used to define an individual as seropositive. A quantitative assay (as opposed to an assay with a binary outcome) used on a longitudinal set of follow-up samples will tell us whether antibodies do or do not wane in the convalescent period immediately following infection. When an antibody response shows no waning at all, an antibody waning rate would be estimated as being close to zero, and we would not be able to use it to time the occurrence of a past infection. Short-lived and transient antibody responses are normally those that wane observably in the post-infection period when a patient is still being monitored or followed up.

Labeling antibody responses as long-lived or short-lived generally implies that some level of antibody waning is taking place. Persistent antibody responses are those that wane to some detectable level and stay constant thereafter. The key characteristic to describe in these dynamics–especially those of short-lived or transient antibody responses–is whether antibody levels wane to a constant and detectable level, or whether the antibody population eventually disappears altogether or becomes undetectable. Simonsen et al. [7,8] show standard models incorporating the persistence level as a parameter in these types of models.

Second, after observing an antibody waning process that appears to persist many years after an infection took place, it is tempting to fit a biphasic decline to these data. A two-phase antibody decay appears to be justified in this situation, with the first phase describing the decay immediately following the infection and the second phase describing the dynamics of the persistence phase. A minimum of three parameters must be inferred here, two slopes and the time point separating the two phases. Another clue that antibody dynamics may not follow a simple exponential decay is a lack of individuals (lower numbers than expected by chance) with high titers in cross-sectional data. This observation suggests that the antibody waning process follows "fast-then-slow" dynamics or "faster-than-exponential" decay, which can be parameterized with two parameters [25]. These descriptions of biphasic or fast-then-slow antibody waning may in fact be accurate reflections of the true process (although the process will differ among pathogens). However, the reality of clinical studies is that they rarely have enough patients and clinical follow-up points to accurately measure a single phase of waning, and almost no studies have enough follow-up to estimate two waning rates. For this reason, most studies simply aim to estimate a single-parameter waning rate, even in cases where long-term persistence is allowed for [7].

Third, follow-up studies are not carried out for the sole purpose of measuring waning rates. They are also carried out for diagnostic purposes, i.e., to determine if an acute-phase or convalescent-phase serum sample can be used to confirm a particular infection.

The most common immunoglobulin classes that are measured are IgG, IgM, and IgA, all of which will have their own dynamics and waning rates after an infection clears. IgG class antibodies are generated in the later stages of an infection (weeks after an infection has established), and they are antigen-specific and typically long-lasting. Antibody waning estimates normally focus on the waning of IgG class antibodies, as IgG can be detected in serum years after an exposure making it a useful tool for determining presence and timing of a past infection. Post-infection follow-up studies do sometimes measure IgM class [1,6,7,9,12, 26–28] and IgA class [1,6,7,9] antibodies, but these generally wane more quickly and are less useful in serological studies aimed at inferring time of past infection. IgM class antibodies are useful clinically for identifying current acute infection or recent acute infection, and thus could in principle be used to time the occurrence of a recent infection; however, the waning rate of IgM antibodies is generally quite fast (days to weeks), and in a general-population cross-section very few individuals would test IgM-positive under most endemicity scenarios.

15.2 Statistical Models for Time of Infection

15.2.1 Minimal model for inferring time of infection

In this section, we present the minimal data set and minimal model for estimating the time of past infection for one individual. For this, we require a longitudinal dataset consisting of n individuals with confirmed recent infection with a particular pathogen. Each of these n individuals is followed up at m post-infection follow-up time points. At each follow-up, antibody titer or antibody concentration is measured. Thus, the longitudinal dataset consists of mn antibody measurements structured as

$$\mathbf{X} = \left\{ x_i^k \right\}_{i=1,\ldots,m \,;\, k=1,\ldots,n} \tag{15.1}$$

where the superscript k runs over individuals, and the subscript i runs over follow-up time points for a single individual. This can be adjusted for missing data or when the sampling times do not match up exactly across individuals. In practice, in observational studies generating longitudinal data like these, loss to follow-up and variation in follow-up times is common.

We ignore any acute-phase time points that would be taken before pathogen-specific IgG antibody is generated. For each individual, the first time point in $\mathbf{X}$ can be viewed as the peak antibody titer, normally measured several weeks after onset of symptoms. The rise in post-infection antibody titer is rapid and there is normally insufficient sampling during this period to determine a true peak time and peak value; nevertheless, mechanistic models have been used for this purpose, and one possible exception where time until peak IgG has been estimated for pertussis infection [5]). In a well-planned study, there will be between four and ten follow-up time points ($4 \leq m \leq 10$), and these follow-ups would occur every few weeks or every few months, as is realistic and appropriate for the pathogen in question and the study setting. We are not considering cases where antibody titers are being measured every day or nearly every day.

The most straightforward analysis of data set $\mathbf{X}$ is done with a simple linear regression on log-transformed titers with a random effect accounting for differences in peak antibody titers among individuals, which in practice can differ by a substantial amount. We assume that the peak titer is normally distributed with mean A and standard deviation σ_A, the log-titer decline has slope λ, and the observation error on a log-scale is σ. These four parameters will be represented by $\Theta = (A, \sigma_A, \lambda, \sigma)$, and the probability model for the longitudinal time series of individual k in a random effects model is

$$P(\mathbf{x}^k \mid \Theta) = \left(\frac{1}{\sqrt{2\pi\sigma^2}}\right)^m \cdot \int_{-\infty}^{+\infty} \prod_{i=1}^m \exp\left[-\frac{(b + \lambda t_i - x_i^k)^2}{2\sigma^2}\right] f(b)\, db \qquad (15.2)$$

where f is the probability density of $\mathcal{N}(A, \sigma_A)$, and t_i is the time at which measurement i was taken. The full probability is obtained by multiplying across all individuals, and the likelihood

$$L(\Theta \mid X) \sim \prod_{k=1}^n P(\mathbf{x}^k \mid \Theta) \qquad (15.3)$$

can be optimized to obtain estimates for the mean peak titer (A), peak titer variance (σ_A), antibody waning rate (λ), and observation error (σ). Recall that all estimates are log-scale, i.e., after titers have been transformed to log-titers.

After obtaining an estimate for the rate of antibody waning, the next goal is to obtain an estimate for the time of infection or the time of peak antibody concentration of a new individual $n + 1$ observed to have titer x^{n+1} with no other information on infection history. Normally, the time of peak IgG concentration occurs just a few weeks after infection, and it is simpler to infer the time of peak IgG. If the time of peak IgG is τ time units ago, then the probability model from Equation (15.2), across all individuals, becomes

$$P(\mathbf{X}, x^{n+1} \mid \Theta, \tau) \qquad (15.4)$$

which is the same inference that is set up by Simonsen et al. (2009, p.1887) [8], with a number of other publications introducing similar analyses [4, 7, 12, 29]. The above equation can be separated into

$$P(\mathbf{X} \mid \Theta) \cdot P(x^{n+1} \mid \Theta, \tau), \qquad (15.5)$$

indicating that the maximum likelihood estimates of Θ will not be influenced by maximum likelihood estimation of τ. And, the right-hand probability above can be written as

$$P(x^{n+1} \mid \Theta, \tau) = \frac{1}{1 - \Phi(x^{n+1} - A)} \frac{1}{\sqrt{2\pi\sigma^2}} \int_{x^{n+1}}^{+\infty} \exp\left[-\frac{(b + \lambda\tau - x^{n+1})^2}{2\sigma^2}\right] f(b)\, db,$$
$$(15.6)$$

where Φ, in the normalization factor in equation 15.6, is a normal cumulative distribution function with variance σ_A^2 and mean 0. Note that in Equation 15.6, we are integrating over the values b of peak titer with a lower integration limit of $b = x^{n+1}$. Assuming that the likelihood optimization in Equation (15.3) resulted in a negative value for the slope $\hat{\lambda}$, we can safely assume that the peak titer is higher than the currently observed titer. In both Equations (15.2) and (15.6) above, x_i^k and x^{n+1} are already presented as log-scale antibody measurements.

Confidence intervals for $\hat{\tau}$ will not be symmetric and cannot be constructed using standard likelihood theory and assumptions of normality. Confidence intervals for $\hat{\tau}$ require profiling the likelihood, which will require re-optimization of Θ for each fixed value of τ in the profile.

15.2.2   Censored values

It is common for antibody measurement to be recorded as right-censored values, i.e., values which are above the limit of detection L of a particular immunological assay. To account for the fact that censoring will influence the inference of λ and τ, we can use cross-sectional data to examine what proportion of data points normally would appear as censored in the population. A typical analysis of cross-sectional ELISA data or titer data involves mixture-distribution fits that are meant to uncover the major sero-status groups in the population (traditionally, seropositives and seronegatives), and the largest component in a mixture distribution fit of antibody titers usually will describe how a censored titer relates to its true uncensored value, see Chapter 19 and [30–34]. In a K-component mixture fit with normal densities $g_1, g_2, \ldots, g_K$ (ordered by increasing mean), the expected true titer based on an observed censored titer of L is

$$\frac{1}{1 - \Phi(L - \mu_K)} \int_L^\infty z\, g_K(z)\, dz\,. \tag{15.7}$$

To estimate the time of infection of an individual with a censored titer, we modify Equation (15.6) to obtain

$$P(\,x^{n+1} \geq L \mid \boldsymbol{\Theta}, \tau\,) \;=\; \frac{1}{1 - \Phi(L - \mu_K)} \int_L^\infty P(\,z \mid \boldsymbol{\Theta}, \tau\,)\, g_K(z)\, dz\,, \tag{15.8}$$

where z runs over all the potential true titer values of the observed censored value L; censored titers can be similarly replaced in Equation (15.2) for individuals in the longitudinal cohort used to measure the rate of antibody waning. When a single individual in this cohort has all of their titers censored, they should be removed from the dataset as their follow-up time points are not informative for inferring waning.

15.3 Application to *Salmonella enterica* IgG Measurements

We start with one of the better-described datasets on antibody waning, 154 Danish patients with culture-confirmed *Salmonella enterica* serovar Enteritidis (hereafter *S.* Enteritidis) as described by Strid et al. [6] and Simonsen et al. [7]. A subset of 138 patients was taken here, removing individuals with insufficient follow-up or missing data at the first visit. Patients were followed up at four time points ($m = 4$) with samples being taken shortly after infection (several weeks), as well as 3, 6, and 12 months post-infection. The median times of sampling were 21, 106, 202, and 417 days post-infection. Optical density (OD) values from an IgG ELISA ranged from 0.0421 to 4.304, and for the purposes of this analysis, we do not consider any of the OD values to be censored. Some of the patients appeared to have non-monotonic decay of IgG antibody, and these are shown in the bottom four panels of Figure 15.2. The panels are grouped by quartiles of starting OD value.

Optimizing likelihood Equation (15.3) with a Nelder-Mead routine and profiling the likelihood, the estimated rate of decline in the optical density measurement (OD) is $\hat{\lambda} = -0.991\ \log_2$–OD units/year (95% CI: $-1.168 - -0.799$). This result means that the half-life of the OD value is approximately 1 year. The estimated peak optical density, several weeks after infection, is $\hat{A} = 2.372$ (95% CI: 2.218–2.536). And, the estimated standard deviation in $\log_2$-peak OD is $\hat{\sigma}_A = 0.374$ (95% CI: 0.273–0.476). The error estimate is $\hat{\sigma} = 0.394$. Figure 15.3 shows the antibody decline for all 138 patients, together with the predicted pattern of decay for the "mean" individual whose OD value after infection is 2.372 OD units.

The goal now is to infer the time of past infection (by way of inferring τ, the time of peak IgG concentration) for a randomly sampled individual in the population, one for whom we have no knowledge of past infection. Figure 15.3 shows visually the individuals for whom we will be able to most confidently predict τ. Inferring a τ value within the past 15 months gives us more certainty in our estimate than an inferred τ value larger than 15 months,

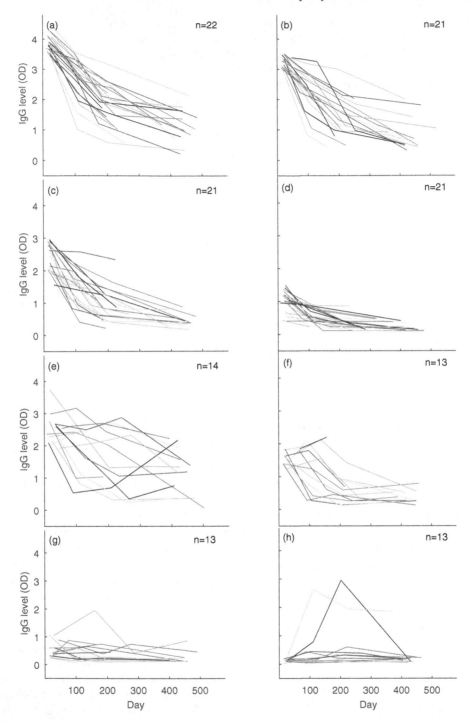

FIGURE 15.2
Declines of IgG antibody to *S*. Enteritidis for 138 individuals after confirmed infection.
Panels (a) through (d) show individuals with monotonic declines over time. The four panels
are broken up into quartiles according to the first antibody measurement (the peak antibody
level). Panels E through H show individuals with non-monotonic declines. The four panels
are broken up into quartiles according to the first antibody measurement.

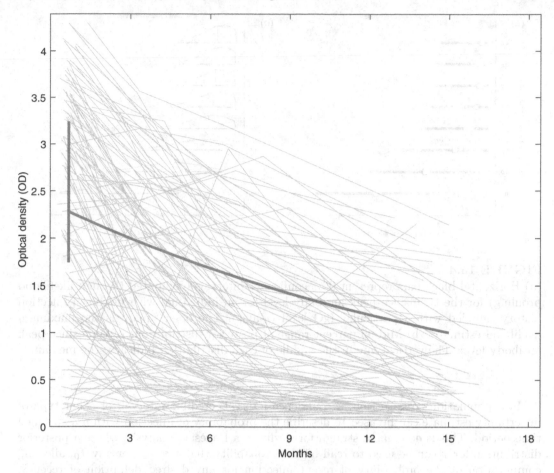

FIGURE 15.3
Antibody decay for 138 individuals with confirmed infection to *S.* Enteritidis. Vertical gray line shows the estimated range (± one standard deviation) of ELISA OD values shortly after infection. The gray curve is the estimated decay for the mean individual with post-infection OD value equal to 2.372.

as the patient data had approximately 15 months of follow-up. This result means that we will have less confidence in our inference for individuals who are sampled with OD values below 1.0. In addition, individuals with an OD-value larger than $\hat{A} = 2.372$ will result in similar maximum-likelihood estimates $\hat{\tau}$, as the data contain very little information as to when these individuals' infections occurred other than "very recently."

Figure 15.4a shows the estimates $\hat{\tau}$ and 95% confidence intervals for eight hypothetical individuals with OD values ranging from 0.5 to 4.0. For field or clinical applications, the confidence intervals are too wide to be useful. As an example, an individual with an OD measurement of 2.0 is more informatively described as "probably having been infected in the past 16 or 17 months" rather than "most likely infected 4.4 months ago" since the uncertainty around the maximum likelihood estimator (MLE) of 4.4 months is substantial. The confidence interval, therefore, is the more useful entity to emerge from this analysis. The maximum-likelihood time of infection estimates $\hat{\tau}$ are valid, but it is the confidence interval or credible interval (Figure 15.4b) that will allow useful epidemiological questions to be answered.

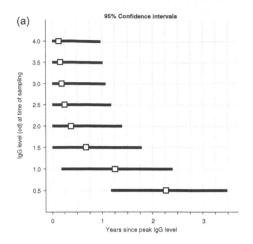 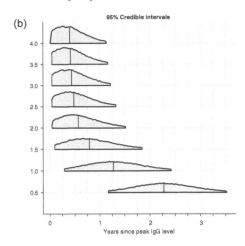

FIGURE 15.4

(a) Horizontal black bars represent 95% confidence intervals (computed through likelihood profiling) for the time since peak antibody level for an individual with unknown infection history sampled with a particular IgG level (y-axis). The open square is the maximum likelihood estimate. (b) Mid-95 percent range of posterior distributions of time since peak antibody level. The vertical line in the middle of each distribution indicates the median.

In a population cross-section, a confidence interval, credible interval, or other type of uncertainty estimate can be used to describe the probability of infection within a specified time period. This is done most straightforwardly in a Bayesian analysis, where a posterior distribution for τ can be used to read off the probability that $\tau \leq T_0$, for any T_0, allowing computation of the probability of recent infection for any desired definition of recency. Questions of bias will need to be answered when the posterior distribution is used to generate an estimator of a population attack rate, and these likely will need to be separately evaluated for every epidemiological scenario.

Bias in $\hat{\tau}$. As with any estimator of a strictly positive quantity, we need to investigate potential bias in $\hat{\tau}$ when the true value of τ is close to zero. In practice, this will be a concern for high OD-values, and all values where the observed optical density is higher than the estimate $\hat{A}$ of peak OD-value. As no analytical expression exists for $\hat{\tau}$, we simulate the antibody decay for a group of independent individuals, with a starting peak OD-value sampled from $N(\hat{A}, \hat{\sigma}_A)$, a decay rate of $\hat{\lambda}$ over a pre-determined time span, and a normally-distributed observation error $\hat{\sigma}$.

Estimates of time of infection are shown in Figure 15.5 for 15 sets of 1,000 individuals, with each individual having one sampling time between 30 days and 450 days after their peak IgG level. Note that these estimates are specific to the particular observed reference cohort of 138 individuals infected with S. Enteritidis and their subsequent IgG waning. Thirty days past peak titer, $E(\hat{\tau})$ is 149 days as computed across 1,000 independent individuals. Clearly, for recently infected individuals, this estimate $\hat{\tau}$ is substantially biased upwards. The reason for the upward bias (when averaging arithmetically over non-transformed data) is that approximately half of infected individuals will have an OD-value smaller than $\hat{A}$ at thirty days, and with a large enough standard deviation (σ_A) in peak IgG this will cause the inferred τ-values to range from 30 days to 700 days; negative τ-values cannot be inferred, and this right skew in the distribution of estimates biases $E(\hat{\tau})$ upwards. The modal estimate for individuals 30 days past their peak IgG level is 64 days, much closer to the true value.

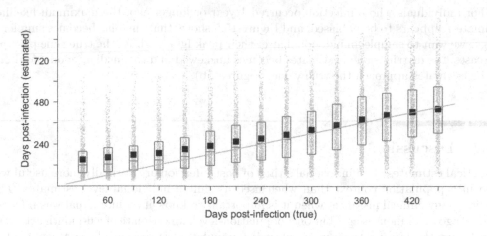

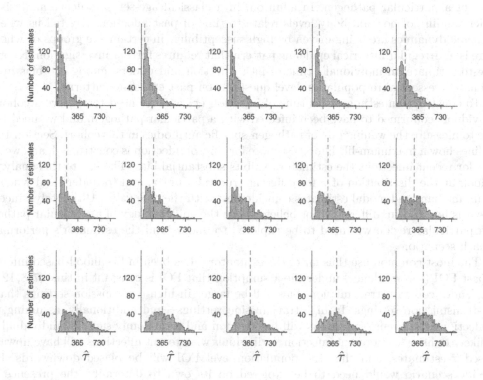

FIGURE 15.5

Individual antibody declines were simulated independently for 15 sets of 1,000 individuals and observed 30 days, 60 days, etc. post infection (top panel, x-axis), taking into account variation in peak antibody level (σ_A) and observation error (σ). In the top panel, light gray dots in the background show the maximum-likelihood estimates $\hat{\tau}$ for each individual, and the boxes show the interquartile range of the estimates. The black square is the arithmetic mean over all the estimates $\bar{\hat{\tau}}$. The gray line shows where the true value would be equal to the mean of the estimates. The bottom panels show the distribution of 1,000 estimates $\hat{\tau}$ for each true value of τ shown by the gray dashed line. The true values of τ range from 30 days to 450 days.

For individuals whose infection occurred 1 year or longer ago, the maximum-likelihood estimate $\hat{\tau}$ appears to be unbiased, and Figure 15.5 shows that the bias becomes smaller the longer we wait to sample an individual after their peak IgG level. As the true time post-peak increases, the distribution of estimates becomes unskewed and the median, mode, and mean of the estimates approach the true value (Figure 15b).

15.4   Discussion

Statistical estimates of an individual's time of past infection are normally more useful when used in a population context than when used as simple individual-level estimates. There are not many clinical instances when it is important to know if an individual was infected 6 months ago or 12 months ago, but on a population-level, an estimate of a 6-month attack rate or a 12-month attack rate [7] may tell us if a population is susceptible to a new epidemic wave of a particular pathogen. In addition, in a classical age-seroprevalence analysis, an understanding of how antibody levels relate to time of past infection may tell us whether epidemic dynamics are being driven by high susceptibility in certain age groups or whether there is an irregular historical epidemic pattern that requires further investigation. Knowing how to estimate an individual's time of past infection and understanding the bias in this estimate is essential to population-level questions on past epidemic patterns.

To construct an estimator for time of infection (τ) we first need to observe a cohort of individuals confirmed to have been infected with a particular pathogen, and we need to be able to measure the waning rate of pathogen-specific antibodies in this cohort. Section 15.2.1 outlines how a maximum-likelihood estimate for time of infection is constructed, and we note that for recent infections the estimator exhibits substantial bias. The key to this analysis is to look at the distribution of $\hat{\tau}$ for different true values of τ, and to understand when the mean, median, and modal estimates coincide best with the true value. Ultimately, since the true τ is not known, different prior beliefs about the epidemiology of a particular pathogen in a particular region will need to be explored to understand the estimator's performance in each scenario.

The most common use thus far of the estimator $\hat{\tau}$ has been in likelihood-based inference of past FOI (seroincidence) under the assumption that FOI is constant in time [7, 8, 12, 35–37]. Under constant transmission, bias will be larger in high-transmission settings than in low-transmission settings. In high-transmission settings—and additionally, assuming that reinfections can occur—infections will be common and a randomly sampled individual will be likely to have had a recent infection. Individuals with recent infections will have upwardly biased $\hat{\tau}$-estimates, and thus the population-level FOI will be biased downwards. Each specific scenario would need to be explored on its own to determine the presence and strength of bias. In low-transmission settings, most individuals will not have any marker of past infection, and a small fraction of individuals with signs of past infection will have signs of recent infection. The time-of-infection estimates for these individuals will be biased upwards, but they will represent a small proportion of all individuals sampled from the general population. Again, for each epidemiological scenario, bias will need to be evaluated accordingly. Simonsen et al. [8] investigated this bias for the Danish general population and their exposure to non-typhoidal Salmonella (using the same cohort data as presented in this chapter). They found that their inferred incidence of 0.09 cases per person per year was likely low enough to be unbiased, as a simulated data set with this FOI showed little bias using the same inference.

In populations where past FOI is known to be non-constant, an additional source of bias will need to be evaluated. When the goal of the analysis is reconstructing past seroincidence, we must be aware of adjacent time periods which have large differences in true incidence. For example, an analysis of time-to-infection for influenza virus (in a temperate region) should place most times of infection in the winter months as this is when influenza epidemics are known to occur. Because of error in the estimates, some of these infection times will be placed (incorrectly) in spring or autumn. However, as there are typically very few true influenza infections the spring/autumn months, there will be almost no re-classification of spring/autumn infections as winter infections. Thus, wintertime incidence will be underestimated (downward bias) and spring/autumn infections will be overestimated (upward bias). This effect is not observed when incidence is constant throughout the year. This concern was discussed by Borremans et al. [29] who attempted reconstruction of non-constant past FOI on simulated data sets of Morogoro virus infection in mouse populations. When using quantitative antibody data (rather than presence/absence) or when including multiple data types in the analysis (presence of virus, age), the authors were able to reconstruct accurate time series of past incidence. One reason for the success of their incidence reconstructions is that their data showed little variation in peak antibody level, substantially reducing the error in the time-of-infection estimate for each individual. Similarly, Vinh and Boni [25] evaluated inference on the timing and strength of an influenza epidemic using a serological time series, and inference was shown to be unbiased for larger sample sizes and more frequent sampling, partly due to a deterministic model of antibody acquisition and antibody waning. When sample sizes are small and/or variation in peak titer is large, the inference will be more biased. Simonsen et al. [8] (p. 1893) and Vinh and Boni [25] (their Figure 6) both note that the "seasonality of seroresponses will be less pronounced than those of outbreaks" [8].

To reduce uncertainty in time-of-infection estimates, one potential approach is adding more antibody, pathogen, or age measurements into the statistical model used to estimate τ. IgM and IgA class antibodies are the next obvious measurements to take from an available serum sample, and these may in fact be critical in helping estimate recent times of infection, potentially reducing the bias present in IgG-only models. For infections with predictable dynamics of viral or bacterial load, the pathogen population size may also serve as an indicator of time of infection [29]. However, this generally will not be possible for acute self-limiting infections, and for chronic or longer-duration infections the interdependent dynamics of the pathogen and immune system would need to be well understood, as the pathogen population size normally will not follow the simple exponential decay we have assumed here for IgG antibody.

Time-of-infection estimates can have great public health value both in outbreak investigations and in routine surveillance. They may be able to address the challenge that most surveillance systems are affected by underreporting and with considerable uncertainty surrounding the number of known cases. Therefore, serological surveys may be important in obtaining independent estimates of the FOI and thus crucial for risk assessments and scenario predictions in disease outbreaks. Serological surveys on past data may also reveal whether an upsurge in reported cases represents a true emergence or is an artefactual feature of increased awareness. For surveillance purposes, time-of-infection estimates are useful for estimating so-called "multipliers" or "underreporting factors" which are measures of the underestimation of the true disease incidence. This is useful for calibrating different surveillance systems against each other [11, 36–38]. In addition, this approach has been further extended to aid in the estimation of burden of disease for infectious diseases in Europe [39].

Emerging disease and novel outbreak scenarios are a common scenario where research needs are neglected, as the past decade's experience with Zika, Ebola, Chikungunya, and other novel pathogens has taught us. The West African Ebola epidemic of 2014 caused a minimum of 28,000 infections with an approximate 40 percent case fatality. The long epidemic wave of Zika virus in the Americas in 2015–2016 caused millions of infections and thousands of cases of microcephaly in infants. However, with very little data from these epidemics on serology and antibody dynamics (but see [40]), it would be nearly impossible to carry out a population-based serological survey to accurately measure attack rate or overall attack rates, a determination that is critical in all stages of managing an emerging disease outbreak. In the field, perhaps a priority needs to be placed on performing follow-up on recovered individuals in the early stages of an outbreak (creating the cohort **X** described by (15.1)) to calibrate the association between antibody concentration and past infection. For statisticians, the next critical work to be done is in understanding sources of bias and optimizing study designs for individual-level estimates of time-of-infection. For epidemiologists, the next challenge is making this data collection part of the routine investigation process so that the estimates can be put to good use.

Acknowledgments

Thanks to Niel Hens, Ottar Bjørnstad, Ephraim Hanks for many useful statistical comments on this chapter. Thanks to Stephen Baker for conversations on *Salmonella*.

References

[1] Sarah S. Long, Celeste J. Welkon, and Janet L. Clark. Widespread silent transmission of pertussis in families : Antibody correlates of infection and symptomatology. *J. Infect. Dis.*, 161:480–486, 1990.

[2] Sally L. Hodder, James D. Cherry, Edward A. Mortimer, Amasa B. Ford, Jeffrey Gornbein, and Klara Papp. Antibody responses to *Bordetella pertussis* antigens and clinical correlations in elderly community residents. *Clin. Infect. Dis.*, (1):7–14, 2000.

[3] H E de Melker, F G A Versteegh, M A E Conyn-van Spaendonck, L H Elvers, G A M Berbers, A van der Zee, and J F P Schellekens. Specificity and sensitivity of high levels of immunoglobulin G antibodies against pertussis toxin in a single serum sample for diagnosis of infection with Bordetella pertussis specificity and sensitivity of high levels of immunoglobulin G antibodies again. *J. Clin. Microbiol.*, 38(2):800–806, 2000.

[4] P F M Teunis, O G van der Heijden, H E de Melker, J F P Schellekens, F G A Versteegh, and M E E Kretzschmar. Kinetics of the IgG antibody response to pertussis toxin after infection with *B. pertussis*. *Epidemiol. Infect.*, 129:479–489, 2002.

[5] F G A Versteegh, P L J M Mertens, H E de Melker, J J Roord, J F P Schellekens, and P F M Teunis. Age-specific long-term course of IgG antibodies to pertussis toxin after symptomatic infection with *Bordetella pertussis*. *Epid. Infect.*, 133(4):737–748, 2005.

[6] Mette A. Strid, Tine Dalby, Kåre Mølbak, and Karen A. Krogfelt. Kinetics of the human antibody response against *Salmonella enterica* serovars Enteritidis and Typhimurium

determined by lipopolysaccharide enzyme-linked immunosorbent assay. *Clin. Vaccine Immunol.*, 14(6):741–747, 2007.

[7] J Simonsen, M A Strid, K Mølbak, K A Krogfelt, A Linneberg, and P Teunis. Sero-epidemiology as a tool to study the incidence of *Salmonella* infections in humans. *Epidemiol. Infect.*, 136(7):895–902, 2008.

[8] J Simonsen, K Molbak, G Falkenhorst, K A Krogfelt, A Linneberg, and P F M Teunis. Estimation of incidences of infectious diseases based on antibody measurements. *Stat. Med.*, 28:1882–1895, 2009.

[9] Gerhard Falkenhorst, Tina H. Ceper, Mette A. Strid, Kåre Mølbak, and Karen A. Krogfelt. Serological follow-up after non-typhoid salmonella infection in humans using a mixed lipopolysaccharide ELISA. *Int. J. Med. Microbiol.*, 303(8):533–538, 2013.

[10] Tine Dalby, Mette A. Strid, Natasha H. Beyer, Jens Blom, Kare Molbak, and Karen A. Krogfelt. Rapid decay of *Salmonella* flagella antibodies during human gastroenteritis: A follow up study. *J. Micriobiol. Methods*, 62(2):233–243, 2005.

[11] Mette A. Strid, Jorgen Engberg, Lena B. Larsen, Kamilla Begtrup, Kare Molbak, and Karen A Krogfelt. Antibody responses to campylobacter infections determined by an enzyme-linked immunosorbent assay: 2-year Follow-up study of 210 patients. *Clin. Diag. Lab. Immunol.*, 8(2):314–319, 2001.

[12] P. F. M. Teunis, J. C. H. van Eijkeren, C. W. Ang, Y. T. H. P. van Duynhoven, J. B. Simonsen, M. A. Strid, and W. van Pelt. Biomarker dynamics: estimating infection rates from serological data. *Stat. Med.*, 31:2240–2248, 2012.

[13] Frank L. Horsfall Jr. Present status of knowledge concerning influenza. *Am. J. Pub. Health.*, 30(11):1302–1310, 1940.

[14] Frank L. Horsfall Jr and E R Rickard. Neutralizing antibodies in human serum after influenza A: the lack of strain specificity in the immunological response. *J. Exp. Med.*, 74(5):433–439, 1941.

[15] Jill J. Severson, Katelyn R. Richards, John J. M Moran, and Mary S. Hayney. Persistence of influenza vaccine-induced antibody in lung transplant patients and healthy individuals beyond the season. *Hum. Vacc. Immunother.*, 8(12):1850–3, 2012.

[16] Jung Pu Hsu, Xiahong Zhao, Mark I-Cheng Chen, Alex R. Cook, Vernon Lee, Wei Yen Lim, Linda Tan et al., Rate of decline of antibody titers to pandemic influenza A (H1N1-2009) by hemagglutination inhibition and virus microneutralization assays in a cohort of seroconverting adults in Singapore. *BMC Infect. Dis.*, 14(1):414, 2014.

[17] Saranya Sridhar, Shaima Begom, Katja Hoschler, Alison Bermingham, Walt Adamson, William Carman, Steven Riley, and Ajit Lalvani. Longevity and determinants of protective humoral immunity after pandemic influenza infection. *Am. J. Resp. Crit. Care. Med.*, 191:325–332, 2015.

[18] Rosemary Markovic-Delabre, Nicolas Salez, Magali Lemaitre, Marianne Leruez-ville, Xavier De Lamballerie, and Fabrice Carrat. Antibody persistence and serological protection among seasonal 2007 influenza A(H1N1) infected subjects : Results from the FLUREC cohort study. *Vaccine*, 33:7015–7021, 2015.

[19] P Van Damme, S Thoelen, M Cramm, K De Groote, A Safary, and A Meheus. Inactivated hepatitis A vaccine: reactogenicity, immunogenicity, and long-term antibody persistence. *J. Med. Virol.*, 44:446–451, 1994.

[20] Irja Davidkin and Martti Valle. Vaccine-induced measles virus antibodies after two doses of combined measles, mumps and rubella vaccine: A 12-year follow-up in two cohorts. *Vaccine*, 16(20):2052–2057, 1998.

[21] Henry R. Shinefield, Steven B. Black, Brenda O. Staehle, Holly Matthews, Tama Adelman, Kathleen Ensor, Shu Li et al., Vaccination with measles, mumps and rubella vaccine and varicella vaccine: Safety, tolerability, immunogenicity, persistence of antibody and duration of protection against varicella in healthy children. *Pediatr. Infect. Dis. J.*, 21(6):555–561, 2002.

[22] L. Roznovsky, I. Orsagova, A. Kloudova, J. Tvrdik, L. Kabieszova, I. Lochman, J. Mrazek, L. Hozakova, A. Zjevikova, and L. Pliskova. Long-term protection against hepatitis B after newborn vaccination: 20-year follow-up. *Infection*, 38(5):395–400, 2010.

[23] Michael T. White, Philip Bejon, Ally Olotu, Jamie T. Griffin, Kalifa Bojang, John Lusingu, Nahya Salim et al., A combined analysis of immunogenicity, antibody kinetics and vaccine efficacy from phase 2 trials of the RTS,S malaria vaccine. *BMC Med.*, 12(1):1–11, 2014.

[24] Barnaby Young, Xiahong Zhao, Alex R. Cook, Christopher M. Parry, Annelies Wilder-Smith, and Mark Chen I-Cheng. Do antibody responses to the influenza vaccine persist year-round in the elderly? A systematic review and meta-analysis. *Vaccine*, 35(2): 212–221, 2017.

[25] Dao Nguyen Vinh and Maciej F. Boni. Statistical identifiability and sample size calculations for serial seroepidemiology. *Epidemics*, 12:30–39, 2015.

[26] Khairul Anam, Farhat Afrin, Dwijadas Banerjee, Netai Pramanik, Subhasis K Guha, Rama P Goswami, Shiben K Saha, and Nahid Ali. Differential decline in leishmania membrane antigen-specific immunoglobulin G (IgG), IgM, IgE, and IgG subclass antibodies in Indian Kala-Azar patients after chemotherapy. *Infect. Immun.*, 67(12): 6663–6669, 1999.

[27] Metzkor-Cotter, Einat, Yehudith Kletter, Boaz Avidor, Merav Varon, Yoav Golan, Moshe Ephros, and Michael Giladi. Long-Term serological analysis and clinical follow-up of patients with cat scratch disease. *Clin. Infect. Dis.*, 37(9):1149–1154, 2003.

[28] Khin Saw Aye Myint, Timothy P. Endy, Mrigendra P. Shrestha, Sanjaya K. Shrestha, David W. Vaughn, Bruce L. Innis, Robert V. Gibbons, Robert A. Kuschner, Jitvimol Seriwatana, and Robert Mc N. Scott. Hepatitis E antibody kinetics in Nepalese patients. *Trans. R. Soc. Trop. Med. Hyg.*, 100(10):938–941, 2006.

[29] Benny Borremans, Niel Hens, Philippe Beutels, Herwig Leirs, and Jonas Reijniers. Estimating time of infection using prior serological and individual information can greatly improve incidence estimation of human and wildlife infections. *PLoS Comput. Biol.*, 12(5):1–18, 2016.

[30] M. Greiner, C. R. Franke, D. Böhning, and P. Schlattmann. Construction of an intrinsic cut-off value for the sero-epidemiological study of *Trypanosoma evansi* infections in a canine population in Brazil: a new approach towards an unbiased estimation of prevalence. *Acta Trop.*, 56(1):97–109, 1994.

[31] Andrew L. Baughman, Kristine M. Bisgard, Freyja Lynn, and Bruce D. Meade. Mixture model analysis for establishing a diagnostic cut-off point for pertussis antibody levels. *Stat. Med.*, 25(17):2994–3010, 2006.

[32] Dennis te Beest, Erwin De Bruin, Sandra Imholz, Jacco Wallinga, Peter Teunis, Marion Koopmans, and Michiel Van Boven. Discrimination of influenza infection (A/2009 H1N1) from prior exposure by antibody protein microarray analysis. *PLoS One*, 9(11):e113021, 2014.

[33] Dennis E. te Beest, Paul J. Birrell, Jacco Wallinga, Daniela De Angelis, and Michiel van Boven. Joint modelling of serological and hospitalization data reveals that high levels of pre-existing immunity and school holidays shaped the influenza A pandemic of 2009 in the Netherlands. *J. R. Soc. Interface.*, 12(103):20141244, 2015.

[34] Nguyen Thi Duy Nhat, Stacy Todd, Erwin de Bruin, Tran Thi Nhu Thao, Nguyen Ha Thao Vy, Tran Minh Quan, Dao Nguyen Vinh et al., Structure of general-population antibody titer distributions to influenza A virus. *Nat. Sci. Rep.*, 7(1):6060, 2017.

[35] Hester E. de Melker, Florens G. A. Versteegh, Joop F. P. Schellekens, Peter F. M. Teunis, and Mirjam Kretzschmar. The incidence of *Bordetella pertussis* infections estimated in the population from a combination of serological surveys. *J. Infect.*, 53(2):106–113, 2006.

[36] P F M Teunis, G Falkenhorst, C W Anf, M A Strid, H de Valk, M Sadkowska-Todys, L Zota et al., Campylobacter seroconversion rates in selected countries in the European Union. *Epidemiol. Infect.*, 141:2051–2057, 2013.

[37] Hanne D. Emborg, Peter Teunis, Jacob Simonsen, Karen A. Krogfelt, Charlotte S. Jorgensen, Johanna Takkinen, and Kare Molbak. Was the increase in culture-confirmed Campylobacter infections in Denmark during the 1990s a surveillance artefact? *Euro Surveill.* 2015;20(41):pii=30041

[38] Cheryl L. Gibbons, Marie-Josée J. Mangen, Dietrich Plass, Arie H. Havelaar, Russell John Brooke, Piotr Kramarz, Karen L. Peterson, Anke L. Stuurman, Alessandro Cassini, Eric M. Fèvre, and Mirjam EE Kretzschmar. Measuring underreporting and under-ascertainment in infectious disease datasets: a comparison of methods. *BMC Public Health*, 14(1):147, 2014.

[39] Alessandro Cassini, Edoardo Colzani, Alessandro Pini, Marie-Josee J Mangen, Dietrich Plass, Scott A McDonald, Guido Maringhini et al. Impact of infectious diseases on population health using incidence-based disability-adjusted life years (DALYs): Results from the burden of communicable diseases in Europe study, European Union and European economic area countries, 2009 to 2013. *Eurosurveillance*, 23(16):pii=17-00454, 2018.

[40] Robert S. Lanciotti, Olga L. Kosoy, Janeen J. Laven, Jason O. Velez, Amy J. Lambert, Alison J. Johnson, Stephanie M. Stanfield, and Mark R. Duffy. Genetic and serologic properties of Zika virus associated with an epidemic, Yap State, Micronesia, 2007. *Emerg. Infect. Dis.*, 14(8):1232–1239, 2008.

16

The Use of Seroprevalence Data to Estimate Cumulative Incidence of Infection

Benjamin J. Cowling and Jessica Y. Wong

CONTENTS

16.1   Introduction

One of the important uses of serologic studies is to allow estimation of the cumulative incidence of infections (CII) in a population, for example, during or after an epidemic of an emerging infectious disease. This situation is often extremely informative because the cases counted through clinical surveillance will only include a fraction of all of the infections that have occurred. While an effort might be made to extrapolate from confirmed cases to all infections, by making assumptions on the proportion of infections that lead to illness or medical attention, this method can be challenging in most populations. Serologic data provide a more straightforward source of information on the CII. In addition, serologic data can permit assessment of the potential susceptibility of the population to subsequent epidemics, and can be combined with data on severe cases to allow estimation of the severity of infections, as illustrated by the concept of the iceberg of disease (Figure 16.1). In this chapter, we focus on the use of serologic data to estimate the CII.

As a brief note on terminology, epidemiologists are generally careful in the technical usage of terms. The term "attack rate" is commonly used to refer to the CII, but is inappropriate for two reasons. First, most infectious diseases include mild or even asymptomatic infections, and not every infection causes acute clinical disease (an "attack"). In addition, we usually are interested in the cumulative (i.e., over a period of time) estimation of incidence, not the incidence rates, which may vary substantially, increasing and decreasing through an epidemic. It can be possible to estimate incidence rates in addition to cumulative incidence, but serologic studies generally aim to estimate cumulative incidence. Recognizing this, we prefer the term "cumulative incidence of infection".

As described in Chapter 14, humoral immune responses typically appear within a few weeks of an infection (or vaccination) and can be measured for months or even years after that infection (or vaccination). In some infected persons, there may a decay in the level of humoral immunity over time that may or may not correspond to a decay in the degree of

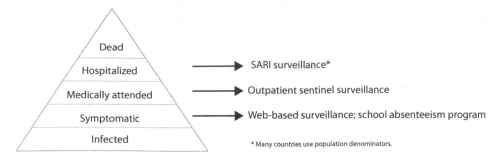

FIGURE 16.1

Left: iceberg of disease showing a large number of individuals infected (the base of the iceberg, often unobserved) while only a smaller number require hospitalization or die (tip of the iceberg, often observed). Right: examples of surveillance programs to capture the corresponding level of disease.

protection against reinfection. These humoral responses can be measured in sera extracted from peripheral blood samples. Figure 16.2 illustrates an epidemic of a new virus in terms of the incidence of infections in a population (the epidemic curve) shown in the upper panel, with the corresponding population seroprevalence of detectable antibodies shown in the lower panel. Note that the seroprevalence increases along with the cumulative number of infections, and reaches a peak soon after the end of the epidemic. In the medium-term there is a gradual decline in seroprevalence, shown on the right-hand side of the lower panel.

Figure 16.2 also indicates six different periods in which serologic samples might be collected, denoted A through F. Sera collected before the peak of the epidemic are classified as pre-epidemic sera (time period A or B in Figure 16.2a), and can provide information on pre-epidemic seroprevalence. Samples collected in period A would be preferable, but in some scenarios the epidemic will have already started before baseline samples can be collected [1]. Sera collected after the peak of the epidemic (time period D or E or F in Figure 16.2a) will provide the best information on post-epidemic seroprevalence. Collection of samples before the epidemic has ended, and while seroprevalence is still increasing (time period D in Figure 16.2a), could lead to underestimation of the total number of infections in the epidemic. Collection of samples relatively later after the end of the epidemic (time period F in Figure 16.2a) also could lead to underestimation of the total number of infections if waning in antibody titers in some infected people leads them to be misclassified as uninfected. These observations are summarized in Table 16.1.

If the pre-epidemic population seroprevalence is estimated as θ_1, and the post-epidemic population seroprevalence is estimated as θ_2, a basic estimate of the cumulative incidence of infection is given by $\theta_2 - \theta_1$. This basic estimate could be improved upon if information is available on (1) antibody dynamics following infection and (2) the timing of the epidemic in relation to sera collection, as will be elucidated in the following sections. If vaccines have been used, inference on the cumulative incidence of infection can be more complex, and this is discussed in the final section of this chapter.

There are various types of serologic study designs, and one basic distinction can be made between cross-sectional studies and longitudinal studies. In cross-sectional studies, sera are collected from a sample of the population, and in general the same person will not be sampled more than once. Cross-sectional studies can include collection of sera before, during, and/or after epidemics. Perhaps the simplest type of cross-sectional study is a study for a novel pathogen, with collection of sera after the epidemic (e.g., time period E in Figure 16.2),

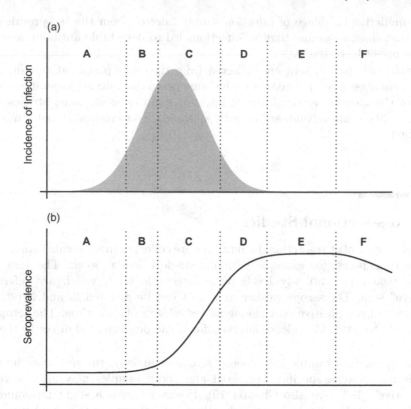

FIGURE 16.2

(a) Epidemic curve (incidence of infections) and periods when sera might be collected, described in more detail in Table 16.1. (b) Corresponding population seroprevalence over the same period of time. The time axis would vary for different diseases; for the first epidemic wave of a novel pandemic influenza virus the epidemic might last around 8 weeks, with serum antibody responses lagging infections by around 2–4 weeks.

TABLE 16.1

Various times of sera collection illustrated in Figure 16.2.

Time period	Timing of the epidemic	Notes
A	Before the start of the epidemic	Ideal pre-epidemic/baseline sera.
B	In the early part of the epidemic when transmission is increasing	Suboptimal pre-epidemic sera. May need to allow for early infections.
C	At the peak of the epidemic	Not preferable because seroprevalence is changing rapidly.
D	As transmission is declining	Suboptimal post-epidemic sera. It may take a few weeks after infection to develop detectable antibody.
E	The epidemic has just ended	Ideal post-epidemic sera.
F	Sometime after the end of the epidemic	Suboptimal post-epidemic sera if antibodies wane after infection.
		Waning may occur more quickly for some infections than others.

with the cumulative incidence of infection simply inferred from the seroprevalence in the sample at that time, assuming that all infections led to detectable antibody and that pre-epidemic seroprevalence was 0.

In longitudinal studies, sera are collected from the same people at two or more time points, with changes in seroprevalence in the same people permitting generally more precise estimates of the cumulative incidence of infection than cross-sectional studies of similar sample sizes. There are advantages of each approach, and cross-sectional studies will be discussed first.

16.2   Cross-sectional Studies

In the simplest type of cross-sectional study, sera are collected from members of a population at a single time point, for example within a single calendar week. The sera from this sample are tested for antibody levels at a detectable level, which are referred to as "seropositive" sera. The seroprevalence at time t can be denoted θ_t and is estimated by the proportion of seropositive sera among all tested sera at that time. The seroprevalence ranges from 0% to 100%. Confidence intervals for θ_t can be calculated direct by the binomial formula.

In some cases, for example in influenza seroepidemiology, the sera may be tested for antibody levels above a specified threshold and those samples may also be referred to as "seropositive" [1–3] (see also Chapter 19). However this is a slight misnomer because "seronegative" samples in which antibody titers are below that threshold may still have detectable antibody. Examples of seropositivity thresholds for various infections are shown in Table 16.2.

As with other types of cross-sectional studies, it is important that the tested sera are representative of the underlying population. This representation can be achieved in theory by random sampling, although in practice it is often challenging to build an appropriate sampling frame and successfully enroll a high proportion of randomly sampled individuals. Many serologic studies use opportunistic sampling, for example, residual sera from hospital

TABLE 16.2

"Seropositivity" thresholds used for different pathogens in the literature.

Pathogen	Threshold	Reference
Human influenza A(H1N1)pdm09	HI titer≥32, HI titer≥40, and MN titer≥40	Van Kerkhove et al. [1]
Avian influenza A(H5N1)	HI titer≥80 and MN titer≥20	Dung et al. [4]
Chlamydia trachomatis	ELISA≥0.57 to 1.95 OD units	Migchelsen et al. [5]
Parvovirus B19	ELISA≥3 OD units	Vyse et al. [6]
Rubella	ELISA≥10 IU	Hyde et al. [7]
Human papillomavirus type 16	ELISA≥0.05 OD units	Silverberg et al. [8]
Epstein-Barr virus	ELISA>0.1 OD unit	Maurmann et al. [9]

Abbreviation: HI = hemagglutination inhibition; MN = microneutralization; ELISA = enzyme linked immunosorben assay; IU = international units; OD = optical density.

laboratories or blood donors. In these studies, it can be important to use weights to ensure estimates are not skewed by a mismatch in age between the sample and the underlying population.

Cross-sectional studies may include samples drawn at multiple time points, or even continuous sampling. In the case of multiple samples, there will be multiple values of θ_t at different points in time. As an illustration of this, Figure 16.3 shows the estimates of seroprevalence of antibodies against influenza A(H2N2) in 1957–1958 in New York. These estimates were made by testing residual sera from the syphilis serology laboratory which received thousands of specimens per day from physicians across the city for prenatal, premarital, and diagnostic purposes. Sera collected between 20 September 1957 and 5 September 1958 and negative for syphilis were screened for antibodies to NYC/1/57 (Asian) influenza A(H2N2) by hemagglutination inhibition assay at a titration of 1:8, and are shown in comparison with the pneumonia and influenza deaths in New York over the same period [10] (Figure 16.3). In this illustration, the CII in the first wave was estimated to be around 35 percent.

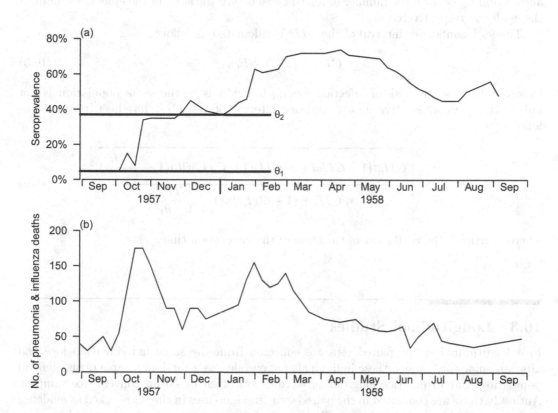

FIGURE 16.3
(a) Seroprevalence of antibodies against influenza A(H2N2) at titers of 1:8 or higher in weekly pools of residual sera. (b) Pneumonia and influenza deaths based on data extracted and redrawn for this illustration from Widelock et al. 1959 [10]. A clear rise in seroprevalence occurs towards the end of October 1957, corresponding to the first wave of A(H2N2) infections and deaths. A second rise occurs in February 1958, corresponding to the second wave of A(H2N2) infections and deaths. Waning in seroprevalence is also apparent between May and September 1958. An estimate of the cumulative incidence of infection based on pre-epidemic and post-epidemic seroprevalence is illustrated in (a).

When there are two samples, one before and one after the epidemic, the CII can be estimated as follows:

$$CII_c = \theta_2 - \theta_1 \qquad (16.1)$$

where θ_1 and θ_2 denote the seroprevalence before the start of the epidemic and after the epidemic respectively.

Their corresponding standard errors are often estimated based on the normal approximation to the binomial proportion, indicated by the following equations:

$$SE_1 = \sqrt{\theta_1(1 - \theta_1)/n_1} \qquad (16.2)$$

$$SE_2 = \sqrt{\theta_2(1 - \theta_2)/n_2} \qquad (16.3)$$

$$SE_{CII} = \sqrt{SE_1^2 + SE_2^2} \qquad (16.4)$$

where SE_1, SE_2 and SE_{CII} denotes the standard error for the θ_1, θ_2, and CII, respectively, and n_1 and n_2 denotes the number of tested cases before the start of the epidemic and after the epidemic respectively.

The 95% confidence interval of the $CIIc$ is calculated as follows:

$$CII_c \pm 1.96 \times SE_{CII} \qquad (16.5)$$

However, because the risk of infection among individuals in the same population is not independent, an alternative 95% confidence interval of the CII_c has been proposed as follows [3]:

$$CII_c \pm 1.96 \times \sqrt{\frac{CII_c^3(1 - CII_c) + \gamma^2 CII_c(1 - CII_c)^2[ln(1 - \frac{CII_c}{1 - \theta_1})]^2}{n[CII_c + (1 - CII_c)ln(1 - \frac{CII_c}{1 - \theta_1})]^2}} \qquad (16.6)$$

where γ denotes the coefficient of variation of the generation time.

16.3 Longitudinal Studies

In a longitudinal study, paired sera are collected from the same individuals before and after an epidemic. Ideally, these individuals are enrolled as a random sample of the general population, but in practice longitudinal studies are often based on convenience samples. Antibody titers are compared in the paired sera, and increases in titers are taken as evidence of recent infection (or vaccination). To allow for measurement error in titers and increase specificity, many studies specify a minimum rise to be counted as evidence of infection. For influenza, this is typically a 4-fold or greater rise in titer [11]. The CII of a longitudinal study (CII_{long}) in the population is calculated as the proportion of participants having a rise in antibody titer that meets the relevant criteria.

The 95% confidence interval of the CII_{long} is calculated as follows:

$$CII_{long} \pm 1.96 \times SE_{long} \qquad (16.7)$$

$$SE_{long} = \sqrt{CII_{long}(1 - CII_{long})/n} \qquad (16.8)$$

where SE_{long} denotes the standard error for the CII, and n denotes the number of paired sera.

Riley et al. [12] estimated the CII of H1N1pdm09 in Hong Kong in 2009 retrospectively from paired serologic data of a cohort of households. First, they defined individuals as conversions as at least 4-fold increase in antibody titer in paired sera. Then, they estimated CII as the proportion of converted between baseline and follow-up.

A challenge of this study design is that serologic data collected do not bracket the epidemic (i.e., collection of sera after the start and/or before the end of the epidemic). Tsang et al. [13] estimated the CII of H1N1pdm09 in 2009 from local influenza surveillance data and paired serologic data in Hong Kong in 2009 using a 3-level Bayesian hierarchical model which accounted for non-bracketing.

16.4   Childhood Diseases

In additional to estimate cumulative incidence of infection of various epidemic diseases, serologic data also can be valuable in determining the dynamics of common childhood infections. In these cases, rather than examining seroprevalence before and after an epidemic, seroprevalence is examined by calendar age. Understanding this age-specific infection information can help in informing control measures and vaccination programs.

Measles is a highly infectious disease, which is characterized by symptoms including fever and rash. Unvaccinated children are at the highest risk of being infected when compared with adults. To illustrate this finding, Farrington and colleagues [14] obtained age-specific seroprevalence data for mumps in the UK between November 1986 and December 1987, before the introduction of routine vaccination with the combined measles, mumps and rubella vaccine (Figure 16.4). These data were used to estimate the cumulative incidence of infection by age. Almost all children had been infected by the age of around 10 years.

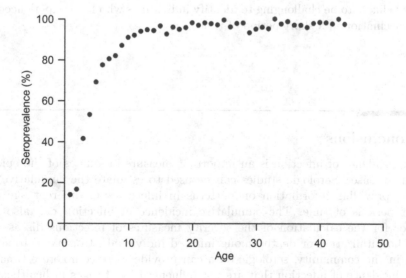

FIGURE 16.4
Seroprevalence of mumps in the United Kingdom 1986–1987 by age based on data extracted from [14, 15] and redrawn.

16.5   Accounting for Vaccination in Serologic Studies

In serologic studies, it can be challenging to distinguish antibodies that are a result of vaccination versus antibodies that are a result of natural infection [16]. If the aim of the study is to determine levels of protective antibodies regardless of whether they occurred as a result of vaccination or infection, there is no problem, and the prevalence of antibodies could be used to estimate the level of immunity in the population. However, it is often the case that we would like to estimate specifically the incidence of natural infections. Ideally, vaccination history would be recorded and included in the analytic dataset, so that analysis could be stratified by vaccination status. Cumulative incidence of infections in unvaccinated individuals then could be estimated as described earlier in this chapter. However, in vaccinated individuals it can be difficult to determine whether they have also been infected, particularly in cross-sectional serologic studies. If the epidemic period occurs after the vaccination period, and paired sera are collected to cover the epidemic period but some time after the vaccinations, it may be possible to identify infections provided that serologic responses are strong enough to detect. In influenza, serologic responses to infection can be reduced in vaccinated individuals, partly because of longer term declines in antibody titers after vaccination [17].

It is more challenging to analyze serologic data if vaccination history is unknown. One example of this is using blood bank studies, or residual blood samples from hospital laboratories, when age and sex are recorded but vaccination history may not be recorded [2, 18]. In some scenarios, it may be possible to identify vaccinations based on the characteristics of the antibody titers. For example, in studies of hepatitis B, the presence of antibody only against the surface protein indicates that the individual has been vaccinated, whereas the presence of antibody to the core protein as well indicates that the individual has been naturally infected [16]. In influenza, because vaccines are trivalent or quadrivalent and generate rises in antibody titers against multiple strains, but infections occur with one particular strain and generally only increase titers against that infecting strain, it may be possible to distinguish infections from vaccinations using a multivariate inferential model. However, it is likely to be challenging to identify individuals who have experienced infection as well as vaccination in a short period of time.

16.6   Conclusions

Cumulative incidence of infection is an important measure in studies of the epidemiology of infectious diseases. Serologic studies can be used to estimate the cumulative incidence of infection, providing information on patterns in infections in different age groups or in different periods of time. The cumulative incidence of infection can also provide a denominator for the calculation of the severity measures of infectious disease including the risk of hospitalization or death among infected individuals. Compared to surveillance of illnesses in the community, serologic data can provide more complete estimates of the cumulative incidence of infection that are not influenced by changes in healthcare-seeking behavior, and capturing mild and subclinical infections [19]. However, it can be difficult to collect blood samples, and serological studies typically require particular laboratory capacity and expertise.

References

[1] Maria D Van Kerkhove, Siddhivinayak Hirve, Artemis Koukounari, and Anthony W Mounts. Estimating age-specific cumulative incidence for the 2009 influenza pandemic: A meta-analysis of a (H1N1) pdm09 serological studies from 19 countries. *Influenza and Other Respiratory Viruses*, 7(5):872–886, 2013.

[2] Joseph T Wu, Andrew Ho, Edward SK Ma, Cheuk Kwong Lee, Daniel KW Chu, Po-Lai Ho et al. Estimating infection attack rates and severity in real time during an influenza pandemic: Analysis of serial cross-sectional serologic surveillance data. *PLoS Medicine*, 8(10):e1001103, 2011.

[3] Hiroshi Nishiura, Gerardo Chowell, and Carlos Castillo-Chavez. Did modeling overestimate the transmission potential of pandemic (H1N1-2009)? Sample size estimation for post-epidemic seroepidemiological studies. *Plos One*, 6(3):e17908, 2011.

[4] Tham Chi Dung, Pham Ngoc Dinh, Vu Sinh Nam, Luong Minh Tan, Nguyen Le Khanh Hang, Le Thi Thanh, and Le Quynh Mai. Seroprevalence survey of avian influenza a (h5n1) among live poultry market workers in northern Viet nam, 2011. *Western Pacific Surveillance and Response Journal: WPSAR*, 5(4):21, 2014.

[5] Stephanie J Migchelsen, Diana L Martin, Khamphoua Southisombath, Patrick Turyaguma, Anne Heggen, Peter Paul Rubangakene et al. Defining seropositivity thresholds for use in trachoma elimination studies. *PLoS Neglected Tropical Diseases*, 11(1):e0005230, 2017.

[6] Andrew J Vyse, Nick J Andrews, Louise M Hesketh, and Richard Pebody. The burden of parvovirus b19 infection in women of childbearing age in England and Wales. *Epidemiology & Infection*, 135(8):1354–1362, 2007.

[7] Terri B Hyde, Deanna Kruszon-Moran, Geraldine M McQuillan, Cynthia Cossen, Bagher Forghani, and Susan E Reef. Rubella immunity levels in the United States population: Has the threshold of viral elimination been reached? *Clinical Infectious Diseases*, 43(Supplement_3):S146–S150, 2006.

[8] Michael J Silverberg, Michael F Schneider, Barbara Silver, Kathryn M Anastos, Robert D Burk, Howard Minkoff, Joel Palefsky, Alexandra M Levine, and Raphael P Viscidi. Serological detection of human papillomavirus type 16 infection in human immunodeficiency virus (HIV)-positive and high-risk HIV-negative women. *Clinical and Vaccine Immunology*, 13(4):511–519, 2006.

[9] Susanne Maurmann, Lutz Fricke, Hans-Joachim Wagner, Peter Schlenke, Holger Hennig, Jürgen Steinhoff, and Wolfram J Jabs. Molecular parameters for precise diagnosis of asymptomatic Epstein-Barr virus reactivation in healthy carriers. *Journal of Clinical Microbiology*, 41(12):5419–5428, 2003.

[10] Daniel Widelock, Sarah Klein, Olga Simonovic, and Lenore R Peizer. A laboratory analysis of the 1957–1958 influenza outbreak in New York City. II. A seroepidemiological study. *American Journal of Public Health and the Nations Health*, 49(7):847–856, 1959.

[11] Simon Cauchemez, Peter Horby, Annette Fox, Pham Quang Thai, Nguyen Tran Hien, Neil M Ferguson et al. Influenza infection rates, measurement errors and the interpretation of paired serology. *PLoS Pathogens*, 8(12):e1003061, 2012.

[12] Steven Riley, Kin O Kwok, Kendra M Wu, Danny Y Ning, Benjamin J Cowling, Joseph T Wu et al. Epidemiological characteristics of 2009 (H1N1) pandemic influenza based on paired sera from a longitudinal community cohort study. *PLoS Medicine*, 8(6):e1000442, 2011.

[13] Tim K Tsang, Vicky J Fang, Ranawaka APM Perera, Dennis KM Ip, Gabriel M Leung, Joseph S Malik Peiris, Simon Cauchemez, and Benjamin J Cowling. Interpreting sero-epidemiological studies for influenza in a context of non-bracketing sera. *Epidemiology (Cambridge, Mass.)*, 27(1):152, 2016.

[14] C Paddy Farrington, Mona N Kanaan, Nigel J Gay. Estimation of the basic reproduction number for infectious diseases from age-stratified serological survey data. *Journal of the Royal Statistical Society: Series C (Applied Statistics)*, 50(3):251–292, 2001.

[15] Heather J Whitaker and C Paddy Farrington. Estimation of infectious disease parameters from serological survey data: The impact of regular epidemics. *Statistics in Medicine*, 23(15):2429–2443, 2004.

[16] C Jessica E Metcalf, Jeremy Farrar, Felicity T Cutts, Nicole E Basta, Andrea L Graham, Justin Lessler, Neil M Ferguson, Donald S Burke, and Bryan T Grenfell. Use of serological surveys to generate key insights into the changing global landscape of infectious disease. *Lancet*, 388(10045):728–730, 2016.

[17] Joshua G Petrie, Suzanne E Ohmit, Emileigh Johnson, Rachel T Cross, and Arnold S Monto. Efficacy studies of influenza vaccines: Effect of end points used and characteristics of vaccine failures. *Journal of Infectious Diseases*, 203(9):1309–1315, 2011.

[18] Elizabeth Miller, Katja Hoschler, Pia Hardelid, Elaine Stanford, Nick Andrews, and Maria Zambon. Incidence of 2009 pandemic influenza a H1N1 infection in England: A cross-sectional serological study. *Lancet*, 375(9720):1100–1108, 2010.

[19] Vernon J Lee, Mark I Chen, Jonathan Yap, Jocelyn Ong, Wei-Yen Lim, Raymond T P Lin et al. Comparability of different methods for estimating influenza infection rates over a single epidemic wave. *American Journal of Epidemiology*, 174(4):468–478, 2011.

17

The Analysis of Serological Data with Transmission Models

Marc Baguelin

CONTENTS

17.1 Interpreting Serological Data in the Light of Disease Transmission

The involvement of at least three complex competing biological processes occurring in parallel renders serological data difficult to interpret. The first process is the continuous change of health status among the individuals in the host population. This change may result from disease transmission where susceptible individuals become infected following contacts with other infected individuals and then (potentially) recover to become immune, but also potentially involve other demographical/sociological processes such as, e.g., aging, spatial movement, economic status, or change of behaviors. The second process is the immunodynamics. The immune systems of the hosts "memorize" some features of past infections and immunizations to protect the host from future infection. Finally, the third process is the genetic evolution of the pathogen population. Pathogen genomes accumulate mutations during replication in the host. The mutations are filtered out during transmission between hosts or through selection pressure. A schematic of the interaction between pathogen evolution, epidemiology of the host, and immunodynamics is given in Figure 17.1.

Although each of these processes might be important for interpreting serological data, no modeling framework can embed all the complexity of the disease ecosystem, and as such models have to rely on simplifying assumptions. We will be considering in this chapter variations of the so-called SIR model (for Susceptible-Infectious-Recovered).

In its original and most simple form (see Equation 17.1), the SIR model, proposed by Kermack and McKendrick in 1927 [2], abstracts the host population in two health states (with or without disease) and two immunity states (protected or susceptible) leading to three classes (or compartments):

- x or S, the susceptible group, not protected but healthy,

- y or I, the infectious group, protected but with disease,

- z or R, the removed group, protected and without disease (whether recovered and back to "normal" health or dead).

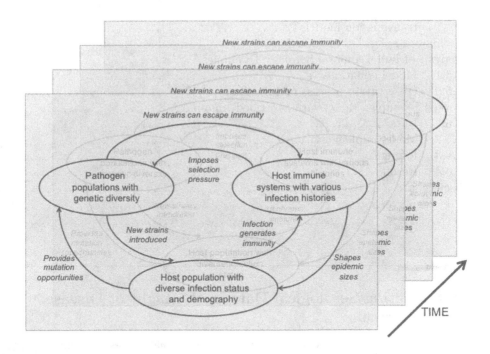

FIGURE 17.1

Disease dynamics result from a complex interaction between pathogen and host populations, and the immune systems of the hosts. These three components of this ecosystem constantly evolve with time. The variation of infectious status in the host population constitutes epidemics, the change of diversity in the pathogen population is genetic evolution, and the changes in the immune systems constitute immunodynamics. Models can reduce the complexity of the system by assuming some of these components to be time invariant. Figure adapted from Kucharski and Baguelin [1].

No evolutionary traits are included. This is thus a very parsimonious model:

$$\left. \begin{array}{rcl} \dfrac{dx}{dt} &=& -\kappa xy \\[2mm] \dfrac{dy}{dt} &=& \kappa xy - ly \\[2mm] \dfrac{dz}{dt} &=& ly \end{array} \right\} \tag{17.1}$$

with $x + y + z = N$, the size of the population given in absolute numbers, and κ and l two constants.

The protected individuals in the R class permanently escape infections and do not revert to the susceptible S class. They are assumed to remain indefinitely immune or dead. This binary structure of immunity often is equated to a bimodal nature of antibody titer distributions found in a population. A common mental representation is that individuals have either low or high levels of antibody and there exists a "correlate of protection," a threshold value at which it can be considered that an individual switches from susceptibility to protection.

Another version of the SIR model, probably more relevant to analyze serological data, can be found in Hens et al. [3]. This more general model builds on the classical model given in the Equation system (17.1) but integrates further biological processes. In particular, the equations include an aging component (as partial derivatives with respect to age a) and a natural death rate $\mu(a)$. The force of infection $\lambda(a,t)$ can follow the mass action principle (i.e., being proportional to the proportion of the infectious population $I(a,t)$) or another more appropriate form. The recovery rate ν is equivalent to l in the system of Equations (17.1). The initial conditions $S(a,0) = \tilde{S}(a)$, $I(a,0) = \tilde{I}(a)$, and $R(a,0) = \tilde{R}(a)$ are functions of the age a. $S(0,t) = B(t)$ represents the number of newborns at time t.

We have chosen to present this model rather than the traditional model to show the concurrent structure of time and age variation in the population. One way of representing this dual dynamic is by using a set of partial differential equations:

$$\left\{ \begin{array}{rcl} \dfrac{\partial S(a,t)}{\partial a} + \dfrac{\partial S(a,t)}{\partial t} &=& -(\lambda(a,t) + \mu(a))S(a,t), \\[3mm] \dfrac{\partial I(a,t)}{\partial a} + \dfrac{\partial I(a,t)}{\partial t} &=& \lambda(a,t)S(a,t) - (\nu + \mu(a))I(a,t), \\[3mm] \dfrac{\partial R(a,t)}{\partial a} + \dfrac{\partial R(a,t)}{\partial t} &=& \nu I(a,t) - \mu(a)R(a,t), \end{array} \right. \tag{17.2}$$

where a is the age of individuals in the population and t is time. $S(a)$, $I(a)$, and $R(a)$ are thus functions of time giving the evolution over time of the proportions in the modeled population of susceptible, infected and recovered individuals, respectively.

Most of the mathematical analysis of serological data is done using models where the time derivative is removed by assuming endemic equilibrium. Patterns observed in the age distribution of the serological profile of the relevant antibodies can be explained by an age-dependent-only force of infection $\lambda(a)$. In contrast, most outbreak data is analyzed using models where the age derivative is removed by assuming whether

1. The period considered is short and thus that the population is not aging.

2. The model can be broken down into discrete age classes, and can be run sequentially, with all individuals aging together from one season to the other.

The time derivative in the case of an outbreak is essential to capture the dynamics of diseases transmission.

There are a number of situations where it is necessary to link serological data with outbreak data and/or disease dynamics. We want to show in this chapter that, in such situations, transmission models can help interpret serology. This method is particularly relevant in the context of public health when serological surveillance can be used to inform prediction and control of the disease dynamics. Examples of use of transmission modes alongside serology is given in the case of the calculation of secondary attack rates in households (Section 17.2), the prediction of the potential for large outbreaks (Section 17.3), or the tracking in real-time of the course of an epidemic (Section 17.4).

We also want to show that the traditional SIR type of models do not fully exploit the information provided by serological data and that a new type of model including a representation of stratified immunity as measured by serology can be developed and fitted to data. In Section 17.5 of this chapter, we present such a model where stratified immunity is incorporated into the model structure. We develop it further into a worked example and code (Section 17.6).

17.2   Final Size—Household Model

Historically, serology has been used as a way of providing an infection attack rate against specific pathogens during a certain time window (see Chapter 16). It has been in particular seen as a way of observing the circulation of pathogens directly in the community rather than through the attendance at healthcare services (e.g., general practices or hospitalization). To measure a serological attack rate (SAR), households with one initial index case need typically to be recruited and sera collected from household members at the beginning and the end of the period of study.

A naive way of interpreting the resulting serological data is to compute SAR directly from these data as follows:

$$\text{SAR} = \frac{\text{No. of infected household members} - 1}{\text{No. of initial susceptible household members} - 1} \times 100$$

with the numerator, the number of infected household members derived from a case definition, typically a certain magnitude rise between the early and late paired sera collections. For example, for influenza, a fourfold antibody titer rise is considered a marker of infection. The denominator also can be derived from the baseline sera, assuming that individuals are susceptible below an agreed threshold.

Additionally to these relatively crude assumption on infection and susceptibility, the implicit additional assumption is made that none of the new infections can be attributed to a reintroduction from outside of the household and that all the secondary cases were infected by the index case rather than being potential tertiary or quaternary infections.

17.2.1   The 1982 Longini and Koopman model of secondary attack rates

Early in the history of computer simulations, transmission models have been proposed as tools to infer how much of the transmission can be attributed to community transmission and chains of transmission inside the household. In their seminal work, Longini at al. [4] use data gathered between 1975 and 1979 for two studies, the Tecumseh Respiratory Illness Study and the Seattle flu study. The authors' objective was to derive the "true" SAR for influenza in the community and compare the transmission potential of B, A/H1N1, and A/H3N2 virus strains.

Longini and Koopman first developed their approach in [5] based on theoretical results from the final size distributions of epidemics derived by Ludwig [6]. These results permit removal of time from the equations modeling transmission and are thus particularly suited for serological data that do not provide any information about timing of infection. We will sketch here the results from Longini and Koopman; all of the technical details from their modeling approach can be found in [5].

The final size of an epidemic involving households can be computed by solving the following system of recursive equations:

$$m_{jk} = \binom{k}{j} m_{jj} B^{k-j} Q^{j(k-1)}, \quad j < k \tag{17.3}$$

and

$$m_{kk} = 1 - \sum_{j=0}^{k-1} m_{jk}.$$

where m_{jk} is the probability that at the end of the epidemics there are j infected among k initial susceptible individuals at the start of the epidemics, B is the probability that a susceptible individual is not infected from the community during the observation period, and Q is the probability that a susceptible person in a household escapes infectious contacts from an infected household member during their entire infectiousness period.

Let a_{jk} be the observed frequencies of households with j infected from k original susceptibles. Given serological data of the form a_{jk} the likelihood of the parameter B and Q of the model is given by

$$L(Q, B) = \prod_k \prod_j m_{jk}^{a_{jk}},$$

which can be merged with (17.3) and written in log form:

$$\ln L = c + \sum_k \sum_j a_{jk} \{\ln m_{jj} + (k-j) \ln B + j(k-j) \ln Q\},$$

with c a constant term which does not depend on Q and B, the parameters of the model.

The maximum-likelihood (ML) estimator then can be found by differentiating $\ln L$ with respect to Q and B. Thus, the ML estimators of $\hat{Q}$ and $\hat{B}$ are given by the solution of

$$0 = \left.\frac{\partial \ln L}{\partial Q}\right|_{\hat{Q},\hat{B}} = \sum_k \sum_j a_{jk} \left\{ \frac{1}{m_{jj}} \left(\frac{\partial m_{jj}}{\partial Q} \right) + \frac{j(k-j)}{Q} \right\},$$

$$0 = \left.\frac{\partial \ln L}{\partial B}\right|_{\hat{Q},\hat{B}} = \sum_k \sum_j a_{jk} \left\{ \frac{1}{m_{jj}} \left(\frac{\partial m_{jj}}{\partial B} \right) + \frac{(k-j)}{B} \right\}.$$

which can be solved numerically.

17.2.2   Some more modern development of interpreting paired sera

As shown in this section, the interpretation of paired sera to derive SARs is challenging as it is necessary to disentangle SARs from reinfections from the community and chains of transmission inside the household. Another complication is the potential bias introduced by the seroconversion algorithm used to detect past infections. Traditionally, the value chosen to confirm infection is chosen to be sufficiently specific and thus avoid false positives. While this selection makes sense at an individual level in order to confirm infection, at a population level, in the setting of a survey, it has the potential to bias estimation by rejecting low increases of antibody which can be both measurement error and genuine antibody increase (e.g., a two-fold increase for influenza hemagglutination inhibition (HI) assays). A rigorous but more involved way of removing such bias is to model the measurement error as part of the estimation process. Using Bayesian techniques, it then is possible to estimate the probability that a rise in titer is due to infection or to a measurement error [7].

The attraction of serology to measure the burden of disease in the community resides in its ability to obtain pathogen specific estimates unbiased by clinical presentation. However, this method is at the price of several hurdles, including logistic challenges as most of serological tests involve taking blood samples from a large number of individuals, ethical considerations, especially for younger children and other persons who are not competent to give consent, or costs as immunological assays are potentially expensive and time consuming. As a consequence, serology to study transmission in the community has been replaced increasingly by syndromic surveillance coupled with regular swabbing and testing for a particular pathogen by RT-PCR. Surveillance based on genetic sequencing is less invasive and provides more specific information about the pathogen [8]. The development of non-invasive immunological tests, such as based on oral fluids (used, e.g., during the West African 2014–2016 ebola outbreak [9]) might provide in the near future an easier way of integrating serology-like tests as a tool for routine surveillance.

Although the analysis of serological data using transmission models and sophisticated statistical methods of linking model parameters with observations (or observation models) has improved our understanding of immune response as measured by serological assays, much remains to be done regarding interpreting cross reactivity (immune response of an individual exposed to a different but closely related pathogen [1, 10–12]). Another challenge for the interpretation of serology is to develop methods (whether in terms of assays or statistical tools based of several data sources) to distinguish between immune response induced by vaccination and natural infection [13].

17.3   Serology as Background Immunity

Most epidemic diseases are modulated by the existing remanent immunity in the host population. This remanent immunity is a result of past infections from previous epidemics or from earlier immunization campaigns. Using the terminology of an age-stratified SIR modeling framework, this means that the age profile of the final number of cases (in terms of size and distribution) will depend on the distribution of susceptible and protected individuals in each age group at the start of the outbreak. This "immunity landscape" constantly changes over time following the dynamics of infection in the population, potential recurring immunization campaigns, the waning of antibodies present in the population, the drift of the pathogen, and the renewal of the susceptible cohort through birth and death.

As a result of these changes, a controlled disease ($R \ll 1$) can resurge progressively. This risk of a resurgence can develop in a relatively short period of time, especially in the case of a disease with a high basic reproduction number R_0 or a fast evolving pathogen. To monitor the potential for resurgence of a particular disease and decide which age group to target, serological surveillance has been implemented for some vaccine-preventable diseases with a high R_0 (e.g., measles [14]) and/or potential complications linked with acquisition at an older age (e.g., rubella [15] which can cause congenital rubella syndrome or miscarriage if contracted during early pregnancy). Setting up serobanks is challenging and therefore not used as widely in human epidemiology as it is for its veterinary counterpart. Despite these potential difficulties, there are increasing calls to set up a global surveillance through a World Serology bank [16]. The issue is that serology alone is difficult to interpret and thus need to be harnessed with the predictive power of transmission modeling.

17.3.1   The 1994 measles catch-up campaign in England

Measles is one of the most highly contagious human infections. When, in 1968, vaccination first became available in England, measles was causing an estimated 100 deaths annually, with entire birth cohorts rapidly becoming infected. However, due to an initial low coverage, high endemic transmission continued. In 1988, a new vaccine was introduced with higher coverage protecting against measles, mumps and rubella (MMR). As a result of these campaigns, measles transmission nearly stopped and notifications were in 1993 at their lowest historical levels [14].

However, because of the interrupted transmission associated with the new vaccine, a cohort of susceptibles had started building up from individuals who had not been immunized by the new program and were not exposed to natural infection anymore. These type of dynamical phenomena had been predicted by mathematical modeling as a consequence of mass vaccination [17] and had triggered the setting up of a serological surveillance program. As predicted, the sera collected in 1991 for routine surveillance were showing a significant increase in levels of susceptibility detected over a 5-year period (see Figure 17.2). The question was raised of the potential resurgence of a large outbreak of measles in the coming years.

In a pioneering work [18], Gay et al. used the serological surveillance data from the 1991 season in England in conjunction with a mathematical model to demonstrate that large outbreaks of measles would be expected if a catch-up immunization campaign was not initiated. As a result of this study a large catch-up campaign was launched in November 1994 [19], in which 92 percent of children aged 5–16 years were vaccinated [20].

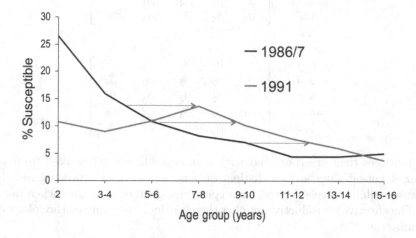

FIGURE 17.2
Proportion of children susceptible to measles in 1986/7 and 1991 as measured by serological surveillance in England. Samples were tested by haemagglutination inhibition (HI). Titers ≥ 8 were considered positive; titers < 4 negative. Samples with titers $= 4$ were retested with enzyme-linked immunosorbent assay (ELISA) and categorized according to ELISA results [18]. The ageing of a birth cohort less vaccinated and not exposed to natural infection raises the question of a potential resurgence of large outbreaks of measles when this cohort reaches school age. (Graph courtesy of Professor Elisabeth Miller)

To demonstrate the likely resurgence of large outbreaks of measles, Gay and co-authors calculated the effective reproduction number under different assumptions of the structure of contacts (referred to as mixing) in the population. These mixing matrices were fitted to pre-vaccination case notification data in England and Wales from 1956 to 1965.

Gay and co-authors built their analysis on two then recently developed techniques, the Who Acquired Infection From Whom (WAIFW) matrices [21] and techniques to calculate reproductive numbers from a heterogeneously mixing model [22]. Given the number of uncertain parameters resulting in particular from the 5×5 mixing matrix, the authors relied on "epidemiogical arguments" to explore a wide variety of scenarios. For example, for the transmission matrix, two options are explored. Option 1 is based on a matrix from the literature whose shape was largely determined for mathematical convenience in terms of derivation of the matrix components from case notifications (matrix (17.4) below). Gay and co-authors propose to use also a second form of matrix with more details in the structure of contacts in the school children age band (i.e., 5- to 14-year-old) as more epidemiologically plausible. They argue that contacts in 10- to 14-year-olds are likely to be higher that for the 5- to 9-year-old children and that as a result the level of contact within the 10- to 14-year-old age group (key in term of resurgence of measles as this cohort had a lower vaccination coverage) should be considered higher than in the 5- to 9-year-old by a factor $\alpha > 1$ varied in the exploration of scenarios (matrix 17.5). More direct derivation of α was not possible from available pre-vaccination notification data as due to the epidemiology of measles, too few cases in the 10- to 14-age group were present as almost all children were infected at an earlier age.

$$
\begin{array}{c}
\begin{array}{cccccc}
\text{Age Group} & 0-1 & 2-4 & 5-9 & 10-14 & 15+
\end{array} \\
\begin{array}{c}
0-1 \\ 2-4 \\ 5-9 \\ 10-14 \\ 15+
\end{array}
\left[
\begin{array}{ccccc}
\beta_1 & \beta_1 & \beta_1 & \beta_4 & \beta_5 \\
\beta_1 & \beta_2 & \beta_2 & \beta_4 & \beta_5 \\
\beta_1 & \beta_2 & \beta_3 & \beta_4 & \beta_5 \\
\beta_4 & \beta_4 & \beta_4 & \beta_4 & \beta_5 \\
\beta_5 & \beta_5 & \beta_5 & \beta_5 & \beta_5
\end{array}
\right]
\end{array}
\tag{17.4}
$$

$$
\begin{array}{c}
\begin{array}{cccccc}
\text{Age Group} & 0-1 & 2-4 & 5-9 & 10-14 & 15+
\end{array} \\
\begin{array}{c}
0-1 \\ 2-4 \\ 5-9 \\ 10-14 \\ 15+
\end{array}
\left[
\begin{array}{ccccc}
\beta_1 & \beta_1 & \beta_1 & \beta_1 & \beta_5 \\
\beta_1 & \beta_2 & \beta_2 & \beta_2 & \beta_5 \\
\beta_1 & \beta_2 & \beta_3 & \beta_4 & \beta_5 \\
\beta_1 & \beta_2 & \beta_4 & \alpha\beta_3 & \beta_5 \\
\beta_5 & \beta_5 & \beta_5 & \beta_5 & \beta_5
\end{array}
\right]
\end{array}
\tag{17.5}
$$

These matrices then are combined with a susceptibility level derived from serological data (using a cut-off threshold to distinguish susceptible from protected individuals) or plausible susceptibility levels derived from epidemiological assumptions when data was not available. The effective reproductive number then is calculated using methodology developed in Diekmann et al. [22].

The analysis shows that in many scenarios, the effective reproductive number would exceed 1 in the next 2 years, which would likely trigger large outbreaks in England. The final size of these predicted outbreaks is derived by doubling the number of cases necessary to bring the effective number back to 1 (thus assuming symmetry of the incidence curve during the pre- and post-peak periods).

This work predates the use of contact survey data as a proxy for intensity of transmission in a heterogeneously mixing population [23]. Since then, a number of studies have shown that contact surveys can help to elucidate the spread of infectious disease and that it is possible to fit the transmission matrix by fitting one parameter assuming that the intensity of transmission between age groups is proportional to measured contacts (the "social contact hypothesis") [24, 25]. More work also has been done trying to improve linkage between antibody titers and reduced risk of infection (see Section 17.3.2) and many difficulties remain as briefly discussed in Section 17.3.3.

17.3.2   Correlate of protection and cross-reaction

An important step into the interpretation of serological data as baseline immunity for a transmission model is to translate a measured antibody titer into a susceptibility/protected status with respect to risk of infection from the disease. The most simple (and widely used) approach is to use a threshold value which splits individuals between susceptible (for the individuals having lower titer than the threshold) and protected (for the individuals with titers equal to or above the threshold, see Chapter 19). Although convenient to map data into the SIR scheme, as noted by Longini et al. [4] this approach is somewhat arbitrary and in any case simplistic. While individuals with no antibodies generally become infected if challenged and individuals with very high titers usually are protected, individuals with intermediate levels of antibody titers might or might not develop the disease with a probability inversely related to titer.

Dunning [26] designed a probability model linking an individual measured titer with the increased risk for this individual of developing a disease during a certain period of observation (typically during a vaccine trial). The probability $P_{\text{disease}}(T)$ of developing a disease during a given period of time is given by

$$P_{\text{disease}}(T) = \lambda(1 - \pi(T)), \tag{17.6}$$

where λ is the probability for a fully susceptible individual to develop this disease during the given period and $\pi(T)$ is a scaled logit model of the protection conferred by antibodies:

$$\pi(T) = \frac{1}{1 + e^{-(\alpha + \beta T)}} \tag{17.7}$$

with T the titer of protective antibodies (in log scale) of the considered individual, α and β the parameters of the logit model.

Although the model proposed by Dunning has been applied to several pathogens (pertussis [26] and enterovirus 71 [27], for example), most citations referring to the work to date are related to influenza viruses [24, 29, 30].

17.3.3   Difficulties with integrating background immunity into transmission models

As seen in Section 17.3.1, while deriving the impact in terms of resurgence is challenging, the interpretation of serology as susceptibility is relatively direct for stable pathogens like measles [31] with life-long induced immunity following infection. For other viruses, with fast evolving antigenic properties, the derivation of immunity from serology is hampered by cross reactivity. Indeed, an individual can present the same titer against a given strain of virus following, e.g., exposure to that particular strain with a weak rise of titer, exposure to a related strain with strong cross-reaction, or vaccination with an inactivated form of the tested virus. Due to the complex and multi-dimensional nature of immunity, one assay only is thus unlikely to provide a sufficient statistic for deriving protection. Understanding how immunity measured by different assays enables reconstruction of the past infection history and prediction of future protection against cross reacting strains is an area of active research [1, 10, 11, 32].

Serology also can be used as part of more complex models in an evidence synthesis framework where it can provide a prior distribution for the immunity landscape. The structure of the SIR model implies that, when fitting a time series of cases from surveillance data, estimation of the background immunity, the proportion of undetected cases (e.g., asymptomatic), and the basic reproduction number will be correlated and renders the reconstruction of the disease dynamics difficult. Serology thus can be used to derived a prior distribution for the susceptibility profile in the population (using, e.g., Dunning's model with a pathogen-specific study like the Coudeville's [29] for influenza). Such an approach has been used by several authors in the context of pandemic and seasonal influenza [28, 33, 34].

Complications in interpreting data linked to cross reactivity increases with the history of multiple infections and vaccination in the host population. One case thus where most of the conditions for using serology might be considered optimal is the case of emerging or newly circulating pathogens. With no pre-existing vaccination, no previous infections history, only potential cross-reactive immunity can interfere with the interpretation of serology. During the 2009 A/H1N1 pandemic in England, background serology was used to provide an estimate of background immunity for a real-time transmission and economical model measuring the impact of potential vaccination policies [35]. The transmission model in turn helped validate a contemporaneous cross-sectional serological survey [36].

17.4　Serology as a Tracker of Infection

The two previous historical examples (Sections 17.2 and 17.3.1) of using serology with transmission models were taking advantage of theoretical results allowing the removal of time from the dynamical equations representing transmission. Longini and co-authors et al. (Section 17.2) compares observations with theoretical derivation of the final size from household transmission models, while Gay and co-authors (Section 17.3.1) use the threshold value of the initial effective reproduction number. None of these models use the potential information from temporal patterns of sequential serological data.

National public agencies routinely use syndromic surveillance to monitor the circulation of infectious diseases. This surveillance relies on the collection of health-related data mainly from patients seeking care. Often these proxy measurements do not capture the entirety of all the ongoing infections in the community. In addition, these quantities are partially dependent on individual behaviors that might vary during an epidemic or between seasons. Serology on the contrary is a direct and potentially unbiased measure of biological markers that only depends on the antibody dynamics in the host following infection.

Thus, the change of seroprevalence with time is a function of current seroprevalence in the population and the ongoing transmission occuring in the population. Sequential sera can thus be used alongside hospitalization cases to track the course of infection and potentially infer the influenza infection attack rate [37].

The relationship between the evolution over time of seroprevalence $p_i^\theta(t)$ in age group i and the disease incidence over time is given by the following equation:

$$p_i^\theta(t) = p_i^0 + \int_0^t \int_0^s Z_i^\theta(s-u)A(u)\,du\,ds$$

where p_i^0 is the background seroprevalence at the start of the outbreak in age group i with $Z(0) = 0$, $A(t)$ the distribution of time from onset of symptoms to seroconversion and $Z_i^\theta(t)$ the incidence of disease for a given model with set of parameters θ. This model assumes that a threshold is used as a marker of seroconversion, $A(t)$ represents thus the distribution of the time that antibodies take to pass the threshold. The time is measured from onset of symptoms.

Assuming independence of the samples, the likelihood of observing the data D given the incidence Z_i^θ is given by

$$L(D|\theta, i) = \prod_{j \in J^+} p_i^\theta(t_j) \prod_{j \in J^-} \left(1 - p_i^\theta(t_j)\right)$$

with J^+ denoting the set of positive samples, J^- the set of negative samples, and t_j the time of collection of sample j.

$Z_i^\theta(t)$ can be given by any model under a set of parameters θ. Baguelin et al. [38] designed the method to link sequential serology with an estimation of cases from statistical modeling, thus working out the proportion of cases missed by national surveillance during the 2009 influenza pandemic, Wu et al. [37] showed that this method could be coupled with a transmission model to improve real-time estimation of disease transmission during a pandemic.

17.5 Analysis of Full Temporal Serology Dynamics

All the models described in this chapter reduce the information from the serological data into a binary output mapping the S (susceptible) and R (protected) compartments of the SIR modeling framework. This reduction is done using a threshold or probabilistically using, e.g., Equation (17.7). These models do not thus fully integrate the information from immunological assays in the form of continuous or stratified concentration of antibodies (expressed as titers). Another way of integrating serological data in a transmission model is to include the dynamic of antibodies alongside the dynamics of infection and protection. This approach is more intricate and for that reason has been less explored. We present here a framework developed by Yuan at al. [30] and based on a modification of an SIRS model (where individuals are allowed to go back to the susceptible class from R). The version we present here is slightly modified from [30] for reasons of clarification of the model and consistency of behavior of the infectious class with the highest titer. As individuals with the highest titers are assumed to be protected, the difference in practice should be small.

Additionally to the S, I, and R grouping, the model further stratifies individuals by age and titers. Susceptible (respectively, infectious and recovered) individuals within an age group a and with titers i thus will belong to compartment $S_i(a)$ (respectively, $I_i(a)$ and $R_i(a)$). Following infection, individuals experience a short-lived period of full protection and as a result move to the R compartement for a duration $1/\omega$. The move to the R is accompanied with an increase in titer.

This short-lived immunity eventually wanes and the individuals revert to being susceptible to infection but retain partially protective titers. Re-infection is thus possible following recovery; however, it is assumed that, following infection, the antibody titers against the infective strain are boosted and that consequently the individuals have higher titers conferring them a lower susceptibility to future infections.

17.5.1   Model equations

The system of ordinary differential equations describing the model is presented in (17.8), and more details on the original model can be found in [30]:

$$
\begin{cases}
\dfrac{dS_i(a)}{dt} & = \quad -S_i\rho_a(i)\lambda(a) + \omega R_i(a) \\[2mm]
\dfrac{dI_i(a)}{dt} & = \quad S_i\rho_a(i)\lambda(a) - \frac{1}{T_g}I_i(a) \\[2mm]
\dfrac{dR_i(a)}{dt} & = \quad \dfrac{1}{T_g}\sum_{j=1}^{i} I_j(a)g_{ij} - \omega R_i(a)
\end{cases}
\tag{17.8}
$$

with $\lambda(a)$ the force infection on age group a, $\rho_a(i)$ the age specific susceptibility for individuals of age a, ω the waning rate for short-lived transient immunity, T_g the duration of infection, and g_{ji} the probability of immunity being boosted from titers i to j.

The force of infection is given by

$$
\lambda(a) = \beta \sum_{b=1}^{a_{\max}} \left\{ m_{ab} \sum_{i=1}^{i_{\max}} f_b I_i(b) \right\}
$$

where m_{ab} is the contact rate between individuals in age groups a and b, $a_{\max}$ and $i_{\max}$ are, respectively, the highest age group and titer level, f_b is the age specific infectivity, and β is a constant dependent on the transmissibility of the virus.

The age specific susceptibility $\rho(i)$ of an individual with titer i is given by

$$
\rho(i) = \frac{1}{1 + e^{\gamma(i - TP50)}}
$$

which is the same equation as Equation (17.7) but with a slightly different parameterization. $TP50$ represents the titer level (possibly non integer) at which an individual has 50 percent protection and γ is a parameter setting how the protection increases with increasing titers (the bigger γ, the stiffer the increase). For $\gamma \gg 1$, the function acts as a threshold function with $\rho(i) \approx 0$ for $i < TP50$ and $\rho(i) \approx 1$ for $i > TP50$. Coudeville et al. [29] have estimated γ to be equal to 2.102 in the case of influenza viruses with titers measured by HI assays.

When recovering, individuals get their antibody levels boosted. The antibody boosting g_{ji} is the probability that an individual with antibody level i (log scale) reaches antibody level j is given by a renormalized truncated Poisson distribution:

$$
\begin{cases}
h_{ji} & = \quad \dfrac{Abb^{\delta} e^{-Abb}}{\delta!} \\[4mm]
g_{ji} & = \quad \dfrac{h_{ji}}{\displaystyle\sum_{j=i+1}^{i_{\max}} h_{ji}}
\end{cases}
\tag{17.9}
$$

with Abb the parameter of the truncated renormalized Poisson distribution, $\delta = j - i$ the difference in log-titer, and $j > i$. For $i = j$, we have $g_{ii} = 0$ for all $i < i_{\max}$ and $g_{i_{\max} i_{\max}} = 1$. This result means that all individuals have antibody boosted following infection by at least one log-titer increase. Individual with the highest titers remain at the same level (supposed to provide near full protection).

17.5.2   Observation process and likelihood

An observation error is included, with the probability of observing a sample with titer e given by

$$f(e) = \sum_{i=1}^{i_{max}} \{S_i(a) + I_i(a) + R_i(a)\} P_{\text{error}}(e|i) \tag{17.10}$$

where $P_{\text{error}}(e|i)$ is the probability of observing titer e given that the true titer is i.

In the original paper, the probability of observational error was uniformly distributed as 0.005 for each titer i not equal to e. The sum of all observation errors including i equal to e was 1. The i_{max} was set to 10 i=1 are individuals with no detectable antibodies i=2 corresponds to a titer of 10 i=3, and 20 doubling until i=10 associated with the 2,560 titer.

The likelihood of observing the cross-sectional titers is

$$L(\theta|e_{t1}, e_{t2}, ..., e_{tN}) = \prod_{n=1}^{N} f(e_{t_n}) \tag{17.11}$$

where N is the total number of the samples, $f(e_{tn})$ is the frequency of observing titer e of the individual n from the model output with the parameter values θ at time t.

17.6   Worked Example: Model with Stratified Immunity

17.6.1   Data

We use a set of sera collected during the 2009 A/H1N1 pdm in Hong Kong [39]. From this dataset, we use the sera collected during the "baseline" collection and the first follow up as Yuan et al. [30]. These are 994 sera collected between July 2009 and February 2010 [30]. The data is aggregated in four age groups (see Figure 17.3).

17.6.2   Model implementation

We implemented the model described in Section 17.5 using R [40] and the package odin[1] which provides a friendly way of coding ordinary differential equation (ODE) models based on the deSolve package. The code used to reproduce this worked example can be downloaded.[2]

17.6.3   Inference

In this particular example, we are infering the initial states of the population in terms of $S_i(a)_{|t=0}$, $I_i(a)_{|t=0}$, and $R_i(a)_{|t=0}$. Here we have $a_{max} = 4$ and $i_{max} = 10$. Given that

$$\sum_{i=1}^{i_{max}} S_i(a) + I_i(a) + R_i(a) = N(a)$$

is constant with $N(a)$ the size of age group a, we have 116 initial parameters to infer. In addition to these 116 parameters, we infer the age specific $Abb(a)$ parameters (4, one for

---

[1] https://github.com/mrc-ide/odin
[2] https://github.com/MJomaba/immunodyn

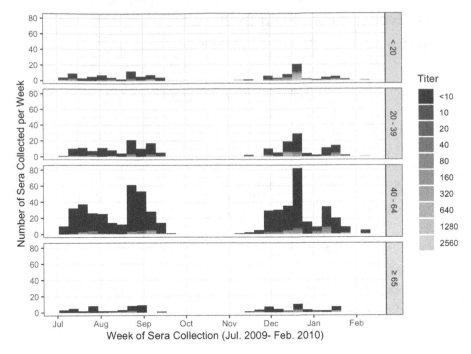

FIGURE 17.3

Detail of the collection of sera from the 2009 A/H1N1pdm in Hong Kong used to fit the stratified immunity model. The two first periods of data collection are used. The data is stratified in four age groups (< 20, 20–39, 40–64, ≥ 65) and ten titers (from titer < 10 for individuals with undetectable antibodies to 2560 the highest titer).

each age group) and the age specific $TP50$ (also 4 with one for each age group). Finally, we infer β and $f_{<20}$ the children specific infectivity. Following [30], we assume that the prior on $f_{<20}$ is normally distributed with mean 4 and standard deviation 0.5. We constraint the prior distribution of the $S_i(a)_{|t=0}$, $I_i(a)_{|t=0}$, and $R_i(a)_{|t=0}$ by assuming that the total number of infections is small at the start of the outbreak:

$$\frac{\sum_{i=1}^{i_{max}} I_i(a) + R_i(a)}{N(a)} \sim Beta(1, 10e6).$$

The TP50 are given exponential priors of parameter 0.25. All the other prior are uninformative.

We use the function adaptive.mcmc from the fluEvidenceSynthesis package [41] to perform an adaptive Markov chain Monte Carlo MCMC. To use the adaptive algorithm with the values bounded by $[0, 1]$, we have transformed the proportion of the population with different titers using a logit transformation.

17.6.4   Results

The result from the fitting of the model to the data can be seen in Figure 17.4 and 17.5. The rest of the fitted parameters can be found in Table 17.1.

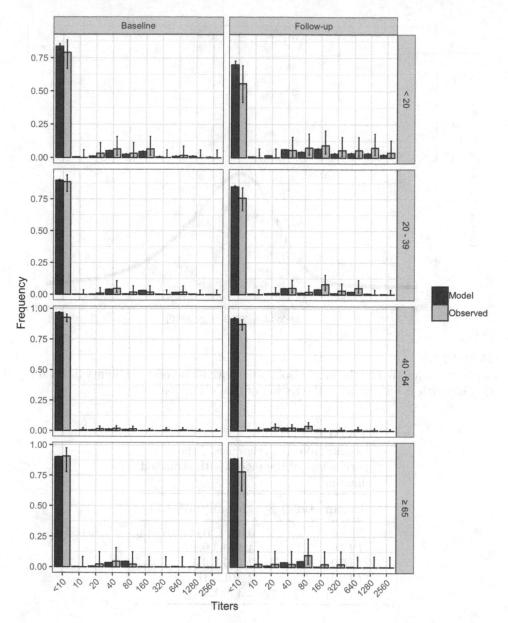

FIGURE 17.4

Proportion of the age groups with given titers. The bars show the proportion inferred from the model and the observed proportion, respectively. The sera are grouped to present the results as "Baseline" and "Follow-up" but the exact dates are used in the likelihood used to fit the model.

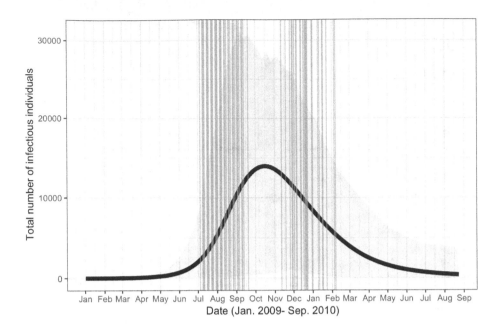

FIGURE 17.5
Epidemic curve inferred by the model (solid line) with 95 percent credibility interval (shaded area). The vertical lines indicate the timing of sera collection.

TABLE 17.1
Results from the inference of the parameters of the model with stratified immunity

Parameter	Mean[95% CrI]
β	0.0011 [0.0089,0.014]
$TP50_1$	4.4 [0.3,9.1]
$TP50_2$	2.1 [0.1,6.3]
$TP50_3$	2 [0.1,6.1]
$TP50_4$	2.3 [0.1,6.7]

17.7   Discussion

Transmission models are a particularly handy tool to analyze serological data. In particular, in the case of household studies, they make possible quantifying how much of the infection is due to the index case, household transmission, or reintroduction from the community. Transmission models also can be used to assess the potential for resurgence of pathogens by analyzing the serological profile of protective antibodies in a population. When sampled sequentially, they can be used to assess the amount of undetected transmission occurring in a population. Finally, a new generation of models also can designed tracking explicitly the level of immunity in a population.

Nevertheless, many challenges remain regarding interpreting serological data in the context of disease transmission. Immunological assays do provide a measurement correlating with protection. However, these assays might also captures cross reactive antibodies (e.g., from a related but drifted strain of influenza and also related pathogens such in the case of the interaction between Zika virus transmission and dengue induced immunity [12]) and cannot distinguish between antibodies resulting from vaccination and natural infections. The interpretation of serology is likely to be linked with the health status of the individual being sampled, and such phenomenon as immunosenescence are likely to be important for disease and need to be included in models.

This multi-dimensionality of disease transmission and immunodynamics imply that the future of using serology lies probably in the use of integrative evidence synthesis approach, where multiple data streams are linked through mathematical models. Multiple immunological assays might allow for better reconstruction of individual immunity landscape [10], which might allow for reconstruction of past infection history [11].

Acknowledgements

I would like to thank Adam Kucharski, Hsiang-Yu (Sean) Yuan, Edwin van Leeuwen, John Edmunds and Steven Riley for constructive discussions regarding the use of serology with transmission models. I am also grateful to Liz Miller for giving me comments after reading this chapter and talking me through the genesis of the measles 1994 catch-up campaign "from the horse's mouth." The writing of this chapter also has been considerably smoothened with the help from Cristina's parents Manolo and Teresa with childcare at a critical time. We finally thank the UK Medical Research Council (www.mrc.ac.uk) for Centre funding (MR/R015600/1).

The author thanks the MRC Centre for Global Infectious Disease Analysis (grant MR/R015600/1) and the UK National Institute for Health Research Health Protection Research Unit (NIHR HPRU) in Modelling Methodology at Imperial College London in partnership with Public Health England (PHE) (grant HPRU-201210080) for funding.

References

[1] A. J. Kucharski and M. Baguelin. The role of human immunity and social behavior in shaping influenza evolution. *PLoS Pathogens*, 13(8):e1006432, 2017.

[2] W. O. Kermack and A. G. McKendrick. A contribution to the mathematical theory of epidemics. *Proceedings of the Royal Society A: Mathematical, Physical and Engineering Sciences*, 115(772):700–721, 1927.

[3] N. Hens, Z. Shkedy, M. Aerts, C. Faes, P. Van Damme, and P. Beutels. *Modeling Infectious Disease Parameters Based on Serological and Social Contact Data*, volume 63 of *Statistics for Biology and Health*. Springer, New York, New York, 2012.

[4] I. M. Longini, J. S. Koopman, A. S. Monto, and J. P. Fox. Estimating household and community transmission parameters for influenza. *American Journal of Epidemiology*, 115(5):736–751, 1982.

[5] I. M. Longini and J. S. Koopman. Household and community transmission parameters from final distributions of infections in households. *Biometrics*, 38(1):115–126, 1982.

[6] D. Ludwig. Final size distribution for epidemics. *Mathematical Biosciences*, 23(1–2):33–46, 1975.

[7] S. Cauchemez, P. Horby, A. Fox, L. Q. Mai, L. T. Thanh, P. Q. Thai, L. N. M. Hoa, N. T. Hien, and N. M. Ferguson. Influenza infection rates, measurement errors and the interpretation of paired serology. *PLoS Pathogens*, 8(12):e1003061, 2012.

[8] S. Cauchemez, C. A. Donnelly, C. Reed, A. Ghani, C. Fraser, C. Kent, L. Finelli, and N. Ferguson. Household transmission of 2009 pandemic influenza A (H1N1) virus in the United States. *The New England Journal of Medicine*, 361(27):2619–2627, 2009.

[9] C. F. Houlihan, C. R. McGowan, S. Dicks, M. Baguelin, D. A. J. Moore, D. Mabey, C. H. Roberts, A. Kumar, R. Tedder, and J. R. Glynn. Ebola exposure, illness experience, and Ebola antibody prevalence in international responders to the West African Ebola epidemic 20142016: A cross-sectional study. *PLoS Medicine*, 14(5):e1002300, 2017.

[10] J. M. Fonville, S. H. Wilks, S. L. James, A. Fox, M. Ventresca, M. Aban, L. Xue et al., Antibody landscapes after influenza virus infection or vaccination. *Science*, 346(6212):996–1000, 2014.

[11] A. J. Kucharski, J. Lessler, D. A. T. Cummings, and Steven Riley. Timescales of influenza A/H3N2 antibody dynamics. *PLoS Biology*, 16(8):e2004974, 2018.

[12] I. Rodriguez-Barraquer, F. Costa, E. J. M. Nascimento, N. Nery, P. M. S. Castanha, G. A. Sacramento, J. Cruz et al., Impact of preexisting dengue immunity on Zika virus emergence in a dengue endemic region. *Science*, 363(6427):607–610, 2019.

[13] P. Hardelid, N. J. Andrews, K. Hoschler, E. Stanford, M. Baguelin, P. A. Waight, M. Zambon, and E. Miller. Assessment of baseline age-specific antibody prevalence and incidence of infection to novel influenza A/H1N1 2009. *Health Technology Assessment*, 14(55):115–192, 2010.

[14] M. Ramsay, N. Gay, E. Miller, M. Rush, J. White, P. Morgan-Capner, and D. Brown. The epidemiology of measles in England and Wales: Rationale for the 1994 national vaccination campaign. *Communicable Disease Report. CDR Review*, 4(12):R141–R146, 1994.

[15] A. Nardone, E. Miller, and on behalf of the ESEN2 Group. Serological surveillance of rubella in Europe: European Sero-Epidemiology Network (ESEN2). *Eurosurveillance*, 9(4):5–6, 2004.

[16] C. J. E. Metcalf, J. Farrar, F. T. Cutts, N. E. Basta, A. L. Graham, J. Lessler, N. M. Ferguson, D. S. Burke, and B. T. Grenfell. Use of serological surveys to generate key insights into the changing global landscape of infectious disease. *The Lancet*, 388(10045):728–730, 2016.

[17] A. R. Mclean and R. M. Anderson. Measles in developing countries. Part II. The predicted impact of mass vaccination. *Epidemiology and Infection*, 100(03):419–442, 1988.

[18] N. J. Gay, L. M. Hesketh, P. Morgan-Capner, and E. Miller. Interpretation of serological surveillance data for measles using mathematical models: Implications for vaccine strategy. *Epidemiology and Infection*, 115(1):139–156, 1995.

[19] E. Miller. The new measles campaign. *BMJ (Clinical research ed.)*, 309(6962): 1102–1103, 1994.

[20] N. Gay, M. Ramsay, B. Cohen, L. Hesketh, P. Morgan-Capner, D. Brown, and E. Miller. The epidemiology of measles in England and wales since the 1994 vaccination campaign. *Communicable Disease Report. CDR Review*, 7(2):R17–21, 1997.

[21] R. M. Anderson and R. M. May. Age-related changes in the rate of disease transmission: Implications for the design of vaccination programmes. *The Journal of Hygiene*, 94(3):365–436, 1985.

[22] O. Diekmann, J. A. P. Heesterbeek, and J. A. J. Metz. On the definition and the computation of the basic reproduction ratio R 0 in models for infectious diseases in heterogeneous populations. *Journal of Mathematical Biology*, 28(4):365–382, 1990.

[23] J. Mossong, N. Hens, M. Jit, P. Beutels, K. Auranen, R. Mikolajczyk, M. Massari et al., Social contacts and mixing patterns relevant to the spread of infectious diseases. *PLoS medicine*, 5(3):e74, 2008.

[24] A. Melegaro, M. Jit, N. Gay, E. Zagheni, and W. J. Edmunds. What types of contacts are important for the spread of infections? Using contact survey data to explore European mixing patterns. *Epidemics*, 3(3–4):143–151, 2011.

[25] J. Wallinga, P. Teunis, and M. Kretzschmar. Using data on social contacts to estimate age-specific transmission parameters for respiratory-spread infectious agents. *American Journal of Epidemiology*, 164(10):936–944, 2006.

[26] A. J. Dunning. A model for immunological correlates of protection. *Statistics in Medicine*, 25(9):1485–97, 2006.

[27] P. Jin, J. Li, X. Zhang, F. Meng, Y. Zhou, X. Yao, Z. Gan, and F. Zhu. Validation and evaluation of serological correlates of protection for inactivated enterovirus 71 vaccine in children aged 6-35 months. *Human Vaccines & Immunotherapeutics*, 12(4):916–921, 2016.

[28] M. Baguelin, S. Flasche, A. Camacho, N. Demiris, E. Miller, and W.J. Edmunds. assessing optimal target populations for influenza vaccination programmes: An evidence synthesis and modelling study. *PLoS Med.*, 10(10):e1001527, 2013.

[29] L. Coudeville, F. Bailleux, B. Riche, F. Megas, P. Andre, and R. Ecochard. Relationship between haemagglutination-inhibiting antibody titres and clinical protection against influenza: Development and application of a bayesian random-effects model. *BMC Medical Research Methodology*, 10(1):18, 2010.

[30] H.-Y. Yuan, M. Baguelin, K. O. Kwok, N. Arinaminpathy, E. van Leeuwen, and S. Riley. The impact of stratified immunity on the transmission dynamics of influenza. *Epidemics*, 20:84–93, 2017.

[31] B. O. Fulton, D. Sachs, S. M. Beaty, S. T. Won, B. Lee, P. Palese, and N. S. Heaton. Mutational analysis of measles virus suggests constraints on antigenic variation of the glycoproteins. *Cell Reports*, 11(9):1331–1338, 2015.

[32] A. J. Kucharski, J. Lessler, J. M. Read, H. Zhu, C. Q. Jiang, Y. Guan, D. A. T. Cummings, and S. Riley. Estimating the life course of influenza A(H3N2) antibody responses from cross-sectional data. *PLoS Biology*, 13(3):e1002082, 2015.

[33] P. J. Birrell, G. Ketsetzis, N. J. Gay, B. S. Cooper, A. M. Presanis, R. J. Harris, A. Charlett, X.-S. Zhang, P. J. White, R. G. Pebody, and D. De Angelis. Bayesian modeling to unmask and predict influenza A/H1N1pdm dynamics in London. *Proceedings of the National Academy of Sciences of the United States of America*, 108(45):18238–18243, 2011.

[34] I. Dorigatti, S. Cauchemez, and N. M. Ferguson. Increased transmissibility explains the third wave of infection by the 2009 H1N1 pandemic virus in England. *Proceedings of the National Academy of Sciences of the United States of America*, 110(33):13422–13427, 2013.

[35] M. Baguelin, A. J. Van Hoek, M. Jit, S. Flasche, P. J. White, and W. J. Edmunds. Vaccination against pandemic influenza A/H1N1v in England: A real-time economic evaluation. *Vaccine*, 28(12):2370–2384, 2010.

[36] E. Miller, K. Hoschler, P. Hardelid, E. Stanford, N. Andrews, and M. Zambon. Incidence of 2009 pandemic influenza A H1N1 infection in England: A cross-sectional serological study. *Lancet*, 375(9720):1100–1108, 2010.

[37] J. T. Wu, K. Leung, R. A. P. M. Perera, D. K. W. Chu, C. K. Lee, I. F. N. Hung, C. K. Lin et al., Inferring influenza infection attack rate from seroprevalence data. *PLoS Pathogens*, 10(4):e1004054, 2014.

[38] M. Baguelin, K. Hoschler, E. Stanford, P. Waight, P. Hardelid, N. Andrews, and E. Miller. Age-specific incidence of A/H1N1 2009 influenza infection in England from sequential antibody prevalence data using likelihood-based estimation. *PloS One*, 6(2):e17074, 2011.

[39] S. Riley, K. O. Kwok, K. M. Wu, D. Y. Ning, B. J. Cowling, J. T. Wu, L.-M. Ho et al., Epidemiological characteristics of 2009 (H1N1) pandemic influenza based on paired sera from a longitudinal community cohort study. *PLoS Medicine*, 8(6):e1000442, 2011.

[40] R Core Team. *R: A Language and Environment for Statistical Computing*. R Foundation for Statistical Computing, Vienna, Austria, 2018.

[41] E. van Leeuwen, P. Klepac, D. Thorrington, R. Pebody, and M. Baguelin. fluEvidenceSynthesis: An R package for evidence synthesis based analysis of epidemiological outbreaks. *PLoS Computational Biology*, 13(11):e1005838, 2017.

18

The Analysis of Multivariate Serological Data

Steven Abrams

CONTENTS

18.1 Introduction

Cross-sectional serosurvey collections are used commonly to study the epidemiology of infectious diseases. Serological survey data is obtained by testing blood serum samples, derived from an age-specific cross-sectional sample, for the presence of infection-specific immunoglobulin G (IgG) antibodies which are formed by the immune system in response to an infecting organism. More specifically, IgG antibody concentrations are determined by means of a biochemical technique called enzyme-linked immunosorbent assay (ELISA). Hence, the presence of antibody levels indicates whether infection or vaccination occurred in the past. After determining the antibody titer concentrations, individuals typically are classified as either being seropositive, i.e., the individual has been infected/vaccinated before, or seronegative based on a pre-specified cut-off level (or range) proposed by the manufacturer of the test. Consequently, serological data provide information on the age-specific prevalence of past infection in a population in the absence of an immunization program, at least when a serological correlate of protection for the infection under study is agreed upon (see Chapter 14).

Blood serum samples often are tested for more than one antigen at once due to economical reasons. Modeling these multivariate serological data altogether can provide new insights regarding joint disease dynamics and similarity in infection-specific transmission routes for the pathogens under investigation. As well, individuals differ in susceptibility to infection, infectiousness upon infection, and propensity to make contacts relevant to the transmission of diseases (e.g., activity levels representing individual sociability). Such sources of individual heterogeneity may have important effects on the dynamics of ongoing epidemics, and consequently, on the design of control strategies [1]. Multivariate frailty models provide a convenient framework to model the association among multiple infection times explicitly, and to investigate the presence of unobserved heterogeneity in the acquisition of these infections [2, 3]. Individual frailty terms are assumed to act multiplicatively on a baseline force of infection, and infection times are considered independent given the frailty level. Although attention is restricted to the analysis of two infections throughout this chapter, the frailty methodology presented herein is readily generalizable towards three or more infections.

First, we introduce the marginal bivariate Dale model as well as conditional approaches to describe association in multivariate serological data in Section 18.2. In Section 18.3, we introduce compartmental transmission models describing immunizing and non-immunizing infection dynamics. In Section 18.4, we ascribe the association between infections to heterogeneity in the acquisition thereof. We link the deterministic expressions for the seroprevalence in Section 18.3 to the frailty methodology in Section 18.4. In Section 18.5 two data applications are presented on (1) parvovirus B19 and varicella zoster virus serology and (2) hepatitis A and B serological data. Finally, avenues for further research are provided in Section 18.6.

18.2 Modeling Association

Consider bivariate serological data denoted by (y_{1j}, y_{2j}, t_j), $j = 1, \ldots, n$, where y_{ij} represents the immunological status for the jth individual of age t_j with regard to infection $i = 1, 2$. More specifically, y_{ij} equals one in case of past/current infection with pathogen i and zero, if individual j is still susceptible to infection i at time t_j. Let $p_{y_{1j}, y_{2j}}(t_j) = \Pr(Y_{1j} = y_{1j}, Y_{2j} = y_{2j} | t_j)$ denote the joint multinomial probabilities for Y_{1j} and Y_{2j}. One way to model such multivariate categorical data is by means of a marginal bivariate Dale model [4, 5] consisting of the following three models which are considered simultaneously:

$$\text{logit}\{\pi_1(t_j)\} = h_1(t_j),$$

$$\text{logit}\{\pi_2(t_j)\} = h_2(t_j),$$

$$\log\{\text{OR}(t_j)\} = h_3(t_j),$$

where $\pi_1(t_j) \equiv p_{1,+}(t_j)$ and $\pi_2(t_j) \equiv p_{+,1}(t_j)$ are the marginal probabilities (seroprevalence) $\Pr(Y_{1j} = 1 | t_j)$ and $\Pr(Y_{2j} = 1 | t_j)$, respectively, $\text{logit}(x) = \log\{x/(1-x)\}$, $h_i(t_j)$, $i = 1, 2, 3$

smooth differentiable functions entailing (parametric or non-parametric) functional forms for the age-effects, and $OR(t_j)$ represents the age-dependent odds ratio defined as

$$OR(t_j) = \frac{p_{11}(t_j)p_{00}(t_j)}{p_{10}(t_j)p_{01}(t_j)}.$$

Modeling the age-dependent odds ratio allows for studying the (time-varying) association between both diseases. More specifically, an odds ratio equal to 1 implies that both disease processes behave independently, whereas $OR \neq 1$ indicates an association between both infections. Note that it is straightforward to write down the multinomial likelihood function in terms of $h_i(t_j)$, $i = 1, 2, 3$, thereby enabling a maximum likelihood (ML) estimation. See [6] for more details on a multivariate extension of the smoothing spline approach, known as vector generalised additive models, in order to ensure a flexible estimation of the unknown functions $h_i(t_j)$.

Although the temporal strength of association in bivariate serological data can be studied by estimating a non-local age-specific odds ratio, [7] demonstrated that it can vary with age even in the absence of any age-dependent effects. As an alternative, we could consider the cross-ratio function (CRF) which is a local association measure that was introduced by [2], i.e.,

$$\theta(t_{1j}, t_{2j}) = \frac{\lambda\left(t_{1j}|T_2^* = t_{2j}\right)}{\lambda\left(t_{1j}|T_2^* > t_{2j}\right)} = \frac{p_{00}\left(t_{1j}, t_{2j}\right) \partial_{12}^2 p_{00}\left(t_{1j}, t_{2j}\right)}{\partial_1 p_{00}\left(t_{1j}, t_{2j}\right) \partial_2 p_{00}\left(t_{1j}, t_{2j}\right)},$$

where $\lambda(t_{1j}|T_2^* = t_{2j})$ and $\lambda(t_{1j}|T_2^* > t_{2j})$ are the conditional hazard functions for the time to first infection T_1^* given that the time to the second infection T_2^* equals t_{2j} or is larger than t_{2j}, respectively. In addition, $\partial_{12}^2 = \partial^2/\partial t_{1j}\partial t_{2j}$, $\partial_1 = \partial/\partial t_{1j}$, and $\partial_2 = \partial/\partial t_{2j}$ denote partial derivatives. In case of single (or univariate) monitoring times t_j for both infections, the CRF is not directly estimable as we only have information about $p_{00}(t_j)$. However, the CRF, and equivalently the age-varying association, can be modeled based on parametric assumptions related to the survival probability $p_{00}(t_{1j}, t_{2j})$ and its partial derivatives which can be imposed through the specification of latent frailty terms (see, e.g., Section 18.4).

In contrast with the marginal Dale model, conditional models focus on the association by looking at one variable conditional on the other one. Examples of conditional models include the baseline category logits model in which one of the joint probabilities is used as baseline and the other probabilities are modeled in relation to the baseline probability using a log-link function and smooth differentiable functions $\tilde{h}_i(t_j)$, $i = 1, 2, 3$. For more details regarding this approach and differences with the marginal Dale model, referred to [6].

18.3 Mathematical Transmission Models

Mathematical infectious disease epidemiology typically involves the study of deterministic compartmental models describing the flows of individuals between mutually exclusive states. Throughout this chapter, we rely on such mathematical transmission models while developing tools for the estimation of important epidemiological parameters in the presence of observed and unobserved individual heterogeneity inherent to the spread of infectious diseases (in endemic equilibrium) in large populations. One of the simplest compartmental models mimicking disease spread of infections conferring life-long immunity is the so-called

Susceptible-Infected-Recovered (SIR) model. First, individuals are born in the susceptible compartment S. Under time homogeneity, individuals flow from a susceptible compartment S to an infectious compartment I at an age-dependent rate $\lambda(a)$ (i.e., the so-called time-homogeneous force of infection). Furthermore, individuals are 'removed' from the at-risk population and move to the R state at rate $\varphi(a)$. In the absence of disease-related mortality, individuals are subject to natural mortality rates $\mu(a)$ in each of the compartments. The SIR model is graphically depicted by the solid lines in Figure 18.1. Note that the dashed line in Figure 18.1 describes replenishment of the S compartment at rate $\sigma(a)$, which is not part of the SIR dynamics discussed first. Details on this extension of the SIR model will be provided afterwards.

In a time-homogeneous setting (i.e., endemic equilibrium), the flows in an SIR model can be described using the following set of ordinary differential equations (ODEs) in terms of the age-dependent proportions of individuals in each compartment, i.e., dividing the number of individuals in each compartment by the (stationary) population age distribution $N(a)$ in demographic equilibrium:

$$\frac{dS(a)}{da} = -\lambda(a)S(a),$$

$$\frac{dI(a)}{da} = \lambda(a)S(a) - \varphi(a)I(a),$$

$$\frac{dR(a)}{da} = \varphi(a)I(a).$$

Consequently, solving the set of ODEs produces an age-dependent expression for the (conditional) proportion of susceptible individuals in the population under the constraint $S(0) = 1$:

$$S(a) = \exp\left(-\int_0^a \lambda(u)du\right). \tag{18.1}$$

Note that maternal immunity is not accounted for since $S(0) = 1$, albeit that similar expressions can be derived when newborns have maternal immunity.

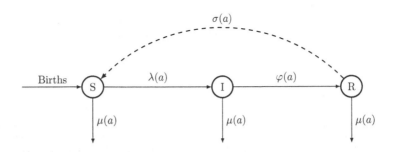

FIGURE 18.1

Flow diagram for the time-homogeneous mathematical SIR(S) model: Individuals are born into the susceptible class S and move to the infected state I at rate $\lambda(a)$, after which they recover and move to R at rate $\varphi(a)$. In an SIRS setting, individuals loose protective immunity and move back from R to S at replenishment rate $\sigma(a)$ (dashed line). All individuals are subject to natural mortality at rate $\mu(a)$.

Furthermore, expressions for the proportion of infectious and recovered individuals are obtained by applying the method of variation of parameters:

$$I(a) = \int_0^a \lambda(u) \exp\left(-\int_u^a \varphi(v)dv\right) \exp\left(-\int_0^u \lambda(v)dv\right) du,$$

$$R(a) = \int_0^a \varphi(u)I(u)du,$$

with initial conditions $I(0) = R(0) = 0$.

One natural extension of the simple SIR model for infections that do not confer life-long immunity upon recovery is the SIRS model. The SIRS model allows for loss of disease-acquired immunity and thus potential reinfections. Individuals are assumed to move from R back to the susceptible state S at a replenishment rate $\sigma(a)$ (see dashed line in Figure 18.1). The set of ODEs describing the flow of individuals between the compartments can be formulated as (in case of demographic and endemic equilibrium):

$$\frac{dS(a)}{da} = -\lambda(a)S(a) + \sigma(a)R(a),$$

$$\frac{dI(a)}{da} = \lambda(a)S(a) - \varphi(a)I(a),$$

$$\frac{dR(a)}{da} = \varphi(a)I(a) - \sigma(a)R(a).$$

Solving the set of ODEs and making use of $R(a) \approx 1 - S(a)$, we obtain the following expressions for the proportions of susceptibles and seropositives of age a:

$$S(a) = \exp\left(-\int_0^a \{\lambda(u) + \sigma(u)\} du\right) +$$

$$\int_0^a \sigma(u) \exp\left(-\int_u^a \{\lambda(v) + \sigma(v)\} dv\right) du, \tag{18.2}$$

$$R(a) = \int_0^a \lambda(u) \exp\left(-\int_u^a \{\lambda(v) + \sigma(v)\} dv\right) du.$$

For the endemic infections under consideration in this chapter, the proportion of infected and infectious individuals of age a is small compared to the proportion of individuals in compartments S and R, implying that the assumption $R(a) \approx 1 - S(a)$ is tenable.

Other compartmental models, such as, e.g., SIRW models, allowing for waning of disease-acquired antibodies without loss of protective ('cellular') immunity, could be considered as well. However, throughout this chapter, we will limit ourselves to the SIR and SIRS models to describe disease dynamics for infections conferring life-long immunity (immunizing) and infections with temporary immunity (non-immunizing).

18.4   Frailty Models in Infectious Disease Epidemiology

It has been understood for a long time that individual heterogeneity with respect to factors that may enhance or inhibit the transmission of infectious diseases affects the effectiveness of control strategies [8]. In general, the greater the heterogeneity in the population, the greater the epidemic potential of an infection and the more difficult to contain it. When unobserved heterogeneity is not appropriately accounted for, we potentially end up with biased estimates for important epidemiological parameters such as the basic reproduction number and criticial vaccination coverage [1]. As some people will experience infection earlier than others due to a different susceptibility level, the age-dependent force of infection can be expressed as $\lambda(a, Z)$ where Z represents an individual-specific random variable or frailty term expressing to what extent an individual has a lower or higher infection risk [9, 10]. In epidemic theory, [11] were the first to systematically treat heterogeneity in the acquisition of infections. Building upon their work, [1] demonstrated the use of shared gamma frailty models to quantify variation in activity levels for bivariate current status data on measles and mumps in the UK. More recently, [12] illustrated that the restrictive assumption of a common frailty for both infections can be relaxed by using a correlated gamma frailty model, albeit at the cost of specifying a parametric baseline hazard function. From an epidemiological point of view, these traditional frailty models assume life-long immunity after recovery, which is untenable for some diseases. In the following subsections, we consider age- or time-invariant frailty models, implying that individuals have a constant 'frailty' level during their entire life, and time-varying extensions thereof, implying that individual frailties – and hence the correlations they induce – may vary with age, for infections with different underlying disease dynamics.

18.4.1   Time-invariant Frailty Models

Individuals are dissimilar in the way they acquire infections and consequently transmit these pathogens. Some individuals are more susceptible to infection than others, and therefore will experience infection earlier. Multivariate frailty models allow us to model multisera data, which are mostly used to infer this unobserved heterogeneity, and to describe the association between multiple infection times. Consider bivariate serological data denoted by $(y_{1j}, t_{1j}, y_{2j}, t_{2j})$, $j = 1, \dots, n$, where y_{ij} represents the immunological status for the jth individual with regard to infection $i = 1, 2$ and t_{ij} denotes the corresponding cross-sectional sampling time. Typically, univariate monitoring times $t_{1j} = t_{2j} \equiv t_j$ are observed referring to the individual's age at sampling (see Section 18.5), at least for infections under endemic equilibrium. In general, we have

$$(Y_{ij}|T_{ij} = t_{ij}) = \begin{cases} 1 & \text{if } T_{ij}^* \leq t_{ij} \text{ (seropositive)}, \\ 0 & \text{if } T_{ij}^* > t_{ij} \text{ (seronegative)}, \end{cases}$$

where T_{ij}^* is the true unknown infection time and $(Y_{ij}|T_j = t_{ij}) \sim B(1, \pi_i(t_{ij}))$ with $\pi_i(t_{ij}) = 1 - S_i(t_{ij})$. The proportion of susceptible individuals $S_i(t_{ij})$ at time t_{ij} is termed the marginal survival or survivor function in survival analysis. Differences in susceptibility (and social activity levels) can be expressed in terms of the infection-specific age-dependent force of infection $\lambda_i(t_{ij}, Z_{ij})$ for infection $i = 1, 2$, where Z_{ij} represents the latent or random 'frailty' level expressing to what extent individual j has a lower or higher infection risk for infection i [9, 10]. For identifiability reasons, we typically assume that $\mathrm{E}(Z_{ij}) = 1$. Under the proportional hazards assumption, we have

$$\lambda_i(t_{ij}, Z_{ij}) = Z_{ij}\lambda_{i0}(t_{ij}),$$

where $\lambda_{i0}(t_{ij})$ is the baseline force of infection. The corresponding conditional susceptible proportion for an immunizing infection is obtained by introducing $\lambda_i(t_{ij}, Z_{ij})$ in (18.1):

$$S_i(t_{ij}|Z_{ij}) = \exp\left(-\int_0^{t_{ij}} \lambda_i(u, Z_{ij})du\right) = \exp\left(-Z_{ij}\int_0^{t_{ij}} \lambda_{i0}(u)du\right).$$

The marginal or unconditional susceptible proportion is derived by integrating out the random frailty terms Z_{ij} and can therefore be expressed in terms of the so-called Laplace transform $\mathcal{L}_{Z_{ij}}(\cdot)$ of Z_{ij} as follows:

$$S_i(t_{ij}) = \mathrm{E}\left\{S_i(t_{ij}|Z_{ij})\right\} = \mathcal{L}_{Z_{ij}}\left(\int_0^{t_{ij}} \lambda_{i0}(u)du\right). \tag{18.3}$$

For an infection with SIRS dynamics, the unconditional proportion of susceptible individuals can be derived based on equation (18.2):

$$S_i(t_{ij}) = \exp\left(-\int_0^{t_{ij}} \sigma_i(u)du\right)\mathcal{L}_{Z_{ij}}\left(\int_0^{t_{ij}} \lambda_{i0}(u)du\right) +$$

$$\int_0^{t_{ij}} \sigma_i(u)\exp\left(-\int_u^{t_{ij}} \sigma_i(v)dv\right)\mathcal{L}_{Z_{ij}}\left(\int_u^{t_{ij}} \lambda_{i0}(v)dv\right)du. \tag{18.4}$$

Bivariate frailty distributions for (Z_{1j}, Z_{2j}), such as, e.g., a bivariate gamma distribution, impose a specific dependence structure in the sense that a correlation parameter ρ describes the strength of the dependency among the two infection-specific frailties and thus describes the association in acquisition of both infections. Some commonly made choices with respect to the implied association structure are:

- Univariate frailty model: Z_{1j} and Z_{2j} are independent random variables
- Shared frailty model: a common frailty $Z_{1j} = Z_{2j} \equiv Z_j$
- Correlated frailty model: $Z_{1j} = \gamma_1\left(Y_{0j}^* + Y_{1j}^*\right)$; $Z_{2j} = \gamma_2\left(Y_{0j}^* + Y_{2j}^*\right)$,

where γ_i denotes the frailty variance with respect to infection i, and the additive components Y_{lj}^*, $l = 0, 1, 2$, are independent random variables with mean and variance equal to $\omega_l > 0$. Therefore, direct calculation of the frailty variances results in the equality $\gamma_i = 1/(\omega_0 + \omega_i)$ ascertaining unit frailty means. The additive decomposition of the frailty terms in the correlated frailty model is proposed by [13] and applied to infectious disease modeling by [12]. The correlated frailty model extends the restrictive shared frailty model in the sense that the implied correlation between the infection times is allowed to differ from unity. Needless to say, the correlated frailty model offers a more general approach to account for individual heterogeneity. However, the implied correlation coefficient ρ is restricted due to the additive decomposition as follows:

$$0 \le \rho \le \min\left(\sqrt{\frac{\gamma_1}{\gamma_2}}, \sqrt{\frac{\gamma_2}{\gamma_1}}\right).$$

The shared frailty model is a special case of the correlated frailty model in which the infection-specific components Y_{lj}^*, $l = 1, 2$, are identical, i.e., $Y_{1j}^* = Y_{2j}^*$. The proportion of individuals susceptible to both infections under study can be derived relying on the conditional independence assumption of the infection times given the frailties. More specifically, $S(t_{1j}, t_{2j}|Z_{1j}, Z_{2j}) = S_1(t_{1j}|Z_{1j})S_2(t_{2j}|Z_{2j})$, where $S_i(t_{ij}|Z_{ij})$ refers to the conditional susceptible proportions for which formulas were presented previously. An expression for the marginal $S(t_{1j}, t_{2j})$ can be obtained by integrating over the bivariate frailty distribution for (Z_{1j}, Z_{2j}). Depending on the specific choice of the (bivariate) frailty distribution, either an explicit expression can be given for the unconditional univariate or bivariate proportion of susceptible individuals or numerical integration is required. Here, we consider the gamma (frailty) distribution due to its computational and analytical convenience which owes to the closed form expression for the Laplace transform. Furthermore, it is well-established that in a time-invariant bivariate setting the gamma distribution implies a constant association between two infection times, and therefore it could serve as a useful starting point. Independent gamma distributed components Y_{lj}^* with equal scale parameters result in infection-specific gamma frailties Z_{ij}. The Laplace transform corresponding to a gamma distributed random variable with mean one and variance γ_i is given by $\mathcal{L}(s) = (1 + \gamma_i s)^{-1/\gamma_i}$, for $s > -1/\gamma_i$.

18.4.2   Time-varying Frailty Models

In the previous subsection, individual- and infection-specific frailty terms Z_{ij} do not vary over time (or with age). Hence, individuals are assumed to have a constant frailty level. However, time-varying frailty models offer a way to allow these individual frailty terms to vary with time which could reflect time-dependent changes in humoral immunity responses to pathogen exposure. Suppose that the infection hazard at time t_{ij} under the proportional hazards assumption is given by

$$\lambda_i\{t_{ij}, Z_{ij}(t_{ij})\} = Z_{ij}(t_{ij})\lambda_{i0}(t_{ij}),$$

where $Z_{ij}(t_{ij})$ denotes a time-varying frailty term.

18.4.2.1   Piecewise Constant Model

[14] and [15] proposed the use of a piecewise constant frailty model on disjoint intervals $[t_{[m]}, t_{[m+1]}[$ which can be obtained as follows:

$$Z_{ij}(t_{ij}) = \sum_{m=1}^{M} I_m(t_{ij}) Z_{ijm}^*,$$

where $I_m(t_{ij})$ is a function indicating whether $t_{ij} \in [t_{[m]}, t_{[m+1]}[$. The components Z_{ijm}^* are independent non-negative random variables with unit mean and variance γ_{im}. A time-dependent piecewise constant shared gamma frailty model (TDPCSGF) is derived under the constraint $Z_{jm}^* = Z_{1jm}^* = Z_{2jm}^*$, $m = 1, \ldots, M$, and Z_{jm}^* follows a gamma distribution with unit mean and variance $\gamma_{.m}$. Although the piecewise constant model for $Z_{ij}(t_{ij})$ is straightforward and simple, a disadvantage of this model is the subjective choice of the M time-intervals in which the frailties Z_{ijm}^* are assumed constant. In addition, the frailty components are assumed to be independent such that heterogeneity in subsequent time-intervals is unrelated which seems counter-intuitive.

18.4.2.2   Multiplicative Model

An alternative model was introduced by [16] and further exploited by [17] in the context of shared frailty models for immunizing infections. This model overcomes the disadvantages of the piecewise constant model. In line with the work by these authors, a bivariate frailty model is proposed with time-varying frailty terms given by

$$Z_{ij}(t_{ij}) = \prod_{m=1}^{M} \{1 + (Z_{ijm}^* - 1) h_{im}(t_{ij})\}, \qquad 0 \le h_{im}(t_{ij}) \le 1,$$

where Z^*_{ijm}, $m = 1, \ldots, M$ are independent random variables with unit mean and variance γ_{im}, and $h_{im}(\cdot)$ is a deterministic function describing the frailty evolution over time. We can easily verify that the frailty terms $Z_{ij}(t_{ij})$ have unit mean and time-varying frailty variance equal to

$$\gamma_i(t_{ij}) = \left[\prod_{m=1}^{M}\left\{1 + h^2_{im}(t_{ij})\gamma_{im}\right\}\right] - 1.$$

Suppose that $h_{im}(t_{ij})$ is a deterministic exponential decay function defined as follows:

$$h_{im}(t_{ij}) = \exp\left\{-\left(\phi_{im}t_{ij}\right)^k\right\},$$

where the exponential decay parameter $\phi_{im} > 0$ and k is a non-negative integer. In the case studies, we assume that $k = 2$ and gamma distributed frailty components Z^*_{ijm} leading to various two-component gamma frailty models (i.e., taking $M = 2$):

1. Two-component time-dependent shared gamma frailty model (TDSGF-2C):

$$Z_{ij}(t_{ij}) = \left\{1 + \left(Z^*_{j1} - 1\right)h_{i1}(t_{ij})\right\}Z^*_{j2},$$

$$Z^*_{j1} \equiv Z^*_{1j1} = Z^*_{2j1}, \quad Z^*_{j1} \sim \Gamma\left(\gamma^{-1}_{\cdot 1}, \gamma^{-1}_{\cdot 1}\right),$$

$$Z^*_{j2} \equiv Z^*_{1j2} = Z^*_{2j2}, \quad Z^*_{j2} \sim \Gamma\left(\gamma^{-1}_{\cdot 2}, \gamma^{-1}_{\cdot 2}\right),$$

$$\gamma_i(t_{ij}) = \gamma_{\cdot 2} + h^2_{i1}(t_{ij})\gamma_{\cdot 1}\left(1 + \gamma_{\cdot 2}\right),$$

$$\rho(t_{1j}, t_{2j}) = \frac{\gamma_{\cdot 2} + h_{11}(t_{1j})h_{21}(t_{2j})\gamma_{\cdot 1}\left(1 + \gamma_{\cdot 2}\right)}{\sqrt{\left\{\gamma_{\cdot 2} + h^2_{11}(t_{1j})\gamma_{\cdot 1}\left(1 + \gamma_{\cdot 2}\right)\right\}\left\{\gamma_{\cdot 2} + h^2_{21}(t_{2j})\gamma_{\cdot 1}\left(1 + \gamma_{\cdot 2}\right)\right\}}}$$

2. Two-component time-dependent correlated gamma frailty model (TDCGF-2C):

$$Z_{ij}(t_{ij}) = \left\{1 + \left(Z^*_{ij1} - 1\right)h_{i1}(t_{ij})\right\}Z^*_{ij2},$$

$$Z^*_{ij1} = \gamma_{i1}\left(Y^*_{0j1} + Y^*_{ij1}\right), \quad Y^*_{lj1} \sim \Gamma\left(\omega_{l1}, 1\right),$$

$$Z^*_{ij2} = \gamma_{i2}\left(Y^*_{0j2} + Y^*_{ij2}\right), \quad Y^*_{lj2} \sim \Gamma\left(\omega_{l2}, 1\right),$$

$$\gamma_{i1} = \left(\omega_{01} + \omega_{i1}\right)^{-1}, \quad \gamma_{i2} = \left(\omega_{02} + \omega_{i2}\right)^{-1}$$

$$\gamma_i(t_{ij}) = \gamma_{i2} + h^2_{i1}(t_{ij})\gamma_{i1}\left(1 + \gamma_{i2}\right),$$

$$\rho(t_{1j}, t_{2j}) = \frac{\omega_{02}\gamma_{12}\gamma_{22} + h_{11}(t_{1j})h_{21}(t_{2j})\left(\omega_{01}\gamma_{11}\gamma_{21}\right)\left(1 + \omega_{02}\gamma_{12}\gamma_{22}\right)}{\sqrt{\left\{\gamma_{12} + h^2_{11}(t_{1j})\gamma_{11}\left(1 + \gamma_{12}\right)\right\}\left\{\gamma_{22} + h^2_{21}(t_{2j})\gamma_{21}\left(1 + \gamma_{22}\right)\right\}}}$$

These two-component models simplify to one-component time-dependent shared gamma frailty (TDSGF-1C) and time-dependent correlated gamma frailty (TDCGF-1C) models, if Z^*_{j2} and Z^*_{ij2}, $i = 1, 2$, follow degenerate distributions with unit mean ($\gamma_{\cdot 2} = 0$ and $\gamma_{12} = \gamma_{22} = 0$), respectively. Unconditional proportions of susceptible individuals are obtained using a combination of analytical and numerical integration techniques (not shown here).

18.4.3   Maximum Likelihood Estimation

The frailty methodology described in this chapter is applied to bivariate current status data $(y_{1j}, t_{1j}, y_{2j}, t_{2j})$. The individual log-likelihood contributions can be expressed in terms of joint probabilities $p_{y_{1j}, y_{2j}}(\cdot, \cdot)$ as follows [18]:

$$
ll_j\left(\boldsymbol{\theta}, \boldsymbol{\psi}|y_{1j}, t_{1j}, y_{2j}, t_{2j}\right) = y_{1j}y_{2j} \log\left[p_{11}(t_{1j}, t_{2j}|\boldsymbol{\theta}, \boldsymbol{\psi})\right]
$$
$$
+ y_{1j}\left(1 - y_{2j}\right) \log\left[p_{10}(t_{1j}, t_{2j}|\boldsymbol{\theta}, \boldsymbol{\psi})\right]
$$
$$
+ \left(1 - y_{1j}\right) y_{2j} \log\left[p_{01}(t_{1j}, t_{2j}|\boldsymbol{\theta}, \boldsymbol{\psi})\right]
$$
$$
+ \left(1 - y_{1j}\right)\left(1 - y_{2j}\right) \log\left[p_{00}(t_{1j}, t_{2j}|\boldsymbol{\theta}, \boldsymbol{\psi})\right],
$$

where $\boldsymbol{\theta}$ and $\boldsymbol{\psi}$ represent vectors of parameters associated with the baseline hazard functions and frailty distribution, respectively, and $p_{y_{1j}, y_{2j}}(t_{1j}, t_{2j}|\boldsymbol{\theta}, \boldsymbol{\psi}) = \Pr(Y_{1j} = y_{1j}, Y_{2j} = y_{2j}|t_{1j}, t_{2j}, \boldsymbol{\theta}, \boldsymbol{\psi})$ are the multinomial probabilities associated with the distribution of (Y_{1j}, Y_{2j}). In general, we have

$$
p_{y_{1j}, y_{2j}}(t_{1j}, t_{2j}|\boldsymbol{\theta}, \boldsymbol{\psi}) = y_{1j}y_{2j} + (y_{2j} - 2y_{1j}y_{2j}) S_1(t_{1j}, t_{2j}|\boldsymbol{\theta}, \boldsymbol{\psi})
$$
$$
+ (y_{1j} - 2y_{1j}y_{2j}) S_2(t_{1j}, t_{2j}|\boldsymbol{\theta}, \boldsymbol{\psi})
$$
$$
+ (1 - 2y_{1j} - 2y_{2j} + 4y_{1j}y_{2j}) S(t_{1j}, t_{2j}|\boldsymbol{\theta}, \boldsymbol{\psi}),
$$

where y_{ij} is the 'current' immunological status for individual j with respect to infection i. All available serology is included by means of a direct likelihood (DL) approach; individuals with a missing immunological status for one of the infections under consideration contribute to the log-likelihood as follows:

$$
ll_j\left(\boldsymbol{\theta}, \boldsymbol{\psi}|t_{ij}, y_{ij}\right) = y_{ij} \log\left\{\pi_i(t_{ij}|\boldsymbol{\theta}, \boldsymbol{\psi})\right\} + (1 - y_{ij}) \log\left\{1 - \pi_i(t_{ij}|\boldsymbol{\theta}, \boldsymbol{\psi})\right\},
$$

where $\pi_i(t_{ij}|\boldsymbol{\theta}, \boldsymbol{\psi}) = 1 - S_i(t_{ij}|\boldsymbol{\theta}, \boldsymbol{\psi})$ and only information about infection i is available for subject j. In the case studies presented in Section 18.5, the unit of time is the age a_{ij} of individual $j = 1, \ldots, n$ at the cross-sectional sampling time for infection $i = 1, 2$, and univariate monitoring times are present such that $a_{1j} = a_{2j} = a_j$.

18.5   Case Studies

18.5.1   Parvovirus B19 and varicella zoster virus

18.5.1.1   Belgian Serological Data

Serology on parvovirus B19 (PVB19) and varicella zoster virus (VZV) was collected in Belgium between 2001 and 2003, and 3,378 serum samples were tested for the presence of PVB19- and VZV-specific IgG antibodies, albeit some samples did not convey information about the status with respect to one of the two pathogens. Several individual characteristics were collected in addition to the ELISA test results of which age at the time of data collection is relevant for the analyses herein. One of the most well-known clinical presentations of PVB19 is the common childhood rash called fifth disease or slapped cheek syndrome [19]. In children and teenagers, the disease is usually mild, but in adults, especially women, it is often complicated by acute arthritis which may persist [20]. Infection with PVB19 during pregnancy has been associated with intrauterine fetal death, fetal anemia and fetal hydrops [21]. Human PVB19 is primarily transmitted by infected respiratory droplets. VZV causes two clinically distinct diseases, namely varicella and herpes zoster. Primary infection with VZV results in varicella (chickenpox), an extremely contagious acute infection, which mainly occurs during childhood. Chickenpox is characterized by a generalized vesicular rash, and despite the fact that varicella is most often relatively benign, it can cause a range of severe and potentially lethal complications. Transmission of the virus occurs through direct contact with lesions or aerosol contact by saliva and sneezing. The immunological response following primary infection with VZV induces life-long protective immunity against chickenpox, after which the virus becomes dormant in the body. Potential reactivation of latent VZV may occur years to decades later when humoral and cell-mediated immunity levels are compromised, giving rise to so-called herpes zoster (or shingles). Observed multinomial probabilities $p_{y_{1j}, y_{2j}}(\cdot)$ are plotted against age (in years) in Figure 18.2.

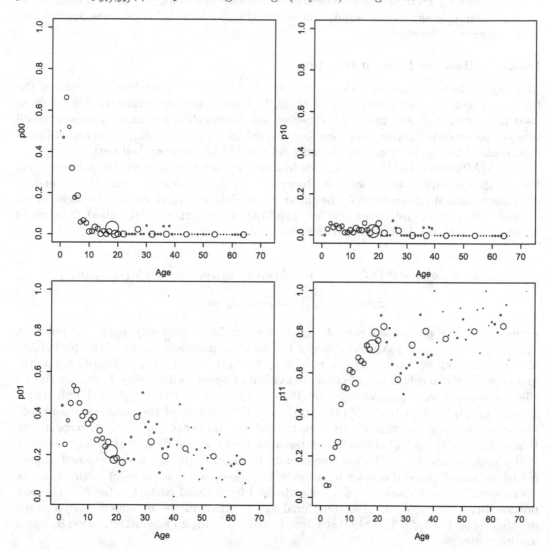

FIGURE 18.2

The observed multinomial probabilities $p_{y_{1j}, y_{2j}}(\cdot)$ with the size of the dots proportional to the number of observations for the bivariate serological survey data on PVB19 and VZV in Belgium (2002–2003) plotted against age (in years): (1) $p_{00}(a_j)$ (left upper panel); (2) $p_{10}(a_j)$ (right upper panel); (3) $p_{01}(a_j)$ (left lower panel); (4) $p_{11}(a_j)$ (right lower panel).

18.5.1.2   Infection Dynamics

Although PVB19-IgG antibodies have been assumed to persist for life [22], in recent years evidence against this hypothesis has been found by several authors [see, e.g., 23, 24]. This hypothesis also is supported by the serological profile which after an initial monotone increase with age, shows a decrease between the ages of 20 and 40 (see Figure 18.2). Since in endemic (and demographic) equilibrium the proportion of seropositives is expected to monotonically increase with age for immunizing infections as the duration of exposure to infection increases with age, the observed phenomenon does not support the life-long immunity assumption for PVB19. [24] argued that PVB19 reinfections are plausible based on an exploration of different compartmental transmission models encompassing different disease dynamics for PVB19. The aforementioned frailty methodology accommodating (time-varying) heterogeneity in the acquisition of PVB19 and VZV infections was applied and results are shown hereunder.

18.5.1.3   Baseline Force of Infection

The baseline infection hazard $\lambda_{i0}(a_j)$ with respect to infection i is modeled by means of the time-homogeneous mass action principle (MAP), being a specific parametric hazard often used in infectious disease modeling. However, our approach is generally applicable to all types of parametric hazards, and therefore it is not mandatory to grasp all complexities of this mechanistic model. Some details concerning the MAP are described next.

The MAP relates the infection hazards to social contact data through the specification of the so-called social contact hypothesis. Recently, several authors argued that the estimation of epidemiological parameters can be informed by data on social contact behavior when dealing with airborne infections [25, 26]. The MAP for infections with a short duration of infectiousness D_i can be formulated as follows:

$$\lambda_i\{a_j, z_{ij}(a_j)\} = ND_iL^{-1}\int_0^\infty\int_0^\infty \beta_i\{a_j, z_{ij}(a_j); a_k, z_{ik}(a_k)\}\lambda_i\{a_k, z_{ik}(a_k)\}$$
$$\times\, S_i\{a_k, z_{ik}(a_k)\}\phi(a_k)da_kdz_{ik}(a_k),$$

where N is the population size, L represents the life expectancy in the population, $\lambda_i\{a_k, z_{ik}(a_k)\} = z_{ik}(a_k)\lambda_{i0}(a_k)$ denotes the force of infection, $\phi(a_k)$ is the probability of being alive at age a_k and $\beta_i\{a_j, z_{ij}(a_j); a_k, z_{ik}(a_k)\} = z_{ij}(a_j)z_{ik}(a_k)\beta_{i0}(a_j, a_k)$ is the 'per-capita' rate at which an infectious individual of age a_k with frailty $z_{ik}(a_k)$ makes an effective contact with a susceptible individual of age a_j with frailty $z_{ij}(a_j)$. Furthermore, $S_i\{a_k, z_{ik}(a_k)\} = S_i\{a_k|z_{ik}(a_k)\}f\{z_{ik}(a_k)\}$, i.e., the product of the conditional susceptible proportion and the joint density function of the components in $Z_{ik}(a_k)$, respectively. Hence, $f\{z_{ik}(a_k)\}dz_{ik}(a_k)$ abbreviates integration over the joint density of the age-invariant frailty components Z^*_{ikm}. The baseline contact function $\beta_{i0}(a_j, a_k)$ is decomposed according to the so-called social contact hypothesis, i.e., $\beta_{i0}(a_j, a_k) = q_i(a_j, a_k|c) \times c(a_j, a_k)$. The "per-capita" contact rates $c(a_j, a_k)$ are estimated from social contact data [26]. The proportionality factor $q_i(a_j, a_k|c)$ is considered age-invariant in the presented analyses (and denoted by q_i, $i = 1, 2$). The MAP is solved iteratively using an age-discretization in 1-year age-intervals.

For infections transmitted by similar routes, the shared frailty model accounts for variability in individual propensity to make (effective) contacts with others. Consequently, Z_j describes an individual activity level. Individual sociability, variation in sexual activity and personal hygiene are likely relevant factors in the spread of respiratory infections, sexually transmitted infections, and infections transmitted by the feco-oral route, respectively [1]. On the other hand, correlated frailty models enable us to accommodate unshared heterogeneity in susceptibility to infection, and infectiousness after infection, in addition to a shared activity level. The correlation between the frailties Z_{ij} is predictive for the association between the infections, albeit the different sources cannot be disentangled. An important transmission parameter describing the spread of an infection is the so-called basic reproduction number. The basic reproduction number R_0 is defined as the expected number of secondary cases produced by a single typical infectious individual during his/her entire infectious period when introduced into a fully susceptible population. Furthermore, R_0 represents an epidemiological threshold parameter in large populations for which a value larger than 1 implies that an infection can invade the population, whereas the infection will go extinct otherwise. More realistically, the effective reproduction number R_e reflects the actual expected number of secondary cases in a population with pre-existing immunity. The effective reproduction number R_{ie} related to infection i, or alternatively R_{i0} when $S_i(a_j) = 1$, $\forall a_j$, can be calculated as the leading eigenvalue of the next generation matrix [27]:

$$ND_i L^{-1} S_i(a_j) \beta_{i0}(a_j, a_k) \{1 + \gamma_i(a_j)\},$$

where $S_i(a_j)$ is the unconditional proportion susceptible individuals of age a_j with regard to infection $i = 1, 2$, and $\gamma_i(a_j)$ is the age-dependent frailty variance. Moreover, we implicitly assume that there is Type I natural mortality and no disease-related mortality [28]. Hence, adequately accounting for heterogeneity is of importance in the estimation of the basic R0. The mean duration of infectiousness for PVB19 is assumed to be $D_1 = 6/365$ years [19] and for VZV to be $D_2 = 7/365$ years [29]. The life expectancy and population size are taken to be $L = 80$ and $N = 9,943,749$, respectively, based on Belgian demographic data for the reference year 2003.

18.5.1.4 Time-invariant Frailty Models

Table 18.1 links the model definitions to the proposed candidate models. Frailty models relying on the assumption of life-long immunity for both infections are denoted by UGF-1, SGF-1, and CGF-1 for univariate, shared, and correlated gamma frailty models, respectively. In addition, UGF-2, SGF-2, and CGF-2 models allow for replenishment of the susceptible compartment for PVB19 at a constant rate σ_1. As advocated previously, infections with VZV are considered to confer life-long immunity leading to $\sigma_2(a_j) = 0$, $\forall a_j$. Despite the general formulation of the frailty models in terms of infection-specific age-dependent proportionality factors $q_{i0}(a_{ij}, a_{ik}|c)$, these terms are considered to be age-invariant, say q_{i0}, in all fitted models as age-dependent proportionality in transmission did not reveal any improvement in model fit.

In Table 18.2, ML estimates for the model parameters in the time-invariant models, derived using the DL approach, are presented together with bootstrap 95% percentile confidence limits based on $B = 500$ bootstrap samples. Results for the time-varying models can be found in Table 18.3 and are discussed herein. Models are compared based on the Akaike Information Criterion (AIC) and Bayesian Information Criterion (BIC). These criteria deal with the trade-off between model fit and model complexity in the sense that they penalize for the number of parameters in the model. The penalization is less strong in AIC compared to BIC. The results in Table 18.2 clearly indicate that the UGF, SGF, and CGF models with SIRS dynamics for PVB19 outperform their SIR counterparts assuming life-long immunity after recovery for both infections. Moreover, based on both information criteria it turns out that the SGF-2 model is the best fitting model. Although more flexible than shared

TABLE 18.1

Definition of the frailty models fitted to the bivariate serological survey data on PVB19 ($i = 1$) and VZV ($i = 2$)

		Dynamics		
Model	Frailty	PVB19	$\sigma_1(a_j)$	Heterogeneity
UGF-1	Univariate	SIR	0	Time-invariant
UGF-2	Univariate	SIRS	σ_1	Time-invariant
SGF-1	Shared	SIR	0	Time-invariant
TDSGF-1-1C	Shared	SIR	0	Time-dependent – 1 component
TDSGF-1-2C	Shared	SIR	0	Time-dependent – 2 components
SGF-2	Shared	SIRS	σ_1	Time-invariant
TDSGF-2-1C	Shared	SIRS	σ_1	Time-dependent – 1 component
TDSGF-2-2C	Shared	SIRS	σ_1	Time-dependent – 2 components
CGF-1	Correlated	SIR	0	Time-invariant
CGF-2	Correlated	SIRS	σ_1	Time-invariant

Note: Simple SIR dynamics are assumed for VZV, giving rise to a replenishment rate $\sigma_2(a_j) = 0$, $\forall a_j$.

frailty models, the use of CGF models shows little advantage over the use of SGF models, at least when accounting for reinfections with PVB19. Given that modeling the underlying infection process decreases the unobserved infection-specific heterogeneity, it is no surprise that the SGF-2 frailty model is preferred over its correlated counterpart (CGF-2). Since the estimated correlation among the infection-specific correlated frailties, implied by the additive decomposition thereof (see Section 18.4), is bounded by the ratio of the frailty standard deviations, the bootstrap-based 95 percent percentile confidence interval for ρ in CGF-2 is asymmetric.

The frailty variances in the UGF models are not comparable with those in the bivariate models since their interpretation differs. In the univariate setting, the frailty variance reflects solely heterogeneity with respect to unobserved factors in the population. By contrast, in any bivariate frailty model, frailty terms impose also a correlation structure among infections. In Figure 18.3, the estimated marginal seroprevalences for PVB19 and VZV are graphically displayed based on the bivariate SGF models (SGF-1: black solid line and SGF-2: gray dashed line). The differences in estimated seroprevalence are more pronounced for PVB19 compared to VZV due to the fact that the models only differ in assumptions regarding PVB19 transmission. Potential reinfections with PVB19 increase the infection hazard which is reflected in an underestimation of the force of infection in the SGF-1 model compared to the SGF-2 model. Note that frailty models with SIRS dynamics for both PVB19 and VZV lead to an equivalent performance in terms of loglikelihood value at the cost of one additional parameter, which is estimated to be not significantly different from zero (not shown here). This result coincides with our previous arguments to settle for SIR features with regard to VZV.

Finally, interest lies in the quantification of the impact of misspecifying the underlying infection process on estimates for the reproduction number R_{i0}, $i = 1, 2$. In Table 18.2, the shared SIR gamma frailty model (SGF-1) yields larger R_0 estimates for both PVB19 and VZV ($\hat{R}_{10} = 3.60$ [3.34, 3.93] and $\hat{R}_{20} = 11.64$ [10.22, 13.26], respectively, with bootstrap 95% confidence limits between squared brackets) as compared to the estimates obtained in the preferred SGF-2 model ($\hat{R}_{10} = 3.18$ [2.99, 3.45] and $\hat{R}_{20} = 8.98$ [8.15, 10.20]), encompassing reinfection dynamics for PVB19. Estimates for R_{i0} in the shared and correlated SIRS models (SGF-2, CGF-2) are almost identical.

TABLE 18.2

ML estimates for the model parameters as well as for the basic reproduction number R_{i0} (PVB19: $i = 1$, VZV: $i = 2$), together with 95% bootstrap percentile confidence intervals in square brackets; AIC- and BIC-values (minima indicated in boldface)

Model				$\hat{R}_0$		AIC	BIC
UGF-1	q_{10}	0.087	[0.080, 0.096]	5.44	[4.73, 6.52]	4900.69	4925.19
	γ_1	0.448	[0.348, 0.580]				
	q_{20}	0.165	[0.159, 0.179]	8.33	[8.02, 9.32]		
	γ_2	1.8e-5	[3.4e-7, 0.044]				
	ρ	0.000	−				
UGF-2	q_{10}	0.070	[0.068, 0.074]	3.05	[2.94, 3.41]	4873.44	4904.06
	σ_1	0.012	[0.008, 0.016]				
	γ_1	3.6e-7	[3.4e-7, 0.077]				
	q_{20}	0.165	[0.159, 0.179]	8.33	[8.02, 9.32]		
	γ_2	1.8e-5	[3.4e-7, 0.044]				
	ρ	0.000	−				
SGF-1	q_{10}	0.072	[0.069, 0.076]	3.60	[3.34, 3.93]	4937.13	4955.51
	q_{20}	0.200	[0.184, 0.220]	11.64	[10.22, 13.26]		
	γ	0.152	[0.101, 0.210]				
	ρ	1.000	−				
SGF-2	q_{10}	0.071	[0.068, 0.075]	3.18	[2.99, 3.45]	**4869.83**	**4894.33**
	σ_1	0.011	[0.008, 0.015]				
	q_{20}	0.172	[0.161, 0.189]	8.98	[8.15, 10.20]		
	γ	0.032	[5.8e-7, 0.082]				
	ρ	1.000	−				
CGF-1	q_{10}	0.087	[0.080, 0.096]	5.42	[4.71, 6.49]	4900.29	4930.91
	q_{20}	0.175	[0.162, 0.192]	9.20	[8.21, 10.51]		
	γ_1	0.446	[0.345, 0.578]				
	γ_2	0.043	[3.7e-7, 0.097]				
	ρ	0.310	[0.001, 0.472]				
CGF-2	q_{10}	0.071	[0.068, 0.075]	3.18	[2.99, 3.50]	4873.83	4910.58
	σ_1	0.011	[0.007, 0.015]				
	q_{20}	0.172	[0.161, 0.189]	8.98	[8.15, 10.22]		
	γ_1	0.032	[3.9e-7, 0.092]				
	γ_2	0.032	[3.9e-7, 0.084]				
	ρ	1.000	[0.689, 1.000]				

Note: UGF, SGF, CGF represent univariate, shared and correlated gamma frailty models, respectively, with versions 1 and 2 referring to immunizing and non-immunizing infection dynamics for PVB19.

18.5.1.5 Time-varying Frailty Models

The results of fitting time-varying bivariate shared frailty models to the Belgian serology on PVB19 and VZV are presented in Table 18.3. In addition to the ML estimates and profile likelihood confidence limits, AIC- and BIC-values are shown for model comparison. Table 18.1 presents an overview of the time-varying models fitted to the Belgian serology

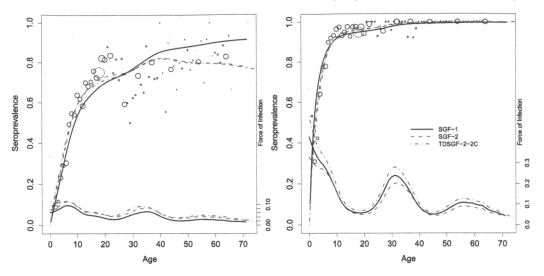

FIGURE 18.3
Observed seroprevalence (dots with size proportional to the number of observations), esti-
mated seroprevalence (upper curves) and corresponding force of infection (lower curves) of
PVB19 (left panel) and VZV (right panel) in Belgium based on bivariate SGF models: the
SGF-1 model (black solid line), the SGF-2 model (gray dashed line), and the TDSGF-2-2C
model (gray dash-dotted line).

on PVB19 and VZV. One- and two-component TDSGF models are considered either with
immunizing (TDSGF-1-1C and TDSGF-1-2C, respectively) or non-immunizing infection
dynamics (TDSGF-2-1C and TDSGF-2-2C, respectively) with regard to PVB19. Although
the SGF-2 and TDSGF-2 frailty models cover more complex disease dynamics, the improved
fit to the data reveals that the assumption of life-long immunity for PVB19 seems questionable. Furthermore, the age-dependent frailty models tend to outperform their age-invariant
counterparts. This result leads to the conclusion that variability is indeed higher in the
younger age groups and decreases with age until a constant frailty variance γ_2 is achieved
(see Figure 18.4).

18.5.2   Hepatitis A and B

18.5.2.1   Flemish Serological Data

In 1993 and early 1994, a sero-epidemiological study on the prevalence of hepatitis A and
B was conducted in the Flemish Community in Belgium [30]. Residual blood samples were
collected from noninfectious disease wards in hospitals. The dataset contains 3,890 and
3,838 individuals with observed immunological statuses for hepatitis A and B, respectively,
and having reported ages ranging from 0 to 100 years. When focusing on individuals with a
known immunological status regarding both diseases, 3,787 complete profiles can be identified. The age-dependent seroprevalence for hepatitis A and B is shown in the left and right
panel of Figure 18.5, respectively. Hepatitis A, formerly known as infectious hepatitis, is
caused by the hepatitis A virus (HAV), resulting in an infection of the liver. Early clinical
manifestations include fatigue, nausea, vomiting, and discomfort in the right upper quadrant
of the torso [31]. Other symptoms of HAV infection are diarrhoea, fever, abdominal pain
and jaundice (yellow skin). HAV is mainly transmitted by food or water contaminated with

TABLE 18.3

ML estimates for the model parameters as well as for the basic reproduction number R_{i0} (PVB19: $i = 1$, VZV: $i = 2$), together with 95% profile likelihood confidence intervals in square brackets; AIC- and BIC-values (minima indicated in boldface)

Model				$\hat{R}_0$		AIC	BIC
TDSGF-1-1C	q_{10}	0.072	[0.069, 0.076]	3.60	[3.22, 3.99]	4939.14	4963.64
	q_{20}	0.200	[0.183, 0.221]	11.64	[9.99,13.49]		
	$\gamma_{\cdot 1}$	0.152	[0.100, 0.210]				
	$\phi_{\cdot 1}$	0.000	[0.000, 0.009]				
TDSGF-1-2C	q_{10}	0.066	[0.062, 0.071]	3.74	[3.15, 4.87]	4912.08	4942.70
	q_{20}	0.235	[0.191, 0.299]	15.65	[11.38, 24.08]		
	$\gamma_{\cdot 1}$	2.918	[1.524, 5.004]				
	$\gamma_{\cdot 2}$	0.233	[0.156, 0.323]				
	$\phi_{\cdot 1}$	0.316	[0.246, 0.425]				
TDSGF-2-1C	q_{10}	0.065	[0.061, 0.070]	2.90	[2.64, 3.49]	4862.93	**4893.56**
	σ_1	0.012	[0.009, 0.016]				
	q_{20}	0.158	[0.141, 0.179]	8.19	[7.15, 10.46]		
	$\gamma_{\cdot 1}$	1.470	[0.415, 3.498]				
	$\phi_{\cdot 1}$	0.330	[0.209, 0.530]				
TDSGF-2-1C unequal frailty variances	q_{10}	0.065	[0.060, 0.070]	2.94	[2.60, 4.97]	4863.83	4900.57
	σ_1	0.013	[0.009, 0.021]				
	q_{20}	0.154	[0.133, 0.175]	7.98	[6.76, 11.83]		
	$\gamma_{\cdot 1}$	1.646	[0.459, 6.443]				
	ϕ_{11}	0.239	[0.141, 0.648]				
	ϕ_{21}	0.377	[0.226, 0.677]				
TDSGF-2-2C	q_{10}	0.066	[0.063, 0.071]	3.30	[2.79, 4.45]	**4859.26**	4896.01
	σ_1	0.011	[0.007, 0.015]				
	q_{20}	0.193	[0.156, 0.257]	11.27	[8.11, 18.90]		
	$\gamma_{\cdot 1}$	2.419	[0.839, 4.960]				
	$\gamma_{\cdot 2}$	0.095	[0.017, 0.186]				
	$\phi_{\cdot 1}$	0.303	[0.226, 0.423]				
TDSGF-2-2C unequal frailty variances	q_{10}	0.066	[0.063, 0.081]	3.40	[2.78, 6.17]	4860.73	4903.60
	σ_1	0.012	[0.007, 0.020]				
	q_{20}	0.188	[0.151, 0.251]	10.98	[7.85, 19.47]		
	$\gamma_{\cdot 1}$	2.554	[0.861, 5.994]				
	$\gamma_{\cdot 2}$	0.095	[0.016, 0.181]				
	ϕ_{11}	0.249	[0.160, 0.706]				
	ϕ_{21}	0.327	[0.228, 0.486]				

Note: TDSGF-1 and TDSGF-2 refer to time-varying shared gamma frailty models with immunizing or non-immunizing infection dynamics for PVB19, respectively, and based on a one- (1C) or two-component (2C) multiplicative model.

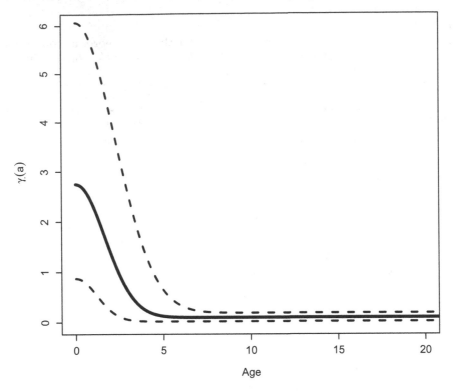

FIGURE 18.4
Age-dependent frailty variance (solid line) for the TDSGF-2-2C model and corresponding
95% confidence limits (dashed lines) when applied to the bivariate serological survey data
on PVB19 and VZV in Belgium.

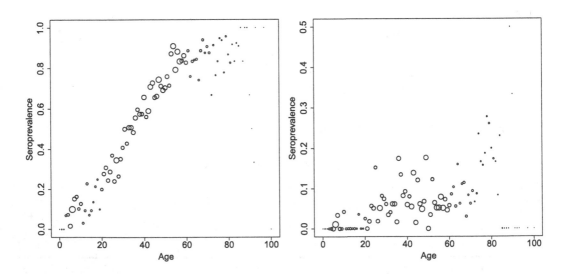

FIGURE 18.5
Seroprevalence of HAV (left panel) and HBV (right panel) in Flanders, Belgium (1993–1994)
with the size of dots proportional to the number of observations.

feces and rarely through the parenteral route, i.e., by injection in case of drug users and hemophiliacs. Transmission is facilitated by poor hygienic living and housing conditions, and HAV is particularly common in developing countries [30]. Hepatitis B or serum hepatitis is caused by the hepatitis B virus (HBV). Infection with HBV leads to chronic infection which is the main cause of death among patients with cirrhosis of the liver, chronic liver inflammation, and hepatocellular carcinoma (liver cancer). Furthermore, chronic hepatitis carriers remain infectious and may transmit the disease for many years [32]. HBV transmission is mainly driven by blood contact via the parenteral route, i.e., blood transfusions, injections, tattoos, contaminated blood products, or through sexual contact.

18.5.2.2 Baseline Force of Infection

Time-invariant and time-dependent SGF and CGF models are fitted to the HAV and HBV serology. Gompertz infection-specific baseline hazard functions $\lambda_{i0}(a_j)$, $i = 1, 2$, are considered here, i.e., $\lambda_{i0}(a_j) = \xi_i \exp(\nu_i a_j)$, where $\xi_i > 0$ and $-\infty < \nu_i < +\infty$. In addition, both infections are presumed to confer life-long immunity, entailing SIR infection dynamics. Fore more details on the models fitted to the Flemish serological survey data on HAV and HBV infections, and their abbreviations, we refer to Table 18.4.

18.5.2.3 Time-invariant and Time-varying Frailty Models

In Table 18.5, ML estimates and standard error estimates for the model parameters are presented. An improvement in model fit is observed when comparing age-invariant frailty models (SGF and CGF) with their age-dependent counterparts, underlining the importance of accommodating time-varying heterogeneity. Leaving aside the piecewise constant model due to its different interpretation, shared frailty models with (TDSGF-1C*) and without unequal frailty variances (TDSGF-1C) provide the best fit among all fitted multiplicative models based on their respective AIC- and BIC-values, respectively. Two-component shared frailty models (TDSGF-2C) with either equal or unequal decay rates for both infections did not improve the model fit. The time-dependent piecewise constant shared gamma frailty (TDPCSGF) model is considered to assess the goodness-of-fit of the imposed variance functions or, equivalently, the exponential decay functions $h_{i1}(t_{ij})$. In the TDPCSGF model, we selected four age-groups [0, 12), [12, 25), [25, 65), 65+ for which independent frailty terms are considered. Note that this model allows for greater flexibility in modeling age-dependent heterogeneity, albeit that the choice of the age-intervals is subjective and influences the model fit. The piecewise constant model outperforms all other presented frailty models based on AIC, albeit that model TDSGF-1C has a smaller BIC value. It is clear that heterogeneity is highest at young ages. Variability decreases with time and increases again

TABLE 18.4

Overview of frailty models fitted to the Flemish seroprevalence data on HAV and HBV; 1C refers to a one-component multiplicative model

Model	Dynamics HAV	Dynamics HBV	Heterogeneity	Z^*_{ijm}
SGF	SIR	SIR	Time invariant	Shared
CGF	SIR	SIR	Time invariant	Correlated
TDSGF-1C	SIR	SIR	Time-dependent $- \phi_{11} = \phi_{21}$	Shared
TDSGF-1C*	SIR	SIR	Time-dependent	Shared
TDCGF-1C	SIR	SIR	Time-dependent $- \phi_{11} = \phi_{21}$	Correlated
TDPCSGF	SIR	SIR	Piecewise constant time-dependent	Shared

TABLE 18.5

ML estimates and standard error estimates for the model parameters with corresponding AIC- and BIC-values (minima indicated in boldface)

Parameter	SGF	CGF	TDSGF-1C $\phi_{11}=\phi_{21}$	TDSGF-1C* $\phi_{11}\neq\phi_{21}$	TDCGF-1C $\phi_{11}=\phi_{21}$	TDPCSGF
ξ_1	0.012 (0.001)	0.007 (0.001)	0.077 (0.029)	0.139 (0.093)	0.151 (0.105)	0.029 (0.006)
ν_1	0.036 (0.005)	0.106 (0.017)	-0.012 (0.007)	-0.021 (0.009)	-0.022 (0.009)	0.009 (0.005)
ξ_2	0.002 (4e$-$4)	0.002 (4e$-$4)	0.003 (0.001)	0.003 (0.001)	0.003 (0.001)	0.002 (4e$-$4)
ν_2	-0.003 (0.008)	-0.001 (0.014)	-0.009 (0.008)	-0.012 (0.009)	-0.008 (0.008)	-0.005 (0.008)
$\sqrt{\gamma_{11}}$	0.725 (0.086)	1.651 (0.176)	5.843 (0.829)	6.444 (1.013)	6.606 (1.020)	3.671 (0.606)
$\sqrt{\gamma_{21}}$	0.725 (0.086)	1.608 (2.272)	5.843 (0.829)	6.444 (1.013)	5.765 (0.831)	3.671 (0.606)
$\sqrt{\gamma_{2}}$	–	–	–	–	–	2.421 (0.504)
$\sqrt{\gamma_{3}}$	–	–	–	–	–	0.012 (0.160)
$\sqrt{\gamma_{4}}$	–	–	–	–	–	8.813 (7.856)
ϕ_{11}	–	–	0.034 (0.005)	0.026 (0.007)	0.025 (0.007)	–
ϕ_{21}	–	–	0.034 (0.005)	0.044 (0.011)	0.025 (0.007)	–
ρ	1.000 (–)	0.497 (0.702)	1.000 (–)	1.000 (–)	0.871 (0.080)	1.000 (–)
AIC	5824.90	5794.89	5756.01	5755.52	5757.04	**5749.01**
BIC	5856.41	5838.99	**5793.82**	5799.62	5807.44	5799.42

Note: SGF and CGF represent shared and correlated gamma frailty models, respectively. TDSGF-1C and TDCGF-1C are time-dependent shared and correlated gamma frailty models based on a one-component multiplicative model; * refers to unequal frailty variances. TDPCSGF is a time-dependent piecewise constant shared gamma frailty model.

in the last age-group, albeit that a limited amount of data is available therein. Although slightly outperforming the TDSGF-1C* model, little evidence against an exponential decay in heterogeneity is obtained from the TDPCSGF model. Despite its improved fit, the biological interpretation of the TDPCSGF model is not straightforward and independence of the frailty components is unrealistic. Nevertheless, fitting this model is useful to investigate the time-varying shape of the frailty variance. The estimated multinomial probabilities for the TDSGF-1C* (black solid line) and TDPCSGF model (gray dotted line) are shown in Figure 18.6 with the observed probabilities (size proportional to the sample size). The TD-PCSGF fit deviates from the TDSGF-1C* fit at higher ages. In Figure 18.7, age-dependent frailty variances for HAV (left panel) and HBV (right panel) are presented, signalling a faster decrease for hepatitis B (TDSGF-1C* model).

Estimating the correlation between infection-specific frailty terms could reflect to what extent latent processes, such as social contact behavior of people, susceptibility to infection,

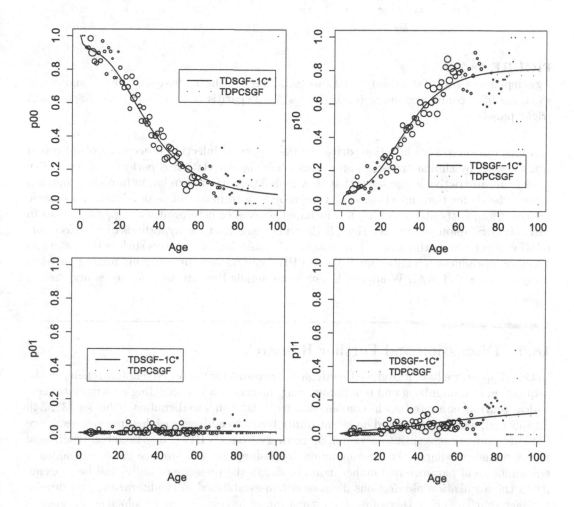

FIGURE 18.6

The observed (dots with size proportional to the number of observations) and estimated multinomial probabilities $\hat{p}_{y_{1j}, y_{2j}}(\cdot)$ for the TDCGF-1C* and TDPCSGF-models when applied to the bivariate serological survey data on hepatitis A and B infections in Flanders, Belgium anno 1993–1994: (1) $\hat{p}_{00}(a_j)$ (left upper panel); (2) $\hat{p}_{10}(a_j)$ (right upper panel); (3) $\hat{p}_{01}(a_j)$ (left lower panel); (4) $\hat{p}_{11}(a_j)$ (right lower panel).

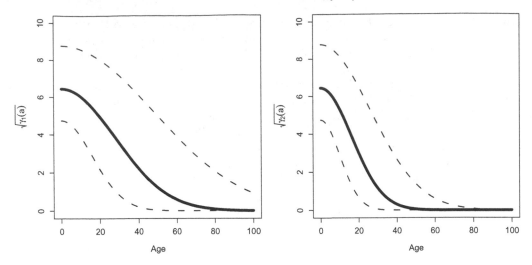

FIGURE 18.7
Age-dependent frailty standard deviations (solid line) in the TDSGF-1C* model and corresponding 95% confidence limits (dashed lines) for hepatitis A (left panel) and hepatitis B
(right panel).

and infectiousness after infection, drive the more general infection process, or could reveal
transmission by similar transmission routes when the correlation is perfect. Shared frailty
models are restrictive in the sense that they assume a perfect correlation implying common
activity levels for both infections, i.e., the propensity to make contacts relevant for disease
transmission, without accounting for unshared sources of heterogeneity, e.g., differences in
susceptibility among infections. Here, little evidence against the hypothesis of a perfect correlation is present. Estimation of important epidemiological parameters such as the basic and
effective reproduction number for HAV and HBV can be done by imposing mixing patterns
using the so-called WAIFW approach. For more details thereon, we refer to [8] and [28].

18.6   Discussion and Further Research

In this chapter, we have introduced strategies to account for unobserved heterogeneity in the
acquisition of immunizing and non-immunizing infections when modeling multivariate serological (current status) data in combination with data on social contact behavior [33, 34].
To this end, we mainly focused on latent frailty terms to address such heterogeneities. Since
life-long protection against infection upon recovery from PVB19 is questionable, traditional
frailty models relying on the life-long immunity assumption will produce biased estimates of
epidemiological parameters. Further more, although the presence of individual heterogeneity in the acquisition of infectious diseases is well-established in the literature, and despite
the fact that the effect thereof on the estimation of important epidemiological parameters
has been demonstrated, unmeasured variability is rarely accounted for in epidemiological
and mathematical infectious disease models. Applying the refined frailty methodology to
bivariate serological data on PVB19 and VZV (for which immunizing dynamics could not
be disproved) revealed that secondary infections with PVB19 are likely, thereby invalidating the life-long immunity assumption. As pointed out by [24], we can further differentiate
between long-term processes of waning immunity for PVB19, natural boosting of immunity

upon re-exposure to the pathogen, and secondary infections through the use of various compartmental models. Immunizing and non-immunizing views on the evolution of the PVB19 immune response resulted in altered estimates of the age-specific force of infection and corresponding basic reproduction numbers for both PVB19 and VZV. Unobserved heterogeneity in the observed seroprevalences decreased substantially when adjusting for PVB19 reinfection dynamics, and shared heterogeneity across infections was preferred over a more flexible correlation structure. This result could be explained by similar transmission pathways (activity levels) for these childhood infections. The aforementioned analyses rely on (1) transmission rates being directly proportional to social contact rates estimated from the Belgian POLYMOD survey [35], and (2) endemicity of PVB19 and VZV which seems tenable in industrialized countries such as Belgium. Although dichotomizing (or trichotomizing) infection-specific antibody levels using one (or two) threshold values is common practice, all diagnostic tests classifying subjects based on a single or multiple threshold values, such as an ELISA test, suffer from diagnostic uncertainty and misclassification. More specifically, this approach entails both false negative (seronegative individuals with protective immunity) and false positive (seropositive individuals without protective immunity) cases, leading to biased estimates of the prevalence and force of infection. In recent years, mixture-models have been proposed to model continuous antibody titres directly and to infer important epidemiological parameters thereof while avoiding the specification of threshold values, see Chapter 19 and [36], and relating this approach to the frailty methodology would be an interesting topic for further research.

The application of time- or age-varying frailty models for immunizing and non-immunizing infections has been studied here as well. It has been shown that these models are essential to describe age-dependency in individual heterogeneity, and that these models generally outperform age-invariant counterparts in both case studies at hand. Reinfection dynamics for PVB19 still are supported based on the age-varying frailty methodology. A drawback of the proposed multiplicative frailty models is the time- or age-dependency of the frailty range to ensure positivity of these frailties. It would therefore be interesting to consider frailty decompositions, e.g., power transformations, that overcome this limitation. In addition, heterogeneity is assumed to decay exponentially with age which seems plausible for childhood infections, but could be untenable for other diseases. In future research, it would be interesting to test the goodness-of-fit for the parametric shape of the decay function in multiplicative time-varying frailty models, and to explore different parametric and semi-parametric shapes thereof. Recently the statistical problem of overdispersion has been studied for CS data. [37] developed a combined model accommodating individual heterogeneity and overdispersion at the age stratum level through the specification of individual frailty terms and stratum-specific random effects, respectively. Their flexible conditional approach relies on concepts of partial marginalization. Furthermore, the MAP considered in the PVB19 and VZV case study allows individuals to make contact with each other at different rates depending on observed covariates such as their ages, and unmeasured activity (frailty) levels, but these contacts can occur with whomever in the population. Hence, the mass action concept assumes that there does not exist a predefined relationship or causal circumstance by which certain pairs of individuals are more likely to interact with each other than other pairs of individuals with similar characteristics. Clustering of contacts, hereby extending the MAP, could be important in modeling disease spread.

One of the key assumptions when deriving the expressions for the proportion of individuals in the different compartments of the proposed mathematical models is the assumption of endemic equilibrium. However, when time heterogeneity is present, the mathematical models should be described using a system of partial differential equations rather than ordinary differential equations. Under an SIR scenario, the proportion of recovered individuals (i.e., individuals who acquired humoral immunity) can be related to the age- and time-dependent force of infection [see, e.g., 38, 39]. In the same manner as presented in this chapter, the force of infection can be extended to include individual- and infection-specific frailty terms, which are potentially age- and/or time-varying, acting multiplicatively on a baseline hazard function. Using multivariate serial serological survey data, i.e., serological survey data on different pathogens collected at different cross-sectional time points, and considering parametric or semi-parametric baseline hazard functions, we could estimate the individual heterogeneity and (age- and time-varying) association in the acquisition of multiple pathogens. This is an interesting avenue for further research as presently more serial serological data is collected.

Other applications are also worthwhile to pursue such as quantifying heterogeneity in the acquisition of sexually transmitted infections thereby extending previous work by [40] in the context of HPV to name one or the analysis of trivariate serological data in the presence of vaccination by [41].

References

[1] C. P. Farrington, M. N. Kanaan, and N. J. Gay. Estimation of the basic reproduction number for infectious diseases from age-stratified serological survey data. *Journal of the Royal Statistical Society, Series C (Applied Statistics)*, 50(3):251–292, 2001.

[2] D. G. Clayton. A model for association in bivariate life tables and its application in epidemiological studies of familial tendency in chronic disease incidence. *Biometrika*, 65(1):141–151, 1978.

[3] P. Hougaard. *Analysis of Multivariate Survival Data*. Statistics for Biology and Health. Springer, New York, 2000.

[4] J. R. Dale. Global cross-ratio models for bivariate, discrete, ordered responses. *Biometrics*, 42:909–917, 1986.

[5] J. Palmgren. Regression models for bivariate binary responses. Technical report, Technical Report 101, Department of Biostatistics,University of Washington, Seattle, WA, 1989.

[6] N. Hens, M. Aerts, Z. Shkedy, H. Theeten, P. Van Damme, and P. Beutels. Modelling multi-sera data: The estimation of new joint and conditional epidemiological parameters. *Statistics in Medicine*, 27(14):2651–2664, 2008.

[7] S. Unkel and C. P. Farrington. A new measure of time-varying association for shared frailty models with bivariate current status data. *Biostatistics*, 13(4):665–679, 2012.

[8] R. M. Anderson and R. M. May. *Infectious Diseases of Humans; Dynamics and Control*. Oxford University Press, Oxford, UK, 1991.

[9] J. Vaupel, K. Manton, and E. Stallard. The impact of heterogeneity in individual frailty on the dynamics of mortality. *Demography*, 16(3):439–454, 1979.

[10] O. O. Aalen. Heterogeneity in survival analysis. *Statistics in Medicine*, 7(11):1121–1137, 1988.

[11] F. A. B. Coutinho, E. Massad, L. F. Lopez, M. N. Burattini, C. J. Struchiner, and R. S. Azevedo-Neto. Modelling heterogeneities in individual frailties in epidemic models. *Mathematical and Computer Modelling*, 30(1–2):97–115, 1999.

[12] N. Hens, A. Wienke, M. Aerts, and G. Molenberghs. The correlated and shared gamma frailty model for bivariate current status data: An illustration for cross-sectional serological data. *Statistics in Medicine*, 27(14):2785–2800, 2009.

[13] A. I. Yashin, J. W. Vaupel, and I. A. Iachine. Correlated individual frailty: An advantageous approach to survival analysis of bivariate data. *Mathematical Population Studies*, 5(2):145–159, 1995.

[14] M. C. Paik, W.-Y. Tsai, and R. Ottman. Multivariate survival analysis using piecewise gamma frailty. *Biometrics*, 50(4):975–988, 1994.

[15] C. M. A. Wintrebert, H. Putter, A. H. Zwinderman, and van Houwelingen J. C. Centre-effect on survival after bone marrow transplantation: Application of time-dependent frailty models. *Biometrical Journal*, 46(5):512–525, 2004.

[16] C. P. Farrington, S. Unkel, and K. Anaya-Izquierdo. The relative frailty variance and shared frailty models. *Journal of the Royal Statistical Society, Series B (Statistical Methodology)*, 74(4):1–24, 2012.

[17] S. Unkel, C. P. Farrington, H. J. Withaker, and R. Pebody. Time varying frailty models and the estimation of heterogeneities in transmission of infectious diseases. *Journal of the Royal Statistical Society, Series C (Applied Statistics)*, 63(1):141–158, 2014.

[18] J. Sun. *The Statistical Analysis of Interval-Censored Failure Time Data*. Statistics for Biology and Health. Springer, New York, 2006.

[19] M. Anderson and J. D. Cherry. *Textbook of Pediatric Infectious Diseases*, chapter 17, page 1796. Saunders (Elsevier), Philadelphia, PA, 5th ed., 2004.

[20] B. J. Cohen. Parvovirus B19: An expanding spectrum of disease. *British Medical Journal*, 311(7019):1549–1552, 1995.

[21] T. Tolfvenstam, N. Papadogiannakis, O. Norbeck, K. Petersson, and K. Broliden. Frequency of human parvovirus B19 in intrauterine fetal death. *The Lancet*, 357(9267):1494–1497, 2001.

[22] N. S. Young and K. E. Brown. Mechanisms of disease: Parvovirus B19. *The New England Journal of Medicine*, 350(6):586–597, 2004.

[23] J. P. Nascimento, M. M. Buckley, K. E. Brown, and B. J. Cohen. The prevalence of antibody to human parvovirus B19 in Rio De Janeiro, Brazil. *Revista do Instituto de Medicina Tropical de Sao Paulo*, 32(1):41–45, 1990.

[24] N. Goeyvaerts, N. Hens, M. Aerts, and P. Beutels. Model structure analysis to estimate basic immunological processes and maternal risk for parvovirus B19. *Biostatistics*, 12(2):283–302, 2011.

[25] J. Wallinga, P. Teunis, and M. Kretzschmar. Using data on social contacts to estimate age-specific transmission parameters for respiratory-spread infectious agents. *American Journal of Epidemiology*, 164(10):936–944, 2006.

[26] N. Goeyvaerts, N. Hens, B. Ogunjimi, M. Aerts, Z. Shkedy, P. Van Damme, and P. Beutels. Estimating infectious disease parameters from data on social contacts and serological status. *Journal of the Royal Statistical Society, Series C (Applied Statistics)*, 59(2):255–277, 2010.

[27] C. P. Farrington, S. Unkel, and K. Anaya-Izquierdo. Estimation of basic reproduction numbers: Individual heterogeneity and robustness to perturbation of the contact function. *Biostatistics*, 14(3):528–540, 2013.

[28] N. Hens, Z. Shkedy, M. Aerts, C. Faes, P. Van Damme, and P. Beutels. *Modeling Infectious Disease Parameters Based on Serological and Social Contact Data: A Modern Statistical Perspective*. Springer, New York, 2012.

[29] M. E. Halloran, S. L. Cochi, T. A. Lieu, M. Wharton, and L. Fehrs. Theoretical epidemiologic and morbidity effects of routine varicella immunization of preschool children in the United States. *American Journal of Epidemiology*, 140(2):81–104, 1994.

[30] M. Beutels, P. Van Damme, W. Aelvoet, J. Desmyter, F. Dondeyne, C. Goilav, R. Mak et al. Prevalence of hepatitis A, B and C in the Flemish population. *European Journal of Epidemiology*, 13(3):275–280, 1997.

[31] S. M. Lemon. Type A viral hepatitis: Epidemiology, diagnosis, and prevention. *Clinical Chemistry*, 43(8):1494–1499, 1997.

[32] E. J. Aspinall, G. Hawkins, A. Fraser, S. J. Hutchinson, and D. Goldberg. Hepatitis B prevention, diagnosis, treatment and care: A review. *Occupational Medicine*, 61(8): 531–540, 2011.

[33] S. Abrams and N. Hens. Modeling individual heterogeneity in the acquisition of recurrent infections: An application to parvovirus B19. *Biostatistics*, 16(1):129–142, 2015.

[34] S. Abrams, A. Wienke, and N. Hens. Modelling time varying heterogeneity in recurrent infection processes: An application to serological data. *Journal of the Royal Statistical Society: Series C (Applied Statistics)*, 67:687–704, 2018.

[35] J. Mossong, N. Hens, M. Jit, P. Beutels, K. Auranen, R. Mikolajczyk, M. Massari et al. Social contacts and mixing patterns relevant to the spread of infectious diseases. *PLoS Medicine*, 5(3):381–391, 2008.

[36] K. Bollaerts, M. Aerts, Z. Shkedy, C. Faes, Y. Van der Stede, P. Beutels, and N. Hens. Estimating the population prevalence and force of infection directly from antibody titres. *Statistical Modelling*, 12(5):441–462, 2012.

[37] S. Abrams, M. Aerts, G. Molenberghs, and N. Hens. Parametric overdispersed frailty models for current status data. *Biometrics*, 73:1388–1400, 2017.

[38] N. G. Becker. *Analysis of Infectious Disease Data*. Chapman and Hall, London, UK, 1989.

[39] N. Keiding. Age-specic incidence and prevalence: a statistical perspective (with discussion). *Journal of the Royal Statistical Society*, Series A 154(3):371–412, 1991.

[40] M.A. Vink, J. Berkhof, J. van de Kassteele, M. van Boven, and J. A. Bogaards. A bivariate mixture model for natural antibody levels to human papillomavirus types 16 and 18: Baseline estimates for monitoring the herd effects of immunization. *PLoS One*, 2016.

[41] J. G. Wood, N. Goeyvaerts, C. R. MacIntyre, R. I. Menzies, P. B. McIntyre, and N. Hens. Estimating vaccine coverage from serial trivariate serologic data in the presence of waning immunity. *Epidemiology*, 26(3):381–389, 2015.

19

Mixture Modeling

Emanuele Del Fava and Ziv Shkedy

CONTENTS

19.1 Introduction

The prevalence of immune (or seroprevalence or, simply, prevalence) and the force of infection (FOI) are critical factors in the epidemiology of infection. The prevalence, π, is the proportion of immune individuals at a specific time in a specific population, and the FOI, λ, is the instantaneous per capita rate at which susceptible individuals acquire infection [1]. For many airborne infections, both the prevalence and the FOI are assumed to be dependent on the age of the host a and on the calendar time t [2]. For the analyses presented in this chapter, we assume that the disease is in a steady state, i.e., the FOI and the transmission parameters are time-independent. We further assume that the disease is irreversible, meaning that immunity is assumed to be life long and that the mortality caused by the infection is negligible and can be ignored. The prevalence and the FOI are commonly estimated using current status data [3, 4] from cross-sectional serological surveys. It is assumed that the current infection status Z_i of the ith subject aged $a_i, i = 1, \ldots, n$, is known and has Bernoulli distribution,

$$Z_i = \begin{cases} 0, & \text{if } Y_i < \phi_l, \quad 1 - \pi(a_i), & \text{susceptible,} \\ 1, & \text{if } Y_i > \phi_u, \quad \pi(a_i), & \text{immune,} \end{cases} \tag{19.1}$$

where $\pi(a_i)$ is the population prevalence for age group a. The variable Z_i is obtained by dichotomizing the individual antibody count Y_i using the set of cut-off points ϕ_l and ϕ_u. Antibody titers higher than ϕ_u are considered as the signal (evidence of past infection), while antibody titers lower than ϕ_l are considered as noise (residual of maternal protection, giving no evidence of past infection). Finally, the antibody titers encompassed by the cut-offs are deemed as inconclusive (or equivocal) and are usually discarded from the serological analysis (Figure 19.1a). The prevalence $\pi(a_i)$ is defined as $\pi(a_i) = P(Z_i = 1|a_i) = P(Y_i > \phi_u|a_i)$. Therefore, in each age group, the observed prevalence is the proportion of individuals in the sample for which the antibody titers are higher than the cut-off ϕ_u (Figure 19.1b). For example, Figure 19.1c shows the observed prevalence of varicella-zoster virus (VZV) in Belgium.

Methods for the estimation of $\pi(a)$ assume that the current status of the disease Z_i is known, given the set of fixed cut-off points ϕ_l and ϕ_u. These cut-offs are often arbitrarily chosen and given as fixed thresholds by the assay's manufacturer based on some conventions, e.g., mean plus three-fold standard deviation [5, 6]. Defining the sensitivity as the probability to correctly identify the true antibody-positive cases and the specificity as the probability to correctly identify the true antibody-negative cases [7], it has been argued that conventional cut-offs imply that test specificity is larger than test sensitivity [8–10]. This situation happens since assays are primarily designed for diagnostic purposes, where the focus is on the detection of true negative cases (susceptible), to exclude with a higher probability that a person is infected. Such an approach allows to have a high positive predictive value (i.e., the proportion of cases, classified as positive, that are true positive), which is appropriate in a diagnostic setting [9]. However, the focus of population serological surveys is more on the detection of true positive cases (immune), as the main interest is not the individual patient management (as in diagnoses), but rather the estimation of the seroprevalence in the population. For this purpose, a larger sensitivity, rather than a larger specificity,

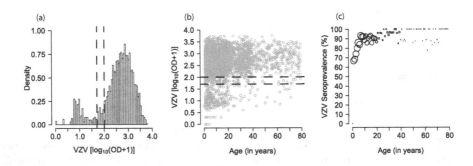

FIGURE 19.1
VZV in Belgium, 2001–2003. (a) Histogram of the antibody titers (after a log-10 plus one transformation) with conventional cut-off points (dashed lines). (b) Scatter plot of the antibody titers (after a log-10 plus one transformation of with conventional cut-off points (dashed lines). (c) Proportions seropositive by age determined using the cut-off points.

is necessary. Indeed, the use of conventional thresholds would lead to underestimating the prevalence because many seropositive cases with low antibody response would likely be classified as seronegative. Moreover, the use of a fixed set of cut-off points exposes to the risk of misclassification of observations, such as false negative (immune individuals classified as seronegative) and false positive (susceptible individuals classified as seropositive), and inconclusive classification (when the individual antibody count is included between the two manufacturer's thresholds) [11, 12].

In this chapter, we focus on an alternative approach in which we consider, for the purpose of the analysis, the entire distribution of the antibody titers, thus assuming that individuals with different infection status (susceptible or immune) arise from different antibody titer distributions.

Figure 19.1 shows the distribution of the concentration of the antibody titers (optical density (OD)) for VZV in Belgium in 2001–2003 [13], after a common logarithm plus one transformation (to avoid issues with negative values when the OD is zero). The figures reveal two groups in the distribution of the log10(OD+1). The group to the left accounts for the antibody levels of the susceptible people, while the group on the right accounts for the antibody levels of the immune. The determination of the current status of infection depends on the subpopulation to which the ith subject belongs, namely,

$$Z_i = \begin{cases} 0, & \text{if } Y_i \sim H_1(\mu_1), \quad 1 - \pi(a_i), \quad \text{susceptible,} \\ 1, & \text{if } Y_i \sim H_2(\mu_2), \quad \pi(a_i), \quad \text{immune.} \end{cases} \tag{19.2}$$

Here, H_1 and H_2 are the distributions of log10(OD+1) for the susceptible and the immune, respectively, and μ_1 and μ_2 are the mean log10(OD+1) in the two groups. We aim to estimate μ_1 and μ_2, as well as $\pi(a)$, the probability that the ith subject belongs to the immune group, i.e., the prevalence.

Estimation of the unknown parameters in (19.2) can be achieved using a mixture modeling approach [5, 14]. Assuming that a specific population can be divided into K subpopulations, mixture modeling is a data-driven approach that aims to assign the observations to these K subpopulations (components) and that allows us to characterize their distribution within the obtained component. In the context of serological data, the primary approach assumes a two-component mixture model stratified by age class, with one component for the susceptible (H_1) and one for the immune (H_2), as shown in (19.2) [8, 14]. Different distributions can be used, such as symmetric distributions as the normal or skewer distributions as the truncated normal, the Gamma, or the Student's t. Developing models for vaccine-preventable infections, other authors did not constrain the mixture to two components only, but considered the number of sub-populations as an additional parameter of the model to be estimated [9, 10, 15–17].

In all these mixture models, the component with the lower mean antibody level represents the distribution of the log antibody titers of the susceptible individuals, while the remaining components account for increasing levels of antibodies, arising either from vaccination or from natural infection. The prevalence can be estimated by summing up the mixture probabilities (i.e., the probability of belonging to a specific component) of all the components labeled as immune [18]. A different approach consists in estimating the true prevalence and the FOI combining the use of a mixture model (for the estimation of the means of the components) and a flexible regression model (for the estimation of the age-dependent mean of the antibody titers) [11].

In this chapter, we focus on a hierarchical Bayesian finite mixture model [19], estimated using Markov chain Monte Carlo (MCMC) methods. The mixture probability is assumed to be age-dependent. Several models, either parametric or nonparametric, are used to model the dependence of the mixture probability on age. In contrast with earlier work, which focused on the estimation of the prevalence, the methods discussed in this chapter allow

Handbook of Infectious Disease Data Analysis

the modeling of both the prevalence and the FOI, the latter for pre-vaccination serological data only.

The chapter is structured as follows. In Section 19.2, we introduce the data used in the analysis. We discuss the hierarchical Bayesian mixture models and the criteria for model selection in Section 19.3. In Section 19.4, we present the results of the analysis of two pre-vaccination serological samples, i.e., parvovirus B19 (B19) in Belgium and VZV in England and Wales, and a post-vaccination serological sample of measles (MeV) in Italy. Finally, we discuss the findings in Section 19.5.

19.2   Case Studies

19.2.1   Parvovirus B19 in Belgium

Parvovirus B19 is a human virus that causes a childhood rash called fifth disease or slapped cheek syndrome. The virus is spread primarily by infected respiratory droplets. Symptoms usually begin around six days after exposure and last around a week. Infected individuals with normal immune systems are infective before they become symptomatic, but probably not afterwards [20]. Individuals with B19 IgG antibodies generally are considered immune to recurrent infection, although re-infection is possible in a minority of cases [21]. There is currently no vaccine available against this virus [22].

Serological samples were collected and tested for antibodies to B19 for five European countries (Belgium, England and Wales, Finland, Italy, and Poland) between 1995 and 2004 [23]. Data from Belgium are used for illustration of the methodology discussed in this chapter. The analysis sample consists of 3,098 residual sera collected between 2001 and 2003 during routine laboratory testing from people aged 1–82 years. For each subject, the antibody titers (expressed as $\log_{10}$ (OD+1)) and the age are available. Figure 19.2 shows a scatter plot by age (a) and a histogram (b) of the log antibody titers, respectively, with the given set of cut-offs.

19.2.2   Varicella zoster virus in England and Wales

VZV is transmitted by airborne droplets and direct contact [24]. VZV is responsible for two clinical manifestations, namely, varicella (chickenpox) and herpes zoster (shingles) (HZ). Varicella is a highly transmissible infection occurring early in childhood, with 90 percent of European children becoming immune by age 12 in the absence of vaccination [25]. After recovery, the virus remains latent in the sensory ganglia and can reactivate at later ages causing HZ, a skin disease yielding serious morbidity. Safe and effective varicella vaccines have been available since 1970s and are recommended by the World Health Organization (WHO). Currently, due to the unclear impact of varicella vaccination on the epidemiology of HZ, only a few European countries have introduced varicella vaccination into their national programs [26].

Serological samples were collected and tested for antibodies to VZV as part of the European Sero-Epidemiology Network (ESEN2) [25]. Data from England and Wales are used for illustration of the methodology discussed in this chapter. In particular, samples of 2,091 specimens (collected in 1996 from residual sera) from persons aged 1–20 years were used. For each subject, the antibody titers (expressed as $\log_{10}(OD+1)$) and the age are available. Figure 19.2 shows a scatter plot by age (c) and a histogram (d) of the log antibody titers, respectively, with the given set of cut-offs.

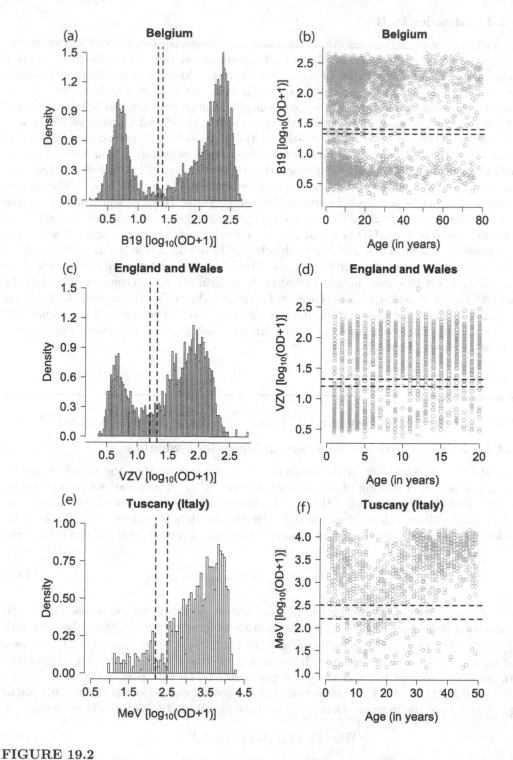

FIGURE 19.2
Scatter plot and histogram of $\log_{10}(OD + 1)$ with over imposed the set of cut-off points given by the assay's manufacturer (dashed lines): (a and b) B19 in Belgium, (c and d) VZV in England and Wales, (e and f) MeV in Tuscany (Italy).

19.2.3 Measles in Italy

Measles is a very contagious infection transmitted by the measles virus (MeV). The disease is characterized by a red, flat rash that usually starts on the face, then spreads to the rest of the body, and appears about 14 days after exposure. Measles is an airborne infection transmitted primarily from person to person by large respiratory droplets, but also by aerosolized droplet nuclei. Infected people are usually contagious from four days before until four days after rash onset. Measles has been preventable since 1963 through vaccination.

Data from Italy are used for illustration of the methodology discussed in this chapter. According to the Italian vaccination schedule, the vaccine is usually administered, in combination with mumps and rubella through the MMR vaccine, in two doses, the first one between 12 and 15 months of age, the second one between 5 or 6 years of age. The sample consists of residual sera collected between 2005 and 2006 in Tuscany, Italy, during routine laboratory testing from 927 subjects aged 1–49 years [27]. For each subject, the antibody titers (expressed as $\log_{10}(\text{OD}+1)$) and the age are collected. Since the analyzed sera were anonymous, it was not known whether subjects had been vaccinated for measles or not.

The analysed specimens were taken right after the implementation of a supplementary immunization activity that involved children from primary and secondary school (7–14 years). During that period, regional coverage for the first dose of MMR vaccine, administered within 24 months of age, passed from 89.3 percent in 2005 to 91.3 percent in 2006. Figure 19.2 shows a scatter plot by age (e) and a histogram (f) of the log antibody titers, respectively, with the given set of cut-offs.

19.3 Hierarchical Bayesian Mixture Models for Serological Data

19.3.1 Mixture models with age-independent weights

To model the heterogeneity in the antibody titers, we assume that the sample is drawn from a population consisting of an unknown number of K subpopulations (components), resulting in a density function g that can be represented as a mixture distribution of K unobserved densities. Thus, given a sample of antibody titers for subject i, Y_i, $i = 1, \ldots, n$, we aim to estimate the parameters of a finite K-component mixture distribution of the form

$$g(Y_i) = \sum_{k=1}^{K} \pi_k f(Y_i | \boldsymbol{\xi}_k), \tag{19.3}$$

where $f(Y_i | \boldsymbol{\xi}_k)$ is the distribution of the kth mixture component (and whose choice will be discussed in Section 19.3.4), π_k are the mixture weights (or mixture probabilities) with $\sum_{k=1}^{K} \pi_k = 1$, and $\boldsymbol{\xi}_k$ are the vectors of density parameters to be estimated [28]. In particular, we focus on a hierarchical Bayesian mixture model [29–31] of two components with possibly different location and scale parameters. The first component is the distribution of $\log_{10}(OD + 1)$ of the susceptible and the second component is the distribution of $\log_{10}(OD + 1)$ of the immune. Hence, the mixture model in (19.3) can be rewritten as

$$g(Y_i) = (1 - \pi)f(Y_i | \boldsymbol{\xi}_1) + \pi f(Y_i | \boldsymbol{\xi}_2). \tag{19.4}$$

We introduce a latent indicator variable Z_i that represents the individual unknown infection status [19], assumed to be Bernoulli distributed,

$$Z_i = \begin{cases} 0, & 1 - \pi, & \text{individual } i \text{ is susceptible,} \\ 1, & \pi, & \text{individual } i \text{ is immune.} \end{cases} \tag{19.5}$$

We can then reformulate the mixture model in (19.4) in terms of Z_i:

$$g(Y_i) = (1 - Z_i)f(Y_i|\boldsymbol{\xi}_1) + Z_i f(Y_i|\boldsymbol{\xi}_2). \tag{19.6}$$

The probabilities π and $1 - \pi$ are the mixture weights of the infected and the suscepti-ble components, respectively. In particular, π is the probability that an individual in the population belongs to the "immune" component and can be interpreted as the prevalence of the infection in the population [32]. Under the Bayesian framework, we assume for the probability π a prior beta distribution, namely,

$$\pi \sim \text{Beta}(\alpha, \beta). \tag{19.7}$$

In case both α and β are specified equal to 1, the beta prior turns into a uniform distribution between 0 and 1.

The specification of the prior distributions for the mixture parameters $\boldsymbol{\xi}_k$ will be dis-cussed in Section 19.3.4.

19.3.2 Mixture models with age-specific weights for pre-vaccination data

It is widely documented that the prevalence of childhood infections depends on the age of individuals [2]. Therefore, we express the mixture probabilities as a function of the age and we consequently rewrite the mixture model of (19.4) as

$$g(Y_i) = (1 - \pi(a_i))f(Y_i|\boldsymbol{\xi}_1) + \pi(a_i)f(Y_i|\boldsymbol{\xi}_2). \tag{19.8}$$

As we mentioned previously, $\pi(a_i)$, which is the age-dependent probability governing the Bernoulli distribution of $Z_i(a_i)$, is interpreted as the population prevalence. Note that the FOI can be estimated by

$$\lambda(a) = \frac{d\pi(a)}{da} \frac{1}{1 - \pi(a)}. \tag{19.9}$$

The prevalence and FOI are estimated simultaneously with the mixture parameters and with the latent classification variables $Z_i(a_i)$. The chosen models ought to guarantee a nonnegative FOI; thus, we must constrain the prevalence function to be monotonically non-decreasing.

19.3.2.1 Deterministic model for mixture weights

In this section, we assume a deterministic relationship between age and the prevalence given the parameterization of the mean structure for the prevalence. In particular, we consider a piecewise-constant model for the FOI, which is typically adopted in the applied epidemio-logical practice [2, 33, 34]. Note that this model can be used to estimate the FOI of a simple age-structured susceptible-infected-recovered (SIR) model for transmission under which the data are observed, but other, more complex, transmission models can be taken into account. The piecewise-constant model is based on the idea that the different age groups for indi-viduals in school age are characterized by different FOI levels. Assuming that the FOI is constant in each age class $[a_{j-1}, a_j)$, we formulate the model for the prevalence at age a, with $a \in [a_J, a_{J+1})$, in the following way:

$$\pi(a) = 1 - \exp\left\{-\sum_{j=1}^{J-1} \lambda_j(a_{j+1} - a_j) - \lambda_J(a - a_J)\right\}, \tag{19.10}$$

where λ_j, with $j = 1, \ldots, J$, is the constant FOI in the jth age group. We specify a truncated normal distribution with mean zero and large variance for the constant FOI in each age group, $\lambda_j \sim TN(0, 1000)$. The specification of the prior distributions for the unknown parameter of the mixture components will be discussed in Section 19.3.4. We also can estimate the fraction of people remaining susceptible at old age as $1 - \pi_J$, where J represents the last available age group [1].

Note that other models can be used for the mixture probability instead of the piecewise-constant model specified in (19.10). For example, a log-logistic model for the prevalence, with the relative FOI, is given by

$$\pi(a_i) = \frac{e^{\beta_0} a_i^{\beta_1}}{1 + e^{\beta_0} a_i^{\beta_1}}, \qquad \text{and} \qquad \lambda(a_i) = \frac{e^{\beta_0} \beta_1 a_i^{\beta_1 - 1}}{1 + e^{\beta_0} a_i^{\beta_1}}, \qquad (19.11)$$

where the coefficients β_0 and β_1 are given their own prior distributions (e.g., a normal distribution with large variance).

19.3.2.2 Probabilistic model for mixture weights

Considering $j = 1, \ldots, J$ one-year age groups, we assume that $\boldsymbol{\pi}$ is a right-continuous non-decreasing function defined on $[0, \delta]$, with $\pi_J \leq \delta \leq 1$. In the previous section, we formulated a generalized linear model (GLM) for the mixture weights. In contrast, in this section we do not assume any deterministic relationship between π_j and $a_i = j$, but we rather specify a probabilistic model for π_j at each distinct level of $a_i = j$. For this purpose, we propose the product-beta prior for $\boldsymbol{\pi}$ [35],

$$P_B(\boldsymbol{\pi}|\boldsymbol{\alpha}, \boldsymbol{\beta}) \propto \prod_{j=1}^{J} (\pi_j)^{\alpha_j - 1} (1 - \pi_j)^{\beta_j - 1}, \quad (\alpha_j > 0, \beta_j > 0), \qquad (19.12)$$

where $\boldsymbol{\alpha} = (\alpha_1, \alpha_2, \ldots, \alpha_J)$ and $\boldsymbol{\beta} = (\beta_1, \beta_2, \ldots, \beta_J)$. Note that the product-beta is a conjugate prior for the binomial likelihood. Thus, the posterior distribution of $\boldsymbol{\pi}|\boldsymbol{Y}$ is also beta-distributed.

Since we assume that the prevalence is monotonically non-decreasing, in order to get a non-negative estimate of the FOI, we require that $\pi_1 \leq \pi_2 \leq \cdots \leq \pi_J$. Thus, the J-dimensional parameter vector is a subset S^J of the whole parameter space R^J. This constraint can be defined by using a restricted prior distribution [35]. The ensuing posterior distribution of $\boldsymbol{\pi}$ given the order constraint is the unconstrained posterior distribution normalized such that [36]

$$P(\boldsymbol{\pi}|\boldsymbol{Y}) \propto \frac{P(\boldsymbol{Y}|\boldsymbol{\pi})P(\boldsymbol{\pi}|\boldsymbol{\alpha}, \boldsymbol{\beta})}{\int_{S^J} P(\boldsymbol{Y}|\boldsymbol{\pi})P(\boldsymbol{\pi}|\boldsymbol{\alpha}, \boldsymbol{\beta})d\boldsymbol{\pi}}, \qquad \boldsymbol{\pi} \in S^J \qquad (19.13)$$

Hence, in our setting,

$$\begin{cases} P(\pi_j|\boldsymbol{Y}, \alpha_j, \beta_j, \boldsymbol{\pi}_{-j}) \propto P(\boldsymbol{Y}|\boldsymbol{\pi})P(\boldsymbol{\pi}|\boldsymbol{\alpha}, \boldsymbol{\beta}) & \pi_j \in S_j^J, \\ P(\pi_j|\boldsymbol{Y}, \alpha_j, \beta_j, \boldsymbol{\pi}_{-j}) = 0 & \pi_j \notin S_j^J, \end{cases} \qquad (19.14)$$

where $\boldsymbol{\pi}_{-j} = (\pi_1, \ldots, \pi_{j-1}, \pi_{j+1}, \ldots, \pi_J)$. Therefore, the conditional posterior distribution of $\pi_j|\boldsymbol{Y}, \boldsymbol{\alpha}, \boldsymbol{\beta}, \boldsymbol{\pi}_{-j}$ is the standard posterior distribution $\text{Beta}(y_j + \alpha_j, n_j - y_j + \beta_j)$ restricted to the interval $[\pi_{j-1}, \pi_{j+1}]$ [35]. This result means that during the MCMC simulation, sampling from the full conditional distribution can be reduced to interval-restricted sampling from the standard posterior distribution [36]. In addition to the likelihood of the mixture model specified in (19.6), we assume that the latent current status variable follows an age-dependent binomial distribution given by

$$Z_i(a_i = j) \sim \text{Bin}(n_j, \pi_j),$$

and that a prior for the age dependent mixture probability is given by

$$\pi_j \sim \text{Beta}(\alpha_j, \beta_j) I(\pi_{j-1}, \pi_{j+1}), \tag{19.15}$$

where $I(\pi_{j-1}, \pi_{j+1})$ is an indicator variable which takes the value one if $\pi_{j-1} \leq \pi_j \leq \pi_{j+1}$, and zero otherwise.

In order to complete the specification of the hierarchical model in (19.15), we specify prior distributions for the hyperparameters $\boldsymbol{\alpha}$ and $\boldsymbol{\beta}$. In the special case that $\alpha_j = \beta_j = 1$, the prior distribution of the prevalence in the jth age group is a uniform distribution over the interval $[\pi_{j-1}, \pi_{j+1}]$. In general, for the upcoming analysis presented herein, we specify weakly informative distributions for the hyperparameters, i.e., a Gamma prior distribution with small parameters $\varepsilon = 0.01$ for both $\boldsymbol{\alpha}$ and $\boldsymbol{\beta}$ in each age group j.

We also model the maximum seroprevalence π_J, namely, the seroprevalence at the oldest available age. For this purpose, we use an informative Beta prior with mean 0.95 and standard deviation 0.025. These parameters are chosen in order to have a maximum prevalence ranging in a reasonable interval, for example, between 0.90 and 1. The fraction of remaining susceptible individuals at the oldest age, f, is then estimated by $1 - \pi_J$ [1]. Given the estimate of the seroprevalence, the FOI λ_j is successively estimated as $\pi'_j/(1 - \pi_j)$, where the first derivative of the prevalence at the numerator is approximated by $(4\pi_{j+1} - 3\pi_j - \pi_{j+2})/2$ and then smoothed.

19.3.3 Mixture models with age-specific weights for post-vaccination data

When the interest lies in modeling post-vaccination serological data, there are mainly two issues that the researcher has to take into account. First, it often happens that the information on whether immune individuals acquired their immunity either from natural infection or from vaccination is not available. Hence, it is not possible to estimate the FOI of the natural infection, unless we make an assumption about vaccination coverage or manage to estimate it [37]. On the other hand, if there is no interest in the estimation of the FOI, then it is not necessary to be subjected to the constraint of monotonicity when estimating the prevalence. Second, the presence of individuals who acquired their immunity either from natural infection or from vaccination, with possibly different levels of antibody titer, calls for the relaxation of the assumption of a mixture model with only two components, one for the susceptible and one for the immune. Rather, a mixture model with more than two components might provide a better fit to the data, as the use of multiple components allows to account for increasing levels of antibody titers (even though this does not necessarily imply different immunity levels, as cell-mediated response also plays an important role in protection [38]).

For this setting, we generalize the mixture model with age-dependent weights in (19.8) by considering K mixture components:

$$g(Y_i) = \sum_{k=1}^{K} \pi_k(a_i) f(Y_i | \boldsymbol{\xi}_k), \tag{19.16}$$

where the mixing weight $\pi_k(a_i)$ represents the probability that an individual aged a_i belongs to the kth mixture component. The current status of an individual is described by a binary latent classification random variable T_{ik} that represents the membership of the ith individual to the component k. Since each individual can be classified only into one of the components, we have that $\sum_{k=1}^K T_{ik} = 1$. We also aim to classify each component k either as susceptible or immune. For this purpose, we assume that the sum of the mixture weights of the components that account for different levels of antibody response provides the overall probability that an individual is immune, therefore representing the population prevalence [18].

Under the Bayesian paradigm, for the mixture weights $\pi_k(a)$, we do not assume any deterministic relationship between the probabilities and the age, but we rather assign a flat prior distribution for π_k at each distinct level of the age a, consisting in a uniform distribution between 0 and 1 for each component k [18]. This method is equivalent to assuming a Dirichlet prior for all the mixture probabilities π_k at age a [19]:

$$(\pi_1(a),\ldots,\pi_K(a)) \sim \text{Dir}(\alpha_1,\ldots,\alpha_K). \tag{19.17}$$

All parameters α_k can be set equal to 1 to obtain a uniform prior for all the probabilities $\pi_k(a)$ under the constraint that $\sum_{k=1}^K \pi_k(a) = 1$.

19.3.4 Selecting the distribution for mixture components

To complete the specification of the hierarchical models presented in the previous sections, we need to specify the distribution for the mixture components and, consequently, the prior distributions for the mixture parameters. Usually, the same distribution is chosen for all mixture components. An obvious choice for modeling antibody data is the normal distribution. Other distributions can be considered as well, which can allow either for skewness (skew-normal), or for thick tails (Student's t), or for both (skew-t) [39]. Another possible flexible choice is the Gamma distribution [10]. On the other hand, different distributions can be used for the mixture components, i.e., B19 data for England were modelled with a normal distribution for the seronegative component and a modification of the normal distribution to allow for skewness for the seropositive component [14].

In what follows, we consider two different distributions: (1) a skew-normal distribution for modeling pre-vaccination data to have more flexibility when restricting to two components, and (2) a normal distribution for modeling post-vaccination data, where the flexibility is guaranteed by the use of multiple components.

19.3.4.1 Normal density

A K-component normal mixture model is formulated as follows [19]:

$$g(Y_i|\mu_k,\sigma_k^2) = \sum_{k=1}^K \pi_k(a_i)N(Y_i|\mu_k,\sigma_k^2). \tag{19.18}$$

For the location parameter μ_k, we tried two different prior distributions, all specified in a strictly positive range of values. A first possible prior is a uniform distribution within a large positive range, e.g.,

$$\mu_k \sim U(0,100). \tag{19.19}$$

Another possibility is a truncated normal distribution, with hyperparameters for the mean η and the precision ζ, e.g.,

$$\mu_k \sim TN_{0,}(\eta_k,\zeta_k), \tag{19.20}$$

where η_k is normally distributed with mean 0 and large variance, while the precision ζ_k is given a Gamma distribution with parameter $\varepsilon = 0.01$. The specification of a prior for the mean μ_k over a strictly positive range is chosen as the normal distribution can allow for negative values, while the serological data can only take positive values. Moreover, we specify both prior distributions under the order restriction $\mu_k < \mu_{k+1}$, with $k = 1, \ldots, K$. This order restriction reflects the fact that seropositive individuals show higher average antibody titers than seronegative individuals and, in case of $K > 2$, that there exist groups of seropositive people with increasing average levels of immune response. Moreover, this order restriction is computationally required in order to avoid label switching during MCMC sampling, thus ensuring the identifiability of the parameters [28]. Depending on the model specification, this order constraint can be implemented by sorting the values of μ_k at each MCMC iteration (as required by the software JAGS) or by introducing a new variable, for example δ, which represents the distance between the two location parameters (this is the implementation preferred by softwares such as WinBUGS).

For the prior distribution of the variance σ_k^2, different options are available [40]. A first option is a uniform prior distribution for the standard deviation σ_k on a large range, such as

$$\sigma_k \sim U(0, M), \tag{19.21}$$

where M is a large number, such as 1,000.

Another option is an inverse-Gamma(ϵ, ϵ) prior distribution for the variance σ_k^2, where ϵ is a small value, such as 0.01 or 0.001. Practically, for the implementation of this prior in JAGS, we specify a Gamma distribution for the inverse of the variance, namely, the precision τ_k:

$$\tau_k = 1/\sigma_k^2 \sim \Gamma(0.01, 0.01). \tag{19.22}$$

A drawback of this prior is that, for data with low values of σ_k, inference may influenced by the value of ϵ [40].

Finally, we can use a half-Cauchy distribution as prior distribution for the standard deviation σ_k. This prior is often, in practice, a weakly informative prior, as it usually lets the likelihood be the dominant part of the posterior distribution when a high precision level is chosen [40]. In JAGS, this prior can be implemented by exploiting the equivalence between a Cauchy distribution and a Student's t distribution with one degree of freedom:

$$\sigma_k \sim t(\mu = 0, \tau = 0.01, \nu = 1)I(0,), \tag{19.23}$$

where μ is the location, τ is the precision, ν the degrees of freedom, and $I(0,)$ indicates that the Cauchy is truncated below 0, as only positive values are possible for the standard deviation σ_k.

19.3.4.2 Skew-normal density

We choose the skew-normal distribution [41] for pre-vaccination serology, as this distribution allows for skewness in the components and thus ensures more flexibility when a model with only two components is used. The probability density function (pdf) of this distribution is given by

$$f(X|\mu, \sigma^2, \alpha) = \frac{2}{\sigma}\phi\left(\frac{X - \mu}{\sigma}\right)\Phi\left(\alpha\frac{X - \mu}{\sigma}\right), \tag{19.24}$$

where ϕ and Φ are the pdf and the cumulative density function of the standard normal distribution, respectively.

The parameters μ and σ^2 are the location and the scale parameters, respectively, and α is the skewness parameter, which can lead to a skewness coefficient in the interval

$(-0.9953, 0.9953)$ [39]. In order to fit a hierarchical Bayesian mixture model with this distribution, we use a stochastic representation of the distribution, based on a random-effect model, as suggested by [39]. We define the variable $Y = \mu + \sigma\delta S + \sigma\sqrt{1 - \delta^2}\varepsilon$, where S is a random effect with truncated normal distribution, $S \sim TN_{[0,\infty]}(0,1)$, ε is the measurement error with normal distribution, $\varepsilon\ N(0,1)$, independent from S, and $\delta = \alpha/\sqrt{1 + \alpha^2}$. To implement the model in JAGS, the parameter vector $(\mu_k, \sigma_k\delta_k, \sigma_k\sqrt{1 - \delta_k^2})$ is parameterized as $(\mu_k, \psi_k, \omega_k)$ [39]. Hence, we rewrite (19.16) as the following two-component skew-normal mixture model:

$$g(Y_i|\mu_k, \sigma_k^2, \alpha_k) = \sum_{k=1}^{2} \pi_k(a_i)SN(Y_i|\mu_k + \psi_k S_i, \omega_k^2). \tag{19.25}$$

The parameters σ_k^2 and α_k can be recovered through $\sigma_k^2 = \omega_k^2 + \psi_k^2$ and $\alpha_k = \psi_k/\omega_k$, respectively. The same prior distributions as in Section 19.3.4.1 were specified for μ_k and ω_k. A weakly informative prior can be specified for parameters ψ_k assuming a normal prior distribution with large variance.

19.3.5   Model selection

When fitting mixture models, the problem of model selection is related to the choice of the optimal number of components, which is particular important in our case when dealing with post-vaccination serological data. Choosing the number of components can be based on model selection criteria. This method requires to fit several mixture models, with an increasing number of components, and to use a model selection criterion to select the "best" model in terms of goodness-to-fit to data and parsimony in the number of parameters.

The deviance information criterion [DIC, 42], which is a commonly used model selection criterion within the hierarchical Bayesian framework, cannot be safely used for model selection for mixture models (as well as with other latent data problems) [43]. Indeed, for mixture models, the current status of infection of the individuals, Z_i, is a latent variable. This usage leads to poor estimation of the effective dimension of the model (the effective number of parameters) and therefore the use of DIC can be misleading. Several alternative selection criteria to the DIC were proposed. In this section, we focus on two methods, namely, the penalized expected deviance [PED, 44] and the difference in posterior deviance [45]. The PED can be considered as a loss function when predicting the data Y using the same data Y. The issue of using the data twice (for estimation as well as for prediction) makes the expected deviance (the posterior mean of the deviance), $\overline{D(\theta)}$, too optimistic [44]. Thus, the PED penalizes it with a measure for model complexity, p_{opt}:

$$PED = \overline{D(\theta)} + p_{opt}. \tag{19.26}$$

Even though outside the exponential family it is hard to calculate the optimism parameter p_{opt}, it can be estimated for general models using MCMC methods. The JAGS software uses importance sampling to estimate the parameter p_{opt}. However, the author warns that the estimates may be numerically unstable when the effective number of parameters is high, as it typically occurs with random-effects models [46]. Similarly to the DIC, the smaller the PED, the better.

The difference in posterior deviances [45] permits comparison of pairs of models to select the best one. This approach is based on the observation that models with growing numbers of parameters are automatically penalized by the increasing diffuseness of the posterior distributions in their parameters. Thus, we can base the selection between two models on the difference between the whole posterior distributions of their deviances,

$$\left\{ D_{1,2}^{(m)} = D_1^{(m)} - D_2^{(m)} : m = 1, \dots, M \right\}, \tag{19.27}$$

where M is the length of the MCMC chain. We can derive the posterior probability that Model 1 is better than Model 2,

$$P\left(D_{1,2}^{(m)} < 0\right) = \frac{1}{M} \sum_{m=1}^{M} I\left(D_{1,2}^{(m)} < -2\log 9 = 4.39\right), \qquad (19.28)$$

where the value $-2\log 9$ is calibrated to correspond to a likelihood ratio test favouring Model 1 with a posterior probability of 0.9 [45]. It is also possible to derive 95 percent credible intervals (CI) for the difference in deviances: a totally negative 95 percent CI implies that we favour Model 1 over Model 2.

As a final note, we remark that these selection criteria work at best when interest lies in the choice of the optimal number of components. More caution is needed when the interest lies in choosing the best model for the seroprevalence and FOI, as it is the case of the models for the pre-vaccination data, or for selection of the best data distribution.

19.3.6 Determination of the current status of infection

After obtaining the posterior means of the parameters of interest, $(\bar{\pi}_k(a), \bar{\mu}_k, \bar{\sigma}_k,$ etc.), we need to categorize the components either as susceptible or as immune, and then assign the individuals to one of the components. First, according to the estimated locations $\bar{\mu}_k$, we label each component, based on previous biological knowledge. Usually the component with the lowest value of μ_k is for the susceptible, while the remaining components might describe different levels of immunity. Second, we assign each subject in the sample to one of the components through the posterior mean of the mixture probability $\bar{\pi}_k(a_i)$, i.e., to the component for which $\bar{\pi}_k(a_i)$ is maximal (and larger than 0.5 in case of only two components). If the mixture model has only two components, then we can directly estimate for each subject aged a_i the latent current status of infection, $\bar{Z}(a_i)$. If the mixture model consists of more than two components, a further step is needed. In particular, as we previously mentioned, we have to decide which components can be classified as susceptible and which ones as immune. Hence, if j out of K components are classified as immune (I), then the probability of being immune is $\bar{\pi}^I(a_i) = \sum_{j \in I} \bar{\pi}_j(a_i)$.

When all individuals have been classified, the current status of the infection, $\bar{Z}(a_i)$, is estimated by

$$\bar{Z}(a_i) = \begin{cases} 0, & \bar{\pi}^S(a_i) > \bar{\pi}^I(a_i), \quad \text{individual } i \text{ of age } a \text{ is susceptible,} \\ 1, & \bar{\pi}^S(a_i) < \bar{\pi}^I(a_i), \quad \text{individual } i \text{ of age } a \text{ is immune,} \end{cases} \qquad (19.29)$$

where π^S and π^I are the estimated probability of belonging to one of the susceptible components or to an immune component, respectively.

Finally, when each individual has been classified either as susceptible or immune, we can estimate the proportion of immune individuals per age group by averaging $\bar{Z}_i(a_i)$ in the jth age group,

$$\hat{\pi}^I(a = j) = \frac{\sum_{i=1}^{n_j} \bar{Z}_i(a_i)}{n_j}, \text{ with } j = 1, \ldots, n_j. \qquad (19.30)$$

We remark that $\hat{\pi}^I(a)$ are the estimates of the age-specific proportions seropositive in the serological sample and can be compared with the proportions seropositive in the sample obtained using the conventional cut-off points. In contrast, the mixture probabilities $\bar{\pi}^I(a)$ depend on the chosen model for the prevalence and are an estimate of the age-specific prevalence in the population.

19.4   Application to the Data

The hierarchical Bayesian models for the estimation the mixture parameters, and the age-specific prevalence and FOI were developed in JAGS [46]. The MCMC samples were computed using at least two chains to assess mixing of chains and convergence. For each chain, we discarded the first half of the iterations as burn-in period. Model diagnostic was performed to assess convergence of mixture parameters (mean, standard deviation, and skewness) using three diagnostic tests (available within the R package coda [47]) namely, Geweke's test [48], Gelman and Rubin's test [49], and Heidelberger and Welch's test [50].

19.4.1   Pre-vaccination serology

Hierarchical Bayesian mixture models with age-dependent mixture probabilities were fitted for both B19 antibody data in Belgium and VZV antibody data in England and Wales with MCMC using either two or three chains of at least 20,000 iterations, with the first half discarded as burn-in and using a thinning of 10 (i.e., each 10th iteration was kept). Differences in the number of iterations and in the number of chains among the models for the pre-vaccination data were due to fine tuning of these two parameters to facilitate convergence of the parameters of interest. Figure 19.3a and c show the fit of the skew-normal mixture models to the histograms of the antibody data for B19 and VZV, respectively. For both datasets, the two-component mixture models adequately capture the patterns in the data. In particular, using the skew-normal distribution, we are able to account for the left skewness in the immune component, particularly evident in the B19 data. This is confirmed by the posterior means of the mixture parameters for both models, presented in Table 19.1. The posterior means of the skewness parameter α for both infections are negative (indicating left skewness), with the one for B19 larger in magnitude. The histograms in Figure 19.3 show that, in case of pre-vaccination data, there is usually concordance between the classification achieved by the fixed cut-off approach and the mixture model (see Figure 19.3a, in particular), even though, for the VZV data, we can see a difference between the two classification methods [8], with the mixture model showing a lower threshold (shown in Figure 19.3c by the crossing point between the two mixture components) than the fixed cut-off.

We used the PED and the difference in posterior deviances, shown in Table 19.1, as selection criteria to identify the best model in terms of prevalence and FOI between the probabilistic product-beta model (PB) and the deterministic piecewise-constant FOI model based on the SIR model. We notice a small difference in the PED between the two models, with the criterion favoring model SIR for the B19 data from Belgium and model PB for the VZV data from England and Wales. However, when the difference in posterior deviances is used, we see that the 95 percent CI for the difference $D_{PB,SIR}^{(m)}$ includes zero for both countries, thus indicating that data do not favor any of the models. Similarly, the probability of data supporting model PB rather than model SIR is close to 0.5 for both countries, suggesting that we do not have enough evidence to favor one of the two models [45]. Finally, the proportions of seropositive determined by the mixture model classifcation, the posterior means of the age-specific prevalence and FOI, together with 95 percent CIs for the two models, are shown in Figure 19.3b and d for B19 and VZV, respectively. PB and SIR models differ both in terms of prevalence, and FOI estimates, particularly in case of VZV data. Indeed, the prevalence function from the PB model closely adapts to the pattern shown by the proportions seropositive, which is quite evident from the estimate for VZV data (Figure 19.3d). As a consequence, the FOI estimate shows a high degree of flexibility. On

TABLE 19.1

Posterior means (and 95% CI) for the skew-normal mixture parameters for the susceptible and the immune components (the mean μ, the standard deviation σ, and the skewness parameter α), and for the fraction f of remaining susceptible individuals at older ages, for both PB and SIR models

Country	BE		EW	
Model	PB	SIR	PB	SIR
μ_1	0.56 (0.54, 0.59)	0.56 (0.54, 0.59)	0.38 (0.36, 0.41)	0.38 (0.35, 0.41)
μ_2	2.55 (2.54, 2.56)	2.55 (2.54, 2.56)	2.18 (2.15, 2.21)	2.18 (2.15, 2.21)
σ_1	0.22 (0.20, 0.24)	0.22 (0.19, 0.24)	0.35 (0.31, 0.40)	0.36 (0.32, 0.41)
σ_2	0.47 (0.45, 0.49)	0.48 (0.46, 0.51)	0.49 (0.45, 0.52)	0.50 (0.46, 0.54)
α_1	1.81 (1.35, 2.29)	1.71 (1.24, 2.18)	3.26 (2.31, 4.41)	3.41 (2.44, 4.61)
α_2	−7.86 (−9.58, −6.62)	−8.08 (−9.81, −6.76)	−2.80 (−3.34, −2.28)	−2.91 (−3.55, −2.36)
f	0.15 (0.13, 0.17)	0.09 (0.06, 0.13)	0.07 (0.05, 0.09)	0.06 (0.04, 0.09)
$\bar{D}$	−7523	−7463	−2177	−2162
p_{opt}	19484	19469	11635	11355
PED	11961	12006	9458	9193
$\bar{D}_{PB,SIR}^{(m)}$		−51.69 (−1019.35, 923.85)		68.69 (−550.28, 693.12)
$P(\bar{D}^{(m)} < -2\log 9)$		0.53		0.42

Note: Selection criteria for the choice of the optimal number of components: PED with focus on $\{X, \mu, \sigma, \pi, \lambda\}$ (with mean deviance $\bar{D}$, penalty p_{opt}, and PED); difference in posterior deviance (with posterior mean and 95% CI, and probability that Model PB is better than Model SIR).

the other hand, the prevalence function from the deterministic model provides a smoother fit, when compared to the proportions seropositive, as it guided by the chosen transmission model (here, an SIR model) rather than by data alone (also more evident for VZV data in Figure 19.3d). The FOI estimates from the SIR model, constant within the chosen age groups, are quite consistent with the estimates from the PB model, thereof they represent a kind of average. We notice that the fit provided by the two models is similar, as also indicated by the selection criteria, with the only large difference between PB and SIR evident for B19 between age 20 and 45. Also for the fraction of remaining susceptible at the oldest age (Table 19.1), we did not find any substantial difference between the models.

19.4.2 Post-vaccination serology

Age-dependent Bayesian mixture models with increasing number of components ($K = 2, 3, 4, 5$) were fitted to measles antibody data from Tuscany, Italy. Posterior means for the parameters of interest were calculated using 3,000 samples, obtained running two

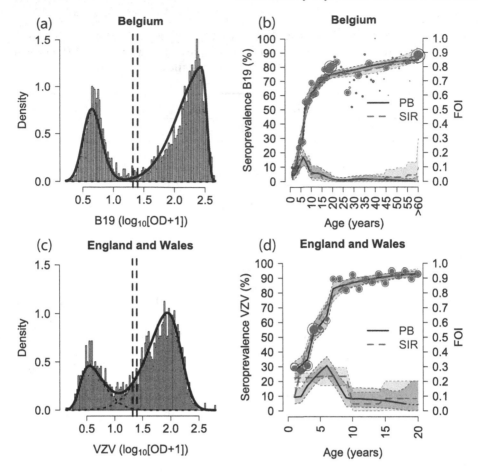

FIGURE 19.3

Histogram of $\log_{10}(OD+1)$ with over imposed the set of cut-off points given by the assay's manufacturer (dashed lines), the fit of the age-independent Bayesian mixture model (solid line), and the fit for the single components (dotted lines). (a) Parvovirus B19 in Belgium. (c) VZV in England and Wales. Posterior mean (with 95% CI) for the seroprevalence (upper lines) and the FOI (lower lines), for the probabilistic model (black lines) and the deterministic model (gray lines), with the proportions seropositive determined by the mixture models (black and gray dots, proportional to age group size). (b) Parvovirus B19 in Belgium. (d) VZV in England and Wales.

independent chains with 30,000 iterations each, with the first half of the chains discarded as burn-in and using a thinning of 10. Table 19.2 reports the model selection criteria for the choice of the optimal number of components. The decisions supported by the two criteria are somehow diverging. The PED, focused on both mixture parameters and data classification, indicates that model M2 should be preferred. This result occurs because the increase in the number of components leads, on the one hand, to a decrease in the posterior mean of the model deviance $\bar{D}$, but, on the other hand, to an increase in the misclassification error of individual data into the components and therefore to an increase in the penalty term p_{opt} added to the expected deviance of the model [44]. For the difference in posterior deviances, model M4 is preferred instead. Indeed, data show more support for model M4

TABLE 19.2

Posterior means (and 95% CI) for the normal mixture parameters (the mean μ and the standard deviation σ) for models with two (M2) up to five components (M5)

Parameter	M2	M3	M4	M5
μ_1	2.67 (2.58, 2.76)	2.35 (2.18, 2.51)	2.24 (2.05, 2.41)	2.12 (1.93, 2.30)
μ_2	3.68 (3.65, 3.72)	3.21 (3.12, 3.31)	3.09 (2.99, 3.19)	2.98 (2.88, 3.12)
μ_3		3.79 (3.75, 3.84)	3.56 (3.47, 3.64)	3.38 (3.22, 3.52)
μ_4			3.92 (3.86, 3.96)	3.66 (3.55, 3.74)
μ_5				3.95 (3.90, 3.98)
σ_1	0.69 (0.64, 0.75)	0.69 (0.62, 0.77)	0.66 (0.56, 0.75)	0.61 (0.50, 0.72)
σ_2	0.28 (0.26, 0.31)	0.33 (0.28, 0.39)	0.32 (0.26, 0.38)	0.29 (0.22, 0.39)
σ_3		0.21 (0.18, 0.24)	0.23 (0.19, 0.29)	0.26 (0.17, 0.37)
σ_4			0.14 (0.11, 0.17)	0.20 (0.15, 0.26)
σ_5				0.12 (0.097, 0.15)
$\bar{D}$	1036	603	273	67
p_{opt}	3397	5049	8279	9723
PED	4433	5652	8552	9789
$\bar{D}^{(m)}$		$D^{(m)}_{M3,M2}$ −430.66 (−602.59, −264.90)	$D^{(m)}_{M4,M3}$ −323.40 (−592.69, −89.80)	$D^{(m)}_{M5,M4}$ −202.73 (−550.36, 140.10)
$P(\bar{D}^{(m)} < -2\log 9)$		1	0.995	0.87

Note: Selection criteria for the choice of the optimal number of components: PED with focus on $\{X, \mu, \sigma, \pi, \lambda\}$ (with mean deviance $\bar{D}$, penalty p_{opt}); difference in posterior deviances (with posterior mean and 95% CI, and probability that Model ℓ, $\ell = 3, 4, 5$, is better than Model 1-1).

with respect to models M3 and, indirectly, M2 (both CIs are completely negative). On the other hand, data do not allow us to confidently choose between models M5 and M4, as the CI for the difference in posterior deviances includes zero and the proportion of simulations with lower deviance for M5 is smaller than 90 percent [45]. We present in Figure 19.4 the fit of both models M2 and M4 to the histogram of the data and the respective posterior mean of the age-dependent prevalence. From Figure 19.4a and c, we notice that the mixture model with four components (M4) fits more closely the histogram of the data, with a larger concordance to the fixed cut-off, than the model with only two components (M2). The mixture model that is over imposed on the histogram shows that the increase in the number of components leads to a more accurate fit to the higher antibody titers. On the other hand, under model M2, the second component, with the higher value of μ, manages

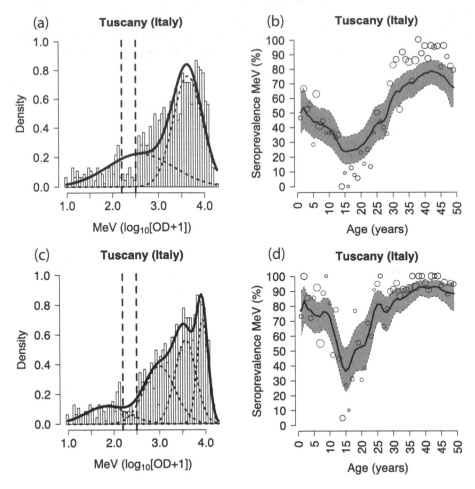

FIGURE 19.4

Histogram of $\log_{10}(OD+1)$ with over imposed the set of cut-off points given by the assay's manufacturer (dashed lines), the fit of the age-independent Bayesian mixture model (solid line), and the fit for the single components (dotted lines), in Tuscany (Italy), 2005. (a) Mixture model with 2 components. (c) Mixture model with four components. Posterior mean (with 95% CI) for the seroprevalence of measles, obtained as the sum of the age-dependent mixture weight for all components but the first one (the one with the lower value for μ), with over imposed the proportions seropositive determined by the mixture models (with dots proportional to age group size). (b) Mixture model with two components. (d) Mixture model with four components.

to capture only the individuals with very high antibody titers. The difference between the two models is also reflected by the estimates of the prevalence (Figure 19.4b and d). Model M2, in particular, captures those individuals with a stronger immune response and it tends, therefore, to predict a lower prevalence than model M4, mostly in the age group of children, adolescents, and young adults (the group of those aged 10–20 years old shows, under each model, the lowest prevalence, as these people went through in a period characterized by low vaccination coverage and low virus circulation).

19.5 Discussion

In this chapter, it was assumed that the log antibody titers of susceptible and infected individuals in the population arose from two (or more) distributions of the antibody titers. We, therefore, presented hierarchical Bayesian mixture models for the estimation of the prevalence and the FOI of an infection directly from the antibody titers, rather than using the current status data obtained from the dichotomization of the antibody titers using the assay's set of fixed cut-off points (see also Chapter 14).

Compared to standard methods to estimate prevalence and FOI based on the cut-off, mixture models present many advantages. The main one is that they allow us to use all the available information provided by the antibody titers for the estimation of the parameters of interest. Different models for the prevalence and the FOI can be incorporated into the hierarchical Bayesian mixture model. For illustration, we presented two possible approaches for modeling the pre-vaccination data, and one for the post-vaccination data. First, we presented a probabilistic model, based on a product-beta prior distribution for each age group. This model neither assumed any parametric relationship with the age, nor was based on a theoretically grounded transmission model, but rather yielded the prevalence estimates for each age group under a common order-constraint for monotonicity. Second, we presented a piecewise-constant FOI model, which was a parametric model based on a specific transmission model for the infection (here, an SIR model). It was nonetheless a flexible model, as it assumed independent constant regimes of the FOI for each age group. Moreover, more complex and realistic transmission models for the infection under investigation can be assumed. It is also possible to include data on social contact patterns to account for social mixing behaviors, at the cost of being more computer-intensive [51]. Hence, a multiplicity of models can be used; what matters is that the constraint of non-decreasing monotonicity is respected, whenever the assumption of strictly positive FOI must hold.

For the post-vaccination data, when we do not have information to distinguish between immunity induced by vaccination or by natural infection and, therefore, the FOI of the natural infection cannot be simply estimated, there is more freedom in the model choice. An alternative to the probabilistic model that we used for the MeV data is the use of a P-splines model, defined as a mixed model, which provides a flexible fit to data, despite being more computer intensive [52].

Other possible extensions to the applications presented in this chapter regard the addition of more than one covariate in the model and the use of bivariate mixture models. In the first case, other information, such as the sex or the geographical area, can be included to differentiate the mixture parameters and/or the mixture probabilities [10, 52]. In the second case, bivariate mixture models allow to model co-infections within the the same subject. These bivariate models can be used to classify each subject as susceptible or immune with respect to each of the considered infections, and to eventually estimate the prevalence for each infection, taking into account their association at the individual level [53].

Finally, in our application, we highlighted possible issues with the methods to select the best models. We introduced two possible selection criteria based on the posterior distribution of the model deviance, namely, the PED and the difference in the posterior model deviances. We found that conclusions based on the two criteria can differ, as the PED considers the predictive ability of the model while the difference in posterior deviances penalizes for excessively parameterized models. It is, therefore, up to the researcher to eventually decide which model provides the most useful fit to the data in terms of the research question under analysis. Further research is definitely needed on this matter. A possible recent solution is the use of the widely applicable information criterion (WAIC), a measure of the pointwise out-of-sample prediction accuracy of the model [54], available for JAGS with the R package loo [55].

19.6 Conclusions

The hierarchical mixture model approach presented in this chapter proved to be flexible enough to incorporate both the pre- and the post-vaccination settings. Since the prevalence in the mixture model is "translated to the mixture probability, the different vaccination policies in the population (pre/post) are taken into account when the model for the mixture probability is formulated. We have shown that a variety of models can be formulated, and that model flexibility and theoretically grounded models can coexist, at the price of being more computer-intensive with respect to methods based on current status data. Hence, more research is needed in order to allow a more straightforward and faster implementation of these models.

Acknowledgements

We thank Paolo Bonanni and Angela Bechini of the University of Florence, Italy, for providing us with the measles serological data from Tuscany used in the analysis and for their permission to make the dataset available. We also thank Piero Manfredi of the University of Pisa for the fruitful discussion of the methodology and, in particular, for the definition of the mathematical SIR transmission model.

References

[1] C.P. Farrington. Modeling forces of infection for measles, mumps and rubella. *Statistics in Medicine*, 9:953–967, 1990.

[2] R.M. Anderson and R.M. May. *Infectious Diseases of humans, Dynamic and Control*. Oxford University Press, Oxford, UK, 1991.

[3] N. Keiding, K. Begtrup, T.H. Scheike, and G. Hasibeder. Estimation from current status data in continuous time. *Lifetime Data Analysis*, 2:119–129, 1996.

[4] N.P. Jewell and M.J. van der Laan. Current status data: Review, recent developments and open problems. In Balakrishnan N. and Rao C.R., ed., *Advances in Survival Analysis*, pp. 625–643. Elsevier, Amsterdam, The Netherlands, 2004.

[5] M. Greiner, C.R. Franke, D. Böhning, and P. Schlattmann. Construction of an intrinsic cut-off value for the sero-epidemiological study of *Trypanosoma evansi* infections in a canine population in Brazil: A new approach towards an unbiased estimation of prevalence. *Acta Tropica*, 56:97–109, 1994.

[6] M. Greiner, T.S. Bhat, R.J. Patzelt, D. Kakaire, G. Schares, E. Dietz, D. Böhning, K.H. Zessin, and D. Mehlitz. Impact of biological factors on the interpretation of bovine trypanosomosis serology. *Preventive Veterinary Medicine*, 30:61–73, 1997.

[7] A.G. Lalkhen and A. McCluskey. Clinical tests: Sensitivity and specificity. *Continuing Education in Anaesthesia, Critical Care & Pain*, 8:221–223, 2008.

[8] A.J. Vyse, N.J. Gay, L.M. Hesketh, P. Morgan-Capner, and E. Miller. Seroprevalence of antibody to varicella zoster virus in England and Wales in children and young adults. *Epidemiology & Infection*, 132:1129–1134, 2004.

[9] A.J. Vyse, N.J. Gay, L.M. Hesketh, R. Pebody, P. Morgan-Capner, and E. Miller. Interpreting serological surveys using mixture models: The seroepidemiology of measles, mumps and rubella in England and Wales at the beginning of the 21st century. *Epidemiology & Infection*, 134:1303–1312, 2006.

[10] P. Hardelid, D. Williams, C. Dezateux, P. A. Tookey, C. S. Peckham, W. D. Cubitt, and M. Cortina-Borja. Analysis of rubella antibody distribution from newborn dried blood spots using finite mixture models. *Epidemiology & Infection*, 136(12):1698–1706, 2008.

[11] K. Bollaerts, M. Aerts, Z. Shkedy, C. Faes, Y Van der Stede, P. Beutels, and N. Hens. Estimating the population prevalence and force of infection directly from antibody titers. *Statistical Modelling*, 12(5):441–462, 2012.

[12] N. Hens, Z. Shkedy, M. Aerts, C. Faes, P. Van Damme, and P. Beutels. *Modeling Infectious Disease Parameters Based on Serological and Social Contact Data*. Springer, New York 2012.

[13] J. Mossong, N. Hens, M. Jit, P. Beutels, K. Auranen, R. Mikolajczyk, M. Massari et al. Social contacts and mixing patterns relevant to the spread of infectious diseases. *PLoS Medicine*, 5:e74, 2008.

[14] N.J. Gay. Analysis of serological surveys using mixture models: Application to a survey of Parvovirus B19. *Statistics in Medicine*, 15:1567–1573, 1996.

[15] N.J. Gay, A.J. Vyse, F. Enquselassie, W. Nigatu, and D.J. Nokes. Improving sensitivity of oral fluid testing in IgG prevalence studies: Application of mixture models to a rubella antibody survey. *Epidemiology and Infection*, 130:285–291, 2003.

[16] A.L. Baughman, K.M. Bisgard, F. Lynn, and B.D. Meade. Mixture model analysis for establishing a diagnostic cut-off point for pertussis antibody levels. *Statistics in Medicine*, 25:2994–3010, 2006.

[17] M.C. Rota, M. Massari, G. Gabutti, M. Guido, A. De Donno, and M.L. Ciofi degli Atti. Measles serological survey in the Italian population: Interpretation of results using mixture model. *Vaccine*, 26:4403–4409, 2008.

[18] E. Del Fava, Z. Shkedy, A. Bechini, P. Bonanni, and P. Manfredi. Towards measles elimination in Italy: Monitoring herd immunity by Bayesian mixture modelling of serological data. *Epidemics*, 4(3):124–131, 2012.

[19] J. Diebolt and C.P. Robert. Estimation of finite mixture distributions through Bayesian sampling. *Journal of the Royal Statistical Society, Series B*, 56:363–375, 1994.

[20] A. Corcoran and S. Doyle. Advances in the biology, diagnosis and host-pathogen interactions of Parvovirus B19. *Journal of Medical Microbiology*, 53:459–475, 2004.

[21] H.W. Lehmann, P. von Landenberg, and S. Modrow. Parvovirus B19 infection and autoimmune disease. *Autoimmunity Reviews*, 2:218–223, 2003.

[22] J.T. Servey, B.V. Reamy, and J. Hodge. Clinical presentations of Parvovirus B19 infection. *American Family Physician*, 75:373–376, 2007.

[23] J.R. Mossong, N. Hens, V. Friederichs, I. Davidkin, M. Broman, B. Litwinska, J. Siennicka et al. Parvovirus B19 infection in five European countries: Seroepidemiology, force of infection and maternal risk of infection. *Epidemiology & Infection*, 136(08):83–10, 2007.

[24] U. Heininger and J. F. Seward. Varicella. *Lancet*, 368(9544):1365–1376, 2006.

[25] A. Nardone, F. de Ory, M. Carton, D. Cohen, P. van Damme, I Davidkin, M.C. Rota et al. The comparative sero-epidemiology of varicella zoster virus in 11 countries in the European region. *Vaccine*, 25:7866–7872, 2007.

[26] P Carrillo-Santisteve and P.L. Lopalco. Varicella vaccination: A laboured take-off. *Clinical Microbiology and Infection*, 20:86–91, 2014.

[27] A. Bechini, S. Boccalini, E. Tiscione, G Pesavento, F. Mannelli, M. Peruzzi, S Rapi, S Mercurio, and P. Bonanni. Progress towards measles and rubella elimination in Tuscany, Italy: The role of population seroepidemiological profile. *The European Journal of Public Health*, 22(1):133–139, 2012.

[28] G.J. McLachlan and D. Peel. *Finite Mixture Models*. John Wiley & Sons, New York, 2000.

[29] W.R. Gilks, S. Richardson, and D.J. Spiegelhalter. *Markov Chain Monte Carlo in Practice*. Chapman & Hall, London, UK, 1996.

[30] P. Congdon. *Applied Bayesian Modelling*. John Wiley & Sons, Chichester, UK, 2003.

[31] A. Gelman, J.B. Carlin, H.S. Stern, and D.B. Rubin. *Bayesian Data Analysis*. Chapman & Hall, London, UK, 2nd ed., 2004.

[32] R.B. Evans and K. Erlandson. Robust Bayesian prediction of subject disease status and population prevalence using several similar diagnostic tests. *Statistics in Medicine*, 23:2227–2236, 2004.

[33] J.R. Mossong, L. Putz, and F. Schneider. Seroprevalence and force of infection of varicella-zoster virus in Luxembourg. *Epidemiology & Infection*, 132(6):1121–1127, 2004.

[34] J. Wallinga, P. Teunis, and M. Kretzschmar. Using data on social contacts to estimate age-specific transmission parameters for respiratory-spread infectious agents. *American Journal of Epidemiology*, 164:936–944, 2006.

[35] A.E. Gelfand and L. Kuo. Nonparametric Bayesian bioassay including ordered polytomous response. *Biometrika*, 78:657–666, 1991.

[36] A.E. Gelfand, A.F.M. Smith, and T-M. Lee. Bayesian analysis of constrained parameter and truncated data problems. *Journal of the American Statistical Association*, 87:523–532, 1992.

[37] N. Goeyvaerts, N. Hens, H. Theeten, M. Aerts, P. V. Damme, and P. Beutels. Estimating vaccination coverage for the trivalent measles-mumps-rubella vaccine from trivariate serological data. *Statistics in Medicine*, 31(14):1432–1449, 2012.

[38] M.B. Isa, J.V. Pavan, P.S. Don, S. Grutadauria, L.C. Martinez, M.O. Giordano, G. Masachessi, P.A. Barril, and S.V. Nates. Persistence of measles neutralizing antibody related to vaccine and natural infection acquired before HIV infection. *Epidemiology & Infection*, 142(08):1708–1712, 2013.

[39] S. Frühwirth-Schnatter and S. Pyne. Bayesian inference for finite mixtures of univariate and multivariate skew-normal and skew-t distributions. *Biostatistics*, 11:317–336, 2010.

[40] A. Gelman. Prior distributions for variance parameters in hierarchical models. *Bayesian Analysis*, 1(3):515–533, 2006.

[41] A. Azzalini. A class of distributions which includes the normal ones. *Scandinavian Journal of Statistics*, 12:171–178, 1985.

[42] D.J. Spiegelhalter, N.G. Best, B.P. Carlin, and A. van der Linde. Bayesian measures of model complexity and fit. *Journal of the Royal Statistical Society, Series B*, 64:583–640, 2002.

[43] G. Celeux, S. Forbes, C.P. Robert, and D.M. Titterington. Deviance information criteria for missing data models. *Bayesian Analysis*, 1:651–674, 2006.

[44] M. Plummer. Penalized loss functions for Bayesian model comparison. *Biostatistics*, 9(3):523–539, 2008.

[45] M. Aitkin. *Statistical Inference. An Integrated Bayesian/Likelihood Approach*. CRC Press, Boca Raton, FL, 2010.

[46] M. Plummer. rjags: Bayesian Graphical Models using MCMC, 2016. R package version 4-6.

[47] M. Plummer, N. Best, K. Cowles, and K. Vines. Coda: Convergence diagnosis and output analysis for mcmc. *R News*, 6(1):7–11, 2006.

[48] J. Geweke. Evaluating the accuracy of sampling-based approaches to calculating posterior moments. In J.M. Bernado, J.O. Berger, A.P. Dawid, and A.F.M. Smith, ed., *Bayesian Statistics 4*. Clarendon Press, Oxford, UK, 1992.

[49] A. Gelman and D.B. Rubin. Inference from iterative simulation using multiple sequences. *Statistical Science*, 7:457–472, 1992.

[50] P. Heidelberger and P. D. Welch. Simulation run length control in the presence of an initial transient. *Operations Research*, 31(6):1109–1144, 1983.

[51] M. van Boven, J. van de Kassteele, M.J. Korndewal, C.H. van Dorp, M. Kretzschmar, F. van der Klis, H.E. de Melker, A.C. Vossen, and D. van Baarle. Infectious reactivation of cytomegalovirus explaining age- and sex-specific patterns of seroprevalence. *PLoS Computational Biology*, 13(9):1–18, 2017.

[52] M.A Vink, J. van de Kassteele, J. Wallinga, P. F.M. Teunis, and J.A. Bogaards. Estimating seroprevalence of human papillomavirus type 16 using a mixture model with smoothed age-dependent mixing proportions. *Epidemiology*, 26(1):8–16, 2015.

[53] M.A. Vink, J. Berkhof, J. van de Kassteele, M. van Boven, and J.A. Bogaards. A Bivariate mixture model for natural antibody levels to human papillomavirus types 16 and 18: Baseline estimates for monitoring the herd effects of immunization. *PLoS ONE*, 11(8):e0161109, 2016.

[54] S. Watanabe. Asymptotic equivalence of vayes cross validation and widely applicable information criterion in singular learning theory sumio. *Journal of Machine Learning Research*, 11:3571–3594, 2010.

[55] A. Vehtari, A. Gelman, and J. Gabry. Practical Bayesian model evaluation using leave-one-out cross-validation and WAIC. *Statistics and Computing*, 27(5):1413–1432, 2017.

Part V

Analysis of Surveillance Data

20

Modeling Infectious Disease Distributions: Applications of Point Process Methods

Peter J. Diggle

CONTENTS

20.1   Introduction

A *point process* is a stochastic process each of whose realizations is a countable set of points. Each point may be a location in time, space, or both. A *point pattern* is a partial realization of a point process; "partial" in the sense that it is restricted to a finite time-interval, $[a, b]$, and a spatial region, R. We call a point of the process or pattern an *event*, to distinguish it from an arbitrary point in time and space. We shall assume that a spatio-temporal point pattern is observed on a set of the form $R \times [a, b]$, meaning that the recorded events are those that occur anywhere within R and at any time between a and b. In epidemiology, each event denotes a location and time associated with a case of the disease being studied. For example, the location may be place of residence and the time the date of diagnosis or sympton onset.

The major part of this chapter will be concerned with spatio-temporal models and methods, but it is helpful to fix some basic ideas in a purely spatial setting, in which context the events are locations, $x_i : i = 1, ..., n$, in a designated planar region R. A simple but useful initial classification of spatial point patterns is as regular, completely random or aggregated. In a *completely random* pattern, the events form an independent random sample from the uniform distribution on R. In a *regular* or *aggregated* pattern the events are distributed over R more evenly or less evenly than this, respectively. Figure 20.1 illustrates this with three simulated point patterns.

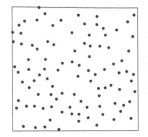 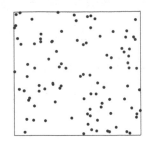 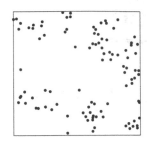

FIGURE 20.1
Three simulated point patterns. Left-hand, middle, and right-hand panels are generated by regular, completely random, and aggregated spatial point processes, respectively.

Aggregated point patterns can arise through either or both of two very different mechanisms: as a consequence of a direct dependence among groups of events; or as a by-product of a heterogeneous environment. To highlight the distinction and illustrate an inherent ambiguity, we use an example given by Bartlett [1] and discussed in more detail in Diggle [2].

Suppose that a set of m "parents" is generated as an independent random sample from the uniform distribution over a designated region R, that each parent produces a random number of "offspring" by independent random sampling from a Poisson distribution, and that offspring are located relative to their parents by independent random sampling from a bivariate distribution with probability density function (henceforth, pdf) $f(\cdot)$. The point process of offspring is called a Poisson cluster process. The name is apt because each "family" of offspring is clustered around their parent to an extent determined by the pdf $f(\cdot)$.

Now suppose, in apparent contrast, that a set of events in R is generated by independent random sampling from a distribution with pdf proportional to $\lambda(x)$, called the *intensity function* of the process, and that $\lambda(x)$ is itself a realization of a non-negative valued stochastic process, $\Lambda(x)$. Processes of this kind are called *Cox processes* (Cox [3]). A legitimate candidate for $\Lambda(x)$ is a mixture,

$$\Lambda(x) = \sum_{j=1}^{m} f(x - U_j),$$

where the U_j are an independent random sample from the uniform distribution over R.

From a mechanistic perspective, a Poisson cluster process and a Cox process are very different entities, but the two examples given here are simply different mathematical representations of the same process (Bartlett [1]). The right-hand panel of Figure 20.1 was generated by this process. The pdf $f(\cdot)$ is a bivariate Normal distribution with uncorrelated components each of which has mean zero and standard deviation 0.05, a value sufficiently large that the 20 clusters are not individually discernible.

In epidemiology, the "location" of an event usually means the place of residence of a person, either a case of the disease being studied or a control. This location is not necessarily the place most relevant to that person's role in the evolution of the disease process, but it is often the best available proxy. We now can identify at least three reasons why we should expect the spatial distribution of a disease to exhibit aggregation. First, population density varies spatially. Second, any individual's risk of contracting a disease depends on a variety of measured and unmeasured factors that may be spatially structured. Finally, the disease may be transmitted directly from person to person, or indirectly through the action of a spatially structured disease-carrying vector. In an infectious disease context, the last of these three is often the one of most interest, but the other two need to be accommodated to avoid drawing false conclusions. Bartlett's example shows that this may be impossible without the imposition of empirically unverifiable assumptions, which is why we prefer the descriptive term "aggregated" to avoid the mechanistic connotations of the more widely used term "clustered."

The discussion so far may convince the reader that so-called "tests of clustering," on which there is an extensive literature, are of limited value, a point made pithily by Rothman [4]. In the author's opinion this is slightly harsh. Tests of clustering, even when they are formally testing a hypothesis that we know to be false, can be useful for exploratory analysis, not least as a minimal hurdle to be overcome before undertaking any more complex analysis. The fitting of a sophisticated model to a dataset that fails to reject the hypothesis of no spatial clustering is more likely to lead to over-interpretation than to yield any useful scientific insights.

To resolve fully the ambiguity between direct dependence among events and environmental heterogeneity as the explanation for observing an aggregated point pattern may be a mathematical impossibility, but we can nevertheless make scientific progress. One way to do so is to incorporate covariates into our point process model. Specifically, if we can capture environmental heterogeneity through a regression model for the intensity function, for example a log-linear model $\lambda(x) = \exp\{d(x)'\beta\}$ where $d(x)$ is a vector of covariates associated with the location x, then any residual clustering might be attributed more plausibly to direct dependence. Another obvious approach when studying an infectious disease is to abandon spatial in favor of spatio-temporal modeling. For example, a spatio-temporal pattern of progressive diffusion from one or more initial foci would favor direct dependence as the underlying mechanism, whereas a region-wide scaling up of the local density of events over time would be more suggestive of environmental heterogeneity as the explanation. In the remainder of the chapter, we describe some of the statistical models and methods that result from the twin strategy of incorporating covariates and taking explicit account of temporal effects.

In Section 20.2 we define some basic properties of a spatio-temporal point process and describe how these can form the basis of an exploratory statistical analysis. In Section 20.3 we draw a distinction between *empirical* and *mechanistic* models, and give examples of each. In Section 20.4 we discuss methods of inference, together with a case-study, for each of the two classes of models. The chapter ends with a short discussion.

A note on style. We use formal mathematical notation throughout and try always to be mathematically correct, while avoiding various technical issues that would be necessary for a rigorous account. In particular, we assume throughout that our point processes are *orderly*, a technical term meaning, essentially, that coincident events cannot occur. In practice, the recorded locations and times of events may coincide because of round-off error, in which case we can break the coincidence by randomly unrounding if necessary. We also assume, unless explicitly stated otherwise, that any directional effects can be modeled as functions of covariates.

Daley and Vere-Jones [5] give a mathematically rigorous treatment of point process theory. Mathematically oriented textbooks that focus on spatial point processes include Møller and Waagepetersen [6] and Ilian et al. [7]. Baddeley and Turner [8] is an encyclopedic account of methods for analyzing spatial point process data and their implementation in the R package `spatstat`. Cressie [9] and Gelfand et al. [10] include extensive material on point processes within a wider treatment of spatial statistical methods in general, including some material on spatio-temporal processes. Cressie and Wikle [11] and Shaddick and Zidek [12] focus primarily on methods for real-valued spatio-temporal processes.

20.2   Moment Properties of Spatio-Temporal Point Processes

In a spatio-temporal point process, the numbers of events, $N(C_1), ..., N(C_m)$, that fall within any designated set of spatio-temporal regions $C_1, ..., C_m$, is a multivariate random variable. Many useful properties of a spatio-temporal point process can be defined conveniently by considering particular cases.

Firstly, let C be a cylinder centered on the point (x, t), with radius u and height v. The *intensity function* of the process, denoted by $\lambda(x, t)$, is the limit of the ratio

$$\frac{\mathrm{E}[N(C)]}{\pi u^2 v} \tag{20.1}$$

as $u \to 0$ and $v \to 0$. Informally, $\lambda(x, t)$ is the expected number of events per unit volume in the immediate vicinity of the point (x, t).

Next, consider a pair of cylinders with common radius u and height v, centered on the points (x, t) and (x', t'). The *second-order intensity function*, $\lambda_2(x, t, x', t')$ is the limit of the ratio

$$\frac{\mathrm{E}[N(C_1)N(C_2)]}{(\pi u^2 v)^2}$$

as $u \to 0$ and $v \to 0$. The function

$$\gamma(x, t, x', t') = \lambda_2(x, t, x', t') - \lambda(x, t)\lambda(x', t')$$

has the character of a covariance and is called the *covariance density*.

Higher-order intensity functions can be defined in the obvious way, but are rarely used in practice. Simplifications of the first-order and second-order intensity functions result from assuming that the point process is *second-order stationary*, meaning that $\lambda(x, t) = \lambda$, a constant, and $\lambda_2(x, t, x', t') = \lambda_2(u, v)$ where u is the distance between x and x', and v is the difference between t and t'. It then follows that for any positive values of u and v, $\gamma(u, v) = \lambda_2(u, v) - \lambda^2$. A less restrictive assumption than second-order stationarity, introduced by Baddeley et al. [13], is *intensity-re-weighted stationarity*. This assumption allows the first-order intensity to vary over space and time but requires the second-order intensity to be of the form

$$\lambda_2(x, t, x', t') = \rho(u, v)\lambda(x, t)\lambda(x', t')$$

The function $\rho(u, v)$ is called the *pair correlation function*, although its values are not correlations in the usual sense. In particular, $\rho(u, v)$ can take any positive value. If the point process is an *inhomogeneous Poisson process*, meaning that the events are distributed independently over the region of interest with pdf proportional to $\lambda(x, t)$, then $\rho(u, v) = 1$. This result is universally accepted as the benchmark for a completely random point process, although it is possible to devise point processes other than the Poisson that also have $\rho(u, v) = 1$, because first-order and second-order properties do not completely define a point process. Baddeley and Silverman [14] give an explicit construction for a non-Poisson spatial point process with $\rho(u) = 1$.

In an extremely influential paper, Ripley [15] introduced a cumulative version of the second-order intensity, called the K-function. The K-function of an intensity-reweighted stationary spatio-temporal point process is

$$K(u,v) = 2\pi \int_0^v \int_0^u \rho(r,s) r \, dr \, ds. \qquad (20.2)$$

For a Poisson process, $K(u,v) = \pi u^2 v$, giving us a second benchmark for complete randomness.

Empirical counterparts of the various intensity functions as defined here can be calculated, in essence, by replacing expectations by observed counts. For example, an estimate of a spatio-temporal intensity can be calculated by a direct analogy with the defining equation (20.1), replacing the expectation in the numerator by the observed number of events in a cylinder of radius u and height v, as the center of its base, (x,t), moves over the region of interest. Second-order functions can be estimated in a similar fashion by considering a moving pair of cylinders. In practice, this approach needs considerable refinement if it is to produce useful results, taking into account issues such as the choices for u and v, the treatment of edge-effects and, in the non-stationary case, the inherent ambiguity between first-order and second-order effects. A good example of this approach is the careful discussion in Baddeley et al. [13] concerning the joint estimation of first-order and second-order intensities of an intensity-reweighted stationary spatial point process.

One way to estimate second-order properties while side-stepping the problem of choosing u and v is to use an empirical version of the K-function, which we obtain by re-expressing equation (20.2) as an expectation and again replacing this expectation by its observed value. We give more details in Section 20.4.

20.3   Models for Spatio-Temporal Point Processes

The word "model" has different connotations in different scientific disciplines. In the mathematical sciences, one clear distinction is between deterministic and stochastic models. Among stochastic models, it is helpful to distinguish between *empirical models*, which claim only to reflect the patterns of variation in a set of data, and *mechanistic models*, which incorporate scientifically informed assumptions that may or may not be empirically verifiable. This distinction is not always clear-cut. Our earlier example of a Poisson cluster process that is also a Cox process shows that a single stochastic model can have more than one mechanistic interpretation. In principle, incorporating context-specific scientific information into the formulation of a model for a set of data should be a good idea, but it is not a free lunch. Adding complexity to a stochastic model increases either the number of parameters, which necessarily leads to inefficient estimation if the additional parameters are redundant (Altham [16]), or the number of assumptions, which risks invalidating the conclusions of an analysis. A pragmatic response is to choose a modeling strategy for each problem according to its scientific context and objectives. Roughly speaking, empirical models are most useful when the objective is prediction and the scientific laws that govern the underlying process are poorly understood. Conversely, mechanistic models give the best value when the objective is explanation and scientific knowledge justifies strong assumptions about the underlying data-generating process.

The scope for defining spatio-temporal point process models is limited only by the ingenuity of the modeler. Here, we describe two classes of model that are widely used: the log-Gaussian Cox process as an example of an empirical model and the more mechanistically oriented strategy of specifying a model through its conditional intensity function.

20.3.1   Log-Gaussian Cox processes

In a *Poisson process* with intensity $\lambda(x,t)$, the number of events in any designated spatio-temporal region $R \times [a,b]$ follows a Poisson distribution with mean $\int_a^b \int_R \lambda(x,t)dxdt$ and the locations of these events form an independent random sample from the distribution on $R \times [a,b]$ with pdf proportional to $\lambda(x,t)$. A *Cox process* (Cox [3]) is a Poisson process whose intensity function is a realization of a stochastic process $\Lambda(x,t)$. A Cox process inherits the first-order and second-order properties of its stochastic intensity $\Lambda(x,t)$ in the sense that the mean and covariance functions of $\Lambda(x,t)$ are also the intensity function and covariance density of the Cox process.

A *Gaussian process* is a real-valued stochastic process $S(x,t)$ with the property that the joint distribution of $S(x_i, t_i) : i = 1, ..., m$ at any finite set of points (x_i, t_i) is multivariate normal. It follows that all properties of a Gaussian process are determined by its mean and covariance structure. Here, we allow the mean to vary, denoting this by $m(x,t) = E[S(x,t)]$, but assume a stationary covariance function, $G(u,v) = \text{Cov}\{S(x,t), S(x-u, t-v)\} = \sigma^2 r(u,v)$.

A *log-Gaussian Cox process* is, as the name implies, a Cox process for which $\log \Lambda(x,t)$ is a Gaussian process (Møller et al. [17]). Standard results for the low-order moments of the log-Gaussian distribution give the mean function, $\lambda(x,t)$, and pair correlation function $\rho(u,v)$, of $\Lambda(x,t) = \exp\{S(x,t)\}$ as

$$\lambda(x,t) = \exp\{m(x,t) + \sigma^2/2\}, \tag{20.3}$$

and

$$\rho(u,v) = \exp\{\sigma^2 r(u,v)\}. \tag{20.4}$$

Gaussian processes can also be derived as solutions to stochastic partial differential equations. This method gives log-Gaussian Cox processes an indirect mechanistic interpretation and leads to computationally efficient algorithms for simulation and inference (Lindgren et al. [18]). However, in the author's opinion the main, and considerable, attraction of the log-Gaussian Cox process is as a flexible class of empirical models for the first-order and second-order structure of aggregated spatio-temporal point patterns. Diggle et al. [19] give several examples.

20.3.2   Conditional intensity models

Note that the events $(x_i, t_i) : i = 1, 2, ...$ of an orderly spatio-temporal point process can be labelled unambiguously in order of increasing event-times t_i. The *history* of the process at time t is the set $H_t = \{(x_j, t_j) : j < t\}$. In Section 20.2, equation (20.1) we defined the intensity of a spatio-temporal process as the limit of the ratio $E[N(C)]/(\pi u^2 v)$ as u and v both tend to zero, where C is a cylinder of radius u and height v, and $N(C)$ is the number of events in C. The *conditional intensity function* of the process, $\lambda(x,t|H_t)$, is similarly defined, but replaces the unconditional expectation of $N(C)$ in the numerator of equation (20.1) by its conditional expectation given H_t. An important theoretical result is that any orderly process is completely specified by its conditional intensity function. Also, *defining* a model by specifying its current properties conditional on its past is a natural approach when the scientific objective is to find a causal explanation for the behaviour of the process being studied.

20.3.2.1 Self-exciting processes

Hawkes [20] introduced a very useful class of models for purely temporal point processes under the name of *self-exciting* point processes. In a self-exciting point process, the conditional intensity function is of the form

$$\lambda(t|\mathcal{H}_t) = \alpha + \int_{-\infty}^{t} g(t-u)dN(u), \qquad (20.5)$$

where $dN(u) = 1$ at each point of the process and zero otherwise, and $g(\cdot)$ is any integrable, non-negative-valued function with, for completeness, $g(v) = 0$ for all $v < 0$.

In the current context a natural extension of equation (20.5) to spatio-temporal point processes is

$$\lambda(x,t|\mathcal{H}_t) = \alpha + \int \int_{-\infty}^{t} g(||x-y||, t-u)dN(y,u), \qquad (20.6)$$

where now $dN(y,u) = 1$ if there is a point of the process at (y,u) and zero otherwise, $||\cdot||$ denotes distance and the outer integral on the right-hand side extends, in principle, to the whole of the Euclidean plane. The first explicit recognition of this extension appears to be in Musmeci and Vere-Jones [21], one of a series of papers by David Vere-Jones and co-authors concerned with statistical modeling in seismology. However, Musmeci and Vere-Jones also noted the strong connection with modeling the spatio-temporal distribution of diseases whose aetiology includes both an endemic (α) and an epidemic ($g(\cdot)$) component.

More recently, Meyer and Held [22] have given a synthesis of work by Leo Held and colleagues formulating and fitting models of this kind to point process data, or to its discrete counterpart in which individual cases are aggregated into counts in spatial regions and time-intervals. The specific point process model that they consider is a version of equation (20.6) proposed by Meyer et al. [23], in which $g(||x-y||, t-u)$ is assumed to be a product of purely spatial and purely temporal functions.

20.3.2.2 Susceptible-Infectious-Recovered processes

Classic stochastic susceptible-infectious-recovered (SIR) models for an infectious disease epidemic assume homogeneous mixing of the population at risk, in which case spatial considerations do not arise (see, for example Britton [24, 25]). The study of spatially structured SIR models dates back at least to the 1960s (Bailey [26]) and gathered pace during the 1970s; a key paper is Mollison [27]. A good point of entry to what is now a very large literature is Keeling and Rohani [28].

The following simple, non-spatial example gives the flavor of this important class of models.

1. At time $t = 0$, a closed population of size n contains one newly infected individual and $n-1$ susceptible individuals.

2. The infectious periods of newly infected individuals are independently and identically distributed with pdf $f(u)$.

3. During their infectious period, an infected individual transmits infection to susceptible individuals in a Poisson process at a rate ρ per susceptible individual.

4. Each infected individual is removed, and plays no further part in the process, at the end of their infectious period.

A realization of this process consists of an ordered sequence of infection times, $t_i : i = 1, ..., m$ where $m \leq n$, as not every member of the population will necessarily become infected.

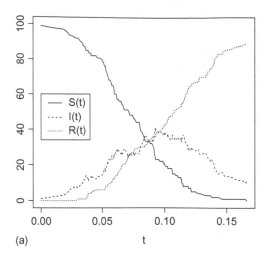 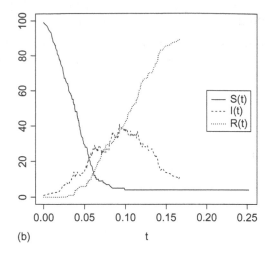

(a)   t   (b)   t

FIGURE 20.2
Panels (a) and (b) show two realizations of a simple SIR model. The plotted functions $S(t)$, $I(t)$, and $R(t)$ are the numbers of infectious, susceptible and removed individuals at time t in a closed population of size 100 (see text for full specification of the model).

The numbers of infectious, susceptible, and removed individuals at time t, denoted by $I(t)$, $S(t)$, and $R(t)$, respectively, then evolve according to the following rules.

1. $S(0) = n - 1, I(0) = 1, R(0) = 0$

2. At all times t, $S(t) + I(t) + R(t) = n$

3. At each infection time, $t = t_i$, $I(t)$ increases by one and $S(t)$ decreases by 1

4. At each removal time, $I(t)$ decreases by one and $R(t)$ increases by 1.

5. The epidemic ends when $I(t) = 0$.

Figure 20.2 shows two realizations of this process when $n = 100$, $\rho = 1.0$, and $f(u) = 20 \exp(-20u) : u \geq 0$. The first realization infects the whole population, while the second leaves four individuals unscathed.

In the simplest spatial version of this SIR model, the single parameter ρ is replaced by a set of quantities ρ_{ij}, the rate at which an infectious individual i transmits infection to a susceptible individual j. These quantities in turn depend on the corresponding spatial locations x_i and x_j. An example that we will re-visit in Section 20.4 specifies $\rho_{ij} = \alpha + \beta \exp\{-(u_{ij}/\phi)^\kappa\}$, where u_{ij} is the distance between x_i and x_j.

20.4   Inference

20.4.1   Inference for Log-Gaussian Cox processes

Equations (20.3) and (20.4) form the basis of moment-based methods of estimation for the parameters of a log-Gaussian Cox process. A convenient re-parameterization of the intensity process $\Lambda(x,t)$ is to

$$\Lambda(x,t) = \lambda(x,t) \exp\{S(x,t)\} \tag{20.7}$$

where now the Gaussian process $S(x,t)$ has mean $-\sigma^2/2$ and variance σ^2 so that $E[\exp\{S(x,t)\}] = 1$ and $\lambda(x,t) = E[\Lambda(x,t)]$, as required.

Suppose that our data consist of n events (x_i, t_i) in a spatio-temporal region $R \times [a,b]$. In the stationary case, $\lambda(x,t) = \lambda$ and a natural estimator for λ is

$$\hat{\lambda} = n/\{|R|(b-a)\}, \tag{20.8}$$

where $|R|$ denotes the area of R. More generally, a log-linear regression model of the form $\lambda(x,t) = \exp\{d(x,t)'\beta\}$, where $d(x,t)$ is a vector of covariates available at all points (x,t) in $R \times [a,b]$, can be fitted by maximizing the Poisson process log-likelihood,

$$L(\beta) = \sum_{i=1}^{n} \log \lambda(x_i, t_i) - \int_R \int_a^b \lambda(r,s)dsdr. \tag{20.9}$$

We can then estimate the parameters of $S(x,t)$ using the K-function as follows. Gabriel and Diggle [29] extend to the spatio-temporal setting a result for intensity-reweighted stationary spatial point processes in Baddeley et al. [13], to give the following approximately unbiased estimator for $K(u,v)$. Assume that the events (x_i, t_i) are ordered by increasing values of t. Denote by u_{ij} the distance between x_i and x_j and by $n(v)$ the number of $t_i \leq b-v$. Finally, denote by w_{ij} the proportion of the circumference of the circle with center x_i and radius u_{ij} that lies within R. Then,

$$\hat{K}(u,v) = \frac{1}{|R|(b-a)} \frac{n}{n(v)} \sum_{i=1}^{n(v)} \sum_{j=i+1}^{n(v)} \frac{1}{w_{ij}} \frac{1}{\hat{\lambda}(x_i,t_i)\hat{\lambda}(x_j,t_j)} I(u_{ij} \leq u)I(t_j - t_i \leq v). \tag{20.10}$$

As noted earlier, jointly estimating first-order and second-order properties from a single dataset is potentially problematic, but the difficulties are alleviated if either the imposition of a parametric model or some other structural simplification on $\lambda(x,t)$ can be justified. In the example below, Diggle et al. [30] assumed a product form, $\lambda(x,t) = \lambda(x)\mu(t)$. They estimated $\lambda(x)$ by applying a nonparametric smoother to the marginal distribution of case-locations and $\mu(t)$ by fitting a parametric log-linear model to the time series of daily case-counts. They then plugged these estimates into the right-hand side of equation (20.10) and minimized a quadrature approximation to the integrated squared difference between $\hat{K}(u,v)$ and the theoretical K-function obtained by substitution of equation (20.4) into equation (20.2).

Likelihood-based estimation, whether frequentist or Bayesian, is generally preferable to moment-based estimation but requires computationally intensive Monte Carlo methods to circumvent the analytical intractability of the likelihood function. Specifically, both Monte Carlo maximum likelihood (Geyer, [31]) and Bayesian estimation rely on a Markov chain Monte Carlo (MCMC) algorithm to draw samples from the required conditional distributions. These methods are discussed in detail in Diggle et al. [19] and Taylor and Diggle [32].

Integrated Nested Laplace Approximations (INLA, Rue et al. [33]) provide a non-Monte Carlo implementation of Bayesian inference through an analytical approximation to the Bayesian posterior that is accessible for a wide-ranging class of models including log-Gaussian Cox processes. The author's experience from using INLA to fit log-Gaussian Cox process models is that carefully tuned MCMC and INLA algorithms require comparable computational effort to deliver comparable accuracy (Taylor and Diggle [32]).

We end this section by summarizing a previously published application in which a log-Gaussian Cox process model was used to address an empirical prediction problem. Diggle et al. [30] give a more detailed account.

Non-specific gastro-intestinal (GI) disease is defined as "any disease of an infectious or toxic nature caused by, or thought to be caused by, the consumption of food or water" (Joint FAO/WHO Expert Committee on Food safety [34]). In the United Kingdom (UK), the pattern of occurrence of non-specific GI disease is traditionally monitored through the reporting by general practitioners of suspected cases, only a proportion of which are followed up with laboratory analysis of a fecal sample. Among the cases that are followed up in this way, confirmation of the responsible pathogen can take 2 weeks or more. In 2000, it was estimated that as few as 1 percent of clinical cases reached national surveillance systems (Food Standards Agency [35]). In March 1998, the UK National Health Service (NHS) launched a 24-hour 7-day phone-in health triage service, NHS Direct. Each call to NHS Direct was logged with, among other things, the date, full post-code of the caller's residence, and a code giving the primary reason for the call. This information presented an opportunity to monitor non-specific GI case incidence more rapidly, and at fine spatial resolution (in urban settings, a UK full post-code typically identifies a single street).

The aim of the project was to develop a real-time spatial surveillance system in which the geocoded post-codes of each day's NHS Direct calls in the southern English county of Hampshire that were coded as "vomiting, diarrhea, or both" with no record of recent out-of-area travel would be processed overnight using a spatio-temporal statistical model to produce daily predictive incidence maps for putative non-specific gastro-intestinal disease. These maps then could be used by public health professionals as aids to public health decision-making.

The first stage of the project consisted of formulating and fitting a spatio-temporal log-Gaussian Cox process model to the data on locations and dates, $(x_i, t_i) : i = 1, ..., n$ over the 2-year period 1 January 2001 to 31 December 2002. The model for the stochastic intensity was formulated as

$$\Lambda(x, t) = \lambda(x)\mu(t)\exp\{S(x, t)\}, \tag{20.11}$$

where $\lambda(x)$ and $\mu(t)$ are deterministic functions of place and time, respectively, and $S(x, t)$ is a stationary Gaussian process. The rationale for this model was as follows. First, the intensity of calls is expected to vary spatially, reflecting the spatial distribution of the user-population for NHS Direct. Second, the intensity is expected to vary temporally for a combination of biological and social reasons: risks associated with common food-borne infections in the UK are known to vary seasonally, use of the then-new NHS Direct service increased over the 2 years in question, and the service was more heavily used during weekends when access to traditional health-care services was more limited. Finally, departures from expectation are, by definition, stochastic in nature and, for GI disease in the UK, are typically localized in both space and time. The purpose of real-time surveillance is to identify these departures from expectation, which we call "anomalies," in a timely manner.

So as to make all three terms on the right-hand side of equation (20.11) identifiable, we imposed the following constraints. Firstly, $\int_A \lambda(x)dx = 1$, where A denotes the study-region (Hampshire). Secondly, $S(x, t)$ has expectation $-\sigma^2/2$ where $\sigma^2 = \text{Var}\{S(x, t)\}$ so that $\text{E}[\exp\{S(x, t)\}] = 1$ for all (x, t), as in equation (20.7). Consequently, $\mu(t)$ is the expected number of cases on day t.

Representing the expected incidence as a product of purely spatial and purely temporal terms was a pragmatic choice, without which it would have been impossible to distinguish empirically between expected and unexpected patterns of spatio-temporal incidence. As a consequence, it cannot be over-emphasized that an anomaly as here defined, however large, need not have any public health significance. The purpose of its detection was to alert public health professionals to an unusual feature that may or may not, in context, have an innocent explanation.

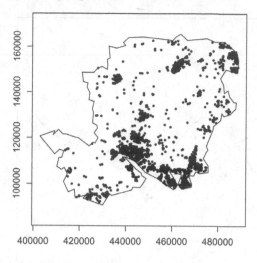
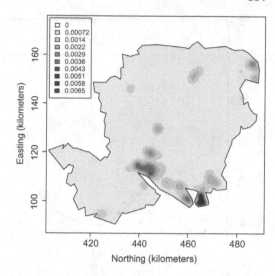

FIGURE 20.3

Left-hand panel: Locations (residential post-codes) of 1 year of cases (i.e. calls to NHS Direct Hampshire recorded as vomiting, diarrhea, or both with no record of out-of-area travel. Right-hand panel: adaptive kernel estimate of spatial intensity $\lambda(x)$ calculated from case locations over 2 years.

The observed spatial point pattern of case-locations (residential post-codes) primarily reflected the distribution of the population of Hampshire, with obvious concentrations in urban areas (Figure 20.3, left-hand panel). However, we knew (but could not quantify) that the uptake of the NHS Direct service was not demographically uniform. To estimate $\lambda(x)$ we therefore used an adaptive kernel estimator as defined in equations (20.4) and (20.5) of Diggle et al. [30], Figure 20.3, right-hand panel.

Daily cases-counts showed the expected pattern of higher numbers at weekends, a seasonal peak in early summer and a generally increasing trend over time. For this component of the model, we fitted a parametric log-linear model,

$$\log \mu(t) = \delta_{d(t)} + \alpha_1 \cos(\omega t) + \beta_1 \sin(\omega t) + +\alpha_2 \cos(2\omega t) + \beta_2 \sin(2\omega t) + \gamma t, \qquad (20.12)$$

where $d(t) = 1, 2, ..., 7$ identifies day-of-week, $\omega = 2\pi/365$, and t is time in days (see Figure 20.4).

Another pragmatic decision was to assume a separable correlation structure for the Gaussian process $S(x, t)$,

$$\text{Corr}\{S(x, t), S(x', t')\} = r_1(||x - x'||)r_2(|t - t'|),$$

where $|| \cdot ||$ denotes distance. From a theoretical perspective, this is a strong and arguably unattractive assumption (see, for example, Section 23.5 of Gneiting and Guttorp [36] but it has a number of compensatory attractions: it eases exploratory data analysis, simplifies computation, and leads to a parsimonious model. Also, we do not agree with Gneiting and Guttorp's statement, citing Kyriakidis and Journel [37] and Cressie and Huang [38], that separable models "do not allow for space-time interaction" at least as we understand that term. Specifically, separable correlation structure for a process $S(x, t)$ is implied by, but does not imply, that the corresponding Cox process is the product of independent spatial and

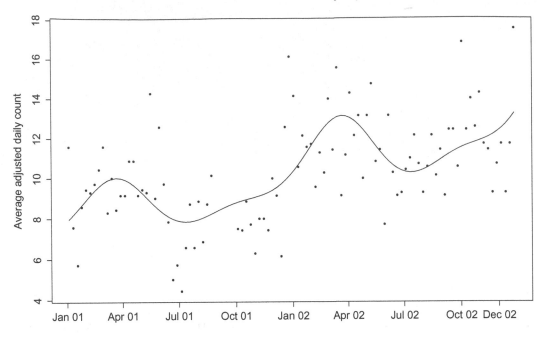

FIGURE 20.4
Weekly-averaged cases per day over the 2-year period 1 January 2001 to 31 December 2002 (solid dots) and fitted model (20.12, solid line).

temporal component processes, the latter being the null hypothesis for a test of space-time interaction (see, for example, Knox [39], Mantel [40] or Besag and Diggle [41].

The two panels of Figure 20.5 compare empirical and fitted spatial pair correlation functions for the intensity-adjusted case-locations and temporal autocovariance functions for the mean-adjusted daily case-counts, for the separable model with $r_1(u) = \exp(-u/\phi_1)$ and $r_2(v) = \exp(-v/\phi_2)$. The empirical estimate of the spatial pair correlation function is a non-parametric estimate based on binned counts of the distances between pairs of case-locations, ignoring their times of occurrence. The empirical estimate of the temporal autocovariance function is the standard time series estimate based on the sequence of daily case-counts ignoring their locations. The parametric fits used the method of moments as described in Diggle et al. [30].

Recall that the aim of the project was to enable more timely detection of unusual patterns of incidence as an early warning system for public health surveillance. Translated into statistical language, the aim was predictive inference about the current state of the latent process $S(x, t)$ using incidence data up to and including time t.

The solution advocated in Diggle et al. [30] was to flag an *anomaly* at location (x, t) when there is a high predictive probability that the incidence at (x, t) exceeds expectation by a factor of at least c, with the value of c chosen to represent a relative increase large enough to be of public health concern. Accordingly, the daily web-report included a set of maps of the predictive *exceedance probabilities*,

$$p(x, t) = \mathrm{P}[\exp\{S(x, t)\} > c|H_t],$$

where, in this discrete-time setting, H_t denotes all case-locations on all days up to and including day t. Figure 20.6 shows an example for 22 February 2002 with $c = 2$. The map is predominantly light gray, switching to gray and dark gray only when $p(x, t)$ exceeds 0.95,

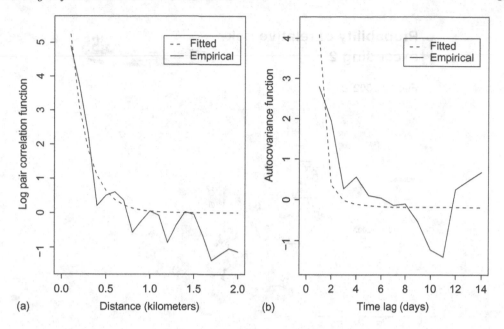

FIGURE 20.5
(a) Empirical (non-parametric) and (b) fitted (parametric) spatial and temporal correlation functions for the Hampshire NHS Direct data.

and 0.99, respectively. In this context, $c = 2$ would generally be considered too small a value to be of public health significance. We have chosen it here simply to illustrate the general approach.

The predictive exceedance probabilities $p(x, t)$ were calculated by MCMC sampling from the predictive distribution of $S(x, t)$ on each day t at a fine grid of locations x to cover the study region; the grid is clearly visible on each of the insets to Figure 20.6. Using plug-in estimates of $\lambda(x)$ and $\mu(t)$, the algorithm drew sampled values from the predictive distribution of $S(x, t)$ and calculated each value of $p(x, t)$ as the proportion of sampled values that were greater than $\log c$. The computation on each day t used a Metropolis-adjusted Langevin MCMC algorithm, incorporating case locations and times over a fixed-length moving time-window to avoid storage problems. The algorithm is described fully in Brix and Diggle [42].

20.4.2 Inference for conditional intensity models

Recall from Section 20.3.2 that the conditional intensity function, $\lambda(x, t|H_t)$ completely specifies an orderly point process, and from equation (20.9) that the log-likelihood of an inhomogeneous spatio-temporal Poisson process observed on $R \times [a, b]$ is

$$L(\beta) = \sum_{i=1}^{n} \log \lambda(x_i, t_i) - \int_R \int_a^b \lambda(r, s) ds dr.$$

The log-likelihood function of a conditional intensity model, or indeed of any orderly spatio-temporal process similarly is given by

$$L(\theta) = \sum_{i=1}^{n} \log \lambda(x_i, t_i|H_{t_i}) - \int_R \int_a^b \lambda(r, s|H_s) ds dr. \qquad (20.13)$$

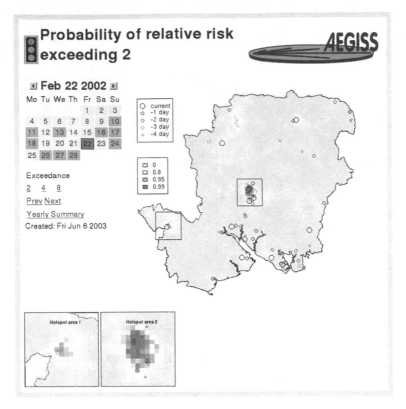

FIGURE 20.6
Hampshire NHS Direct web-report for 22 February 2002 using an anomaly threhold of 2 for
illustrative purposes.

The Poisson log-likelihood (20.9) is recovered as a special case, because a spatio-temporal
Poisson process has no memory, hence $\lambda(x,t|H_t) = \lambda(x,t)$. Conversely, an intuitive justi-
fication for equation (20.13) is that the conditional intensity function acts as a real-time
re-scaling of the current intensity function of a Poisson process in response to its observed
history.

When, as in Section 20.3.2, the conditional intensity function of the model under consideration is explicit, equation (20.13) provides an obvious basis for conducting likelihood-based
inference. The simplicity and generality of equation (20.13) is beguiling, but evaluation of
the integral term can become a serious obstacle as the integrand evolves dynamically over
time. Meyer et al. [23] and Meyer and Held [22] use a sophisticated quadrature method
to evaluate the likelihood for a self-exciting process with a product form for the function
$g(||x - y||, t - u)$ in equation (20.6). This leads to a conditional intensity of the form

$$\lambda(x,t|H_t) = \alpha + \sum_{j:t_j<t} \beta_j g_1(t - t_j)g_2(||x - x_j||). \tag{20.14}$$

Additionally, they allow the endemicity parameter α and the infectivity parameters β_j to
follow log-linear regression models with explanatory variables relating to space-time and to
individual characteristics of the jth case, respectively.

Computational difficulties in evaluation of equation (20.13) also can be eased by adapting
the concept of partial likelihood introduced in a famous paper by Cox [43] for the analysis of

time-to-event data. The partial likelihood is the likelihood of the observed time-ordering of the events $(x_i, t_i) : i = 1, ..., n$. To derive the partial likelihood for a spatio-temporal point process, we first define the *risk-set* at time t, denoted by $\mathcal{R}(t)$, as the set of all locations x at which an event could have occurred at time t. In the setting of an infectious disease affecting a finite population, $\mathcal{R}(t)$ is the set of locations of the susceptible members of the population at time t. Then, the probability that the ith time-ordered event occurred at its observed location x_i is

$$P_i(\theta) = \lambda(x_i, t_i | H_{t_i}) / \sum_{x \in \mathcal{R}(t_i)} \lambda(x, t_i | H_{t_i}). \tag{20.15}$$

In other settings, $\mathcal{R}(t)$ can be the whole of the region R, in which case the summation on the right-hand side of equation (20.15) is replaced by an integral to give

$$P_i(\theta) = \lambda(x_i, t_i | H_{t_i}) / \int_R \lambda(x, t_i | H_{t_i}) dx. \tag{20.16}$$

In either case, the partial log-likelihood is

$$PL(\theta) = \sum_{i=1}^n \log P_i(\theta). \tag{20.17}$$

In the first scenario, the partial likelihood avoids the awkward spatio-temporal integral in expression (20.13) altogether. In the second, the integral is replaced by a discrete set of spatial integrals that, depending on the specification of the conditional intensity, may or may not be materially simpler to compute.

For illustration, we revisit an application from Diggle [44] in which a spatially explicit SIR model previously proposed by Keeling et al. [45] was fitted to data from the epidemic of foot-and-mouth disease (FMD) that affected large parts of the UK in 2001.

The model relates to a finite set of farm-locations $x_i : i = 1, ..., N$, each of which is holding susceptible livestock at the start of the epidemic, and the first n of which become infected at times $t_1, t_2, ..., t_n$. Figure 20.7 shows this scenario as it applied to the northern English county of Cumbria in 2001; of the approximately 5,000 farms that were at risk at the start of the epidemic, 657 reported cases of FMD between 28 January 2001 and 17 July 2001.

FMD is transmitted primarily by the exhalation of air-borne particles by an infectious animal and their subsequent inhalation by a susceptible animal. Within the UK farming system, the two main species affected were cows and sheep. Cumbrian farms are predominantly hill-farms whose stock grazes outdoors for most of the year. The core assumption of the Keeling et al. [45] model is that at time t, the rate of transmission between an infected farm i and a susceptible farm j can be expressed as a product,

$$\lambda_{ij}(t) = \lambda_0(t) a_i b_j f(||x_i - x_j||). \tag{20.18}$$

The terms on the right-hand side of equation (20.18) have the following interpretations. First, $\lambda_0(t)$ is the underlying force of infection of the epidemic; for example, in the FMD epidemic the force of infection depended on current weather conditions. Second, a_i and b_j reflect farm-specific characteristics that determine their inherent infectivity and susceptibility, respectively; in the FMD epidemic model, these depended on a farm's stockholding. Finally, $f(\cdot)$, the *transmission kernel*, describes the mechanism by which infection is transmitted.

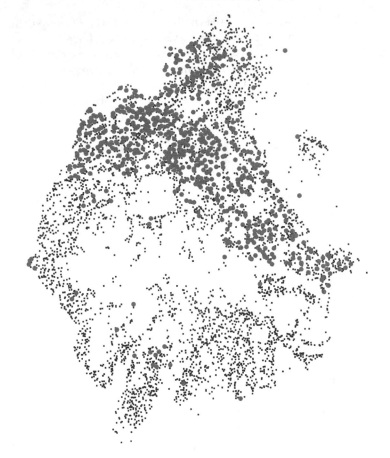

FIGURE 20.7
End-point of the 2001 foot-and-mouth epidemic in the county of Cumbria, UK. Small black
dots show the locations of susceptible stock-holding farms that escaped the epidemic, large
gray dots show case-farms.

It follows from eqution (20.18) that the rate at which a susceptible farm at time t is
infected is $\lambda_j(t) = \sum_{i \in I(t)} \lambda_{ij}(t)$, where $I(t)$ is the set of farms that are infectious at time t.
The partial log-likelihood of the model is $PL(\theta) = \sum_{j=1}^{n} P_j(\theta)$, where

$$P_j(\theta) = \lambda_j(t_j) / \sum_{k \in \mathcal{R}(t_j)} \lambda_k(t_j). \tag{20.19}$$

Note that any term that depends only on time, here $\lambda_0(t)$, cancels in equation (20.19) and
therefore cannot be estimated from the partial likelihood. Also, for the application to the
2001 FMD epidemic, the infection-sets $I(t)$ and risk-sets $\mathcal{R}(t)$ required careful calculation
in order to take account of the pre-emptive culling policy that was implemented during
the epidemic; when a case was notified, stock from the case farm and from uninfected
near-neighboring farms were slaughtered as a control strategy.

Diggle [44] fitted the model to the data from Cumbria and from the southern English
county of Devon, which was the second most highly affected county, with 137 out of

approximately 8,000 farms infected during the epidemic. To parameterize the model, the farm-specific infectivities were specified as

$$a_i = \alpha n_{1i}^\gamma + n_{2i}^\gamma, \tag{20.20}$$

where n_{1i} and n_{2i} denote the numbers of cows and sheep held on farm i. Farm-specific susceptibilities similarly were specified as

$$b_j = \beta n_{1j}^\gamma + n_{2j}^\gamma, \tag{20.21}$$

The parameters α and β represent the relative infectiousness and susceptibility, respectively, of cows to sheep; both parameters would be expected to be greater than 1. We included γ in the model specifically to challenge the hypothesis that the effects of stock-size are linear, which in effect assumes that the whole of a farm's stock is held at a single location whereas, as noted above, stock routinely graze outdoors. Finally, the transmission kernel was specified as

$$f(u) = \exp\{-(u/\phi)^\kappa\} + \rho. \tag{20.22}$$

In equation (20.22) ϕ measures the spatial scale over which transmission decays with increasing distance, while κ controls the shape of the kernel: $\kappa = 1$ gives exponential decay, values $\kappa < 1$ give faster-than-exponential decay at short distances counterbalanced by a longer upper tail, and conversely for $\kappa > 1$. The literal interpretation of the parameter ρ is that infection can be transmitted over arbitrarily large distances at a non-vanishing rate. In practice, including ρ in the model was necessary to prevent estimation of ϕ and κ being influenced by occasional, apparently spontaneous incident cases far from all prevalent cases; these may have resulted from accidental transmission of infected material on vehicles, equipment or clothing.

The above model proved over-parameterized, in the sense that the partial likelihood surface was very flat, particularly in the (κ, ρ) plane. With hindsight, this is unsurprising. Keeling et al.'s modeling choice was for a sharper-than-exponential decay in transmission at short distances, which in our parametric model corresponds to $\kappa < 1$. However, this choice gives a thicker-than-exponential tail, which is hard to distinguish empirically from a positive value of ρ. To deal with this, we decided to keep ρ in the model, but fix $\kappa = 0.5$. Table 20.1 shows the resulting maximum partial likelihood estimates and approximate 95% confidence intervals for the model parameters. Figure 20.8 shows the fitted transmission kernel. The estimates and confidence intervals reported in Table 20.1 show first that the spatial scale has been relatively well estimated. Figure 20.8 shows how this estimate translates into a set of point-wise confidence intervals for $f(\cdot)$. The estimate of ρ, although significantly different from zero, makes a negligible contribution to the estimate of $f(\cdot)$. As noted previously, its role is to prevent an occasional outlying incident case from

TABLE 20.1

Parameter estimation for the Five-Parameter Model
Fitted to Data from the 2001 FMD Epidemic in Cumbria
and Devon

Parameter	Estimate	95% Confidence Interval
α	1.42	1.13 to 1.78
β	36.17	0.19 to 692.92
ϕ	0.41	0.36 to 0.48
$\rho \times 10^4$	1.30	0.85 to 2.10
γ	0.13	0.09 to 0.21

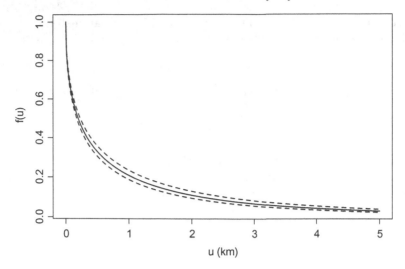

FIGURE 20.8
Fitted transmission kernel (solid line) and 95 percent point-wise confidence intervals (dashed lines) for the 2001 FMD epidemic.

distorting the estimate of ϕ. The estimate and confidence interval for γ confirm that the effect of stock-size is strongly sub-linear. This result, in turn, affects the precision of estimation for α and β. Both point estimates are greater than one, as expected, but the confidence interval for β is very wide. For comparison, Keeling et al. estimated $\alpha = 1.61$ and $\beta = 15.2$, but with γ fixed at 1.

Incidentally, one advantage of a likelihood-based approach is that it makes available all the standard inferential machinery available for likelihood-based testing and estimation. Minimally, this availability discourages over-interpretation of confidence intervals. Perhaps more interestingly, it enables formal comparison between models. In the current example, we justified pooling the data from Cumbria and Devon by first fitting separate models (with $\gamma = 1$) to the data from the two counties, then re-estimating a common set of parameters. The likelihood ratio statistic was 2.98 on 4 degrees of freedom ($p = 0.56$).

To complete this case-study, recall that the partial likelihood gives no information about the underlying force of infection, $\lambda_0(t)$. However, if this is of interest it can be estimated using an adaptation of the Nelson-Aalen estimator (see Chapter 4 of Andersen et al. [46]. Writing $\lambda_{ij}(t) = \lambda_0(t)\rho_{ij}(t)$, the Nelson-Aalen estimate of $\Lambda_0(t) = \int_0^t \lambda_0(u)du$ is

$$\hat{\Lambda}_0(t) = \sum_{i:t_i \leq t} \hat{\rho}(t_i)^{-1}, \tag{20.23}$$

where $\hat{\rho}(t) = \sum_{i \in I(t)} \sum_{j \in \mathcal{R}(t)} \hat{\rho}_{ij}(t)$. Figure 20.9 shows the Nelson-Aalen estimates for the two counties. The larger estimate for Cumbria is consistent with its higher rate of case-incidence over the course of the epidemic.

Another scenario in which a partial likelihood approach may be a useful way to circumvent computational difficulties is when analyzing a multivariate process for which the focus of interest is in the relative intensities of the component processes. Consider a bivariate process with conditional intensties $\lambda_k(t|H_t) : k = 1, ..., m$, where $H_t = \{(x_i, t_i, y_i) : t_i < t\}$,

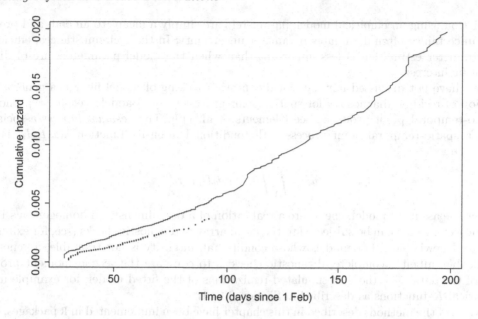

FIGURE 20.9
Estimates of the cumulative hazard, $\Lambda_0(t) = \int_0^t \lambda_0(u)du$, for the UK FMD epidemic in Cumbria (solid line) and Devon (dotted line).

and y_i indicates the label of the ith event. Then, conditional on H_t the labels y_i are realizations of independent multinomials with probabilities

$$p_k(t_i) = \lambda_k(t_i|H_{t_i})/\sum_{j=1^m} \lambda_j(t_i|H_{t_i}) : k = 1,...,m \qquad (20.24)$$

and the partial log-likelihood follows as the sum of the $\log p_{y_i}(t_i)$. The analogue of equation (20.24) for multivariate spatial Poisson point processses has been used for at least 20 years (see, e.g., Kelsall and Diggle [47]) but, to the author's knowledge, has not previously been proposed in the current context.

20.5 Discussion

Likelihood-based methods of inference are now available for a wide range of spatio-temporal point process models. For confirmatory analysis, we recommend their use whenever possible, for a number of reasons. First, likelihood-based methods generally deliver efficient parameter estimators with associated estimates of precision. Second, they provide a way of formally comparing the fits of different models to the data. Finally, and importantly in the author's opinion, a flat likelihood surface gives a warning that a candidate model is over-elaborate. For models whose full likelihood is intractable, partial likelihood methods retain the second and third of the given properties and, although potentially inefficient, do at least deliver estimates of precision.

Because likelihood-based methods can be computationally burdensome, simpler *ad hoc* methods of estimation are useful for exploratory analysis. When the goal of an analysis is prediction using an empirical model, parameters are simply a means to an end, and prediction uncertainty often dominates parameter uncertainty. In these circumstances, efficiency of parameter estimation is less important than when the model parameters are of direct scientific interest.

We have not discussed methods for diagnostic checking of model fit. For a general discussion of residual diagnostics for spatial point processes, see Baddeley et al. [48], and for spatio-temporal point processes see Clements et al. [49]. The *residual process* associated with a spatio-temporal point process with conditional intensity function $\lambda(x,t|H_t)$ is the sequence

$$u_i = \int_A \int^{t_i} \lambda(x,t|H_t)dxdt.$$

Under the assumed model, the u_i are a realization of a one-dimensional homogeneous Poisson process, which can be subjected to the usual array of diagnostic checks (see, for example, Cox and Lewis [50]). For models whose conditional, intensity is not tractable, a generally applicable, albeit incomplete, diganostic check is to compare the second moment properties of the data with those of simulated realizations of the fitted model, for example using empirical K-functions as described in Section 20.4.1.

Most of the methods described in this chapter have been implemented in R packages. The `sttp` package (Gabriel et al. [51]) provides functions for dynamic display of spatio-temporal point process data, simulation of some spatio-temporal point process models, and estimation of the spatio-temporal K-function. The `lgcp` package (Taylor et al. [52]) implements likelihood-based inference for log-Gaussian Cox processes. The `PtProcess` package (Harte [53]) and the `surveillance` package (Meyer et al. [54]) implement maximum likelihood estimation for models of the form of equation (20.14). To the best of my knowledge, at the time of writing this chapter there is no packaged implementation of partial likelihood methods for analyzing spatio-temporal point process data.

References

[1] M.S. Bartlett. The spectral analysis of two-dimensional point processes. *Biometrika*, 51:299–311, 1964.

[2] P.J. Diggle. *Statistical Analysis of Spatial and Spatio-Temporal Point Patterns, Third Edition*. Boca Raton, FL: Chapman and Hall/CRC Press, 2013.

[3] D.R. Cox. Some statistical methods related with series of events (with discussion). *Journal of the Royal Statistical Society B*, 17:129–157, 1955.

[4] K.J. Rothman. A sobering start for the cluster busters conference. *American Journal of Epidemiology*, 132:6–13, 1990.

[5] D.J. Daley and D. Vere-Jones. *An Introduction to the Theory of Point Processes: General Theory and Structure*. New York: Springer, 2005.

[6] J. Møller and R.P. Waagepetersen. *Statistical Inference and Simulation for Spatial Point Processes*. London, UK: Chapman and Hall, 2004.

[7] J. Ilian, A. Penttinen, H. Stoyan, and D. Stoyan. *Statistical Analysis and Modelling of Spatial Point Patterns*. Chichester, UK: Wiley, 2008.

[8] A.J. Baddeley and T.R. Turner. *Spatial Point Patterns: Methodology and Applications with R*. Boca Raton, FL: Chapman and Hall/CRC Press, 2016.

[9] N.A.C. Cressie. *Statistics for Spatial Data*. New York: Wiley, 1991.

[10] A. Gelfand, P.J. Diggle, M. Fuentes, and P. Guttorp. *Handbook of Spatial Statistics*. Boca Raton, FL: CRC Press, 2010.

[11] N. Cressie and C.K. Wikle. *Statistics for Spatio-Temporal Data*. Hoboken, NJ: Wiley, 2011.

[12] G. Shaddick and J.V. Zidek. *Spatio-Temporal Methods in Environmental Epidemiology*. Boca Raton, FL: CRC Press, 2016.

[13] A.J. Baddeley, J. Møller, and R. Waagepetersen. Non and semi parametric estimation of interaction in inhomogeneous point patterns. *Statistica Neerlandica*, 54:329–350, 2000.

[14] A.J. Baddeley and B.W. Silverman. A cautionary example on the use of second-order methods for analyzing point patterns. *Biometrics*, 40:1089–1093, 1984.

[15] B.D. Ripley. Modelling spatial patterns (with discussion). *Journal of the Royal Statistical Society B*, 39:172–212, 1977.

[16] P.M.E. Altham. Improving the precision of estimation by fitting a model. *Journal of the Royal Statistical Society B*, 46:118–119, 1984.

[17] J. Møller, A. Syversveen, and R. Waagepetersen. Log-Gaussian Cox processes. *Scandinavian Journal of Statistics*, 25:451–482, 1998.

[18] F. Lindgren, H. Rue, and J. Lindström. An explicit link between Gaussian fields and Gaussian Markov random fields: The stochastic partial differential equation approach (with discussion). *Journal of the Royal Statistical Society B*, 73:423–498, 2011.

[19] P.J. Diggle, P. Moraga, B. Rowlingson, and B.M. Taylor. Spatial and spatio-temporal log-Gaussian Cox processes: Extending the geostatistical paradigm. *Statistical Science*, 28:542–563, 2013.

[20] A.G. Hawkes. Spectra of some self-exciting and mutually exciting point processes. *Biometrika*, 58:83–90, 1971.

[21] F. Musmeci and D. Vere-Jones. A space-time clustering model for historical earthquakes. *Annals of the Institute of Statistical Mathematics*, 44:1–11, 1992.

[22] S. Meyer and L. Held. Power law models for infectious disease spread. *Annals of Applied Statistics*, 8:1612–1639, 2014.

[23] S. Meyer, J. Elias, and M. Höhle. A spacetime conditional intensity model for invasive meningococcal disease occurrence. *Biometrics*, 68:607–616, 2012.

[24] T. Britton. Stochastic epidemic models: A survey. *Mathematical Biosciences*, 225: 24–35, 2010.

[25] T. Britton. Basic stochastic transmission models and their inference. In L. Held, N. Hens, P. O'Neill, and J. Wallinga, eds., *Handbook of Infectious Disease Data Analysis*, pages XXX–YYY. Boca Raton, FL: CRC Press, 2019.

[26] N.T.J. Bailey. The simulation of stochastic epidemics in two dimensions. *Proceedings of the Fifth Berkeley Symposium on Mathematical Statistics and Probability*, 4:237–257, 1967.

[27] D. Mollison. Spatial contact models for ecological and epidemic spread (with discussion). *Journal of the Royal Statistical Society B*, 39:283–326, 1977.

[28] M.J. Keeling and P. Rohani. *Modelling Infectious Diseases in Humans and Animals*. Princeton, NJ: Princeton University Press, 2008.

[29] E. Gabriel and P.J. Diggle. Second-order analysis of inhomogeneous spatio-temporal point process data. *Statistica Neerlandica*, 63:43–51, 2009.

[30] P. Diggle, B. Rowlingson, and T-L. Su. Point process methodology for on-line spatio-temporal disease surveillance. *Environmetrics*, 16:423–434, 2005.

[31] C. J. Geyer. Markov chain Monte Carlo maximum likelihood. In *Proceedings of the 23rd Symposium on the Interface*. Interface Foundation of North America. Retrieved from the University of Minnesota Digital Conservancy, http://hdl.handle.net/11299/58440, 1991.

[32] B.M. Taylor and P.J. Diggle. INLA or MCMC? A tutorial and comparative evaluation for spatial prediction in log-Gaussian Cox processes. *Journal of Computational and Graphical Statistics*, 84:2266–2284, doi: 10.1080/00949655.2013.788653, 2014.

[33] H. Rue, S. Martino, and N. Chopin. Approximate Bayesian inference for latent Gaussian models by using integrated nested Laplace approximations (with discussion). *Journal of the Royal Statistical Society B*, 71:319–392, 2009.

[34] Joint FAO/WHO Expert Committee on Food Safety. *The Role of Food Safety in Health and Development: Report of a Joint FAO/WHO Expert Committee on Food Safety*. Technical Report Series 705. Geneva, Switzerland: WHO, 1984.

[35] Food Standards Agency. *A Report on the Study of Infectious Disease in England*. London, UK: Food Standards Agency, 2000.

[36] T. Gneiting and P. Guttorp. Continuous parameter spatio-temporial processes. In A. Gelfand, P.J. Diggle, M. Fuentes, and P. Guttorp, eds., *Handbook of Spatial Statistics*, pages 427–436. Boca Raton, FL: CRC Press, 2010.

[37] P.C. Kyriakidis and A.G. Journel. Geostatistical space-time models: A review. *Mathematical Geology*, 31:651–684, 1999.

[38] N. Cressie and H-C. Huang. Classes of non-separable spatio-temporal stationary covariance functions. *Journal of the American Statistical Association*, 94:1330–1340, 1999.

[39] G. Knox. Epidemiology of childhood leukaemia in Northumberland and Durham. *British Journal of Preventive and Social Medicine*, 18:17–24, 1964.

[40] N. Mantel. The detection of disease clustering and a generalized regression approach. *Cancer Research*, 27:209–220, 1967.

[41] J. Besag and P.J. Diggle. Simple Monte Carlo tests for spatial pattern. *Applied Statistics*, 26:327–333, 1977.

[42] A. Brix and P.J. Diggle. Spatio-temporal prediction for log-Gaussian Cox processes. *Journal of the Royal Statistical Society B*, 63:823–841, 2001.

[43] D.R. Cox. Regression models and life tables (with discussion). *Journal of the Royal Statistical Society B*, 34:187–220, 1972.

[44] P.J. Diggle. Spatio-temporal point processes, partial likelihood, foot-and-mouth. *Statistical Methods in Medical Research*, 15:325–336, 2006.

[45] M.J. Keeling, M.E.J. Woolhouse, D.J. Shaw, L. Matthews, M. Chase-Topping, D.T. Haydon, S.J. Cornell, J. Kappey, J. Wilesmith, and B.T. Grenfell. Dynamics of the 2001 UK Foot and Mouth epidemic: Stochastic dispersal in a heterogeneous landscape. *Science*, 294:813–817, 2001.

[46] P.K. Andersen, O. Borgan, R.D. Gill, and N. Keiding. *Statistical Models Based on Counting Processes*. New York: Springer, 1992.

[47] J.E. Kelsall and P.J. Diggle. Spatial variation in risk: A nonparametric binary regression approach. *Applied Statistics*, 47:559–573, 1998.

[48] A. Baddeley, T.R. Turner, J. Møller, and M. Hazelton. Residual analysis for spatial point processes (with discussion). *Journal of the Royal Statistical Society B*, 67: 617–666, 2005.

[49] R.A. Clements, F.P. Schoenberg, and D. Schorlemmer. Residual analysis methods for spacetime point processes with applications to earthquake forecast models in California. *Annals of Applied Statistics*, 5:2459–2571, 2011.

[50] D.R. Cox and P.A.W. Lewis. *The Statistical Analysis of Series of Events*. London, UK: Chapman and Hall, 1966.

[51] E. Gabriel, B. Rowlingson, and P.J. Diggle. STPP: Plotting, simulating and analysing spatio-temporal point patterns. *Journal of Statistical Software*, 53:1–29, 2013.

[52] B.M. Taylor, T.M. Davies, B.S. Rowlingson, and P.J. Diggle. lgcp: Inference with spatial and spatio-temporal log-Gaussian Cox processes in R. *Journal of Statistical Software*, 52:1–40, 2013.

[53] D. Harte. Pt Process: An R package for modelling marked point processes indexed by time. *Journal of Statistical Software*, 35:1–32, 2010.

[54] S. Meyer, L. Held, and M. Höhle. Spatio-temporal analysis of epidemic phenomena using the R package surveillance. *Journal of Statistical Software*, 77, doi: 10.18637/jss.v077.i11, 2017.

21

Prospective Detection of Outbreaks

Benjamin Allévius and Michael Höhle

CONTENTS

An essential aspect of infectious disease epidemiology is the timely detection of emerging infectious disease threats. To facilitate such detection, public health authorities maintain surveillance systems for the structured collection of data in humans, animals and plants. In this chapter we focus on the *prospective* (i.e., as-data-arrive) detection of outbreaks in such data streams obtained as part of the routine surveillance for known diseases, symptoms, or other well-defined events of interest. The organization of this chapter is as follows: In Section 21.2 we briefly present methods for outbreak detection in purely temporal data streams, which is followed by a more extensive presentation of methods for spatio-temporal detection in Section 21.3.

21.1 Motivation and Data Example

Surveillance data currently is collected in vast amounts to support the analysis and control of infectious diseases. As a consequence, the data volume, velocity, and variety exceeds the resources to look at each report individually and thus statistical summaries, insightful visualizations, and automation are needed (Höhle, 2017). In response to this, semi-automatic systems for the screening and further investigation of outbreaks have been developed. This screening typically consists of identifying emerging spikes in the monitored data streams and flagging particular cases for further inspection. For foodborne diseases, for example, this inspection could consist of attempts to identify and remove the food source consumed by all cases.

Our aim is thus to develop data mining tools to support the sequential decision making problem (to react or not) for pathogens with quite heterogeneous features, differing in, for example, data collection, prevalence, and public health importance. As an example, even a single Ebola case constitutes a serious public health threat, whereas only larger clusters of *Campylobacter jejuni* infections will trigger public health actions. It is worthwhile also to point out that large accumulations of cases in a short time period are almost surely noticed at the local level. Automatic procedures nonetheless provide a safety net ensuring that nothing important is missed, but the added value lies predominantly in the detection of dispersed cross-regional outbreaks. Another added value is that the quantitative nature of the algorithms allows for a more objective approach, which can be a helpful addition to epidemiological intuition. However, alarms are useless if they are too frequent for proper investigation. On the other hand, missing an important outbreak is fatal.

21.1.1   Invasive meningococcal surveillance in Germany

As an illustration we use 2002–2008 data from the routine monitoring of invasive meningococcal disease (IMD) by the National Reference Center for Meningococci (NRZM) in Germany[1] as motivating example. Figure 21.1 shows the number of new cases of two particular finetypes described in more detail in Meyer et al. (2012) and available as dataset `imdepi` in the R package `surveillance` (Salmon et al., 2016b; Meyer et al., 2017).

From the figure and its context we observe a number features that make the statistical modeling and monitoring of surveillance time series a challenge. From the time series in the figure we see that we are dealing with a low integer number of reported cases, which can contain secular trends, seasonality, as well as past outbreaks. In the IMD example a

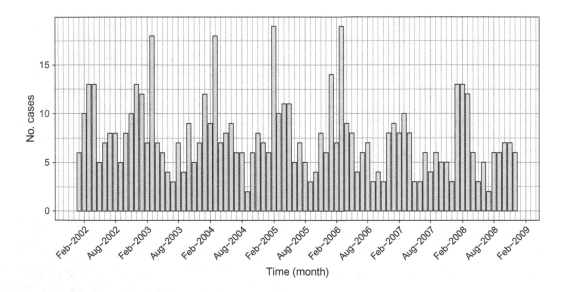

FIGURE 21.1
Time series of monthly number of IMD cases of the two finetypes.

---

[1] http://www.meningococcus.de

microbiological investigation provides a pretty clear definition; however, having a clear case definition can otherwise be a challenge. Furthermore, it is common to report only positive test outcomes with no information on how many tests actually were performed. Spikes in the incidence of new cases might very well be due to an increased testing behavior. This situation brings us to the important issues of under-ascertainment and under-reporting often reflected as stages in a surveillance pyramid of which only the top stage are the reported cases. Another issue, which we will ignore in this chapter, is the problem of reporting delays; depending on the aims it can be necessary to adjust the detection for these phenomena (c.f. Chapter 22 of this book). Instead, we move on to a statistical description and solution of the detection problem.

21.2 Univariate Surveillance Methods

We assume data have been pre-processed such that a univariate time series of counts is available. We then denote by $y_1, \ldots, y_t$ the time series of cases with the time index representing, for example, daily, weekly, or monthly time periods, and y_t being the observation under present consideration. Different statistical approaches then can be used to detect an outbreak at the last instance t of the series. Such approaches have a long tradition and comprehensive review articles exist (Farrington and Andrews, 2003; Sonesson and Bock, 2003; Le Strat, 2005; Woodall, 2006; Höhle and Mazick, 2011; Unkel et al., 2012). An implementational description of many of these algorithms can be found in the R package surveillance (Salmon et al., 2016b). We therefore keep this account short and just present two of the most commonly used algorithms in particular because their approach fits well into that of the multivariate approaches covered in Section 21.3. Both algorithms presented compute a prediction for y_t based on a set of historic values under the assumption that there is no outbreak at y_t, and then assess how extreme the actually observed value is under this assumption.

21.2.1 Early aberration detection system algorithm

The Early Aberration Detection System (EARS) method of the Centers for Disease Control and Prevention (CDC) as described in Fricker et al. (2008) is a simple algorithm convenient in situations when little historic information is available and, hence, trends and seasonality are not of concern. In its simplest form, the baseline is formed by the last $k = 7$ timepoints before the assessed timepoint t, which is particularly meaningful when monitoring a time series of daily data. The simplest version of the method is based on the statistic $C_t = (y_t - \bar{y}_t)/s_t$, where

$$\bar{y}_t = \frac{1}{7} \sum_{s=t-7}^{t-1} y_s \quad \text{and} \quad s_t^2 = \frac{1}{k-1} \sum_{s=t-k}^{t-1} (y_s - \bar{y}_t)^2$$

are the usual unbiased estimators for the mean and variance of the historic values. For the null hypothesis of no outbreak, it is assumed that $C_t \sim N(0,1)$. The threshold for an extreme observation, under the assumption of no outbreak, is now defined as $U_t = \bar{y}_t + 3 \cdot s_t$. Consequently, an alarm is raised if the current observation y_t exceeds this upper limit.

The simplicity of the method makes it attractive, and variants of this Gaussian approach can be found in different contexts, for example as an approximation when the underlying distribution is binomial (Andersson et al., 2014). However, from a statistical point of view the method has a number of shortcomings. In particular the distributional $N(0,1)$ assumption is likely to be inaccurate in case of counts below 5–10, because the distribution is discrete, non-negative, and hence right skewed. As easy as the three times standard deviation is to remember, the appropriate comparison of y_t should be with the upper limit of a prediction interval. Assuming that the y values are identical and independent variables from a Gaussian distribution with both mean and standard deviation unknown, such a one-sided $(1 - \alpha) \cdot 100\%$ interval has an upper limit

$$\bar{y}_t + t_{1-\alpha}(k - 1) \cdot s_t \cdot \sqrt{1 + \frac{1}{k}}, \tag{21.1}$$

where $t_{1-\alpha}(k-1)$ denotes the $1-\alpha$ quantile of the t-distribution with $k-1$ degrees of freedom. Note that for k larger than 20–30, this quantile is very close to that of the standard normal distribution, which is why some accounts, for example, Farrington and Andrews (2003), use $z_{1-\alpha}$ instead. However, when $k = 7$, the α corresponding to a multiplication factor of 3 is not $\alpha = 1 - \Phi(3) = 0.0013$, as one might think, but $\alpha = 1 - F(3/\sqrt{1 + 1/k}) = 0.0155$, where F denotes the cumulative distribution function of the t-distribution with $k - 1$ degrees of freedom. In other words, using a factor of 3 means that the probability of false discoveries is notably higher than possibly expected. From an epidemiologist's point of view, this might seem as yet another instance of statistical nitpicking; however, in the next section we provide an example illustrating how misaligned the $3 \cdot s_t$ rule can be in the case of few and low count data.

The more historical values that are available, the larger k we can choose in practice. However, seasonality and secular trends then become an issue. A simple approach to handle seasonality suggested by Stroup et al. (1989) is to pick time points similar to the currently monitored time point. For example, when working with weekly data and looking at week 45 in year 2017, we could take the values of, for example, weeks 43 to 47 of the previous years as historical values. Another approach is to handle seasonality and trends explicitly in a linear regression model framework,

$$\mu_t = \mathbb{E}(y_t) = \beta_0 + \beta_1 \cdot t + \sum_{l=1}^{L} \left\{ \beta_{2l} \sin\left(\frac{2\pi lt}{P}\right) + \beta_{2l+1} \cos\left(\frac{2\pi lt}{P}\right) \right\},$$

where P is the period, for example, 52 for weekly data. This method has the advantage that *all* historical values are used to infer what is expected. As an alternative to the above superposition of harmonics previous could instead use (penalized) cyclic splines (Wood, 2006) or factor levels for the individual months or days.

21.2.2 Farrington algorithm

An extension of the above approaches is the so-called Farrington algorithm (Farrington et al., 1996; Noufaily et al., 2013), which explicitly uses an underlying count data distribution and handles possible trends through the use of an (over-dispersed) Poisson regression framework. The algorithm is particularly popular at European public health institutions because it is easy to operate and handles a large spectrum of time series with different characteristics without the need of particular tuning.

Assuming, as before, that we want to predict the number of cases y_t at time t under the assumption of no outbreak by using a set of historical values from a window of size $2w + 1$ up to b periods back in time. With weekly data and assuming 52 weeks in every year the set of historical values would be $\cup_{i=1}^{b} \cup_{j=-w}^{w} y_{t-i \cdot 52+j}$. We then fit an over-dispersed Poisson generalized linear model (GLM) with $\mathbb{V}(y_s) = \phi \cdot \mu_s$ and log-linear predictor

$$\mathbb{E}(y_s) = \mu_s, \quad \text{where} \quad \log(\mu_s) = \beta_0 + \beta_1 \cdot s$$

to the historical values. In the previous expression, s denotes the $b(2w + 1)$ time points $t - i \cdot 52 + j$ of the historic values and $\phi > 0$ is the over-dispersion parameter. If the dispersion parameter in the quasi-Poisson is estimated to be smaller than one, then a Poisson model (i.e. $\phi = 1$) is used instead. Based on the estimated GLM model, we compute the upper of limit of a $(1 - \alpha) \cdot 100\%$ one-sided prediction interval for y_t by

$$U_t = \hat{\mu}_t + z_{1-\alpha} \cdot \sqrt{\mathbb{V}(y_t - \hat{\mu}_t)}, \tag{21.2}$$

where $\mathbb{V}(y_t - \hat{\mu}_t) = \mathbb{V}(y_t) + \mathbb{V}(\hat{\mu}_t) - 2\operatorname{Cov}(y_t, \hat{\mu}_t) = \phi\mu_t + \mathbb{V}(\hat{\mu}_t)$, because the current observation is not used as part of the estimation. We know that asymptotically $\hat{\beta} \overset{a}{\sim} N(\beta, I^{-1}(\beta))$, where I^{-1} denotes the inverse of the observed Fisher information. Therefore, $\hat{\eta}_t = \log(\hat{\mu}_t)$ is normally distributed with variance $\mathbb{V}(\hat{\eta}_t) = \mathbb{V}(\hat{\beta}_0) + t^2\mathbb{V}(\hat{\beta}_1) + 2t\operatorname{Cov}(\hat{\beta}_0, \hat{\beta}_1)$. Through the use of the delta method, we find that $\mathbb{V}(\hat{\mu}_t) \approx \exp(\hat{\eta}_t)\mathbb{V}(\hat{\eta}_t)$.

Figure 21.2 displays the fitted GLM and the limits of a corresponding two-sided $(1 - 2\alpha) \cdot 100\%$ prediction interval for the first observation in 2008 when $b = 3$, $w = 3$ and $\alpha = 0.00135$. Because the upper limit 21.1 of the prediction interval is larger than the observed value of 13 no alarm is sounded.

Note that the previous discussion is a somewhat simplified description of the Farrington procedure. For example, a trend is included only if the following three conditions are met: it is significant at the 0.05 level, there are at least 3 years of historical values, and it does not lead to an over-extrapolation (i.e., $\hat{\mu}_t$ is smaller than the maximum of the historical values). Additional refinements of the algorithm include the computation of the prediction interval in equation (21.2) on a $\sqrt{y}$ or $y^{2/3}$ power transformation scale and then back-transform the result. This would for example fix the obvious problem in equation (21.2) that the prediction includes negative values—using the 2/3-power transformation the resulting upper limit would be 24.5 instead. If the historical values contain outliers in form of previous outbreaks, the Farrington algorithm suggests instead to base the prediction on a re-weighted second fit with weights based on Anscombe residuals. Noufaily et al. (2013) suggest a number of additional improvements to the algorithm. Instead of using the window-based approach to select the historical values, all past data are used in the regression model by adding a cyclic 11-knot zero-order spline consisting of a 7-week historical period and nine 5-week periods. Furthermore, better results seem to be obtained when computing the prediction interval directly on a negative binomial assumption (i.e., by assuming $y_t \sim \operatorname{NegBin}(\mu_t, \mu_t/(\phi - 1))$

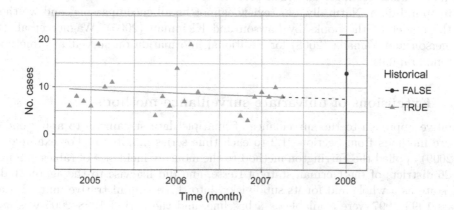

FIGURE 21.2

The historical values, fitted mean, and prediction interval of the simplified Farrington procedure for the observation in January 2008.

where the first argument denotes the mean and the second argument denotes the dispersion parameter of the distribution. By plug-in of the estimates $\hat{\mu}_t$ and $\hat{\phi}$ we obtain that the $1 - \alpha$ quantile of the negative binomial distribution in the example of Figure 21.2 is 24.

For comparison, had we taken the seven observations corresponding to Farrington's $b = 1$ and $w = 3$ as historical values for the EARS approach, we would get $\overline{y}_t = 7.1$, $s_t = 2.6$, and an upper limit of 15.0. When using equation (21.1) with $\alpha = 1 - \Phi(3)$ for the same historical values, the upper limit is 20.8. The corresponding upper limit of the Farrington procedure are 15.7 (untransformed), 17.2 (2/3-power transformation), and 16 (Poisson quantile) for the quasi-Poisson approach. If we assume that a Po(7.1) is the correct null-distribution (the output of the Farrington algorithm in the example), the three times standard deviation rule thus produces too many false alarms—in this particular setting about 0.681 percent instead of the nominal 0.135 percent. Continuing this further, if the seven observations would instead have been a quarter of their value (i.e., 2×1 and 5×2), the corresponding false alarm probability of the $3 \cdot s_t$ approach would raise as high as 9.53 percent, whereas the Farrington procedure with quantile threshold by construction keeps the nominal level. This comparison illustrates the importance of using count response distributions when counts are small.

21.3   Multivariate Surveillance Methods

Surveillance of univariate data streams typically involves some type of spatial or temporal aggregation. For example, many of the detection algorithms discussed in the previous section assume the disease cases are counted on a daily or weekly basis, or monitor just the total sum of all cases that occur in a municipality, a county, or even a whole nation. If this aggregation is too coarse, it could result in the loss of information useful for the detection of emerging threats to public health. Similarly, the failure to monitor secondary data sources such as over-the-counter medicine sales may equate to a forfeiture of the same. These problems motivate the use of *multivariate* methods, which offer a means to treat data at a finer spatial or temporal scale, or to include more sources of information. We start this section by reviewing some of the available extensions of univariate methods to multivariate settings, and then proceed to cover methods for cluster detection in spatio-temporal data. Naturally, our review cannot be all-encompassing, and we therefore direct the reader to the books by Lawson and Kleinman (2005), Wagner et al. (2006), and Rogerson and Yamada (2008) for additional information on surveillance methods for spatio-temporal data.

21.3.1   Extensions of univariate surveillance methods

An intuitive approach to the surveillance of multiple data streams is to apply one of the univariate methods from Section 21.2 to each time series monitored. For example, Höhle et al. (2009) applied the Farrington method to the monthly incidence of rabies among foxes in the 26 districts of the German state of Hesse, and did likewise to the aggregated cases for the state as a whole and for its subdivision into three administrative units. Data from the years 1990–1997 were available as a baseline, and the period 1998–2005 was used for evaluation. The authors were able to to pinpoint the districts in which an outbreak occurred in March of 2000. Höhle et al. (2009) argue that using multiple univariate detectors in this hierarchical way is often a pragmatic choice, because many of the analogous multivariate changepoint detection methods used in the literature (see, e.g., Rogerson and Yamada,

2004) assume continuous distributions for the data; an assumption hardly realistic for the low count time series often seen after partitioning the total number of cases by region, age, serotype, and so on.

The parallel application of univariate methods does have its downsides, however. Univariate methods such as the Farrington algorithm require either a false alarm probability (significance level) α or a threshold c to be set prior to an analysis. These values are often set to achieve some maximum number of false alarms per month or year (see, e.g., Frisén, 2003, for other optimality criteria). If the same conventional α is used for $p \gg 1$, detection methods run in parallel; in the absence of an outbreak, the probability of raising at least one false alarm will be much greater than α. On the other hand, lowering α will make outbreaks harder to detect. Multivariate methods, considered next, do not suffer from the same issues.

21.3.1.1 Scalar reduction and vector accumulation

In the multivariate setting, we suppose that the process under surveillance can be represented as a p-variate vector $\boldsymbol{Y}_t = (Y_{t,1}, Y_{t,2}, \ldots, Y_{t,p})'$, where $t = 1, 2, \ldots$ are the time points under consideration. Each component $Y_{t,i}$ could represent the disease incidence (as a count) of a given region at time t, for example. One of the earliest *control chart* methods of multivariate surveillance is the use of *Hotelling's T^2 statistic* (Hotelling, 1947). Under the null hypothesis for this method, $\boldsymbol{Y}_t$ is assumed to follow a multivariate normal distribution with mean vector $\boldsymbol{\mu}$ and covariance matrix $\boldsymbol{\Sigma}$, both typically estimated from the data. Hotelling's method then reduces the multivariate observation at each timepoint to a scalar statistic, given by

$$T_t^2 = (\boldsymbol{Y}_t - \hat{\boldsymbol{\mu}})' \hat{\boldsymbol{\Sigma}}^{-1} (\boldsymbol{Y}_t - \hat{\boldsymbol{\mu}}), \quad t = 1, 2, \ldots, n. \tag{21.3}$$

The Hotelling T^2 statistic is thus the squared Mahalanobis distance, which measures the distance between the observed data and the null hypothesis distribution while accounting for the different scales and correlations of the monitored variables. When properly scaled, the T^2 statistic has an $F_{p,n-p}$-distribution under the null hypothesis of no outbreak; hence a detection threshold is given by a suitable quantile from this distribution. When dealing with disease count data, however, we know beforehand that the $Y_{t,j}$s should *increase* in case of an outbreak. This prior knowledge is not reflected in the T_t^2 statistic, which penalizes deviations from the mean in either direction. With this motivation, O'Brien (1984) proposed several parametric and non-parametric tests that accomodate alternative hypotheses for consistent departures from the null hypothesis.

A problem with Hotelling T^2 statistic, and likewise the methods proposed by O'Brien (1984), is that they will fail to accumulate evidence for an outbreak over time. As noted by Sonesson and Frisén (2005) (in regard to the T^2 statistic), this failure will render the methods ineffective at detecting small to moderate changes in the monitored process. A solution suggested by Crosier (1988) is to first calculate the Hotelling T_t^2 statistic for each timepoint t in the surveillance period, take its square root T_t, and then apply a CUSUM (Page, 1954) scheme $S_t = \max\{0, S_{t-1} + T_t - k\}$, where $S_0 \geq 0$ and $k > 0$ are chosen together with a threshold c to achieve a certain false positive rate, for example. Similarly, Rogerson (1997) devised a CUSUMized version of the Tango (1995) retrospective spatial statistic, which assumes a Poisson distribution for the data, and calculates a quadratic form statistic using a distance matrix.

The parallel surveillance and scalar reduction methods can be combined by first calculating the ordinary alarm statistics for each data stream, and then applying a scalar reduction method to the vector of such statistics. A few such approaches are reviewed in Sonesson and Frisén (2005). We also point the reader to the important review papers by Frisén (1992),

Sonesson and Bock (2003), Frisén et al. (2010), and Unkel et al. (2012). Finally, for a more general introduction to statistical quality control and the CUSUM method in particular, we recommend the book written by Montgomery (2008).

21.3.1.2 Illustration of Hotelling's T^2 statistic

We now calculate the Hotelling T^2 statistic for the (monthly) meningococcal data introduced in Section 21.1. Because this method assumes that the data follows a multivariate normal distribution, it is at an immediate disadvantage when applied to case data with low counts. We therefore aggregate this data, first over time to form monthly counts for all 413 districts of Germany, and then over space to obtain the corresponding time series for each of the country's 16 states (i.e., $p = 16$). For the purposes of illustration, rather than epidemiological correctness, we also combine the cases across the two different finetypes B (MenB) and C (MenC). In Figure 21.3, we show the calculated T^2 statistics and the critical values at significance level corresponding to an ARL_0 of 3 years. The years 2002–2003 were used as a baseline period for the estimation of the mean vector and covariance matrix using the standard sample formulas (see, e.g., Rencher and Christensen, 2012), and these parameter estimates were updated based on *all* available data at each time step. Note that it may be advisable to use robust estimators of the mean vector and covariance matrix in practice; we chose the standard estimators here because parameter estimation is not the focus of this illustration. Reinhardt et al. (2008) analyzed the meningococcal disease data for the years 2004–2005 using the EpiScanGIS software and found one cluster in the period. For comparison, we therefore run our analysis in the same time interval. Figure 21.3 shows the monthly time series of the T^2 statistic (solid line), along with a critical value (dashed line).

As can be seen in Figure 21.3, Hotelling's method fails to detect any outbreak at the chosen significance level (here $\alpha = 1/36$, corresponding to one expected false detection every 3 years). An apparent flaw is that the detection threshold, which is based on an F distribution with one of the degrees of freedom parameters increasing with n, will decrease monotonically with time, eventually reaching its asymptote. This happens regardless of significance level, and it may therefore be useful to explore other ways of obtaining detection thresholds—simulation-based, perhaps. Another drawback, which is not exclusive to Hotelling's method, is that even if a detection is made, the method does not inform us of *where* (or which variables) the threshold was caused to be exceeded. Methods that remedy this problem are the topic of the next section.

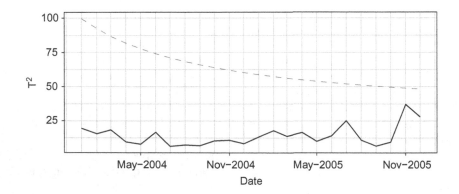

FIGURE 21.3
Hotelling's T^2 statistic (solid) and critical values (dashed), calculated monthly for the years 2004–2005 for the German meningococcal disease data.

21.3.2   Spatio-temporal cluster detection

For some diseases, it may suffice to monitor the univariate time series of cases aggregated across a country using the methods described in Section 21.2. A detection signal then may prompt further investigation into the time, location, and cause of the potential outbreak. For many diseases, however, a large increase in the case count of a small region can be drowned out by the noise in the counts of other regions as they are combined. To detect emerging outbreaks of such diseases before they grow large, the level of aggregation needs to be smaller, perhaps even at the level of individual cases—a tradeoff between variability and detecting a pattern. Despite the possibilities of long-range transmission enabled by modern means of transportation, transmission at a local level is still the dominant way in which most infectious diseases spread (Höhle, 2016). Thus, the statistical methods used to detect the *clusters* that arise should take into account the spatial proximity of cases in addition to their proximity in time. We begin this section by describing methods for *area-referenced* discrete-time data, in which counts are aggregated by region and time period. This topic is followed by Section 21.3.2.2, which discusses methods for continuous space, continuous time data.

21.3.2.1   Methods for area-referenced data

Aggregation by region and time period may in some cases be required by public health authorities due to the way the data collection or reporting works, or for privacy reasons. Legislation and established data formats thus may determine at what granularity surveillance data is available. For example, the CASE surveillance system (Cakici et al., 2010) used by the Public Health Agency of Sweden is limited to data at county (*län*) level, with the least populous of the 21 counties having a population of about 58,000 people. The monitored data in the area-referenced setting is typically of the form $\{y_{it}\}$, where $i = 1, \ldots, N$ denotes the number of (spatial) regions, such as counties, and the index $t = 1, \ldots, T$ denotes time intervals of equal length. Cluster detection in this setting involves identifying a set Z of regions in which a disease outbreak is believed to be emerging during the $D = 1, 2, \ldots$ most recent time periods (weeks, for example). We will denote such a space-time *window* by W, and its complement by $\overline{W}$. A well-established methodology for cluster detection for this task is that of *scan statistics*, which dates back to the 1960s with work done by Naus (1965), and that took on its modern form after the seminal papers by Kulldorff and Nagarwalla (1995) and Kulldorff (1997). These methods, which were extended from the spatial to the spatio-temporal context by Kulldorff (2001), are widely used among public health departments thanks to the free software SATSCAN™ (Kulldorff, 2016).

21.3.2.1.1   Example: Kulldorff's Prospective Scan Statistic

To illustrate the typical procedure of using a scan statistic designed for space-time cluster detection, we work through the steps of calculating and applying of the most popular of such methods, often simply referred to as *Kulldorff's (prospective) scan statistic* (Kulldorff, 2001). This method assumes that the count Y_{it} in region i and time t follows a Poisson distribution with mean $q_{it} \cdot b_{it}$. Here, b_{it} is an "expected count" or "baseline", proportional to the population at risk in region i at time t. For example, these values could be constrained such that the sum of the expected counts over all regions and time periods equals the total of the observed counts during the time period under study. That is, $\sum_{it} b_{it} = \sum_{it} y_{it}$. The factor $q_{it} > 0$, often called the *relative risk*, is assumed to be the same $q_{it} = q$ for all i and t provided there is no outbreak. This method constitutes the null hypothesis. In the case of an outbreak, however, it is assumed that the relative risk is higher inside a space-time window $W = Z \times \{T - D + 1, \ldots, T\}$, consisting of a subset of regions $Z \subset \{1, \ldots, N\}$ and stretching over the most recent time periods, D. That is, for $i \in Z$ and $t > T - D$, we have $E[Y_{it}] = q_W b_{it}$, while for $i \notin Z$ or $t \leq T - D$, it holds that $E[Y_{it}] = q_{\overline{W}} b_{it}$ with $q_W > q_{\overline{W}}$. Here, $\overline{W}$ is the complement of W. This multiplicative increase in the baseline parameters inside a space-time window is typically how outbreaks are modeled for scan statistics. For scan statistics applied to prospective surveillance, it is important to note that all potential space-time clusters have a temporal duration that stretches from the most recent time period backwards, without interuptions. This temporal duration means that no inactive outbreaks are considered, and that any space-time window included in an analysis can be thought of as a cylinder with a base formed by the perimiter of the geographical regions covered by the window, and a height equal to its length in time.

21.3.2.1.2　Definition and Calculation of the Scan Statistic

Of course, there could be many space-time windows W for which the alternative hypothesis is true. If we would conduct hypothesis tests for each window separately—and the number of such windows could well be in the thousands or hundreds of thousands in typical applications—this would result in a very large number of false positives for standard significance levels such as 0.05. This problem could be counteracted by lowering the nominal significance level to a miniscule value, or by using some other repeated testing strategy, but this would in turn allow only very large outbreaks (in terms of q_W relative to $q_{\overline{W}}$) to be captured. The solution proposed by Kulldorff (2001) is to focus only on the window W that stands out compared to the others, as measured by the size of likelihood ratio statistics calculated for all windows W of interest. By calculating the maximum of all such statistics, and using the distribution of this maximum to calculate P-values, the "most anomalous" space-time cluster can be identified. To calculate a likelihood ratio for a given space-time window $W = Z \times \{1, 2, \ldots, D\}$, we must first calculate the maximum likelihood estimates of the relative risks q_W and $q_{\overline{W}}$. For Kulldorff's Poisson scan statistic, these are easily computed as

$$\hat{q}_W = \frac{Y_W}{B_W}, \quad \hat{q}_{\overline{W}} = \frac{Y - Y_W}{Y - B_W} = \frac{Y_{\overline{W}}}{B_{\overline{W}}}, \tag{21.4}$$

where

$$Y_W = \sum_{(i,t) \notin W} y_{it}, B_W = \sum_{(i,t) \in W} b_{it}, \text{ and } Y = \sum_{i=1}^{N} \sum_{t=1}^{T} y_{it} = \sum_{i=1}^{N} \sum_{t=1}^{T} b_{it}. \tag{21.5}$$

Thus, the likelihood ratio statistic conditional on the window W is then given by

$$\lambda_W = \left(\frac{Y_W}{B_W}\right)^{Y_W} \left(\frac{Y - Y_W}{Y - B_W}\right)^{Y - Y_W} \mathbf{1}_{\{Y_W > B_W\}}, \tag{21.6}$$

up to a multiplicative constant not dependent on q_W or $q_{\overline{W}}$. Here, $\mathbf{1}_{\{.\}}$ is the indicator function. This statistic is then calculated for all space-time windows W of interest, and the *scan statistic* is defined as the maximum of all such statistics: $\lambda^* = \max_W \lambda_W$. The corresponding window W^*, often called the *most likely cluster* (MLC), is thus identified.

21.3.2.1.3　Hypothesis Testing

Because the distribution of λ^* cannot be derived analytically, a Monte Carlo approach to hypothesis testing often is taken, whereby new data for each region i and time t is simulated under the null hypothesis using the expected counts b_{it}. For Kulldorff's scan statistic, the sampling is made conditional on the total observed count C, leading to a multinomial distribution over regions and time intervals for the new counts. This sampling is repeated R times, and for each sample r, a new scan statistic λ_r^* is computed. A Monte Carlo P-value for the observed scan statistic then can be calculated in standard fashion using its rank among the simulated values:

$$P = \frac{1 + \sum_{r=1}^{R} \mathbf{1}\{\lambda_r^* > \lambda_{\mathrm{obs}}^*\}}{1 + R}.$$

Typically, a number such as $R = 999$ or $R = 9999$ is used to get a fixed number of digits for the P-value. For prospective surveillance, past analyses—and potentially future ones—also should be accounted for when conducting hypothesis tests to avoid a greater number of expected false positives than implied by the nominal significance value (i.e., a multiple testing problem). The solution suggested by Kulldorff (2001) is to expand the set of replicates $\{\lambda_r^*\}_{r=1}^{R}$ by including replicates calculated in past analyses. If too many past analyses are included, however, the hypothesis tests could become too conservative. Kulldorff (2001) therefore recommends including only the most recent ℓ analyses, where ℓ could be chosen to achieve a certain false positive rate during a given monitoring period, for example. This practice has been the subject of a heated debate recently, with Correa et al. (2015a) asserting that any nominal significance level α used for prospective surveillance with Kulldorff's scan statistic is unrelated to the average run length (ARL) and recurrence interval (RI), which are commonly used in prospective surveillance. Similar points have been raised earlier by Woodall (2006), Joner et al. (2008), and Han et al. (2010). In a rebuttal, Kulldorff and Kleinman (2015) explain that in one of the three prospective cases considered by Correa et al. (2015a) the simulations performed actually show the expected result, and that in the other two cases the concerns raised are actually misunderstandings. Correa et al. (2015b) later clarify that failure to account for future analyses remain a concern, despite the comments by Kulldorff and Kleinman (2015). In the latest reply to the debate, Tango (2016) states that both of the previous parties are in fact wrong: Correa et al. (2015a) for being unrealistic in their consideration of an indefinite number of future analyses and for focusing on the ARL in a setting for which the spatial component of outbreaks is at least as important as the temporal one (because the ARL does not inform us of the spatial spreading of the disease), and Kulldorff (2001) and Kulldorff and Kleinman (2015) for performing a prospective analysis *conditional* on the total number of observed cases in any given study period. Rather, Tango (2016) reiterates the point made by Tango et al. (2011) that such an analysis should be *unconditional* on the total count. This last point will be expanded upon in the upcoming discussion, but the overall implication for those wishing to apply scan statistics in prospective settings is to carefully weigh the benefits and costs of setting the threshold for "sounding the alarm" at a particular level.

Given that the number of space-time windows to be included in the analysis can range in the thousands or hundreds of thousands, the calculation of Monte Carlo P-values means an R-fold increase of an already high computational cost. One way to reduce this computational cost is to calculate a smaller number of Monte Carlo replicates of the scan statistic, fit an appropriate distribution to these replicates, and then compute the tail probability of the observed scan statistic from the fitted distribution. Abrams et al. (2010) tested such a procedure for a number of different distributions (Gumbel, gamma, log-normal, normal) on Kulldorff's scan statistic and others. The authors found that the Gumbel distribution yielded approximate P-values that were highly accurate in the far tails of the scan statistic distribution, in some scenarios making it possible to achieve the same rejection power with one tenth as many Monte Carlo replicates. Another possibility is to circumvent simulation altogether by comparing the value of the scan statistic computed on the current data to values calculated in the past, provided no outbreaks are believed have been ongoing in the data used for these past calculations. Neill (2009a) compared this approach to Monte Carlo simulation with standard and Gumbel P-values and found that the latter two methods for calculating P-values gave misleading results on three medical data sets, requiring a much lower significance level than originally posited to reach an acceptable level of false positives.

21.3.2.1.4   Cluster Construction

A second way of limiting the computational cost of running a scan statistic analysis is to limit the search to clusters with a compact spatial component (*zone*) Z, in the sense that all regions inside the cluster are close to one another geographically. This method makes sense for both computational and practical reasons, since many of the $2^N - 1$ subsets of all N regions are spatially disconnected and therefore not of interest for detection of diseases that emerge locally. For example, we could limit the search to the k nearest neighbors to each region $i = 1, \ldots, N$, for $k = 0, 1, \ldots, K_{max}$, where K_{max} is some user-defined upper bound (as in Tango et al., 2011), or automatically chosen such that the largest zone with region i as center encompasses regions with a combined population that equals approximately 50 percent of the total population in the whole study area (as in Kulldorff, 2001). The set of zones obtained by these methods will be quite compact, which can be problematic if the true outbreak zone consists of regions that all lie along a riverbank, for example. To capture a richer set of zones, Tango and Takahashi (2005) propose a way to construct "flexibly shaped" zones by considering all connected subsets of the K_{max} nearest neighbors of each region i that still contain region i itself. This method can yield a vastly larger set of zones, but becomes impractical in terms of run-time for $K_{max} > 30$ when the number of regions is about 200 or more.

More data-driven approaches to finding the set of interesting zones also can be taken. For example, Duczmal and Assunção (2004) consider the set of all connected subgraphs as the set of allowable zones, and search the most promising clusters using a simulated annealing approach. Here, the nodes in the graph searched are the spatial regions, and edges exist between regions that share a common border. Another more holistic approach is taken by Neill et al. (2013), who propose a framework in which regions are first sorted by priority based on observed counts and estimated parameters, and the set of zones scanned then taken to be only the top n regions, for $n = 1, 2, \ldots, N$. This method is discussed further in Section 21.3.2.1.

21.3.2.1.5   Illustration of Kulldorff's Scan Statistic

After the set of clusters to be scanned have been determined, the analysis can take place. Here, we apply Kulldorff's prospective scan statistic (Kulldorff, 2001) to the meningococcal data considered earlier, now aggregated to monthly counts for each of Germany's 413 districts (*kreise*). This scan statistic is implemented in the R package `scanstatistics` (Allévius, 2017) as the function `scan_pb_poisson`.

In Figure 21.4, we show the resulting scan statistics for each month of the study period (2004–2005). At each time step, the statistic was calculated using at most the latest 6 months of data, and the b_{it} for each district and time point was estimated as

$$\hat{b}_{it} = \frac{Y}{T} \cdot \frac{\text{Pop}_i}{\text{Pop}_{total}}. \tag{21.7}$$

Here, Y is the total observed count over all districts and time points, $T = 6$ is the length of the study period, and Pop_i and Pop_{total} are the 2008 populations for district i and all of Germany, respectively. Critical values (sample quantiles) for the significance level $\alpha = 1/60$ were obtained from Monte Carlo replication with $R = 99$ replicates, and previously generated replicates were included in the calculation at each new time step.

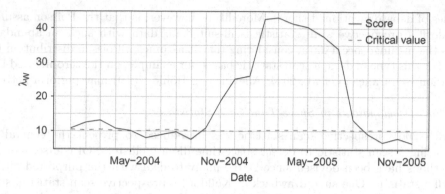

FIGURE 21.4
Observed value of Kulldorff's prospective scan statistic calculated monthly in the years 2004–2005 for the German meningococcal disease data.

The most likely cluster detected by Kulldorff's prospective scan statistic, for most months scanned, corresponds well to the region of highest disease incidence in the years 2004–2005. The core cluster seems to be four districts in North Rhine-Westphalia, one of them the city (urban district) Aachen, and coincides with a confirmed cluster of meningococcal disease discussed in Meyer et al. (2012). This cluster also matches that found by Reinhardt et al. (2008). In Figure 21.5, we show a map of the counties of North Rhine-Westphalia with the detected cluster shaded in gray.

Figure 21.4 shows that the given significance level results in detection signals during much of the study period. This result may not be entirely plausible, and we could see this as an inadequacy of the Monte Carlo method, as discussed in Section 21.3.2.1 (see, in particular,

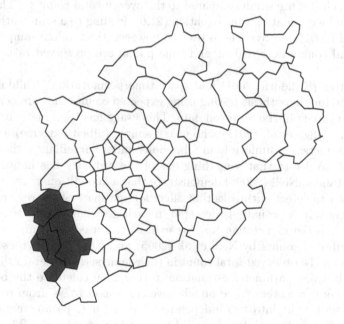

FIGURE 21.5
Districts of North Rhine-Westphalia with the most likely cluster shaded in gray.

the issues of debate mentioned there). More likely, however, is that the Poisson assumption of Kulldorff's prospective scan statistic is ill-suited for data with such an abundance of zeros as the meningococcal data, considering that it assumes a Poisson distribution for the counts. For this type of data, a scan statistic based, for example, on the zero-inflated Poisson distribution (see Cançado et al., 2014; Allévius and Höhle, 2019) may perform better.

21.3.2.1.6 Developments in Space-Time Scan Statistics

Kulldorff's 2001 prospective scan statistic was introduced to present the general procedure of using a scan statistic to detect space-time disease clusters. Of course, many more such methods have been devised since 2001—many to deal with the purported "flaws" of Kulldorff's statistic. One such drawback of Kulldorff's prospective scan statistic is that it requires data on the population at risk and its spatial (and possibly temporal) distribution over the study area. The notion of a population at risk may not be applicable in cases where the surveillance data consists of counts of emergency department visits and over-the-counter medicine sales, for example. Noting this fact, Kulldorff et al. (2005) formulate a *space-time permutation scan statistic*, which uses only the observed counts in the current study period and area to estimate the baselines. Under the assumption that the probability of a case occurring in region i, given that it occurred at time t, is the same for all times $t = 1, \ldots, T$, the baseline (expected value) for the count in region i at time t is estimated by Kulldorff et al. (2005) as

$$b_{it} = \frac{1}{Y} \left(\sum_{j=1}^{N} y_{jt} \right) \left(\sum_{\tau=1}^{T} y_{i\tau} \right). \tag{21.8}$$

The analysis is thus conditional on the marginal counts over regions and time points, leading to a hypergeometric distribution for the total count inside a space-time cluster W. This distribution can in turn be approximated by a Poisson distribution when the marginal counts inside the cluster are small compared to the overall total count C. Thus, a likelihood ratio statistic can be calculated using equation (21.6), leading to a scan statistic of the same form as Kulldorff (2001). For hypothesis testing, however, the random sampling is done such that the marginal counts over regions and time points are preserved rather than just the total count.

The prospective (Kulldorff, 2001) and space-time permutation (Kulldorff et al., 2005) scan statistics conduct hypothesis testing using expected counts that are *conditional* on the total or marginal counts in the observed data. This usage has been met with some critique, particularly from Tango et al. (2011) who give a simple (albeit extreme) example showing that if counts are increased uniformly in all regions under surveillance, these types of scan statistics will fail to detect that something out of the ordinary has happened. Using less extreme circumstances, Neill (2009a) demonstrate that a "conditional" scan statistic of this sort has low power to detect outbreaks that affect a large share of the regions under surveillance. When an outbreak actually is detected in such a scenario, that scan statistic takes longer to do so than the *expectation-based* scan statistics used for comparison. Introduced for Poisson-distributed counts by Neill et al. (2005) and Neill (2006), these scan statistics do not condition on the observed total count in their analysis. Neither do they use the most recent data for baseline parameter estimation; rather they calculate the baselines b_{it} and other non-outbreak parameters based on what we can *expect* to see from past data. In that sense, the analysis is split into two independent parts. First, parameters of the distribution are estimated on historical data believed to contain no outbreaks. This estimation can be done by any method regression preferable; typically by fitting a GLM (McCullagh and Nelder, 1989) or a moving average to the data. Second, the estimated parameters are used for simulating new counts from the given probability distribution and plugged into the calculation of the scan statistic on both the observed and simulated data to conduct Monte Carlo hypothesis testing. Expectation-based scan statistics have been formulated for the Poisson (Neill et al., 2005; Neill, 2009b), Gaussian (Neill, 2006), negative binomial (Tango et al., 2011), and zero-inflated Poisson (Allévius and Höhle, 2019) distributions, among others.

The drawback of these scan statistics, as well as those mentioned at the beginning of this section, is that they scan over a fixed set of space-time windows W. If the true outbreak cluster is not among the windows scanned, the outbreak cannot be exactly identified. As also mentioned, the number of windows to be scanned poses a computational burden, particularly if Monte Carlo hypothesis is to be conducted. To overcome these issues, Neill (2012) proposes a "Fast Subset Scan" framework for making fast searches for the top-scoring cluster, unconstrained by any pre-defined set of windows to be scanned. In particular, Neill introduces a "Linear Time Subset Scanning" (LTSS) property, which is shown to hold for several members of the exponential family of distributions (or rather, scan statistics based thereon). For scan statistics with this property, a *score function* (such as the likelihood ratio in equation (21.6)) is paired with a *priority function* defined, for example, as the ratio of of count to baseline. The latter function is used to sort the data in order of priority, after which the former function only needs to be applied to increasing subsets of the ordered records. This method allows an unconstrained search for the top-scoring subset in linear time (plus the cost of sorting the data records); the method also can be modified to search only for clusters fulfilling spatial constraints, such as subsets of the K nearest neighbors of each region. The Fast Subset Scan framework also can be extended to multivariate space-time data, as covered next.

21.3.2.1.7 *Multivariate Scan Statistics*

Until now, the scan statistics described have been univariate in the sense that the counts $\{y_{it}\}$ typically consist of cases of a single disease or symptoms thereof, each count having both spatial and temporal attributes. In practice, however, public health authorities monitor a multitude of such data streams simultaneously. If each analysis is done without regard for the others, this analysis will undoubtedly yield a number of false positives higher than desirable. Alternatively, if the significance level of each analysis is adjusted for the others, the power to detect an outbreak in any of the data streams diminishes. These issues can be overcome by analyzing all data streams *jointly*, an endeavour that can be particularly fruitful when the streams pertain to the same phenomenon to be detected—typically a disease outbreak. For example, some diseases have multiple symptoms and patients may seek help in different ways. A simultaneous increase in over-the-counter flu medication sales at pharmacies and respiratory symptoms reported at a local clinic may in such a case be indicative of an influenza outbreak, but this signal of an outbreak may be missed if each of the two data streams are considered individually.

With this motivation and inspired by an idea of Burkom (2003), Kulldorff et al. (2007) formulate a multivariate scan statistic based on Kulldorff's prospective scan statistic (Kulldorff, 2001). The data in this setting can be represented as a collection of vector counts $\{\boldsymbol{y}_{it}\}$, where $\boldsymbol{y} = (y_{it}^{(1)}, \ldots, y_{it}^{(M)})'$ are the counts for each of the M data streams monitored. The scan statistic is calculated by first processing each data stream separately, calculating a likelihood ratio statistic using equation (21.6) for each space-time window W, just as is done with the univariate scan statistic. For those windows whose aggregated count exceeds the aggregated baseline, the logarithm of these likelihood ratios are added to form a statistic for the window as a whole. The scan statistic then is defined as the maximum of all such statistics, so that the most likely cluster can be identified as the regions, time intervals, *and* data streams making a positive contribution to the maximum statistic.

Building upon the Fast Subset Scan framework (Neill, 2012) cited earlier, Neill et al. (2013) present two computationally efficient ways to detect clusters in space-time data, with and without spatial constraints on these clusters. The first method, *Subset Aggregation*, is an extension of the work done by Burkom (2003). Subset Aggregation assumes that if an outbreak occurs, it has a multiplicative effect on the baselines b_{it}^m that is equal across all regions, time points, and data streams affected by the outbreak. That is, for those regions, times, and data streams (i, t, m) affected by the outbreak, the expected value of the count $y_{it}^{(m)}$ is $q b_{it}^{(m)}$ rather than $b_{it}^{(m)}$. This method allows the counts and baselines within each *subset* (cluster) to be *aggregated*, so that the Subset Aggregation scan statistic can be reduced to a univariate scan statistic for the cluster. The second method is the one previously proposed by Kulldorff et al. (2007), in which an outbreak affects each data stream separately through a stream-specific multiplicative factor q_m. Neill et al. (2013) then demonstrates how these methods can be combined with the Fast Subset Scan framework for scan statistics satsifying the LTSS property (Neill, 2012), yielding fast, exact detection algorithms when either the number of data streams or the number of regions are small, and fast approximate (randomized) algorithms when there are too many regions and streams for all subsets of each to be scanned. If hypothesis testing is to take place, this testing can be done using Monte Carlo replication as described earlier. Again, such replication can come at a high computational cost, and some efforts have therefore been made to avoid it altogether.

21.3.2.1.8 *Bayesian Scan Statistics*

Neill et al. (2006) introduce the *Bayesian Spatial scan statistic* for cluster detection, based on Kulldorff's 1997 original scan statistic. The method is easily extended to a spatio-temporal setting, which is that described in the following discussion. In Kulldorff's 2001 model, the data $\{y_{it}\}$ are assumed to be Poisson distributed with expected values $q \cdot b_{it}$, the relative risk q varying depending on whether an outbreak is ongoing or not, and estimated by maximum likelihood. In the model of Neill et al. (2006), the parameters q are instead given conjugate gamma distribution priors, with prior probabilities tuned to match the occurrence of an outbreak in each possible outbreak cluster considered. With the conjugate prior for the relative risks, and baselines $\{b_{it}\}$ estimated from historical data, simple analytical formulas can be derived for the marginal probabilities of the data (relative risks integrated out), in the end resulting in the posterior probability of an outbreak for each cluster considered, and for the non-occurrence of an outbreak. Thus, no Monte Carlo replications need to be made.

To examplify the Bayesian scan statistic (Neill et al., 2006), suppose the null hypothesis of no outbreak states that each count is distributed as a Poisson random variable with mean $q \cdot b_{it}$, where b_{it} is fixed and $q \sim \text{Gamma}(\alpha_{\text{all}}, \beta_{\text{all}})$. After marginalizing over the distribution of q, the likelihood under the null hypothesis becomes the negative binomial (also known as gamma-Poisson mixture) probability mass function:

$$\mathbb{P}(\boldsymbol{y}|H_0) = \frac{\Gamma(\alpha_{\text{all}} + Y)}{Y!\,\Gamma(\alpha_{\text{all}})} \left(\frac{\beta_{\text{all}}}{\beta_{\text{all}} + B}\right)^{\alpha_{\text{all}}} \left(\frac{B}{\beta_{\text{all}} + B}\right)^{\alpha_{\text{all}}}, \tag{21.9}$$

where $\boldsymbol{y}$ represents the entire data set, Y is the sum of all counts, and B the sum of all baselines b_{it}. The alternative hypothesis states that an outbreak is occuring in a space-time window W, with a prior distribution placed over all potential windows W. For a given W, it is assumed that counts inside W have a relative risk q distributed as $q \sim \text{Gamma}(\alpha_W, \beta_W)$, while those counts outside have a corresponding distribution for q with parameters $\alpha_{\overline{W}}$ and $\beta_{\overline{W}}$. After marginalizing over the relative risk distributions, the likelihood becomes

$$\mathbb{P}(\boldsymbol{y}|H_1(W)) = \frac{\Gamma(\alpha_W + Y_W)}{Y_W!\,\Gamma(\alpha_W)} \left(\frac{\beta_W}{\beta_W + B_W}\right)^{\alpha_W} \left(\frac{B_W}{\beta_W + B_W}\right)^{\alpha_W}$$

$$\times \frac{\Gamma(\alpha_{\overline{W}} + Y_{\overline{W}})}{Y_{\overline{W}}!\,\Gamma(\alpha_{\overline{W}})} \left(\frac{\beta_{\overline{W}}}{\beta_{\overline{W}} + B_{\overline{W}}}\right)^{\alpha_{\overline{W}}} \left(\frac{B_{\overline{W}}}{\beta_{\overline{W}} + B_{\overline{W}}}\right)^{\alpha_{\overline{W}}}, \qquad (21.10)$$

where Y_W and B_W is the sum of counts and baselines inside W, respectively, $Y_{\overline{W}} = Y - Y_W$, and $B_{\overline{W}} = B - B_W$. With a prior $\mathbb{P}(H_0)$ placed on the null hypothesis, and similarly $\mathbb{P}(H_1(W))$ for each outbreak scenario, we obtain the posterior probabilities

$$\mathbb{P}(H_1(W)|\boldsymbol{y}) = \frac{\mathbb{P}(\boldsymbol{y}|H_1(W))\mathbb{P}(H_1(W))}{\mathbb{P}(\boldsymbol{y})}, \qquad (21.11)$$

$$\mathbb{P}(H_0|\boldsymbol{y}) = \frac{\mathbb{P}(\boldsymbol{y}|H_0)\mathbb{P}(H_0)}{\mathbb{P}(\boldsymbol{y})}, \qquad (21.12)$$

where $\mathbb{P}(\boldsymbol{y}) = \mathbb{P}(\boldsymbol{y}|H_0)\mathbb{P}(H_0) + \sum_W \mathbb{P}(\boldsymbol{y}|H_1(W))\mathbb{P}(H_1(W))$. Neill et al. (2006) gives advice for eliciting the priors $\mathbb{P}(H_0)$ and $\mathbb{P}(H_1(W))$, and also for specification of the hyperparameters of each relative risk distribution.

The space-time extension of the Bayesian spatial scan statistic (Neill et al., 2006) is available as the function `scan_bayes_negbin` in the `scanstatistics` R package (Allévius, 2017). To illustrate, we run this scan statistic on the same data as in the previous illustration of Kulldorff's scan statistic. As hyperparameters, we set b_{it} to the estimate in equation (21.8) and let all gamma distribution parameters $\alpha_{(\cdot)}$ and $\beta_{(\cdot)}$ be equal to 1. The exception is α_W, which we assume to be the same for all W. We give this parameter a discrete uniform prior on equally spaced values between 1 and 15 in the first month, and let subsequent months use the posterior distribution from the previous month as a prior. We also set $\mathbb{P}(H_1) = 1 - \mathbb{P}(H_0) = 10^{-7}$, which is on the order of magnitude of the incidence of meningococcal disease in Germany in 2002–2008. In Figure 21.6, we show the posterior outbreak probability $\mathbb{P}(H_1(W)|\boldsymbol{y})$ at each month of the analysis, for the space-time window W which maximizes this probability.

Figure 21.6 shows clear similarities to the scores calculated for Kulldorff's scan statistic shown in Figure 21.4. Further, half of all most likely clusters (MLCs) reported by each

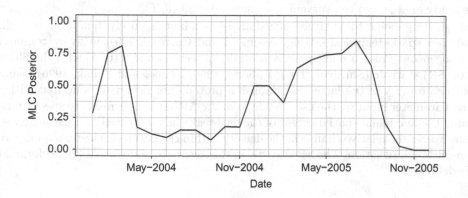

FIGURE 21.6
The posterior outbreak probability $\mathbb{P}(H_1(W)|\boldsymbol{y})$ for the most likely cluster (MLC) W detected in each month of the analysis.

method are the same. The difference, as discussed earlier, is that the output of the Bayesian scan statistic is a posterior probability rather than the maximum of a likelihood ratio.

The Bayesian scan statistic was later extended to a multivariate setting by Neill and Cooper (2010). This *Multivariate Bayesian Scan Statistic* (MBSS) also is capable of detecting multiple event types, thus allowing it, for example, to assign probabilities to outbreaks of different diseases based on records of symptom data. A downside of this method is that the set of clusters to be searched must be specified, and the prior probability of an outbreak in each is (typically) uniform over all clusters regardless of size and shape. To remedy this defect, Neill (2011) modify the MBSS by specifying a hierarchical spatial prior over all subsets of regions to be scanned. This method is shown to be superior to the MBSS in spatial accuracy and detection timeliness, yet remaining computationally efficient. More recently, for univariate data, a Baysian scan statistic based on the zero-inflated Poisson distribution has been proposed by Cançado et al. (2017).

21.3.2.1.9 *Alternative Methods for Cluster Detection in Area-Referenced Data*

Scan statistics are not the only option for cluster detection of the sort we have discussed. To give an example, there is the *What's Strange About Recent Events?* (WSARE; Wong et al., 2005) method, available as software, which can detect outbreaks in multivariate space-time data sets by using a rule-based technique to compare the observed data against a baseline distribution. WSARE uses Bayesian networks, association rules, and a number of other techniques to produce a robust detection algorithm. Other examples with more detail than space allows for here can be found in Rogerson and Yamada (2008).

21.3.2.2 Methods for point process data

The methods discussed in the previous section were applicable to data which has been aggregated over space and time. Athough such an accumulation may be the inherent form of the data, the loss of granularity could impede both the timeliness and spatial accuracy with which outbreaks are detected. When data with exact coordinates and time stamps are available, it may thus be beneficial to analyze data in this format. In this section we therefore assume that the available data is of the form $\{s_i, t_i\}_{i=1}^n$, where $s = (x, y)$ are the coordinates (longitude and latitude) of the event (disease case, typically) and t the time of occurrence. We assume an ordering $t_1 < t_2 < \ldots < t_n$, and that the study region is defined by the study area $\mathcal{A}$ and the surveillance timer interval $(0, \mathcal{T}]$.

One starting point to analyze such data is to adapt a purely temporal surveillance method to a spatio-temporal setting. Assunção and Correa (2009) do so by combining a non-homogeneous Poisson point process partially observed on $\mathcal{A} \times (0, \mathcal{T}]$ with the Shirayev-Roberts (SR) statistic (Shirayev, 1963; Roberts, 1966; Kennet and Pollak, 1996), using the martingale property of the latter to establish a protocol for achieving a desired ARL with minimal parameter input by the user. Aside from the ARL, the user needs to specify a radius ρ defining the maximum spatial extent of the outbreak cluster, as well as a parameter $\epsilon > 0$, which measures the relative change in the density within the outbreak cluster as compared to the non-outbreak situation. The SR statistic in the Assunção and Correa (2009) formulation then is defined as

$$R_n = \sum_{k=1}^n \Lambda_{k,n}, \text{where} \tag{21.13}$$

$$\Lambda_{k,n} = (1 + \epsilon)^{N(Y_{k,n})} I_{Y_{k,n}}(x_y, y_i, t_i) \exp\left(-\epsilon\mu(Y_{k,n})\right). \tag{21.14}$$

Here, $Y_{k,n}$ is the cylinder defined by the ball of radius ρ centered on the location of the kth event and the time interval $(t_k, t_n]$ between the kth and the nth event, $N(Y_{k,n})$ is the number of events inside that cylinder, $\mu(Y_{k,n})$ is the expected number of events inside the cylinder if there is no space-time clustering, and $I_{Y_{k,n}}$ is an indicator taking the value 1 if the kth event is inside $Y_{k,n}$ and 0 otherwise. The outbreak signal goes off if R_n is larger than the specified ARL, and the outbreak cluster is identified as the cylinder $Y_{k,n}$ for which $\Lambda_{k,n}$ is maximized. The quantity $\mu(Y_{k,n})$ requires the specification of two densities related to the intensity function of the process, but since this is too much to ask from the user, $\mu(Y_{k,n})$ is instead replaced by the estimate

$$\hat{\mu}(Y_{k,n}) = \frac{N\left(B(s_k, \rho) \times (0, t_n]\right) \cdot N\left(\mathcal{A} \times (t_k, t_n]\right)}{n}, \qquad (21.15)$$

the product of the number of events within the disk $B(s_k, \rho)$, regardless of time of occurrence, and the number of events that occurred in the time interval $(t_k, t_n]$ anywhere within the whole study region, divided by the total number of events. Every new incoming event thus requires the re-calculation of all terms in equation (21.13), which Assunção and Correa (2009) demonstrate can be done in an efficient iterative procedure.

The method of Assunção and Correa (2009) was later extended by Veloso et al. (2013) to handle the detection of multiple space-time clusters. This detection is accomplished by (randomly) deleting excess events inside the detected clusters and re-running the method with a new ARL threshold corrected for the event deletion.

There also have been attempts to adapt retrospective methods for detection of space-time point event clusters to a prospective setting. For example, Rogerson (2001) formulate a local version of the (retrospective) Knox statistic (Knox, 1964) and combine it with a CUSUM framework to make the method suitable for prospective surveillance. However, Marshall et al. (2007) later concluded that it is certainly not suitable, owing to a number of factors that strongly influence the performance of the method, and which a user has little power to regulate properly. A remedy is offered by Piroutek et al. (2014), who redefine the local Knox statistic by Rogerson (2001) to be prospective rather than retrospective. For a given observation indexed by i, the local Knox statistic $n_{st}(i)$ is defined as the number of observations that are closer than t units of time to t_i, and whose coordinates are less than a distance s away from (x_i, y_i). In Rogerson (2001), the closeness in the temporal dimension is measured in both directions, so that a $n_{st}(i)$ counts nearby events before and *after* the ith event. This account of future events is included in the CUSUM chart, which is not appropriate. Piroutek et al. (2014) instead let only *past* events enter into the calculation of $n_{st}(i)$, which turns out to vastly improve the performance of the method in a prospective setting. As noted by Marshall et al. (2007), there are also problems with the normal distribution approximation made to the statistic calculated for the CUSUM chart. Namely, it can be very poor if the thresholds s and t are small, and this in turn makes it difficult to set the appropriate control limit to achieve a given ARL. Piroutek et al. (2014) instead propose to use a randomization procedure using past data to establish the correct control limit, obviating the need of an approximate distribution.

Paiva et al. (2015) later combine the modified local Knox statistic by Piroutek et al. (2014) with the Cumulative Surface method proposed by Simões and Assunção (2005), allowing for a visualization of clusters in three dimensions. In their method, the local Knox score of each event is smeared using a bivariate Gaussian kernel function, and a threshold for detection is defined through the distribution of the stochastic surfaces formed. In all, the method requires few parameters as input from users, and needs no information of the population at risk.

21.3.2.2.1   Illustration of the Assunção and Correa Shirayev-Roberts statistic

We now illustrate the method by Assunção and Correa (2009) on the meningococcal data (finetype B only) considered previously, however this time using the coordinates and time stamps of each event rather than an aggregated count. The method is implemented as the function stcd in the R package surveillance (Salmon et al., 2016c). As a validation of the method, we run the analysis for approximately the same period as Reinhardt et al. (2008), anticipating that the results will be similar. We guide our choice of the parameter ρ required by this method by the analysis of the meningococcal data by Meyer et al. (2012); Figure 3 of this paper suggests that setting $\rho = 75$ kilometers (km) is adequate. For the choice of the parameter ϵ, which is the relative change of event-intensity within the to-be-detected cluster, we are guided by the simulation study by Assunção and Correa (2009) and set $\epsilon = 0.2$. Finally, we set the desired ARL to 30 days.

In Figure 21.7, the detected cluster is shown with all events up until the point of detection marked as triangles on the map. The cluster detected by the stcd function is centered on the city of Aachen in the state of North Rhine-Westphalia, which corresponds well to the cluster marked in Figure 3 of Reinhardt et al. (2008), and the dates also appear similar. The cluster was detected only 1 day after its estimated start date, showing the potential of the Assunção and Correa (2009) method in terms of timeliness. All in all, the ability to use the spatial and temporal attributes of each individual event for the detection of clusters is an attractive feature when greater exactness in the origins and spatial extent of outbreaks is important.

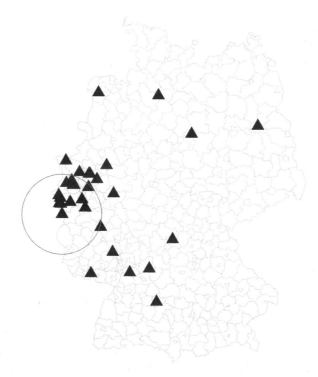

FIGURE 21.7
Detected cluster (gray circle) and observed disease events for the cluster detection method. (From Assunção, R. M. and Correa, T., *Comput. Stat. Data Anal.*, 53, 2817–2830, 2009.)

21.4 Summary and Outlook

This chapter presented temporal and spatio-temporal statistical methods for the prospective detection of outbreaks in routine surveillance data. Such data-driven algorithms operate at the intersection of statistical methodology, data mining, and computational (big) data crunching. Simple methods have their virtues and speed of implementation can be of importance; however, this reason should never be an excuse for ignoring statistical facts when counts get small and sparse—facts that might surprise the non-statisticians uncomfortable beyond the normal distribution.

Despite the many advances in the last 30 years, outbreak detection algorithms will never replace traditional epidemiological alertness. Nevertheless, they offer support for using the digital epidemiologist's time more effectively. From a systems perspective, however, it is our impression that detection algorithms have had limited impact on practical outbreak detection so far. One reason is that, historically, many algorithmic suggestions were not supported by accessible software implementations. Another reason is that their usefulness is questioned by the many false alarms and a misalignment between the users' needs and presentation of the alarms found by the system. Statisticians—as part of interdisciplinary teams—need to worry more about how to roll-out the proposed algorithms to the public health organizations. As a step in this direction, all presented detection methods of this chapter are readily available from open-source packages in R. Examples of software supporting national surveillance systems by increased user focus are the Swedish CASE system (Cakici et al., 2010) and the German avoid@RKI (Salmon et al., 2016a).

Acknowledgements

Benjamin Allévius was supported by grant 2013:05204 by the Swedish Research Council. Michael Höhle was supported by grant 2015-05182_VR by the Swedish Research Council.

References

Abrams, A. M., Kleinman, K., and Kulldorff, M. (2010). Gumbel based *p*-value approximations for spatial scan statistics. *International Journal of Health Geographics*, 9:61.

Allévius, B. (2017). scanstatistics: Space-time anomaly detection using scan statistics. R package version 1.0.0. *The Journal of Open Source Software*, 3(25):515.

Allévius, B. and Höhle, M. (2019). An unconditional space–time scan statistic for ZIP-distributed data. *Scandinavian Journal of Statistics*, 46(1):142–159.

Andersson, T., Bjelkmar, P., Hulth, A., Lindh, J., Stenmark, S., and Widerstrom, M. (2014). Syndromic surveillance for local outbreak detection and awareness: Evaluating outbreak signals of acute gastroenteritis in telephone triage, web-based queries and over-the-counter pharmacy sales. *Epidemiology & Infection*, 142(2):303–313.

Assunção, R. M., and Correa, T. (2009). Surveillance to detect emerging space-time clusters. *Computational Statistics and Data Analysis*, 53(8):2817–2830.

Burkom, H. S. (2003). Biosurveillance applying scan statistics with multiple, disparate data sources. *Journal of Urban Health : Bulletin of the New York Academy of Medicine*, 80 (2, Supplement 1):i57–i65.

Cakici, B., Hebing, K., Grünewald, M., Saretok, P., and Hulth, A. (2010). Case: A framework for computer supported outbreak detection. *BMC Medical Informatics and Decision Making*, 10:14.

Cançado, A. L. F., Da-Silva, C. Q., and da Silva, M. F. (2014). A spatial scan statistic for zero-inflated Poisson process. *Environmental and Ecological Statistics*, 21(4):627–650.

Cançado, A. L. F., Fernandes, L. B., and Da-Silva, C. Q. (2017). A Bayesian spatial scan statistic for zero-inflated count data. *Spatial Statistics*, 20:57–75.

Correa, T., Assunção, R. M., and Costa, M. A. (2015a). A critical look at prospective surveillance using a scan statistic. *Statistics in Medicine*, 34(7):1081–1093.

Correa, T., Assunção, R. M., and Costa, M. A. (2015b). Response to commentary on A critical look at prospective surveillance using a scan statistic. *Statistics in Medicine*, 34(7):1096.

Crosier, R. B. (1988). American society for quality multivariate generalizations of cumulative sum quality-control schemes multivariate generalizations of cumulative Sum quality-control schemes. *Technometrics*, 30(3):291–303.

Duczmal, L. H., and Assunção, R. M. (2004). A simulated annealing strategy for the detection of arbitrarily shaped spatial clusters. *Computational Statistics and Data Analysis*, 45(2):269–286.

Farrington, C., and Andrews, N. (2003). Outbreak detection: Application to infectious disease surveillance. In Brookmeyer, R., and Stroup, D., eds., *Monitoring the Health of Populations*, chapter 8, p. 203–231. New York: Oxford University Press.

Farrington, C., Andrews, N., Beale, A., and Catchpole, M. (1996). A statistical algorithm for the early detection of outbreaks of infectious disease. *Journal of the Royal Statistical Society, Series A*, 159:547–563.

Fricker, R. D., Hegler, B. L., and Dunfee, D. A. (2008). Comparing syndromic surveillance detection methods: EARS versus a CUSUM-based methodology. *Statistics in Medicine*, 27(17):3407–3429.

Frisén, M. (1992). Evaluations of methods for statistical surveillance. *Statistics in Medicine*, 11(11):1489–1502.

Frisén, M. (2003). Statistical surveillance. Optimality and methods. *International Statistical Review*, 71(2):403–434.

Frisén, M., Andersson, E., and Schiöler, L. (2010). Evaluation of multivariate surveillance. *Journal of Applied Statistics*, 37(12):2089–2100.

Han, S. W., Tsui, K. L., Ariyajuny, B., and Kim, S. B. (2010). A comparison of CUSUM, EWMA, and temporal scan statistics for detection of increases in poisson rates. *Quality and Reliability Engineering International*, 26(3):279–289.

Höhle, M. (2016). Infectious disease modelling. In Lawson, A. B., Banerjee, S., Haining, R. P., and Ugarte, M. D., eds., *Handbook of Spatial Epidemiology*, chapter 26, p. 467–490. Boca Raton, FL: Chapman and Hall/CRC, 1st edition.

Höhle, M. (2017). A statistician's perspective on digital epidemiology. *Life Sciences, Society and Policy*, 13:17.

Höhle, M., and Mazick, A. (2011). Aberration detection in R illustrated by Danish mortality monitoring. In Kass-Hout, T. and Zhang, X., eds., *Biosurveillance: A Health Protection Priority*, p. 215–238. Boca Raton, FL: CRC Press.

Höhle, M., Paul, M., and Held, L. (2009). Statistical approaches to the monitoring and surveillance of infectious diseases for veterinary public health. *Preventive Veterinary Medicine*, 91(1):2–10.

Hotelling, H. (1947). Multivariate quality control, illustrated by the air testing of sample bombsights. In Eisenhart, C., Hastay, M. W., and Wallis, W. A., eds., *Techniques of Statistical Analysis*, Chapter 3, p. 111–184. New York: McGraw-Hill, 1st edition.

Joner, M. D., Woodall, W. H., and Reynolds, M. R. (2008). Detecting a rate increase using a Bernoulli scan statistic. *Statistics in Medicine*, 27(14):2555–2575.

Kennet, R. S., and Pollak, M. (1996). Data-analytic aspects of the shiryayevroberts control chart: Surveillance of a non-homogeneos poisson process. *Journal of Applied Statistics*, 1(23):125–138.

Knox, E. G. (1964). The detection of space-time interactions. *Applied Statistics*, 13(1):25.

Kulldorff, M. (1997). A spatial scan statistic. *Communications in Statistics—Theory and Methods*, 26(6):1481–1496.

Kulldorff, M. (2001). Prospective time periodic geographical disease surveillance using a scan statistic. *Journal of the Royal Statistical Society Series a-Statistics in Society*, 164:61–72.

Kulldorff, M. (2016). Satscan^{TM}. https://www.satscan.org. Accessed November 10, 2017.

Kulldorff, M., Heffernan, R., Hartman, J., Assunção, R. M., and Mostashari, F. (2005). A space-time permutation scan statistic for disease outbreak detection. *PLoS Medicine*, 2(3):0216–0224.

Kulldorff, M., and Kleinman, K. (2015). Comments on 'A critical look at prospective surveillance using a scan statistic by T. Correa, M. Costa, and R. Assunção. *Statistics in Medicine*, 34(7):1094–1095.

Kulldorff, M., Mostashari, F., Duczmal, L. H., Yih, K., Kleinman, K., and Platt, R. (2007). Multivariate scan statistics for disease surveillance. *Statistics in Medicine*, 26(8): 1824–1833.

Kulldorff, M., and Nagarwalla, N. (1995). Spatial disease clusters: Detection and inference. *Statistics in Medicine*, 14(8):799–810.

Lawson, A. B., and Kleinman, K. (2005). *Spatial and Syndromic Surveillance for Public Health*. Hoboken, NJ: Wiley.

Le Strat, Y. (2005). Overview of temporal surveillance. In Lawson, A. and Kleinman, K., eds., *Spatial and Syndromic Surveillance for Public Health*, Chapter 3, p. 31–52. Hoboken, NJ: Wiley.

Marshall, B. J., Spitzner, D. J., and Woodall, W. H. (2007). Use of the local Knox statistic for the prospective monitoring of disease occurrences in space and time. *Statistics in Medicine*, 26(7):1579–1593.

McCullagh, P. and Nelder, J. A. (1989). *Generalized Linear Models*. London, UK: Chapman and Hall/CRC Press, 2nd edition.

Meyer, S., Elias, J., and Höhle, M. (2012). A space-time conditional intensity model for invasive meningococcal disease occurrence. *Biometrics*, 68(2):607–616.

Meyer, S., Held, L., and Höhle, M. (2017). Spatio-temporal analysis of epidemic phenomena using the R package surveillance. Also available as vignettes of the R package surveillance. *Journal of Statistical Software*, 77:1–55.

Montgomery, D. C. (2008). *Introduction to Statistical Quality Control*. New York: Wiley, 6th edition.

Naus, J. I. (1965). The distribution of the size of the maximum cluster of points on a line. *Journal of the American Statistical Association*, 60(310):532–538.

Neill, D. B. (2006). Detection of spatial and spatio-temporal clusters. Ph.D. thesis, Carnegie Mellon University.

Neill, D. B. (2009a). An empirical comparison of spatial scan statistics for outbreak detection. *International Journal of Health Geographics*, 8:20.

Neill, D. B. (2009b). Expectation-based scan statistics for monitoring spatial time series data. *International Journal of Forecasting*, 25(3):498–517.

Neill, D. B. (2011). Fast Bayesian scan statistics for multivariate event detection and visualization. *Statistics in Medicine*, 30(5):455–469.

Neill, D. B. (2012). Fast subset scan for spatial pattern detection. *Journal of the Royal Statistical Society. Series B: Statistical Methodology*, 74(2):337–360.

Neill, D. B., and Cooper, G. F. (2010). A multivariate Bayesian scan statistic for early event detection and characterization. *Machine Learning*, 79(3):261–282.

Neill, D. B., McFowland III, E., and Zheng, H. (2013). Fast Subset Scan for multivariate event detection. *Statistics in Medicine*, 32(13):2185–2208.

Neill, D. B., Moore, A. W., and Cooper, G. F. (2006). A Bayesian spatial scan statistic. *Advances in Neural Information Processing Systems*, 18:1003.

Neill, D. B., Moore, A. W., Sabhnani, M., and Daniel, K. (2005). Detection of emerging space-time clusters. In *Proceeding of the Eleventh ACM SIGKDD International Conference on Knowledge Discovery in Data Mining—KDD '05*, p. 218. New York: Association for Computing Machinery.

Noufaily, A., Enki, D. G., Farrington, P., Garthwait, P., Andrews, N., and Charlett, A. (2013). An improved algorithm for outbreak detection in multiple surveillance systems. *Statistics in Medicine*, 32(7):1206–1222.

O'Brien, P. C. (1984). Procedures for comparing samples with multiple endpoints. *Biometrics*, 40(2):1079–1087.

Page, E. S. (1954). Procedures for comparing samples with multiple endpoints. *Biometrica*, 41(1/2):100–115.

Paiva, T., Assunção, R. M., and Simões, T. (2015). Prospective space-time surveillance with cumulative surfaces for geographical identification of the emerging cluster. *Computational Statistics*, 30(2):419–440.

Piroutek, A., Assunção, R. M., and Paiva, T. (2014). Space-time prospective surveillance based on Knox local statistics. *Statistics in Medicine*, 33(16):2758–2773.

Reinhardt, M., Elias, J., Albert, J., Frosch, M., Harmsen, D., and Vogel, U. (2008). EpiScanGIS: An online geographic surveillance system for meningococcal disease. *International Journal of Health Geographics*, 7:33.

Rencher, A. C., and Christensen, W. F. (2012). *Methods of Multivariate Analysis*. Wiley Series in Probability and Statistics. Hoboken, NJ: John Wiley & Sons.

Roberts, S. W. (1966). On the detection of disorder in a manufacturing process. *Technometrics*, 3(8):411–430.

Rogerson, P., and Yamada, I. (2008). *Statistical Detection and Surveillance of Geographic Clusters*. Boca Raton, FL: Chapman and Hall/CRC Press.

Rogerson, P. A. (1997). Surveillance systems for monitoring the development of spatial patterns. *Statistics in Medicine*, 16(18):2081–2093.

Rogerson, P. A. (2001). Monitoring point patterns for the development of space-time clusters. *Journal of the Royal Statistical Society: Series A (Statistics in Society)*, 164(1): 87–96.

Rogerson, P. A., and Yamada, I. (2004). Monitoring change in spatial patterns of disease: Comparing univariate and multivariate cumulative sum approaches. *Statistics in Medicine*, 23(14):2195–2214.

Salmon, M., Schumacher, D., Burman, H., Frank, C., Claus, H., and Höhle, M. (2016a). A system for automated outbreak detection of communicable diseases in Germany. *Eurosurveillance*, 21(13):pii=3018.

Salmon, M., Schumacher, D., and Höhle, M. (2016b). Monitoring count time series in R: Aberration detection in public health surveillance. *Journal of Statistical Software*, 70(10):1–35. Also available as vignette of the R package surveillance.

Salmon, M., Schumacher, D., and Höhle, M. (2016c). Monitoring count time series in R: Aberration detection in public health surveillance. *Journal of Statistical Software*, 70(1):1–35.

Shirayev, A. N. (1963). On the detection of disorder in a manufacturing process. *Theory of Probability and its Applications*, 3(8):247–265.

Simões, T., and Assunção, R. M. (2005). Geoinfo 2005—VII simpósio brasileiro de geoinformática. In *Sistema de vigilância para detecção de interações espaço-tempo de eventos pontuais*, p. 281–291. Instituto Nacional de Pesquisas Espaciais (INPE).

Sonesson, C., and Bock, D. (2003). A review and discussion of prospective statistical surveillance in public health. *Journal of the Royal Statistical Society. Series A: Statistics in Society*, 166(1):5–21.

Sonesson, C. and Frisén, M. (2005). Multivariate surveillance. In *Spatial and Syndromic Surveillance for Public Health*, vol. 3, p. 153–166. Hoboken, NJ: John Wiley & Sons.

Stroup, D., Williamson, G., Herndon, J., and Karon, J. (1989). Detection of aberrations in the occurrence of notifiable diseases surveillance data. *Statistics in Medicine*, 8:323–329.

Tango, T. (1995). A class of tests for detecting "general" and "focused" clustering of rare diseases. *Statistics in Medicine*, 14(21–22):2323–2334.

Tango, T. (2016). On the recent debate on the space-time scan statistic for prospective surveillance. *Statistics in Medicine*, 35(11):1927–1928.

Tango, T., and Takahashi, K. (2005). A flexibly shaped spatial scan statistic for detecting clusters. *International Journal of Health Geographics*, 4(11):15.

Tango, T., Takahashi, K., and Kohriyama, K. (2011). A space-time scan statistic for detecting emerging outbreaks. *Biometrics*, 67(1):106–115.

Unkel, S., Farrington, C. P., Garthwaite, P. H., Robertson, C., and Andrews, N. (2012). Statistical methods for the prospective detection of infectious disease outbreaks: A review. *Journal of the Royal Statistical Society: Series A (Statistics in Society)*, 175(1):49–82.

Veloso, B., Iabrudi, A., and Correa, T. (2013). Towards efficient prospective detection of multiple spatio-temporal clusters. In *Proceedings of the Brazilian Symposium on GeoInformatics*, p. 61–72. São Paulo, Brazil: MCT/INPE (Ministry of Science and Technology/ National Institute for Space Research).

Wagner, M. M., Moore, A. W., and Aryel, R. M. (2006). *Handbook of Biosurveillance*. Boston, MA: Academic Press.

Wong, W.-K., Moore, A. W., Cooper, G. F., and Wagner, M. (2005). What's strange about recent events (WSARE): An algorithm for the early detection of disease outbreaks. *Journal of Machine Learning Research*, 6:1961–1998.

Wood, S. (2006). *Generalized Additive Models: An Introduction with R*. Boca Raton, FL: Chapman & Hall/CRC Press.

Woodall, W. H. (2006). The use of control charts in health-care and public-health surveillance. *Journal of Quality Technology*, 38(2):89–104.

22

Underreporting and Reporting Delays

Angela Noufaily

CONTENTS

22.1 Underreporting

22.1.1 Introduction

Surveillance data are an important tool in public health since they can point to population health issues and give relevant authorities the opportunity to take control measures. Using such data, disease incidences are tracked over time to detect unexpected events or important cases. However, this process often is hindered due to underreporting. Underreporting involves events that have not been reported in a timely fashion for use in surveillance. It includes events that might never be reported but also can include late reports. Reporting sources include clinicians, laboratories, hospitals, and other health care providers who send data at regular intervals of time (daily, weekly, monthly, yearly, or other), depending on the use of data, to health care entities within states or countries. These entities are generally the principle informant on epidemiological figures.

In the USA, the Center for Disease Control (CDC) monitors people's health and collects data on infectious disease from different health sources. Each state in the USA also has its own surveillance department which is run according to the state's procedures. In the UK, Public Health England plays this role and has local units in several areas. UK syndromic data, for example, is received on a daily basis from systems such as the 7-days a week general practitioner in-hours syndromic system (GPIHSS), the 5-days a week general practitioner out-of-hours syndromic system (GPOOHSS), and National Health Service (NHS) 111. Infectious disease data in the UK is, however, lab-based and generally received on a weekly basis. Santé Publique France is the French national public health agency monitoring the country's health along with regional departments while Folkhälsomyndigheten is the public health agency of Sweden and the Robert Koch Institute is Germany's public health hub for surveillance of diseases. These units aim to receive data at the earliest possible time to sway public health decisions.

To understand underreporting and delays in reporting, it is important to understand the underlying process of disease epidemiology that can be described by what is known as a surveillance pyramid, which includes the different stages of the reporting chain. This pyramid has as its base "exposure of a population to a certain infection" moving up to "appearance of symptoms," "seeking primary care," "specimen collection," "laboratory tests," "laboratory case confirmation and subtyping," and at the very top "reporting to surveillance units" (Míkanatha et al., 2013). Underreporting can happen at any of those stages at the level of the patient, clinician, laboratory, or health care body, and reasons for underreporting are diverse. Clinician-based factors frequently arise due to reasons including practitioners' misinformation on the most important diseases, relying on laboratories to report, and ethical matters. Laboratory-based factors include lost cases, testing mistakes, and time for subtyping. The new generation of infectious disease surveillance is heading towards genome sequencing for some organisms and this can happen at the cost of longer delays. Patient-based factors (known as underascertainment) can be due to healthcare costs, minor symptoms, health misinformation, geographical absence of healthcare, and lack of confidence in healthcare suppliers. Finally, department-based underreporting can be due to typing mistakes and staff holidays.

Underreporting and reporting delays in infectious disease surveillance can differ between organisms for reasons related to data aspects such as volume, time, trend, and seasonality. Laboratories across the UK send weekly counts of more than 3000 organisms to Public Health England, and each of the organisms reflect these aspects differently, possibly influencing the delay distribution. Figure 22.1, for example, shows the *Salmonella infantis* and rotavirus weekly counts (from 1991 till 2011) analyzed in Noufaily et al. (2013). *Salmonella infantis* is of low volume and has an annual moderate seasonality with no apparent trend while rotavirus is of high volume and has a very sharp annual seasonality with a slightly increasing trend.

Noufaily et al. (2015) investigated how these factors can influence delays. This investigation was done by analyzing the delay between specimen collection and reporting of 12 representative organisms. Throughout this chapter, we will use the *Salmonella infantis* datasets for counts and delays analyzed in Noufaily et al. (2015) to demonstrate some of the important ideas. Figure 22.1 shows a histogram of the delay distribution of *Salmonella infantis* from 2004 to 2011. It is obvious that most delays range between 0 and 6 months. However, the delay distribution has a heavy right tail and delays can reach more than 1.5 years (573 days, for accuracy). Even longer delays might have existed but it is suggested that some laboratories stop reporting after a certain time. Often, infections are reported

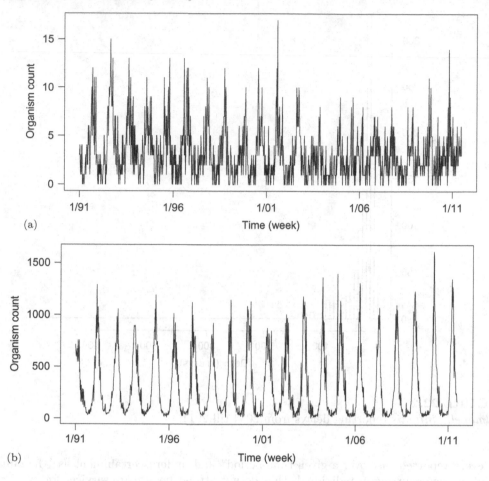

FIGURE 22.1
Salmonella infantis (a) and rotavirus (b) weekly counts from 1991 to 2011.

but after a very long period after the infections, which makes the report somehow irrelevant for action to be taken. For example, the delays of more than 6 months (or possibly even less) seen in Figures 22.1 and 22.2 could be considered as underreported cases. This section investigates cases of underreporting and provides a review of on methods used and obtained results.

22.1.2 Underreporting, underascertainment, and underestimation

Underreporting is particularly common in infectious disease due to the variability of the infection process and the different stages a patient goes through before the final reporting of the incident. Underreporting can be confused with two other situations known as underascertainment and underestimation. Underestimation is the phenomenon in which surveillance data does not reflect reality due to incompleteness. Underascertainment is the phenomenon in which underestimated cases are patient- or community-related. Therefore, underreporting may be assumed as the healthcare-related underestimation. Along those lines, Gibbons et al. (2014) define underreporting as "the number of infections estimated to have occurred in a population that have not been captured by the surveillance system

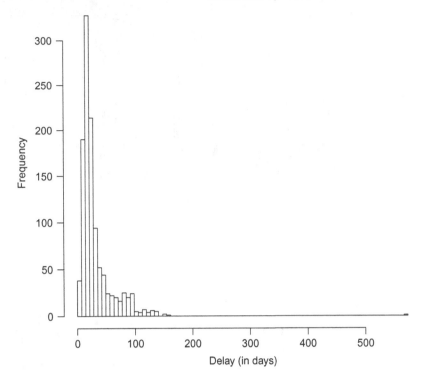

FIGURE 22.2
Salmonella infantis reporting delays from 2004 till 2011.

for every reported case over a given time period" and underascertainment as "the number of infections occurring in individuals that do not attend healthcare services for every case that attends."

22.1.3 Multiplication factors

It is crucial to know the degree of underestimation of surveillance data to account for missing observations and obtain the right picture on the gravity of each disease. Correction methods commonly estimate what is known as "multiplication factors" that compare reported data with reality. In general, multiplication factors should take into account underreporting and underascertainment. In order for correction to be accurate, it also should be geographical- and disease-specific as well as age- and gender-dependent.

In addition, multiplication factors should take into account underreported cases that are either a result of (1) a very long delay or (2) an infinite delay (i.e., cases that will never be reported). Within each case, underreporting occurs as a result of several reasons with different frequencies and hence different weights. Multiplication factors should take into account these weights, which usually can be estimated by performing further investigations such as population surveys. For example, the *Salmonella infantis* delays in in Figure 22.1 have, on average, a reporting delay of 4 weeks and about 90 percent of the cases are reported within 10 weeks. Reports after 10 weeks can lie in the category of underreporting. For the purpose of demonstration, multiplication factors might, for example, weight such reports with very long delays, for example, by 40 percent of the total underreported, and the remaining cases that might never be reported by 60 percent.

22.1.4 Estimation of multiplication factors and correction for underestimation

Several studies have used multiplicative factors for estimation of underreporting for a range of infectious diseases (Bernard et al., 2014; Rosenberg et al., 1977). Undurraga et al. (2013) perform a systematic analysis on the use of such expansion factors to predict the implication of dengue in Southeast Asia. Based on Gibbons et al. (2014), we identify and explain some of the methods for estimating multiplicative factors.

22.1.4.1 Capture-recapture studies

Capture-recapture studies are inspired by studies on wildlife, where animals can be captured more than once and information on the same animal registered a multiple of times. In this case, the main issue is overreporting but a similar logic can be applied for underreporting. These studies are performed in human surveillance in order to identify duplicates so they can be removed for completeness (Hest et al., 2002).

22.1.4.2 Community-based studies

Community-based studies are surveys performed at the level of the people (Grilc and Sočan, 2014) to obtain a clearer idea on the commonness of infectious diseases in the community, in contrast with the reported cases at healthcare departments. The surveys basically trickle down to the very root or starting point of infections, skipping the whole process of reporting from patient to primary care, laboratories, and reporting units. Community-based studies include: (1) population-based studies, (2) serological surveys, and (3) returning travelers studies. These are explained in what follows.

22.1.4.2.1 Population-based surveys

Population-based surveys either follow a cohort of individuals over time or select a random sample of people to identify possible diseases. Health questionnaires are prepared and addressed, in general, to a representative random sample within the population to form an idea on the community's health situation. In practice, surveys are performed by getting in touch with people in the community either by telephone, mail, or internet and questioning them about their health. Serological information can accompany the questionnaires too.

The biggest challenge in such studies is the choice of a representative sample. Therefore, the representative sample are subject to selection bias. For example, certain age groups, ethnicities, socio-economic statuses, or occupations can be missed for several reasons. Measurement bias also can exist since such studies are subject to human error. The media also plays a big role in diverting people's views and introducing bias especially when the situation involves an outbreak. Such studies also rely on modern technology (telephones, internet, and computers) that may incur bias due to the misuse of such tools as well as their lack of availability in certain cases. All these factors might cause biases and hence inaccuracies in results. Given that they involve studies on a large quantity of people, population-based surveys can be time consuming and expensive.

22.1.4.2.2 Serological surveys

Serological surveys are useful mostly when investigating diseases that require vaccination or when looking at the health effects of vaccines. They can inform the level of immunity of a population. They usually involve taking a sample of serum from a representative sample of the population.

Serological surveys are generally accurate as they involve scientific laboratory tests; however, they are subject to bias due to the fact that some vaccines might be hard to detect in serum or can be confused with the natural organism.

22.1.4.2.3 Returning traveler studies

Returning traveler studies compare counts of infected people in a certain populations of travelers to the total counts of this infection in their country of main residence. The aim is to identify the number of infected travelers who were not registered in health departments and to compensate for underreporting. Underreporting is common in travelers since their medical records can be mixed up between countries.

As previously, records for returning travelers can be biased. It is difficult enough to track infections within one country. Records from across borders can be an even more challenging task due to differences in procedures and lack of reporting from abroad.

22.1.4.3 Modeling

Mathematical and statistical methods, applied to simulations or real data, are used to estimate incidence and predict underestimation occurring at several steps of the reporting chain. The predicted estimates then can be used to generate multiplication factors. Several models exist and use different approaches such as catalytic models, decision tree models, probability models, pyramid reconstruction models, Bayesian models, simulation models, and shared component models. Designing representative and consistent models can be challenging since they should take into consideration disease-specific features. For best results, more than one approach can be used, analyzed, and compared.

22.1.4.3.1 Catalytic models

Catalytic models are inspired by chemical reactions whose rates are speeded by the use of a catalyst. The catalyst in our context is the conditions that allow a certain infection to develop and spread at a certain rate. Knowing this rate and the conditions around it allows estimation of the proportion of underreporting. Muench (1959) described the simplest model that can explain infectious disease data as one that should contain one constant representing the rate at which the disease is acquired and one representing the rate at which it is lost. Muench (1959) constructed a catalytic model that fits upon bilharziasis transmission rates. Most existing catalytic models considered for explaining disease paths are deterministic. Presently, it is advised to expand deterministic models to include random factors. More recent probability models introduce an error term that explains natural phenomenon more realistically as will be seen in what follows.

22.1.4.3.2 Probability models

Probability models are often used in epidemiology since they account for uncertainty, by considering nonparametric or parametric probability distributions to explain the randomness that can happen in nature. Parametric models often involve using the negative binomial or Poisson distributions, especially when dealing with discrete counts. Non-parametric models generally use splines or kernels without implying any distributional assumptions. Generalized linear models (GLMs) are an example of probability models used often in infectious disease surveillance.

22.1.4.3.3 Decision tree models

Decision tree models and algorithms (Tanner et al., 2008; Tucker et al., 2008), as the name indicates, are based on a tree-like diagram branching into several events, all linked by a base. They often are used in data mining to represent complex data situations and offer a logical and graphical way to view disease paths and stages. Graphical representations often are clear and easy to interpret. Corrections for underreporting can be considered at each of the different branches and within different levels of the branches.

22.1.4.3.4 Pyramid reconstruction models

Similarly to decision tree models, pyramid reconstruction models (Haagsma et al., 2013; Kumagaia et al., 2015) consider disease-specific corrections at different levels of the surveillance pyramid. Starting at the bottom of the surveillance pyramid, this approach considers the amount of underreporting that may happen, for example, between emergence of symptoms and primary care visits, etc. Corrections at different levels then can be put together for a full picture.

22.1.4.3.5 Bayesian models

Bayesian models have become more and more popular in infectious disease epidemiology (Fernández-Fontelo et al., 2016; Gamado et al., 2013; Yang et al., 2015). Advantages of Bayesian analyses are that they can accommodate a wide range of models; however, they can be computationally complex and time consuming. In the context of modeling underreporting, estimates of infection incidence at several steps of the surveillance pyramid are crucial and Bayesian methods provide a platform that can explain these linked complex situations.

22.1.4.3.6 Simulation models

Simulation models (Rutter et al., 2011), use computer-simulated data based on real-life infections, to assess underreporting. Simulation modeling is increasing and is frequently used currently in epidemiology to explain events and validate methods. The advantage of using simulations is that the underlying model is known. In addition, multiple simulations (as many as necessary) can be generated to obtain more accurate results. Disadvantages include the fact that mistakes can happen while attempting to mimic real-life examples and so producing representative simulations is necessary.

22.1.4.3.7 Shared-component models

Shared-component models, as the name indicates, aim to estimate common elements, ideally to all diseases, explaining the variation in underreporting. Knorr-Held and Best (2001) proposed a model for two diseases. This model was extended for more than two diseases by Held et al. (2005).

22.2 Reporting Delays

22.2.1 Introduction

This section concerns delays that may occur in infectious disease reporting within a certain time limit where they can still be relevant to surveillance. Crucial dates in infectious disease emergence to reporting, as indicated by the surveillance pyramid, include exposure date, date of symptom onset, date of strain isolation, data of reception at public health body, and date of report. Delays in epidemiology generally refer to the time between the moment of infection and the emergence of symptoms, or what is known as the incubation period. Although other delays are also of interest such as the delay that typically occurs between

TABLE 22.1

Isolate counts with start date i (rows) and delay j (columns). Row totals are in the final column

Start date i	delay j							
	$j = 0$	$j = 1$	$j = 2$	$j = 3$	$j = 4$	$j = 5$	...	Total
$i = 1$	$n_{1,0}$	$n_{1,1}$	$n_{1,2}$	$n_{1,3}$	$n_{1,4}$	$n_{1,5}$	...	N_1
$i = 2$	$n_{2,0}$	$n_{2,1}$	$n_{2,2}$	$n_{2,3}$	$n_{2,4}$	$n_{2,5}$	...	N_2
$i = 3$	$n_{3,0}$	$n_{3,1}$	$n_{3,2}$	$n_{3,3}$	$n_{3,4}$	$n_{3,5}$	...	N_3
$i = 4$	$n_{4,0}$	$n_{4,1}$	$n_{4,2}$	$n_{4,3}$	$n_{4,4}$	$n_{4,5}$	...	N_4
$i = 5$	$n_{5,0}$	$n_{5,1}$	$n_{5,2}$	$n_{5,3}$	$n_{5,4}$	$n_{5,5}$	...	N_5
$i = 6$	$n_{6,0}$	$n_{6,1}$	$n_{6,2}$	$n_{6,3}$	$n_{6,4}$	$n_{6,5}$	...	N_6
...				...			...	
$i = M$	$n_{M,0}$	$n_{M,1}$	$n_{M,2}$	$n_{M,3}$	$n_{M,4}$	$n_{M,5}$	...	N_M

the date a specimen is taken in the laboratory and the date it is reported to public health bodies. Reporting delays are also common in other non-infectious disease areas such as cancer registries, death registries, and actuarial sciences. As a matter of fact, delays have been studied over time since at least the late 1960s (Starwell, 1966). The most common analysis of delays is in the area of acquired immunodeficiency syndrome (AIDS). The dangers of this disease and the importance of its timely detection caused the analysis of reporting delays to be more popular and urged more research in this area. Based on Noufaily et al. (2015), in what follows, we introduce some notations that will be used in this section to describe delays and some of the underlying models.

Notations

- d: delay between start date and end date.
- n_{id}: isolates count with start date i and end date $i + d$.
- $N_{id} = \sum_{k=0}^{d} n_{ik}$: isolates count between start date i and end date $i + d$.
- N_i: total isolates count with start date i.

Table 22.1 summarizes counts subject to delay in the reporting process using the given notations. Rows correspond to start dates and columns correspond to the delay that may occur. The total isolate count with start date i is in the final row. Table 22.1 will be referred to for explaining the different procedures used to tackle delays.

22.2.2 Factors affecting reporting delays

As mentioned in the introduction, delays are affected by several factors. Jones et al. (2014) and others investigated these factors of which we include patient age and gender, laboratory category (private or hospital), seasonality, specimen type (urine, blood, etc.), incidence (low, medium, or high), level of subtyping, time (within the week, month, year, or decade), and geographical location. In their study on salmonella delays in France, Jones et al. (2014) found that most of these factors were significantly associated with delays except for seasonality and day of week effects which seemed to vary randomly. Cui and Kaldor (1998) studied such effects within AIDS cases in Australia and found that delays varied significantly with geographical location and time but no general association was found with age and gender. Noufaily et al. (2015) performed a more general study on the delay distribution by looking at a variety of population-representative organisms and simulations.

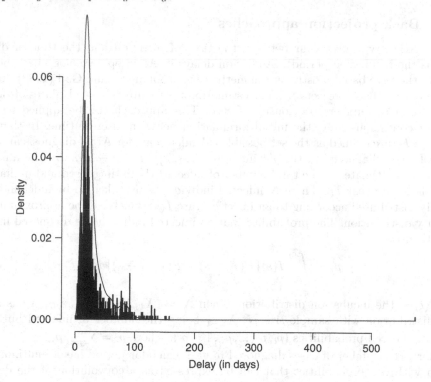

FIGURE 22.3
Time-spline-based model of Noufaily et al. (2015) fitted to the *Salmonella infantis* delays
from 2004 till 2011.

They fitted a continuous time-spline-based model for the hazard of the delay distribution
along with a proportional hazards model to study the effects of time, season, and incidence.
Figure 22.3 shows this model fitted to the *Salmonella infantis* dataset. The model indicated a strong association between delays and time, although season and incidence had less
influence.

22.2.3 Reporting delays in Acquired Immunodeficiency Syndrome epidemiology

In many developed countries, AIDS is considered as one of the main causes of death in
people less than 45 years old (Gebhardt et al., 1998). This problem can get aggravated
when delays in identifying AIDS cases happen. The sooner a syndrome is identified the
quicker measures can be taken to avoid early complications. One of the biggest issues lies in
the fact that the human immunodeficiency virus (HIV) can stay dormant in an individual
for years before it exhibits itself in AIDS. In effect, months or even years can pass by before
AIDS cases are reported. According to Harris (1990), approximately 91,000 AIDS cases
out of the actual 130,000 in March 1989 were reported by that time in the USA. It also is
known that reporting delays are getting longer with time and the actual AIDS incidence
is generally increasing. Given the severity of the disease and the importance of its timely
control, several methods have been introduced in the literature to model the AIDS delay
distribution and incidence. These approaches take into consideration stationary delays and
some are extended to non-stationary delays.

22.2.4   Back-projection approaches

Delays in AIDS typically occur between the time of infection and the time of diagnosis (known as the incubation period). Studies on delays in AIDS epidemiology have been proposed and they are based mostly on the method by Brookmeyer and Gail (1988), known as the technique of "back-projection." The estimation procedure "back-calculates" from AIDS incidence data to numbers previously infected. This approach can be applied to data in discrete or continuous time, the initial formulation being in discrete time. In that framework, $T_0, .., T_L$ are defined as the set possible calender years for AIDS diagnosis and X_j the number of cases diagnosed in the jth interval $[T_{j-1}, T_j]$, $j = j - 1, ..., L$. The aim of this approach is to estimate N, the total number of infected (both diagnosed and undiagnosed) individuals before year T_L. These N infected individuals are taken to be independent and identically distributed according to an infection rate $I(s)$ which can be approximated by a probability distribution. The probability that an infected individual is diagnosed in the jth interval then is

$$p_j = \int_{T_0}^{T_j} I(s)\{F(T_j - s) - F(T_{j-1} - s)\}ds$$

where $F(t)$ is the incubation distribution. Then $X = (X_1, X_2, ..., X_L, X_{L+1})$ has a multinomial distribution with sample size N, X_{L+1} being the number of infected but not yet diagnosed, and cell probabilities $(p_l, p_2, ..., p_L, 1 - p.)$, where $p. = \sum_{j=1}^{L} p_j..$

In short, the number of cases diagnosed in each calendar period has a multinomial distribution with cell probabilities that can be expressed as a convolution of the density of infection times and the incubation distribution. A simple expectation-maximization (EM) algorithm is developed for obtaining maximum likelihood estimates of the size of a multinomial when $I(s)$ is parameterized as a step function. This model has been used and extended in Kalbfleisch and Lawless (1989) and Brookmeyer and Liao (1990).

Kalbfleisch and Lawless (1989) use GLMs to estimate the delay distribution, considering problems of estimation when initiating events occur as a nonhomogeneous Poisson process. A simple form for the likelihood function is obtained and methods of parametric and non-parametric estimation are developed and considered. Regression models also are considered as well as various generalizations of the basic problem. An important practical implication of Kalbfleisch and Lawless (1989) is that it is possible to fit regression models to right-truncated data by using standard computing software for GLMs. Deuffic and Costagliola (1999) also test if a change in incubation time (shortening or lengthening) was observed in France, either globally or in specific transmission groups, using a back-calculation approach. The EM algorithm was used to maximize the likelihood and the best model was selected using the likelihood ratio statistic.

22.2.5   Non-stationary delays

Methods have been formulated to account for delay changes over time. Lawless (1994) model stationary delays but also extend their approach considering a Dirichlet distribution to incorporate random effects for reporting delay distributions that exhibit non-stationary features. Bacchetti (1996) examine the variation in delay according to length of survival after diagnosis. Gebhardt et al. (1998) use a Bayesian GLM on reverse-time hazards to model time trends of the reporting delay distribution and deduce that delays often change (increase or decrease) with time. Cui and Kaldor (1998) and Noufaily et al. (2015) also suggest the use of non-stationary delay distributions to estimate delay data. Generally, it is concluded by most studies that delays cannot be considered stationary and that models should take into account the change of delay distributions over time.

22.2.6   Bayesian estimation methods

Bayesian approaches to model the delay distribution include Markov chain Monte Carlo (MCMC) methods (Höhle and an der Heiden, 2014), approximate Bayesian computation methods (McKinley et al., 2009), and sequential Monte Carlo methods (Ionides et al., 2006). Zeger et al., (1989) propose a Bayesian approach to estimate infectious disease incidence in subgroups, particularly seven risk groups, including AIDS subgroups with modest frequencies. O'Neill et al. (2000) introduce a Bayesian non-parametric method using Gaussian processes to estimate the incidence.

22.2.7   Reporting delays for outbreak detection

Outbreak detection is one of the major aims of infectious disease surveillance. Databases based on reported cases to national public health bodies are arguably the most reliable source for detecting outbreaks in infectious disease surveillance since such data concern laboratory-confirmed cases from different geographical areas. However, such data is subject to reporting delays. A better source for surveillance would be data based on specimen dates, since these also regard confirmed cases but have the advantage of happening at an earlier date, hence being more timely. The disadvantage, though, of such data is that recent counts are incomplete since cases by date of specimen are only known after they are reported. Recent cases whose specimen have been taken but have not been reported yet are not known to public health bodies and thus do not contribute to their databases. Data can hence be seen as received in two forms, one by date of report and another by date of specimen. The delays of interest in this section are the ones resulting from the time elapsed between the date of specimen and the date of report. Based on that, referring to Table 22.1, the start dates i would represent dates of specimen. For example, the current date is $i = 5$, then the cases reported on that date are cases whose specimen was taken at $i = 5$ and reported during the same week, in addition to those whose specimen was taken on $i = 4$ and reported after 1 week and so on; basically, the sum of the diagonal elements $n_{5,0}$, $n_{4,1}$, $n_{3,2}$, $n_{2,3}$, etc. Counts by date of specimen below that diagonal (with a maximum of $i = 5$) are not known yet even though their specimen has been taken. Thus, we say that data above the diagonal (i.e., the upper triangle) are known but the lower triangle is to be estimated in order to complete the counts by date of specimen. Consequently, if $i = 5$ is the current week, then $n_{5,0}$ is the only count known by date of specimen and the remaining counts by date of specimen on row $i = 5$ are to be estimated to complete the picture. Figure 22.4 shows the *Salmonella infantis* dataset with counts based on dates of report as well as counts based on dates of specimen.

Marinovič et al. (2015) attempted to measure the required reduction level in reporting delays which can significantly enhance outbreak detection by monitoring organism proportions until reporting. Methods are required, however, to integrate such knowledge in automated algorithms for outbreak detection. Salmon et al. (2015) and Noufaily et al. (2016) are the two primary attempts known to the author that incorporate reporting delays in outbreak detection algorithms. To use counts by date of specimen, it is essential to complete the missing values in the reporting triangle. Noufaily et al. (2016) attempt this completion by referring to past observations and following a similar pattern for current observations. Salmon et al. (2015) use a Bayesian approach to model this pattern. Both approaches are inspired by the GLM-based modeling framework proposed by Farrington et al. (1996) and extended in Noufaily et al. (2013), but differ in inference methodology for how the predictive distribution is found, as will be described in what follows.

Noufaily et al. (2013) fit a quasi-Poisson regression-based model to weekly organism counts by date of report, with mean μ_i and variance $\phi\mu_i$ at week i. To estimate the current week, the model is fit to the most recent years (usually 5 years) and includes a linear trend

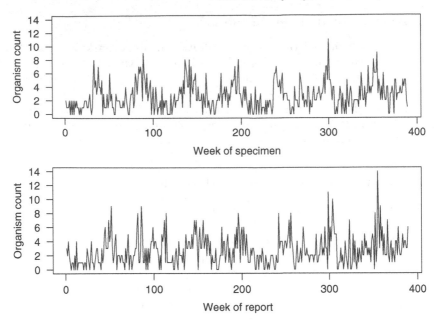

FIGURE 22.4
Salmonella infantis data by week of specimen (top) and week of report (bottom) from 2004 to 2011.

as well as a yearly 10-level factor whose reference period comprises comparable weeks in previous years. The corresponding log-linear model is

$$\log \mu_i = \theta + \beta t_i + \delta_{j(t_i)}, \tag{22.1}$$

where $j(t_i)$ is the seasonal factor level for week t_i, with $j(t_0) = 0$ and $\delta_0 = 0$. In this model, a trend is always fitted except for some special cases where data is very sparse.

A particular week is flagged as being a possible outbreak based on the value of what is known as the exceedance score

$$X = \frac{y_0 - \hat{\mu}_0}{U - \hat{\mu}_0},$$

where y_0 is the current observed count and $\hat{\mu}_0 = \exp\{\hat{\theta} + \hat{\beta} t_0 + \delta_{j(t_0)}\}$ is the current expected count, $\hat{\theta}$ and $\hat{\beta}$ being the estimates of θ and β, respectively. U, the upper threshold, is the $100(1-\alpha)\%$ quantile of a negative binomial distribution with mean μ and dispersion parameter ϕ; α being the type I error. Another suggested approach to compute U uses the 2/3 power transformation of the Poisson distribution that is approximately normal. An alarm is flagged for organism weeks where $X \geq 1$. The exceedance score is conditioned to 0 for particular cases that represent certain data sparsity.

This algorithm is implemented in R Foundation for Statistical Computing (2017) and is available via the function `farringtonFlexible` within the package `surveillance` (Salmon et al., 2016).

22.2.7.1 Bayesian outbreak detection algorithm in the presence of reporting delays

This algorithm is based on the approach by Salmon et al. (2015). It extends the regression model from Noufaily et al. (2013) represented by equation (22.1) to incorporate the delay distribution and then estimate the model using a Bayesian approach based on Manitz and Höhle (2013), using integrated nested Laplace approximation (INLA; Rue et al., 2009). In this sense, estimates of the delay distribution are subject to the necessary uncertainty that results from model fitting. Similarly to the multinomial representation given in Brookmeyer and Gail (1988), for a given week $i = t$, this approach considers $(n_{i,0}, n_{i,1}, ..., n_{i,j})|N_i, \mathbf{p}$ as being multinomial $M(N_i, \mathbf{p})$ with size N_i and probabilities p_i, $(i, j) \in \Omega$, where Ω only contains indices for occurred and reported $n_{i,j}$ at time t. N_i is taken as coming from a negative binomial $NB(\mu_i, \nu)$, with mean μ_i and variance $\mu_i(1 + \mu_i)/\nu$. Then from Schmidt and Wünsche (1998), $n_{i,j} \sim NB(\mu_i p_j, \nu)$ and using Bayes rule, we have

$$f(\psi|n_\Omega) \propto f(n_\Omega|\psi)\pi(\psi),$$

where $f(n_\Omega|\psi)$ is the product of independent negative binomial distributions and $\pi(\psi)$ is the prior, chosen and discussed as in Manitz and Höhle (2013); ψ being the vector of parameters for the covariates.

Two methods were proposed to estimate the posterior: a fully Bayesian procedure using INLA and a better-adaptable approach using an asymptotic normal approximation.

This approach, therefore, tests whether a given week t is a possible outbreak by running the algorithm on what is referred to as "observation" weeks, falling after week t. The most reasonable observation weeks would be weeks t to $t + c$ where c is the maximum reasonable delay for a particular organism. The algorithm was tested by simulation revealing that it detects outbreaks earlier without inflating the type I error. However, the procedure can be cumbersome and not very practical for universal use since the same alarm could be flagged more than once.

Weeks $t = 286$ to 385 (100 weeks) of the *Salmonella infantis* counts by week of specimen were tested for possible alarms using observation weeks t to $t + 4$ for $\alpha = 0.01$ and $b = 4$ (the number of weeks back of the Noufaily et al. [2013] algorithm). No alarms were triggered.

The algorithm corresponding to this approach is implemented in R Foundation for Statistical Computing (2017) and is available via the function `BodaDelay` within the package `surveillance` (Salmon et al., 2016).

22.2.7.2 Regression-based outbreak detection algorithm in the presence of reporting delays

This algorithm is based on the approach by Noufaily et al. (2016). It implements the algorithm in Noufaily et al. (2013) to weekly isolate counts by date of specimen. Informed by the results in Noufaily et al. (2015), only all isolates with delay less than 26 weeks are considered and, for those, the number of specimens in the current and past m weeks are monitored. The big picture is that the delay distribution is estimated using recent data and then used to rescale current expected counts to match the incomplete data by date of specimen. Assuming the current week is t, the delay distribution is calculated using

$$\hat{p}_j = \left(\sum_M^{t-26} n_{ij} + \frac{\epsilon}{26} \right) \bigg/ \left(\sum_M^{t-26} N_i + \epsilon \right); \ \epsilon = \frac{1}{2}$$

where M is the minimum week before $(t - 26)$ for which the sum of N_i for i between M and $(t - 26)$ is at least 100. The algorithm then is as follows:

- Choose a value for m that is close enough to the average delay. Monitoring m "current" weeks (rather than just one) seems crucial when incomplete data is concerned as this reduces the variability in the model. This inflicts though another type of bias.

- Compute the observed isolate count (by specimen date): the total number of isolates with specimen date in the "current" and m previous weeks.

- Estimate the expected counts (by specimen date) for the "current" and m previous weeks using the regression-based approach from Noufaily et al. (2013). For demonstration, if week 389 is the "current" week and $m = 4$, the algorithm should be run for "current" weeks 389, 388, 387, 386, and 385, and the respective expected counts $\hat{\mu}_{389}$, $\hat{\mu}_{388}$, $\hat{\mu}_{387}$, $\hat{\mu}_{386}$, and $\hat{\mu}_{385}$ computed.

- Reweight the expected counts using the computed probabilities of the delay distribution. The combined "current" expected value y_{389} is then $\hat{\nu}_{389} = \hat{\mu}_{389}\hat{f}_0 + \hat{\mu}_{388}\hat{f}_1 + \hat{\mu}_{387}\hat{f}_2 + \hat{\mu}_{386}\hat{f}_3 + \hat{\mu}_{385}\hat{f}_4$, where $\hat{f}_j = \hat{p}_0 + \hat{p}_1 + ... + \hat{p}_j$.

- Compute the test statistic $T^* = y_{389}^{2/3} - \hat{\nu}_{389}^{2/3}$.

- An alarm is triggered if the exceedance score X^* exceeds 1:

$$X^* = \frac{T^*}{U - \hat{\nu}_{389}^{2/3}}. \tag{22.2}$$

This is an approach that can be run universally on organisms with different characteristics. The delay distribution is computed in a simple way, although uncertainty in estimating the delay distribution is not incorporated. Also, a value for m should be pre-specified and is organism- and delay-dependent.

Figure 22.5 shows an application to the *Salmonella infantis* data (excluding the most recent 26 weeks, since before that, data is considered complete) of both the new algorithm with reporting delays (Noufaily et al., 2016) and the standard algorithm (Noufaily et al., 2013).

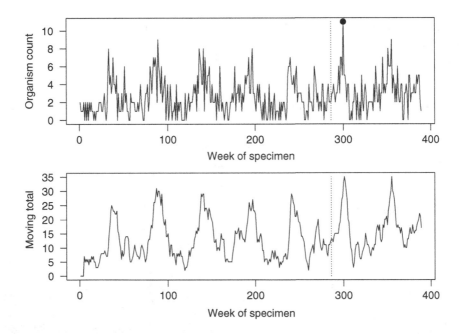

FIGURE 22.5

Salmonella infantis: Time series of organism counts (full lines) and weeks flagged (dots) using the standard algorithm by week of specimen (top) and the new algorithm by week of specimen with $m = 4$ (bottom). The algorithms were applied to the 104 weeks to the right of the vertical dotted line.

The algorithms are applied to the most recent 2 years (weeks 286 to 389) of the *Salmonella infantis* counts by week of specimen (excluding the most recent 26 weeks) for $\alpha = 0.01$ and $b = 4$ (the number of weeks back of the Noufaily et al., 2013 algorithm). The new algorithm – using dates of specimen and $m = 4$ – detects no aberrances, whereas the standard one, using dates of report, detects one. One-week spikes might not be identified by the new algorithm since they are smoothed while using m-week totals. The new algorithm would more probably identify slow moderate rises in organism counts.

22.3 Discussion

This chapter presented some of the most important factors contributing to underreporting and reporting delays, as well as methods used to deal with these issues and results. Underreporting mainly involves incidents that happened but had not been reported or had been reported very late to be useful. Various techniques that tackle underreporting consider incompleteness at every stage of the surveillance chain, starting from the very root of the infections (i.e. from the population itself), by running population surveys. Reporting delays concern data that happened and was reported within a reasonable delay. Early studies on reporting delays have been in the area of AIDS. Two recent promising studies, one Bayesian and another regression-based, incorporate reporting delays in infectious disease outbreak detection algorithms. The Bayesian study explained in Salmon et al. (2015) estimates the delay distribution while incorporating the necessary uncertainty that results from statistical modeling, but is somehow cumbersome to implement in real life. The regression-based algorithm explained in Noufaily et al. (2013) estimates the delay distribution using knowledge from past data, but is more easily applicable in real life. Both algorithms, however, seem to have a reasonable power of detection but such a measure as well as specificity, sensitivity, and false positive rate should be investigated further.

Acknowledgments

Data is from Public Health England's registries for infectious disease surveillance. Help from Dr Maëlle Salmon in implementing the R function `BodaDelay` along with additional comments from Dr Michael Höhle are very much appreciated.

References

Bacchetti, P. (1996). Reporting delays of deaths with aids in the united states. *Journal of Acquired Immune Deficiency Syndromes and Human Retrovirology*, 13:363–367.

Bernard, H., Werber, D., and Höhle, M. (2014). Estimating the under-reporting of norovirus illness in Germany utilizing enhanced awareness of diarrhoea during a large outbreak of Shiga toxin-producing E. coli O104:H4 in 2011 a time series analysis. *BMC Infectious Diseases*, 14:116–121.

Brookmeyer, R., and Gail, M. H. (1988). A method for obtaining short-term projections and lower bounds on the size of the AIDS epidemic. *Journal of the American Statistical Association*, 83:301–308.

Brookmeyer, R., and Liao, J. (1990). The analysis of delays in disease reporting: Methods and results for the acquired immunodeficiency syndrome. *American Journal of Epidemiology*, 132:355–365.

Cui, J., and Kaldor, J. (1998). Changing pattern of delays in reporting AIDS diagnoses in Australia. *Australian and New Zealand Journal of Public Health*, 22:432–435.

Deuffic, S., and Costagliola, D. (1999). Is the AIDS incubation time changing? A back-calculation approach. *Statistics in Medicine*, 18:1031–1047.

Farrington, C. P., Andrews, N. J., Beale, A. D., and Catchpole, M. A. (1996). A statistical algorithm for the early detection of outbreaks of infectious disease. *Journal of the Royal Statistical Society Series A*, 159:547–563.

Fernández-Fontelo, A., Cabaña, A., Puig, P., and Moriña, D. (2016). Under-reported data analysis with INAR-hidden Markov chains. *Statistics in Medicine*, 35:4875–4890.

Gamado, K. M., Streftaris, G., and Zachary, S. (2013). Modelling under-reporting in epidemics. *Journal of Mathematical Biology*, 69:737–765.

Gebhardt, M. D., Neuenschwander, B. E., and Zwahlen, M. (1998). Adjusting AIDS incidence for non-stationary reporting delays: A necessity for country comparisons. *European Journal of Epidemiology*, 14:595–603.

Gibbons, C. L., Mangen, M. J., Plass, D., Havelaar, A. H., Brooke, R. J., Kramarz, P., Peterson, K. L. et al. (2014). Measuring underreporting and under-ascertainment in infectious disease datasets: A comparison of methods. *Journal of the Royal Statistical Society Series A*, 159:147–164.

Grilc, E., and Sočan, M. (2014). Using surveillance data to monitor trends in the AIDS epidemic. *Slovenian Journal of Public Health*, 53:125–132.

Haagsma, J. A., Geenen, P. L., Ethelberg, S., Fetsch, A., Hansdotters, F., Jansen, A., Korsgaard, H. et al. (2013). Community incidence of pathogen-specific gastroenteritis: Reconstructing the surveillance pyramid for seven pathogens in seven European Union member states. *Epidemiology and Infection*, 141:1625–1639.

Harris, J. E. (1990). Reporting delays and the incidence of AIDS. *Journal of the American Statistical Association*, 85:915–924.

Held, L., Natario, I., Fenton, S. E., Rue, H., and Becker, N. (2005). Towards joint disease mapping. *Statistical Methods in Medical Research*, 14:61–82.

Hest, N. A. H. V., Smit, F., and Verhave, J. P. (2002). Underreporting of malaria incidence in the Netherlands: Results from a capturerecapture study. *Epidemiology and Infection*, 129:371–377.

Höhle, M., and an der Heiden, M. (2014). Bayesian nowcasting during the STEC O104:H4 outbreak in Germany, 2011. *Biometrics*, 70:993–1002.

Ionides, E. L., Breto, C., and Yip, A. A. (2006). Inference for non-linear dynamical systems. *Proceedings of the National Academy of Sciences*, 103(49):18438–18443.

Jones, G., Hello, S. L., da Silva, N. J., Vaillant, V., de Valk, H., Weill, F. X., and Strat, Y. L. (2014). The french human salmonella surveillance system: Evaluation of timeliness of laboratory reporting and factors associated with delays, 2007 to 2011. *Eurosurveillance, Surveillance and Outbreak Reports*, 19(1):206–264.

Kalbfleisch, J. D., and Lawless, J. F. (1989). Inference based on retrospective ascertainment: An analysis of the data on transfusion-related AIDS. *Journal of the Royal Statistical Society, Series A*, 84:360–372.

Knorr-Held, L., and Best, N. A. (2001). A shared component model for detecting joint and selective clustering of two diseases. *Journal of the Royal Statistical Society, Series A*, 164:73–85.

Kumagaia, Y., Gilmourb, S., Otac, E., Momosed, Y., Onishie, T., Bilanob, V. L. F., Kasugad, F., Sekizakif, T., and Shibuyab, K. (2015). Estimating the burden of foodborne diseases in Japan. *Bulletin of the World Health Organization*, 93:540–549.

Lawless, J. F. (1994). Adjustments for reporting delays and the prediction of occurred but not reported events. *Canadian Journal of Statistics*, 22:15–31.

Manitz, J., and Höhle, M. (2013). Bayesian outbreak detection algorithm for monitoring reported cases of campylobacteriosis in Germany. *Biometrical Journal*, 55:509–526.

Marinovič, A. B., Swaan, C., van Steenbergen, J., and Kretzschmar, M. (2015). Quantifying reporting timeliness to improve outbreak control. *Emerging Infectious Diseases*, 21:209–216.

McKinley, T., Cook, A. R., and Deardon, R. (2009). Inference in epidemic models without likelihoods. *The International Journal of Biostatistics*, 5(1). Article 24.

Míkanatha, N. M., Lynfield, R., Beneden, C. A. V., and de Valk, H. (2013). *Infectious Disease Surveillance, 2nd ed.* Chichester, UK: Wiley-Blackwell.

Muench, H. (1959). *Catalytic Models in Epidemiology*. Cambridge, MA: Harvard University Press.

Noufaily, A., Enki, D. G., Farrington, C. P., Garthwaite, P., Andrews, N., and Charlett, A. (2013). An improved algorithm for outbreak detection in multiple surveillance systems. *Statistics in Medicine*, 32:1206–1222.

Noufaily, A., Farrington, C. P., Garthwaite, P., Enki, D. G., Andrews, N., and Charlett, A. (2016). Detection of infectious disease outbreaks from laboratory data with reporting delays. *Journal of the American Statistical Association, Applications and Case Studies*, 111:488–499.

Noufaily, A., Weldeselassie, Y. G., Enki, D. G., Garthwaite, P., Andrews, N., Charlett, A., and Farrington, C. P. (2015). Modeling reporting delays for outbreak detection in infectious disease data. *Journal of the Royal Statistical Society, Series A*, 178:205–222.

O'Neill, P. D., Balding, D. J., Becker, N. G., Eerola, M., and Mollison, D. (2000). Analyses of infectious disease data from household outbreaks by markov chain monte carlo methods. *Journal of the Royal Statistical Society Series C*, 49:517–542.

R (2017). *Development Core Team. R: A language for and environment for statistical computing*. R Foundation for Statistical Computing, Vienna, Austria.

Rosenberg, M. L., Marr, J. S., Gangarosa, E. J., Robert, A. P., Wallace, M., Brolnitsky, O., and Marr, J. S. (1977). Shigella surveillance in the United States, 1975. *The Journal of Infectious Diseases*, 136:458–460.

Rue, H., Martino, S., and Chopin, N. (2009). Approximate Bayesian inference for latent Gaussian models by using integrated nested Laplace approximations (with discussion). *Journal of the Royal Statistical Society: Series B (Statistical Methodology)*, 71:319–392.

Rutter, C. M., Knudsen, A. B., and Pandharipande, P. V. (2011). Computer disease simulation models: Integrating evidence for health policy. *Academic Radiology*, 18:1077–1086.

Salmon, M., Schumacher, D., and Höhle, M. (2016). Monitoring count time series in R: Aberration detection in public health surveillance. *Journal of Statistical Software*, 70(10):1–35.

Salmon, M., Schumacher, D., Stark, K., and Höhle, M. (2015). Bayesian outbreak detection in the presence of reporting delays. *Biometrical Journal*, 57:1–17.

Schmidt, K. D., and Wünsche, A. (1998). Chain ladder, marginal sum and maximum likelihood estimation. *Blätter der Deutschen Gesellschaft für Versicherungs und Finanz Mathematik*, 23:267–277.

Starwell, P. E. (1966). The incubation period and the dynamics of infectious disease. *American Journal of Epidemiology*, 175:49–82.

Tanner, L., Schreiber, M., Low, J. G. H., Ong, A., Tolfvenstam, T., Lai, Y. L., Ng, L. C. et al. (2008). Decision tree algorithms predict the diagnosis and outcome of dengue fever in the early phase of illness. *PLoS Neglected Tropical Diseases*, 2:e196.

Tucker, A. W., Haddix, A. C., Bresee, J. S., Holman, R. C., Parashar, U. D., and Glass, R. I. (2008). Cost-effectiveness analysis of a rotavirus immunization program for the United States. *Journal of the American Mathematical Association*, 279:1371–1376.

Undurraga, E. A., Halasa, Y. A., and Shepard, D. S. (2013). Use of expansion factors to estimate the burden of dengue in Southeast Asia: A systematic analysis. *Statistics in Medicine*, 7(2):e2056.

Yang, W., Lipsitch, M., and Shamana, J. (2015). Inference of seasonal and pandemic influenza transmission dynamics. *Proceedings of the National Academy of Sciences of the United States of America*, 112:2723–2728.

Zeger, S. L., See, L. C., and Diggle, P. J. (1989). Statistical methods for monitoring the AIDS epidemic. *Statistics in Medicine*, 8:3–21.

23

Spatio-Temporal Analysis of Surveillance Data

Jon Wakefield, Tracy Qi Dong, and Vladimir N. Minin

CONTENTS

23.1 Introduction

The surveillance of disease statistics is now routinely carried out at the national and sub-national level. For example, in the USA, the Centers for Disease Control and Prevention (CDC) has a National Notifiable Disease Surveillance System (NNDSS) to which case notifications for more than 70 infectious disease are sent from all states. At a more local level, surveillance systems also are implemented by state public health departments.

There are many uses for a surveillance system. Early detection of outbreaks is clearly important to quickly assign resources to minimize the disease burden and hopefully determine the cause(s) of the outbreak. Various approaches, with varying degrees of sophistication, are available. Often, no formal statistical methods are used, but rather astute public health workers notice increased counts. A simple approach is to analyze each area separately and to compare newly collected data with the historic numbers of cases [31]. A more refined approach is to use a scan statistic. For example, Greene et al. [21], describe how the New York City Department of Health and Mental Hygiene carry out automated daily spatio-temporal cluster detection using the SatScan software and discuss the action taken in response to several outbreaks including three common bacterial-caused infections that lead to diarrhea: shigellosis, legionellosis, and campylobacteriosis. This approach does not acknowledge that spread of an infectious disease under examination has complex nonlinear dynamics. The models we describe in this chapter generally have not been used for outbreak detection, but could be, if trained on retrospective data.

Prediction of future disease counts will clearly be of interest in some situations and for this purpose a model that is not built around an infectious process may be adequate. If there is interest in predictions under different scenarios, for example, following different vaccination strategies, then a biologically motivated model is likely to be more useful than a model without a strong link to the underlying science. The same is true of another aim, which is to gain an understanding of disease dynamics, including estimation of fundamental parameters such as R_0.

In a time series only situation in which space is not considered, a number of authors have discussed integer-valued autoregressive (INAR) models in the context of modeling infectious disease data [7, 14, 18]. The epidemic/endemic models [22], which we discuss extensively in this chapter, are closely related to integer-valued generalized autoregressive conditionally heteroscedastic (INGARCH) models that also have been used for modeling infectious data [13, 51]. Since these approaches do not consider spatial modeling, we do not consider them further (although we note that there is no reason that they could not be extended to include a spatial component).

In a surveillance setting the following data are typically available: demographic information on each case (e.g., age and gender), symptom onset date, date of diagnosis, clinical information (e.g., symptoms), laboratory information on virology (perhaps on a subset of cases), and areal (ecological) geographical information. These data usually are supplemented with population information at the areal level. We emphasize that we will be concerned with the usual form in which the data are available, which is *incidence counts*, that is, new cases of disease (as opposed to *prevalence data*, which constitute the total counts).

We structure this chapter as follows. In Section 23.2, we review disease transmission models with brief descriptions of deterministic approaches, discrete time, and continuous time models. Section 23.3 introduces a measles data example, and Section 23.4 describes in detail discrete space-time models. We return to the measles data in Section 23.5 and conclude with a discussion in Section 23.6. On-line materials contain code to reproduce all analyses.

23.2   Overview of Disease Transmission Models

23.2.1   Deterministic models

Historically [28], infectious disease data were analyzed using deterministic models based on differential equations (see Anderson and May [1] for a thorough discussion). As an example, we consider the susceptible-infectious-recovered (SIR) model, which is depicted in Figure 23.1. Models are set up based on a set of compartments in which individuals undergo homogenous mixing. This approach typically is used when the number of disease counts is large, and the integer numbers in the constituent S, I, and R compartments are taken to be continuous. Let $x(t)$, $y(t)$, $z(t)$ be the number of susceptibles, infectives, recovered at time t in a closed population. The *hazard rate (force of infection)* is

$$\underbrace{\lambda^\dagger(t)}_{\text{Hazard}} = \underbrace{c(N)}_{\text{Contact Rate}} \times \underbrace{\frac{y(t)}{N}}_{\text{Prevalence}} \times \underbrace{p_I}_{\text{Infection Prob}} .$$

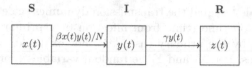

FIGURE 23.1
Susceptible-Infectious-Recovered (SIR) model representation. Solid arrows show the movement from S to I to R.

Two common forms for the contact rate [4] are

$$c(N) = \begin{cases} c_{\mathrm{FD}} & \text{Frequency Dependent,} \\ N c_{\mathrm{DD}} & \text{Density Dependent.} \end{cases}$$

The frequency-dependent model often is used, particularly for childhood infections when the most relevant contact group is the classroom, whose size will be of the same order, regardless of the population size. Under frequency dependency, $\lambda^{\dagger}(t) = \beta y(t)/N$, where $\beta = c_{\mathrm{FD}} \times p_{\mathrm{I}}$.

The deterministic SIR model is defined through classic *mass-action* [1]. With frequency dependent transmission, we have the following set of ordinary different equations:

$$\frac{dx(t)}{dt} = -\frac{\beta x(t) y(t)}{N},$$
$$\frac{dy(t)}{dt} = \frac{\beta x(t) y(t)}{N} - \gamma y(t),$$
$$\frac{dz(t)}{dt} = \gamma y(t),$$

with *infection rate* β and *recovery rate* γ.

To turn these equations into a statistical model there are two important considerations:

1. Given initial states, and values for the parameters β and γ, these differential equations can be solved to find the time trajectories of the three compartments. This solution must be done numerically, but can be achieved very efficiently, which means, in general, that complex compartmental models can be formulated, with the advantage that the transmission parameters are biologically interpretable.

2. More critically, the introduction of an artificial error model is needed. For example, we could assume additive errors with constant variance or a variance that depends on the mean, and then fitting can be performed in a straightforward fashion using ordinary, or weighted, least squares. The arbitrariness of the error model means that inference is dicey. Implicitly considering the inherent stochasticity directly is important for small populations and when the disease is rare. If ordinary least squares is used for fitting, the implicit assumption is of uncorrelated errors with constant variance, see for example [8]. Refined versions of least squares [26] also exist. The arbitrariness of the (implicit) error model is unlikely to result in reasonable uncertainty quantification for parameter estimation. For these reasons, we do not consider these models further here.

23.2.2 Discrete-time stochastic models

We will concentrate on discrete-time models and postpone an in-depth discussion of these models to Section 23.4. The basic idea is to model the current disease counts as a function of previous counts on a regular time scale. For a discrete-time stochastic SIR model we may choose the time scale to equal the transmission dynamics scale (latency plus infectious periods) or the generation time (time from infection of a primary case to infection of a secondary case infected by the primary case) [41]. For example, often, but not always, 2 weeks is used for measles. Let X_t and Y_t be random variables representing the number of susceptibles and infectives at time t, $t = 1, \ldots, T$. In the simplest case, the counts at t depend only on the counts at the previous time $t - 1$. Susceptibles may be reconstructed from, $X_t = X_{t-1} - Y_t$, assuming a closed population (we describe more complex susceptible reconstruction models in Section 23.4). The joint distribution of the counts is

$$\Pr(y_1, \ldots, y_T, x_1, \ldots, x_T | y_0) = \prod_{t=1}^{T} \Pr(y_t | y_{t-1}, x_{t-1}) \times \Pr(x_t | y_t, x_{t-1}),$$

where the second term is deterministic and we have suppressed the dependence on unknown parameters.

23.2.3   Continuous-time stochastic models

The most realistic approach is to build a model that considers infections and recoveries on a continuous time scale. We describe a continuous-time Markov chain for $\{X(t), Y(t), t \geq 0\}$ with frequency dependent transmission. The *transition probabilities* for a susceptible becoming infective and an infective becoming recovered are

$$\Pr\left(\begin{bmatrix} X(t + \Delta t) \\ Y(t + \Delta t) \end{bmatrix} = \begin{bmatrix} x - 1 \\ y + 1 \end{bmatrix} \middle| \begin{bmatrix} X(t) \\ Y(t) \end{bmatrix} = \begin{bmatrix} x \\ y \end{bmatrix}\right) = \frac{\beta x y}{N} \Delta t + o(\Delta t),$$

$$\Pr\left(\begin{bmatrix} X(t + \Delta t) \\ Y(t + \Delta t) \end{bmatrix} = \begin{bmatrix} x \\ y - 1 \end{bmatrix} \middle| \begin{bmatrix} X(t) \\ Y(t) \end{bmatrix} = \begin{bmatrix} x \\ y \end{bmatrix}\right) = \gamma y \Delta t + o(\Delta t),$$

where the remainder terms $o(\Delta t)$ satisfy $o(\Delta t)/\Delta t \to 0$ as $\Delta t \to 0$. From the standpoint of an infective, each can infect susceptibles in Δt with rate $\beta \Delta t x/N$, where x is the number of susceptibles at time t. From the standpoint of a susceptible, each can be infected in Δt with rate $\beta \Delta t y/N$, where y is the number of infectives at time t. This set-up leads to exponential times in each of the S and I compartments. Interpretable parameters are contained in this formulation, but unfortunately this approach is not extensively used as it quickly gets computationally hideous as the populations increase in size, which is the usual case with surveillance data (see the references in [16]). We do not consider these models further here.

23.3   Motivating Data

We analyze a simple measles dataset that has been extensively analyzed using the **hhh4** framework that we describe in Section 23.4.3. The analysis of these data is purely illustrative and for simplicity we do not use the vaccination information that is available with these data (though we do discuss how such data may be included in Section 23.4.5). We also analyze the data on a weekly time scale for consistency with previous analyses of these data using epidemic/endemic models [22, 38]. There is no demographic information on the cases and no information on births; looking at measles post-vaccination in the developed world is unlikely to yield any insight into transmission. Figure 23.2 shows 15 time series of counts in 15 districts (we exclude 2 areas that have 0 counts) and Figure 23.3 shows maps of total cases over 3-month intervals. We see great variability in the numbers of cases over time and area.

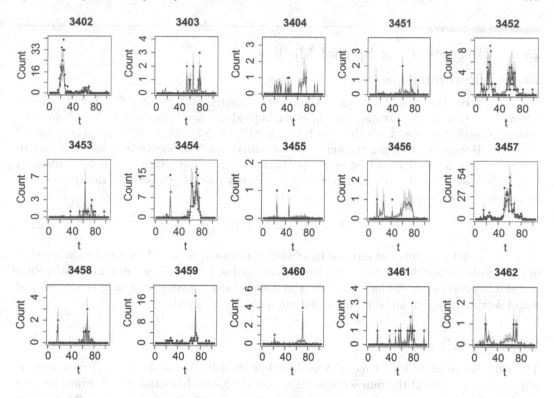

FIGURE 23.2
Observed (black dots) data in the 15 districts with non-zero counts and posterior summaries (2.5%, 50%, 97.5% quantiles) for μ_{it} under the time series SIR (TSIR) model.

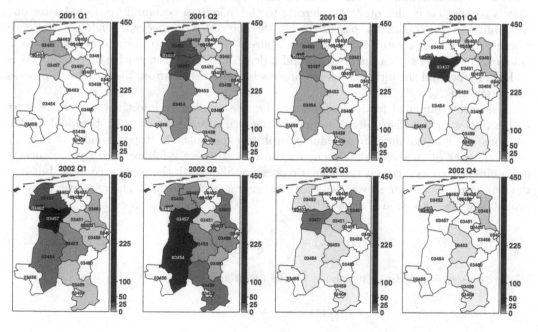

FIGURE 23.3
Average quarterly incidence by city district (per 100,000 inhabitants).

23.4   Discrete-Time Spatial Models

23.4.1   Preliminaries

We will derive the probability that a susceptible individual at time $t - 1$ will become infected by time t. We assume that infected individuals are infectious for one time unit before becoming removed, so that we have an SIR model with a fixed infectious period duration. Hence, we lose the recovery rate parameter and incidence is assumed equal to prevalence. All of the models that we discuss in this section assume that the force of infection is constant over the chosen time interval. A simple discrete-time model for the susceptibles in the context of measles [15] is

$$X_t = X_{t-1} - Y_t + B_{t-d}, \tag{23.1}$$

where B_{t-d} is the number of births d time units previously, with d chosen to be the number of time units for which maternally derived immunity lasts. There is no term for deaths since measles is primarily a childhood disease and deaths from measles are low in the developed world setting in which our data are collected, as is child mortality.

23.4.2   TSIR models

The time series SIR (TSIR) model was first described in [15], and has received considerable attention. The TSIR framework usually uses a negative binomial model, which we now carefully define, since there is some confusing terminology. To quote from [5] (with our own italics added), "Starting with I_t infected individuals, and assuming independence between them, the *birth-death process* will hence be realized according to a negative binomial distribution." In the following, we will consider a simple birth process. Perhaps the death process that is mentioned in this quote is referring to the infectives becoming recovered after one time unit. As [27] comments (page 236), "In the deterministic theory it made no difference whether the intrinsic rate of growth ν was purely reproductive in origin, or was really a balance, $\beta - \mu$, between a birth rate β and a death rate μ. In the stochastic theory this is no longer true, and the birth-and-death process is quite distinct from the pure birth process just described".

A negative binomial model is developed for the number of infectives and so we start with a review of this distribution. In one parameterization of the negative binomial model, the constant r is the number of failures until an experiment is stopped and $k = 0, 1, \ldots$ is the number of successes that occur on the way to these r failures, with p the success probability. It turns out that this scenario does not align with the present context, but it is the standard motivation, so we keep this language for a short while. The negative binomial probability mass function is defined by

$$\Pr(K = k) = \binom{k + r - 1}{k}(1 - p)^r p^k. \tag{23.2}$$

We write as $K \sim \text{NegBin}(\mu, r)$, and state the mean and variance,

$$\mathrm{E}(K) = \frac{rp}{1 - p} = \mu,$$

$$\mathrm{Var}(K) = \frac{rp}{(1 - p)^2} = \mu\left(1 + \frac{\mu}{r}\right).$$

Note that $p = \mu/(\mu + r)$. The overdispersion relative to the Poisson is indexed by r, with greater overdispersion corresponding to smaller r. The negative binomial can be formulated in a number of ways; the total number of trials $K^* = K + r$ may also be described as negatively binomially distributed with $K^* = r, r+1, r+2, \ldots$. We write, $K^* \sim \text{NegBin}^*(\mu^*, r)$, where $\mu^* = r + \mu = r/(1 - p)$.

Moving towards the context of interest, the negative binomial distribution arises as the distribution of the population size in a linear birth process (see, for example, Feller (1950, p. 448) and Cox and Miller (1965, p. 157)). We describe a linear birth process, also known as a Yule-Furry process. Individuals currently in the population each reproduce independently in $(t, t + \Delta t)$ with probability $\alpha \Delta t + o(\Delta t)$. Let $N(t)$ be the number of individuals at time t. Then,

$$\Pr(\text{ birth in } (t, t + \Delta t) \mid N(t) = n) = n\alpha\Delta t + o(\Delta t),$$

with the probability of two or more births being $o(\Delta t)$. Let

$$\Pr(N(t) = n \mid N(0) = n_0) = p_n(t).$$

From the Kolmogorov forward equations,

$$p_n(t + \Delta t) = p_n(t)(1 - n\alpha\Delta t) + p_{n-1}(t)(n - 1)\alpha\Delta t + o(\Delta t),$$

where the $n - 1$ appears in the second term on the right-hand side because any of the $n - 1$ individuals could give birth and each does so with probability α. Hence,

$$p_n'(t) = -n\alpha p_n(t) + (n - 1)\alpha p_{n-1}(t),$$

with $p_n(0) = 1$ for $n = n_0$ and $p_n(0) = 0$ for $n \neq n_0$. It then can be verified directly [12] or using probability generating functions [9] that for $n \geq n_0 > 0$:

$$p_n(t) = \Pr(N(t) = n) = \binom{n-1}{n-n_0} e^{-\alpha t n_0} \left(1 - e^{-\alpha t}\right)^{n-n_0}, \qquad (23.3)$$

with the probability p in (23.2) given by $p_t = 1 - e^{-\alpha t}$ and $N(t) \sim \text{NegBin}^*(\mu_t^*, n_0)$ with $\mu_t^* = n_0 e^{\alpha t}$. This result is also derived for $n_0 = 1$ by Kendall (1949, equation (17)). Note that the total number of trials $N(t)$ corresponds to $r + K$, which fits in with the total population size n (so there are $n - n_0$ births). We also can think of this model as starting with n_0 individuals, each of which independently produces a geometric number of progenies by time t; the probabilities are given by (23.3) with $n_0 = 1$.

Now let $M(t) = N(t) - n_0$ be the number of births since time 0. Then

$$\Pr(M(t) = n) = \binom{n + n_0 - 1}{n} e^{-\alpha t n_0} \left(1 - e^{-\alpha t}\right)^n, \qquad (23.4)$$

so $M(t) \sim \text{NegBin}(\mu_t, n_0)$, with

$$\mu_t = \text{E}(M(t)) = \frac{n_0 p_t}{1 - p_t} = n_0(e^{\alpha t} - 1),$$

and

$$\text{Var}(M(t)) = \frac{n_0 p_t}{(1-p_t)^2} = n_0(e^{2\alpha t} - e^{\alpha t}) = \mu_t\left(1 + \frac{\mu_t}{n_0}\right),$$

so that as $n_0 \to \infty$, we approach the Poisson distribution.

In the context of the SIR model, let y_{t-1} be the number of infectives at time $t-1$ and then assume that each gives rise to infectives with constant rate $x_{t-1}\beta/N$ over the interval $(t-1, t)$ (where we have assumed frequency dependent transmission). Note that the constant hazard is an approximation, because as a new infective appears in $(t-1, t)$ the number of susceptibles x_{t-1} will drop by 1. With respect to the linear birth process derivation, y_{t-1} is the "initial number".

We assume that the previous infecteds are all recovered. Then the total number of infectives is equal to the number of new infectives that are produced, Y_t, and is a negative binomial random variable, $\text{NegBin}(\mu_t, y_{t-1})$, with

$$\Pr(Y_t = y_t \mid Y_{t-1} = y_{t-1}) = \binom{y_t + y_{t-1} - 1}{y_t}\left(e^{-\beta x_{t-1}/N}\right)^{y_{t-1}}\left(1 - e^{-\beta x_{t-1}/N}\right)^{y_t}$$

and

$$E(Y_t \mid Y_{t-1} = y_{t-1}) = \mu_t = y_{t-1}\left(e^{x_{t-1}\beta/N} - 1\right),$$
$$\text{Var}(Y_t \mid Y_{t-1} = y_{t-1}) = \mu_t(1 + \mu_t/y_{t-1}).$$

The latter form is a little strange since the level of overdispersion is not estimated from the data. Note that as $y_{t-1} \to \infty$, the negative binomial tends to a Poisson. If $x_{t-1}\beta/N$ is small,

$$E(Y_t \mid Y_{t-1} = y_{t-1}) \approx y_{t-1}x_{t-1}\beta/N.$$

We now explicitly examine TSIR models, an umbrella term which includes a number of variants. First, note that the susceptibles often are modeled as (23.1), with correction for underreporting. We begin with a single area and the form

$$Y_t \mid Y_{t-1} = y_{t-1}, X_{t-1} = x_{t-1} \sim \text{NegBin}(\mu_t, y_{t-1}),$$

where

$$\mu_t = \beta y_{t-1}^{\alpha} x_{t-1}^{\gamma}/N.$$

The power γ is far less influential than the power α [32] and so in general the case $\gamma = 1$ has been considered, with α set to be just below 1 (which slows down the spread). The rationale for the power α is that it is included to allow for deviations from mass action [15] and to account for the discrete-time approximation to the continuous time model [20]. With the non-linear term y_{t-1}^{α}, the pure birth process approximating the SIR model is no longer linear. As a result, the number of births during a finite time interval are no longer negative binomially distributed, but the TSIR authors still use the negative binomial nonetheless. From the perspective of the infectives, we have a generalized birth process. We stress again that the level of overdispersion is not estimated from the data, but is determined by y_{t-1}.

We now turn to the case where we have incidence counts y_{it} indexed by both time t and area i, $i = 1, \ldots, n$. Consider the model, $Y_{it} \mid y_{i,t-1}, x_{i,t-1} \sim \text{NegBin}(\mu_{it}, y_{i,t-1})$, with

$$\mu_{it} = \beta(y_{i,t-1} + \iota_{i,t-1})^{\alpha} x_{i,t-1}/N_i,$$

where $\iota_{i,t-1}$ are infected contacts from areas other than i [6]. Again, the negative binomial distribution does not arise mechanistically when the hazard is non-linear.

In [50], a "gravity model" is assumed with $\iota_{i,t-1} \sim \text{gamma}(m_{i,t-1}, 1)$, a gamma distribution with mean and variance

$$m_{i,t-1} = \upsilon N_i^{\tau_1} \sum_{j \neq i} \frac{y_{j,t-1}^{\tau_2}}{d_{ij}^{\rho}},$$

where d_{ij} is the distance between areas i and j, and $\rho > 0$ determines the strength of the neighborhood flow, with the limit as $\rho \to 0$ giving equal weight to all neighbors. In practice, at least a subset of these parameters are often fixed. For example, we could take $\tau_1 = \tau_2 = 1$. A simpler model (that we fit in Section 23.5) with these constraints might replace $\iota_{i,t-1}$ by its expectation to give the mean model

$$\mu_{it} = \beta \left(y_{i,t-1} + \upsilon N_i \sum_{j \neq i} \frac{y_{j,t-1}}{d_{ij}^{\rho}} \right)^{\alpha} \frac{x_{i,t-1}}{N_i}, \tag{23.5}$$

$$= \left(e^{\lambda^{\text{AR}}} y_{i,t-1} + e^{\lambda^{\text{NE}}} N_i \sum_{j \neq i} \frac{y_{j,t-1}}{d_{ij}^{\rho}} \right)^{\alpha} \frac{x_{i,t-1}}{N_i}. \tag{23.6}$$

Note that if for some t, $y_{it} = 0$, for all i, then $\mu_{is} = 0$ for $s > t$. To prevent this issue, we might add an endemic term, $e^{\lambda^{\text{EN}}}$, to the mean (23.6). This difficulty has been circumnavigated by randomly simulating a new count from a Poisson distribution with a mean that depends on the under reporting rate (see the supplementary materials of [47]).

In Section 23.5, we fit a TSIR-like model, which takes various components from the epidemic/endemic model. Specifically, we fit the model

$$Y_{it} | \mu_{it} \sim \text{NegBin}(\mu_{it}, \phi)$$

$$\mu_{it} = \left[e^{\lambda_t^{\text{AR}}} y_{i,t-1} + e^{\lambda^{\text{NE}}} N_i^{\tau_1} \sum_{j \neq i} w_{ij} y_{j,t-1}^{\tau_2} \right]^{\alpha} + e^{\lambda^{\text{EN}}} N_i$$

with seasonality included in the autoregressive (AR) component: $\lambda_t^{\text{AR}} = \beta_0^{\text{AR}} + \beta_1^{\text{AR}} t + \gamma \sin(\omega t) + \delta \cos(\omega t)$. We have replaced $y_{i,t-1}$ by ϕ as the overdispersion parameter $\iota_{i,t-1}$ equal to its mean $m_{i,t-1}$, set $x_{i,t-1}$ equal to N_i (that is, approximating the susceptibles by the population), added an endemic term to the model, use normalized weights

$$w_{ij} = \frac{d_{ij}^{-\rho_1}}{\sum_{k \neq i} d_{ik}^{-\rho_1}},$$

and reparameterized the decay parameter as $\rho_1 = \theta_1 / (1 - \theta_1)$, with $0 < \theta_1 < 1$.

A variety of fitting procedures have been used, with various levels of sophistication. A Markov chain Monte Carlo (MCMC) scheme was used for a TSIR model with under reporting and an endemic term (called an influx parameter) appearing in the mean function [39]. The under reporting was accounted for by using an auxiliary variable scheme to impute the unknown true counts. This scheme is natural from a Bayesian persepctive, although computationally prohibitive in large populations.

TSIR models have been used to model data on multiple strains—for dengue without a spatial component [45] and with spatial component for hand, foot and mouth disease [46]. In the latter, the effect of vaccination was examined and the statistical analysis was based on estimated counts for EV71 and CoxA16 pathogens. A standard TSIR area model was used with no neighborhood component.

TSIR models have been used to examine various aspects of disease dynamics. Koelle and Pascual [29] use a nonlinear time series model to reconstruct patterns of immunity for cholera and examine the contributions of extrinsic factors such as seasonality (there are no spatial effects in the model). Seasonality of transmission has been considered by a number of authors, in particular in the context of measles. Climatic conditions that are more or less favorable to transmission might be relevant along with other seasonal factors that might affect the extent of social contacts. In contrast with the epidemic/endemic model, seasonality has been modeled in the autoregressive component in the TSIR framework. Seasonal forcing (the increase in transmission when children aggregate in schools, with a decrease during school holidays) is a particular aspect that has been considered. A local smoothing model has been used on the raw rates [34]. The simple sinusoidal model has been argued against [11] as being too simplistic. The rate β_t has been modeled as a function of month for rubella in Mexico [35], or allowing a unique set of 26 parameters in each year [5].

The TSIR model also may be fitted in R in the `tsiR` package [3], with implementation based on the method described in [15] or a Bayesian implementation (using the `rjags` package). At the time of this writing, the models are temporal only, with no explicit spatial modeling possible (other than fitting separate TSIR models in each area).

23.4.3   Epidemic/Endemic hhh4 models

We now describe a parallel development, originating in [22], with subsequent developments being reported in [19, 23, 36, 37, 42, 43]. For an excellent review of the statistical aspects of infectious disease modeling, and this class of models in particular, see [25]. The epidemic/endemic description is used to denote the addition of a term in the mean function that does not depend on previous counts, while hhh4 is the key function in the **surveillance** package that fits the models we describe in this section.

We will derive the probability that a susceptible individual at time $t - 1$ will become infected by time t. In contrast to the TSIR derivation, in which the process of the infectives infecting susceptibles was modeled (and lead to a negative binomial for the number of new infectives), the derivation here models the process of susceptibles becoming infected (and, as we will see, leads to a binomial distribution for the number of new infectives).

We again assume that infected individuals are infectious for one time unit before becoming removed, so that we have an SIR model with a fixed infectious period duration (and a constant hazard). So the event of a susceptible at $t - 1$ becoming infected in $[t - 1, t)$ is Bernoulli with probability of infection, $1 - \exp(-\beta y_{t-1}/N)$.

Under homogenous mixing and independence of the Bernoulli outcomes of the susceptibles

$$Y_t | y_{t-1}, x_{t-1} \sim \text{Binomial}\left(x_{t-1}, 1 - \exp(-\beta y_{t-1}/N)\right). \qquad (23.7)$$

If we write $\eta = \exp(-\beta/N)$ (which is appropriate given the frequency dependent model we described in Section 23.2.1), we see we have a (Reed-Frost) chain binomial model (e.g., Daley and Gani, 1999, Chapter 4). Under the chain-binomial formulation, a susceptible at time $t - 1$ can remain susceptible by avoiding being infected by all infectives y_{t-1}, and the probability of avoiding being infected by one infective is η. This leads to $Y_t | y_{t-1}, x_{t-1} \sim$ Binomial$(x_{t-1}, 1 - \eta^{y_{t-1}})$

$$\Pr(Y_t = y_t | y_{t-1}, x_{t-1}) = \binom{x_{t-1}}{x_{t-1} - y_t} (\eta^{y_{t-1}})^{x_{t-1}-y_t} (1 - \eta^{y_{t-1}})^{y_t}.$$

Under the assumption of a rare disease, and the approximation $\exp(-\beta y_{t-1}/N) \approx 1 - \beta y_{t-1}/N$, the model (23.7) becomes (suppressing the dependence on x_{t-1}) $Y_t | y_{t-1} \sim$ Poisson $(\beta x_{t-1} y_{t-1}/N)$. A further assumption that is implicitly made is that $x_{t-1} \approx N$ to give,

$Y_t|y_{t-1} \sim \text{Poisson}(\beta y_{t-1})$. Hence, in the epidemic/endemic development, there is an implicit assumption of frequency dependent transmission.

In the original paper [22] a branching process with immigration formulation was taken:

$$Y_t = Y_t^\star + Z_t,$$

with independent components,

$$Y_t^\star|y_{t-1} \sim \text{Poisson}(\beta y_{t-1}),$$
$$Z_t \sim \text{Poisson}(v_t),$$

which are labeled *epidemic* and *endemic*, respectively. The epidemic component corresponds to the branching process, and the endemic component to immigration. To account for overdispersion in the infectives count, the model is,

$$Y_t|y_{t-1} \sim \text{NegBin}(\mu_t, \kappa),$$

with

$$\text{E}(Y_t|y_{t-1}) = \mu_t = \beta y_{t-1},$$
$$\text{Var}(Y_t|y_{t-1}) = \mu_t \left(1 + \frac{\mu_t}{\kappa}\right),$$

where κ is estimated from the data. Unlike the TSIR development, this distribution does not "drop out" of a stochastic process formulation, but is made on pragmatic considerations. Negative binomial distributions also have been used in other infectious disease developments. For example, in [33] it is assumed that individual level reproductive numbers are gamma distributed, with a Poisson distribution for the cases infected by each infective, to give a negative binomial distribution for the number of infectives generated.

The development of the TSIR model was based directly on the number of infectives produced by the current infectives. In contrast, the epidemic/endemic development here determines the risk of each susceptible being infected. The negative binomial distribution derived under the TSIR framework has countably infinite support, whereas the number of susceptibles is bounded, but given the rate drops with the latter, this approximation is unlikely to be problematic. The negative binomial distribution of the TSIR is a continuous time Markov chain (CTMC) approximation, while the epidemic/endemic in this section is a discrete time Markov chain (DTMC).

Now we consider the more usual situation in which we have incident counts y_{it} and populations N_{it} in a set of areas indexed by $i = 1, \ldots, n$. Suppose that new infections can occur:

1. From *self-area* infectives.
2. From *neighboring-area* infectives.
3. From another source, which may be an environmental reservoir, or infectives from outside the study region.

In the case of different possibilities for becoming infected, we can use the classic *competing risks* framework [44], in which the hazard rates (forces of infection) are additive. We let $\lambda_{it}^{\text{TOT}}$ represent the overall hazard for a susceptible in area i at time t, and write

$$\lambda_{it}^{\text{TOT}} = \underbrace{\lambda_{it}^{\text{AR}}}_{\text{Self-Area}} + \underbrace{\lambda_{it}^{\text{NE}}}_{\text{Neighboring-Area}} + \underbrace{\lambda_{it}^{\text{EN}}}_{\text{Environmental}}.$$

Assuming $\lambda_{it}^{\text{TOT}}$ is small, the probability of infection in $(t-1, t)$, for a single susceptible is $1 - \exp(-\lambda_{it}^{\text{TOT}}) \approx \lambda_{it}^{\text{TOT}}$. Following detailed arguments in [2] (including again assuming that $x_{i,t-1} \approx N_{it}$), we obtain the conditional mean,

$$\mu_{it} = \underbrace{\lambda_{it}^{\text{AR}} y_{i,t-1}}_{\text{Self-Area}} + \underbrace{\sum_{j=1}^{n} \lambda_{it}^{\text{NE}} w_{ij} y_{j,t-1}}_{\text{Neighboring Areas}} + \underbrace{N_{it} \lambda_{it}^{\text{EN}}}_{\text{Environmental}} \,,$$

where w_{ij} are a set of weights that define the neighborhood structure. The rates may depend on both space and time to allow covariate modeling, trends in time (including seasonality) and area-specific random effects, which may or may not have spatial structure. In practice, sparsity of information will lead to simplifications. We describe the model for the measles data from Germany. There are only 17 areas, which (along with the low counts) means a simple neighborhood model is considered. Specifically, as in the majority of illustrations of the epidemic/endemic framework, we assume the seasonality model

$$\mu_{it} = \lambda_i^{\text{AR}} y_{i,t-1} + \lambda^{\text{NE}} \sum_{j=1}^{n} w_{ij} y_{j,t-1} + N_{it} \lambda_{it}^{\text{EN}},$$

with

$$\begin{aligned}
\log \lambda_i^{\text{AR}} &= \beta_0^{\text{AR}} + b_i^{\text{AR}}, \\
\log \lambda_{it}^{\text{EN}} &= \beta_0^{\text{EN}} + \beta_1^{\text{EN}} t + \gamma \sin(\omega t) + \delta \cos(\omega t) + b_i^{\text{EN}},
\end{aligned}$$

where $\omega = 2\pi/26$ for biweekly data. Note the contrast with the TSIR framwork, in which seasonality was modeled in the autoregressive term, although we note that seasonality can be incorporated in any of the three terms [23], and this possibility is available in the **surveillance** package.

Originally, the weights were binary corresponding to spatial contiguity. More recently [36], the weights are assumed to follow a power law, with

$$w_{ij} = \frac{m_{ij}^{-\rho_2}}{\sum_{k \neq i} m_{ik}^{-\rho_2}},$$

where m_{ij} is the number of areas that must be crossed when moving between areas i and j, and $\rho_2 \geq 0$ is a power that may be estimated. The normalization ensures that $\sum_{k \neq i} w_{ik} = 1$ for all rows of the weight matrix (infecteds are being allocated to neighbors). The limit $\rho_2 \to \infty$ corresponds to first-order dependency, and $\rho_2 = 0$ gives equal weight to all areas. The power law allows "contact" between areas that are a large distance apart since it is "heavy-tailed." Hence, by analogy with common spatial models, we have two parameters: λ^{NE} that determines the magnitude of the contribution from the neighbors and ρ_2 that determines the extent of the neighbor contributions. We parameterize as $\rho_2 = \theta_2/(1 - \theta_2)$ with $0 < \theta_2 < 1$.

Fitting using maximum likelihood/Bayes is relatively straightforward. The epidemic/ endemic model with random effects is implemented using penalized quasi-likelihood (PQL) in the **surveillance** package in **R**. The computational burden is not impacted greatly by the data size and so infectious disease data from large populations is not problematic. In Section 23.5 we describe a Bayesian approach with implementation in **Stan**.

A very similar model to the one just given also has been independently developed and fitted to data on hand, foot and mouth disease in China [49]. The model allowed for infections from not only the immediately previous time periods, but also for periods further back.

A more complex model in which there is not a fixed latency plus infectiousness period has been considered [30]. In the context of a susceptible-exposed-infectious-recovered (SEIR) model, they develop a discrete-time approximation to a stochastic SEIR model in which there is a data augmentation step that imputes the number of infected over time. Given these numbers, the counts in each compartment are available, and the likelihood is a product of three binomials (one each for infected counts, first symptom counts, and removed counts).

We describe how the approach of [30] could be used for the SIR model. The key difference is that the fixed latency plus infectious period is relaxed and so it is no longer assumed that incidence is equal to prevalence. Consequently, we continue to let X_t, Y_t, Z_t represent the numbers of susceptibles, incident cases, and number who recover at time t, but now let I_t be the prevalence. The model consists of the two distributions:

$$Y_t | I_{t-1} = i_{t-1}, X_{t-1} = x_{t-1} \sim \text{Binomial}\left(x_{t-1}, 1 - \exp(\beta i_{t-1}/N)\right) \tag{23.8}$$

$$Z_t | I_{t-1} = i_{t-1} \sim \text{Binomial}\left(i_{t-1}, 1 - \exp(\gamma)\right), \tag{23.9}$$

so that γ is the recovery rate with $1/\gamma$ the mean recovery time. In this model, the reproductive number is $R_0 = \beta/\gamma$. Further,

$$I_t = I_{t-1} + Y_{t-1} - Z_{t-1}, \tag{23.10}$$

subject to the initial conditions $x_0 = N$ (the population size, for example) and $I_0 = a$. An obvious way to carry out computation is to introduce the unknown counts Z_t into the model as auxiliary variables, from which the series I_t can be constructed from (23.10). With the "full data" the likelihood is simply the product over the binomials in (23.8) and (23.9). This scheme will be computationally expensive for long time series with large numbers of cases.

Summary: Both the TSIR and the epidemic/endemic formulations are approximations. The TSIR formulation (without the α power) is in continuous time and assumes the number of susceptibles remains constant between observation points. The epidemic/endemic formulation assumes the number of infectives is constant between observation time points.

23.4.4 Under reporting

Underreporting is a ubiquitous problem in infectious disease modeling; this topic is covered in detail in Chapter 22. We describe an approach to underreporting that has been used along with TSIR modeling, particularly for measles, leaning heavily on [15]. We let C_t represent the reported cases and Y_t the true number of cases. Then, again using X_t as the number of susceptibles, we generalize (23.1) to,

$$X_t = X_{t-1} - \rho_t C_t + B_{t-d} + U_t, \tag{23.11}$$

where $1/\rho_t$ is the underreporting rate at time t, and u_t are uncorrelated errors with $\text{E}(U_t) = 0$, $\text{var}(U_t) = \sigma_u^2$, that acknowledge the errors that may creep into the deterministic formulation. We write $X_t = \overline{X} + Z_t$, substitute in (23.11) and successively iterate to give

$$Z_t = Z_0 - \sum_{s=1}^{t} \rho_s C_s + \sum_{s=1}^{t} B_{s-d} + \sum_{s=1}^{t} U_s.$$

From this equation, we see that if underreporting is present and not accounted for, the difference between cumulative births and observed cases will grow without bound. Let

$$\widetilde{C}_t = \sum_{s=1}^{t} C_s, \quad \widetilde{B}_t = \sum_{s=1}^{t} B_{s-d}, \quad \widetilde{U}_t = \sum_{s=1}^{t} U_s, \quad R_t = \sum_{s=1}^{t} (\rho_s - \rho) C_s,$$

where $\rho = \mathrm{E}(\rho_t)$ and $R_t \approx 0$ under a constant reporting rate. Then, to estimate ρ it has become common practice in TSIR work to regress the cumulative births on the cumulative cases,

$$\widetilde{B}_t = Z_t - Z_0 + \rho \widetilde{C}_t - \widetilde{U}_t,$$

to estimate ρ as the slope. Note that the cumulative errors $\widetilde{U}_t$ do not have constant variance, since $\mathrm{var}(U_t) = \sigma_u^2$, so a weighted regression is more appropriate.

With an estimate $\widehat{\rho}$, one may estimate the true number of cases as $Y_t = \widehat{\rho} C_t$, and use these cases in a TSIR model. This approach is often followed, although there is no explicit acknowledgement of the additional (beyond sampling) variability in Y_t.

23.4.5   Ecological regression

Ecological bias occurs when individual and aggregate level (with aggregation here over space) inference differ. The key to its understanding is to take an individual-level model and aggregate to the area-level [48]. We report on recent work [17], that examines the implications of ecological inference for infectious disease data. Let Y_{itk} be a disease indicator for a susceptible individual k in area i and week t and z_{itk} be an individual-level covariate, $k = 1, \ldots, N_i$. We present a simple example in which there is an autoregressive term only, and also assume a rare disease. In this case, the individual-level model is

$$Y_{itk} | y_{i,t-1,k} \sim \mathrm{Bernoulli}\left(\lambda_{itk}^{\mathrm{AR}} y_{i,t-1} / N_i \right),$$

with $\lambda_{itk}^{\mathrm{AR}} = \exp(\alpha + \beta z_{itk})$. The implied aggregate hazard rate for area i and time t is then [17],

$$\overline{\lambda}_{it}^{\mathrm{AR}} = \exp(\alpha) \int_{A_i} \exp(\beta z) g_{it}(z) dz,$$

where A_i represents area i and $g_{it}(z)$ is the within-area distribution of z at time t.

As a simple example consider the binary covariate, $z_{itk} = 0/1$ (for example, the vaccination status of individual k in area i at time t). The aggregate consistent model, for $Y_{it} = \sum_{k=1}^{N_i} Y_{itk}$, is

$$Y_{it} | \overline{\lambda}_{it}^{\mathrm{AR}} \sim \mathrm{Poisson}(\overline{\lambda}_{it}^{\mathrm{AR}} y_{i,t-1} / N_i)$$
$$\overline{\lambda}_{it}^{\mathrm{AR}} = N_i \left[(1 - \overline{z}_{it}) \mathrm{e}^{\alpha} + \overline{z}_{it} \mathrm{e}^{\alpha+\beta} \right].$$

A naive model would assume $\overline{\lambda}_{it}^{\mathrm{AR}} = \exp(\alpha^{\star} + \beta^{\star} \overline{z}_{it})$, where $\overline{z}_{it}$ is the area average. This naive model is very different from the aggregate consistent model.

23.5   Analysis of Measles Data

We now return to the measles data and, for illustration, fit a TSIR model and an epidemic/endemic model. We use a Bayesian approach due to its flexibility, and since the `rstan` package allows these models to be fitted with relative ease. The package implements MCMC using the no U-turns version [24] of Hamiltonian Monte Carlo [40]. The code, and comparison of parameter estimates for the epidemic/endemic model with the PQL versions in the `surveillance` package, is included in the supplementary materials.

23.5.1 Time Series Susceptible-Infectious-Recovered model

The TSIR type model we fit is

$$Y_{it}|\mu_{it} \sim \text{NegBin}\left(\mu_{it}, \phi\right),$$

$$\mu_{it} = \left[e^{\lambda_t^{\text{AR}}} y_{i,t-1} + e^{\lambda^{\text{NE}}} N_i^{\tau_1} \sum_{j=1}^{n} w_{ij} y_{j,t-1}^{\tau_2} \right]^{\alpha} + N_i e^{\lambda^{\text{EN}}},$$

where

$$w_{ij} = \frac{d_{ij}^{-\theta_1/(1-\theta_1)}}{\sum_{k \neq i} d_{ik}^{-\theta_1/(1-\theta_1)}},$$

with d_{ij} being the distance between areas i and j, and $\lambda_t^{\text{AR}} = \beta_0^{\text{AR}} + \beta_1^{\text{AR}} t + \gamma \sin(\omega t) + \delta \cos(\omega t)$. Relatively uninformative priors were used (zero mean normals with standard deviations of 10). The deviation from linearity parameter, α, was restricted to lie in $[0.95, 1]$ and was given a uniform prior on this support.

Figure 23.2 shows the fit, and it appears reasonable. Figure 23.4 displays posterior distributions for a few interesting parameters. Notably, the posterior for α is close to uniform, so that the data tell little about this parameter. The posterior for θ_1 is quite peaked and the decay corresponding to this posterior is a swift decrease with increasing distance; τ_1 and τ_2 are relatively well-behaved.

23.5.2 Epidemic/Endemic model

The epidemic/endemic model we fit is

$$Y_{it}|\mu_{it} \sim \text{NegBin}(\mu_{it}, \phi),$$

$$\mu_{it} = e^{\lambda^{\text{AR}}+b_i^{\text{AR}}} y_{i,t-1} + e^{\lambda^{\text{NE}}+b_i^{\text{NE}}} \sum_{j=1}^{n} w_{ij} y_{j,t-1} + N_i e^{\lambda_t^{\text{EN}}+b_i^{\text{EN}}},$$

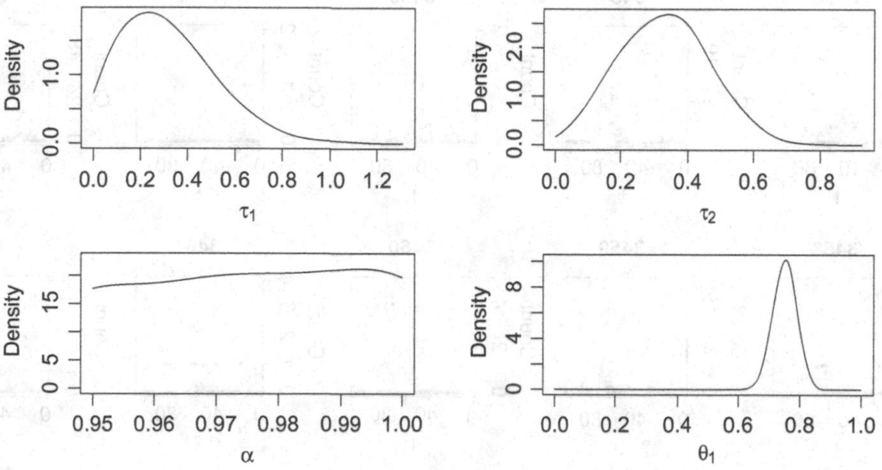

FIGURE 23.4
Density estimates of the posterior marginals for τ_1, τ_2, α, and θ_1, from analysis of the measles data with the TSIR model.

where

$$w_{ij} = \frac{m_{ij}^{-\theta_2/(1-\theta_2)}}{\sum_{k \neq i} m_{ik}^{-\theta_2/(1-\theta_2)}},$$

with m_{ij} the number of boundaries to cross when traveling between areas i and j. Independent normal random effects were used, that is, $b_i^{\mathrm{AR}} \sim N(0, \sigma_{\mathrm{AR}}^2)$, $b_i^{\mathrm{NE}} \sim N(0, \sigma_{\mathrm{NE}}^2)$, $b_i^{\mathrm{EN}} \sim N(0, \sigma_{\mathrm{EN}}^2)$. Seasonality and a linear trend were included in the endemic component:

$$\lambda_t^{\mathrm{EN}} = \beta_0^{\mathrm{EN}} + \beta_1^{\mathrm{EN}} t + \gamma \sin(\omega t) + \delta \cos(\omega t).$$

We assume relatively flat priors, as for the TSIR model, on λ^{AR}, λ^{NE}, β_0^{EN}, β_1^{EN}, γ, and δ. For the random effects precisions $\sigma_{\mathrm{AR}}^{-2}$, $\sigma_{\mathrm{NE}}^{-2}$, $\sigma_{\mathrm{EN}}^{-2}$, we use gamma(0.5,0.1) priors which have prior medians for the standard deviations of 0.66, and (5%, 95%) points of (0.22, 7.1). We used a uniform prior on $0 < \theta_2 < 1$ and a relatively flat prior on the overdispersion parameter ϕ.

Figure 23.5 shows the time series of data in the areas with non-zero counts, along with posterior medians of μ_{it}, with the gray shading representing 95 percent intervals for μ_{it}. Overall, the model appears to be picking up the time courses well. Figure 23.6 displays posterior distributions for a variety of parameters (for illustration), and we see that λ^{AR} and λ^{NE} are left skewed. The neighborhood parameter θ_2 is relatively well estimated and favors a nearest neighbor structure. The posterior medians of σ_{AR} and σ_{EN} were 1.5 and 1.6,

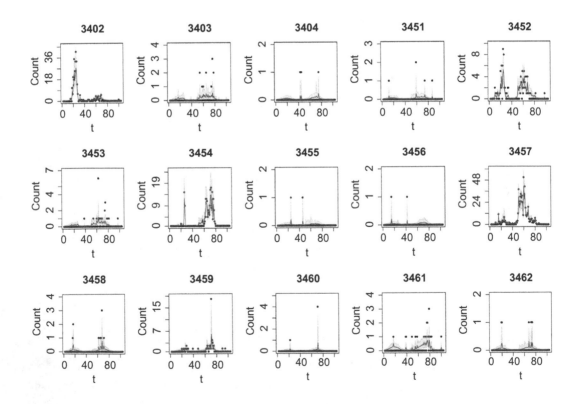

FIGURE 23.5
Observed (black dots) data in the 15 districts with non-zero counts and posterior summaries (2.5%, 50%, 97.5% quantiles) for μ_{it} under the epidemic/endemic model.

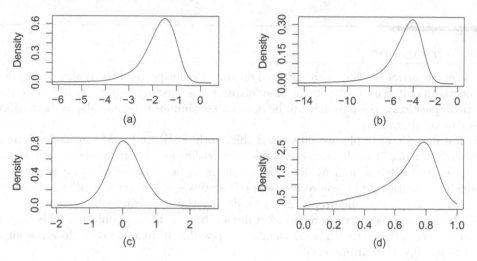

FIGURE 23.6
Density estimates of the posterior marginals for (a) λ^{AR}, (b) λ^{NE}, (c) $\log(\sigma_{\text{AR}})$ and (d) θ_2 from analysis of the measles data with the epidemic/endemic model.

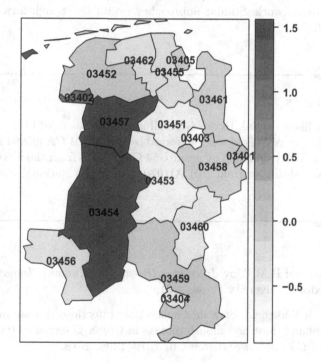

FIGURE 23.7
Posterior medians of autoregressive random effects b_i^{AR}.

respectively (though note that the random effects associated with these standard deviations are acting on different scales, so they are not comparable), while the posterior median of σ_{NE} is 3.3. Posterior medians of the random effects b_i^{AR} are mapped in Figure 23.7, and we see large differences between the areas. In general, the sizes of the random effects show there is large between-area variability.

23.6   Discussion

In this review article we have concentrated on statistical aspects of the models, but perhaps the most difficult part is developing models and interpreting results in order to answer biological questions. Much remains to be done on continuous time models, particularly with respect to computation.

In the measles example, we illustrated that both TSIR and epidemic/endemic models can be fitted using Stan. Residual analysis is underdeveloped for the discrete-time models that we have described, and model comparison in general also requires investigation. We examined conventional Pearson residuals in our analyses, but these are difficult to interpret with small counts. For underreporting, introducing the true counts as auxiliary variables is the obvious approach within a Bayesian model, but for large populations this is computationally very difficult (and also not currently possible in Stan since it does not support inference for discrete parameters).

Contact patterns and disease severity are strongly age dependent, and incorporating age (and gender) in the epidemic/endemic model has been explicitly carried out by Bauer and Wakeeld [2] in the context of modeling hand, foot and mouth disease in China. Meyer and Held [37] constructed contact matrices based on survey data and incorporated these in the epidemic/endemic framework. Similar approaches would be straightforward to include in the TSIR approach.

Acknowledgments

The authors would like to thank Bryan Grenfell and Saki Takahashi for helpful discussions on the TSIR model. Jon Wakefield was supported by grant R01 CA095994 from the National Institutes of Health, Tracy Qi Dong by grant U54 GM111274 from the National Institutes of Health and Vladimir Minin by grant R01 AI107034 from the National Institutes of Health.

References

[1] R.M. Anderson and R.M. May. *Infectious Diseases of Humans: Dynamics and Control.* New York: Oxford University Press, 1991.

[2] C. Bauer and J. Wakefield. Stratified space-time infectious disease modeling: With an application to hand, foot and mouth disease in China. *Journal of the Royal Statistical Society: Series C (Applied Statistics)*, 67:1379–1398, 2018.

[3] A.D. Becker and B.T. Grenfell. tsiR: An R package for time-series Susceptible-Infected-Recovered models of epidemics. *PLoS One*, 12:e0185528, 2017.

[4] M. Begon, M. Bennett, R.G. Bowers, N.P. French, S.M. Hazel, J. Turner, et al. A clarification of transmission terms in host-microparasite models: Numbers, densities and areas. *Epidemiology & Infection*, 129:147–153, 2002.

[5] O.N. Bjørnstad, B.F. Finkenstädt, and B.T. Grenfell. Dynamics of measles epidemics: Estimating scaling of transmission rates using a time series SIR model. *Ecological Monographs*, 72:169–184, 2002.

[6] O.N. Bjørnstad and B.T. Grenfell. Hazards, spatial transmission and timing of outbreaks in epidemic metapopulations. *Environmental and Ecological Statistics*, 15:265–277, 2008.

[7] M. Cardinal, R. Roy, and J. Lambert. On the application of integer-valued time series models for the analysis of disease incidence. *Statistics in Medicine*, 18:2025–2039, 1999.

[8] M.S. Ciupe, B.L. Bivort, D.M. Bortz, and P.W. Nelson. Estimating kinetic parameters from HIV primary infection data through the eyes of three different mathematical models. *Mathematical Biosciences*, 200:1–27, 2006.

[9] D.R. Cox and H.D. Miller. *The Theory of Stochastic Processes*. London, UK: Chapman and Hall, 1965.

[10] D.J. Daley and J. Gani. *Epidemic Modelling: An Introduction*. Cambridge, UK: Cambridge University Press, 1999.

[11] D.J.D. Earn, P. Rohani, B.M. Bolker, and B.T. Grenfell. A simple model for complex dynamical transitions in epidemics. *Science*, 287:667–670, 2000.

[12] W. Feller. *An Introduction to Probability Theory and its Applications, Volume I*. New York: John Wiley & Sons, 1950.

[13] R. Ferland, A. Latour, and D. Oraichi. Integer-valued GARCH process. *Journal of Time Series Analysis*, 27:923–942, 2006.

[14] A. Fernández-Fontelo, A. Cabaña, P. Puig, and D. Moriña. Under-reported data analysis with INAR-hidden Markov chains. *Statistics in Medicine*, 35:4875–4890, 2016.

[15] B.F. Finkenstädt and B.T. Grenfell. Time series modelling of childhood diseases: A dynamical systems approach. *Journal of the Royal Statistical Society: Series C*, 49:187–205, 2000.

[16] J. Fintzi, X. Cui, J. Wakefield, and V.N. Minin. Efficient data augmentation for fitting stochastic epidemic models to prevalence data. *Journal of Computational and Graphical Statistics*, 26:918–929, 2017.

[17] L. Fisher and J. Wakefield. Ecological inference for infectious disease data, with application to vaccination strategies. To appear in *Statistics in Medicine*, 2019.

[18] K. Fokianos and R. Fried. Interventions in INGARCH processes. *Journal of Time Series Analysis*, 31:210–225, 2010.

[19] M. Geilhufe, L. Held, S.O. Skrøvseth, G.S. Simonsen, and F. Godtliebsen. Power law approximations of movement network data for modeling infectious disease spread. *Biometrical Journal*, 56:363–382, 2014.

[20] K. Glass, Y. Xia, and B.T. Grenfell. Interpreting time-series analyses for continuous-time biological models measles as a case study. *Journal of Theoretical Biology*, 223:19–25, 2003.

[21] S.K. Greene, E.R. Peterson, D. Kapell, A.D. Fine, and M. Kulldorff. Daily reportable disease spatiotemporal cluster detection, New York City, New York, USA, 2014–2015. *Emerging Infectious Diseases*, 22:1808, 2016.

[22] L. Held, M. Höhle, and M. Hofmann. A statistical framework for the analysis of multivariate infectious disease surveillance counts. *Statistical Modelling*, 5:187–199, 2005.

[23] L. Held and M. Paul. Modeling seasonality in space-time infectious disease surveillance data. *Biometrical Journal*, 54:824–843, 2012.

[24] M.D. Hoffman and A. Gelman. The No-U-turn sampler: Adaptively setting path lengths in Hamiltonian Monte Carlo. *Journal of Machine Learning Research*, 15:1593–1623, 2014.

[25] M. Höhle. Infectious disease modeling. In A.B. Lawson, S. Banerjee, R.P. Haining, and M.D. Ugarte, eds., *Handbook of Spatial Epidemiology*, p. 477–500. Boca Raton, FL: Chapman and Hall/CRC Press, 2016.

[26] G. Hooker, S.P. Ellner, L.D. V. Roditi, and D.J.D. Earn. Parameterizing state–space models for infectious disease dynamics by generalized profiling: Measles in Ontario. *Journal of the Royal Society Interface*, 8:961–974, 2011.

[27] D.G. Kendall. Stochastic processes and population growth. *Journal of the Royal Statistical Society, Series B*, 11:230–282, 1949.

[28] W.O. Kermack and A.G. McKendrick. A contribution to the mathematical theory of epidemics. *Proceedings of the Royal Society of London Series A, Containing Papers of a Mathematical and Physical Character*, 115:700–721, 1927.

[29] K. Koelle and M. Pascual. Disentangling extrinsic from intrinsic factors in disease dynamics: A nonlinear time series approach with an application to cholera. *The American Naturalist*, 163:901–913, 2004.

[30] P.E. Lekone and B.F. Finkenstädt. Statistical inference in a stochastic epidemic SEIR model with control intervention: Ebola as a case study. *Biometrics*, 62:1170–1177, 2006.

[31] A. Levin-Rector, E.L. Wilson, A.D. Fine, and S.K. Greene. Refining historical limits method to improve disease cluster detection, New York City, New York, USA. *Emerging Infectious Diseases*, 21:265, 2015.

[32] W.-M. Liu, H.W. Hethcote, and S.A. Levin. Dynamical behavior of epidemiological models with nonlinear incidence rates. *Journal of Mathematical Biology*, 25:359–380, 1987.

[33] J.O. Lloyd-Smith, S.J. Schreiber, P.E. Kopp, and W.M. Getz. Superspreading and the effect of individual variation on disease emergence. *Nature*, 438:355, 2005.

[34] W.P. London and J.A. Yorke. Recurrent outbreaks of measles, chickenpox and mumps: I. Seasonal variation in contact rates. *American Journal of Epidemiology*, 98:453–468, 1973.

[35] C.J.E. Metcalf, O.N. Bjørnstad, M.J. Ferrari, P. Klepac, N. Bharti, H. Lopez-Gatell, and B.T. Grenfell. The epidemiology of rubella in Mexico: Seasonality, stochasticity and regional variation. *Epidemiology & Infection*, 139:1029–1038, 2011.

[36] S. Meyer and L. Held. Power-law models for infectious disease spread. *Annals of Applied Statistics*, 8:1612–1639, 2014.

[37] S. Meyer and L. Held. Incorporating social contact data in spatio-temporal models for infectious disease spread. *Biostatistics*, 18:338–351, 2017.

[38] S. Meyer, L. Held, and M. Höhle. Spatio-temporal analysis of epidemic phenomena using the R package `surveillance`. *Journal of Statistical Software*, 77:1–55, 2017.

[39] A. Morton and B.F. Finkenstädt. Discrete time modelling of disease incidence time series by using Markov chain Monte Carlo methods. *Journal of the Royal Statistical Society, Series C*, 54:575–594, 2005.

[40] R.M. Neal. MCMC using Hamiltonian dynamics. In S. Brooks, A. Gelman, G.L. Jones, and X.L. Meng, editors, *Handbook of Markov Chain Monte Carlo*, volume 2, pages 113–162. Boca Raton, FL: Chapman and Hall/CRC Press, 2011.

[41] H. Nishiura, G. Chowell, H. Heesterbeek, and J. Wallinga. The ideal reporting interval for an epidemic to objectively interpret the epidemiological time course. *Journal of the Royal Society Interface*, 7:297–307, 2010.

[42] M. Paul and L. Held. Predictive assessment of a non-linear random effects model for multivariate time series of infectious disease counts. *Statistics in Medicine*, 30:1118–1136, 2011.

[43] M. Paul, L. Held, and A.M. Toschke. Multivariate modelling of infectious disease surveillance data. *Statistics in Medicine*, 27:6250–6267, 2008.

[44] R.L. Prentice, J.D. Kalbfleisch, A.V. Peterson Jr, N. Flournoy, V.T. Farewell, and N.E. Breslow. The analysis of failure times in the presence of competing risks. *Biometrics*, 34:541–554, 1978.

[45] N.G. Reich, S. Shrestha, A.A. King, P. Rohani, J. Lessler, S. Kalayanarooj, I.-K. Yoon, R.V. Gibbons, D.S. Burke, and D.A.T. Cummings. Interactions between serotypes of dengue highlight epidemiological impact of cross-immunity. *Journal of the Royal Society Interface*, 10:20130414, 2013.

[46] S. Takahashi, Q. Liao, T.P. Van Boeckel, W. Xing, J. Sun, V.Y. Hsiao, et al. Hand, foot, and mouth disease in China: Modeling epidemic dynamics of enterovirus serotypes and implications for vaccination. *PLoS Medicine*, 13:e1001958, 2016.

[47] T.P. Van Boeckel, S. Takahashi, Q. Liao, W. Xing, S. Lai, V. Hsiao, et al. Hand, foot, and mouth disease in China: Critical community size and spatial vaccination strategies. *Scientific Reports*, 6:25248, 2016.

[48] J. Wakefield. Ecologic studies revisited. *Annual Review of Public Health*, 29:75–90, 2008.

[49] Y. Wang, Z. Feng, Y. Yang, S. Self, Y. Gao, I.M. Longini, et al. Hand, foot and mouth disease in China: Patterns and spread and transmissibility. *Epidemiology*, 22:781–792, 2011.

[50] Y. Xia, O.N. Bjørnstad, and B.T. Grenfell. Measles metapopulation dynamics: A gravity model for epidemiological coupling and dynamics. *The American Naturalist*, 164:267–281, 2004.

[51] F. Zhu. A negative binomial integer-valued GARCH model. *Journal of Time Series Analysis*, 32:54–67, 2011.

24

Analysing Multiple Epidemic Data Sources

Daniela De Angelis and Anne M. Presanis

CONTENTS

24.1 Introduction

> "A catalogue of the number of deaths induced by the major epidemics of historical time is staggering, and dwarfs the total deaths on all battlefields." [1]

This quote sets the problem of infectious diseases in perspective. Although major historical threats have been defeated [2], new emerging ones continue to challenge humans. It is not surprising that increasing effort has been made by policy makers to assess and anticipate the consequence of epidemics. Evidence-based knowledge of disease burden, including prevalence, incidence, severity, and transmission, in different population strata, in different locations and, if feasible, in real time, is becoming progressively key to the planning and evaluation of public health policies [2]. Direct observation of a disease process hardly ever is possible. However, retrospective and prospective estimation of the key aspects of burden just listed is feasible through the use of indirect information collected in administrative registries. The previous chapters in this handbook (and the rich literature that exists [2, 3] and references therein) provide plenty of examples of how surveillance information, together with statistical models, can be used to reconstruct the disease process underlying the pattern of the observed data, infer the unobserved (latent) characteristics of the epidemic, and forecast its evolution.

Here we focus, in particular, on statistical inference that makes simultaneous use of multiple data sources, including different streams of surveillance data, ad hoc studies, and expert opinion.

This "evidence synthesis" approach is not new in medical statistics. Meta-analysis and network meta-analysis are well established approaches to combine data from studies of similar design, typically clinical trials [4]. The idea has been generalized in the areas of medical decision-making [5], technology assessment [6, 7], and epidemiology (e.g., [8]) to assimilate data from sources of different types and studies of different designs and is becoming popular in other scientific fields as modern technologies enable the collection and storage of ever increasing amounts of information (e.g., [9, 10]). For infectious disease, in the last 10 years there has been a proliferation of papers employing multiple sources of information to reconstruct characteristics of epidemics of blood-borne and respiratory diseases, including estimation of prevalence (e.g., HIV [11], HCV [12, 13], and campylobacteriosis [14]), severity (e.g., [15, 16]), incidence (e.g., toxoplasmosis [17], influenza [18], and pertussis [19]) and, transmission (e.g., influenza [20, 21]).

The use of multiple data sources poses a number of statistical and computational challenges: the combination of various sources, most likely affected by selection and informative observation biases and heterogeneous in type, relevance, and granularity, leads to probabilistic models with complex structures that are difficult to build and fit and challenging to criticize [22].

In this chapter, we will use motivating case studies of influenza to introduce the evidence synthesis setting in infectious diseases, illustrate the building and fitting of relevant models, and highlight the opportunities offered and the challenges posed by the multiplicity of sources. The models we will concentrate on are typically Bayesian as this framework offers a natural setup for the synthesis of information.

The chapter is organized as follows. In Section 24.2, we describe our motivating examples; in Section 24.3, the generic framework for evidence synthesis for infectious diseases is introduced; the models developed for the chosen examples are presented in Sections 24.4 and 24.5; Section 24.6 is devoted to the challenges encountered in the building, fitting, and criticism of models that incorporate multiple sources; and we conclude with a final discussion in Section 24.7.

24.2   Motivating Example: Influenza

Public health responses aimed at mitigating the impact of an outbreak need reliable (and prompt) assessment of the likely severity and spread of the infection. This understanding is particularly key when a new pathogen emerges, potentially causing a pandemic, for example a new influenza strain as in 2009 [23] or more recently, the zika [24] and ebola [25] outbreaks.

We will use examples of influenza severity and transmission estimation, in particular referring to the 2009 A/H1N1 pandemic in the United Kingdom, to illustrate how, in the absence of ideal information, estimation of severity and transmission can be carried out by using data from a multiplicity of sources.

24.2.1 Severity

The severity of an infectious disease, such as influenza, can be thought as a "pyramid" (Figure 24.1), where with increasing severity, there are fewer and fewer infections. A proportion of infected individuals progress to symptoms, then to hospitalization, and the most severe end-points of either intensive care unit (ICU) admission or death. Severity is usually expressed as "case-severity risks" (CSRs); i.e. probabilities that an infection leads to a severe event such as being hospitalized, admitted to ICU, or dying. Quantification of such risks is necessary both prospectively, during an outbreak, to understand the severity and likely burden on health-care of an ongoing epidemic; and retrospectively, to assess the severe burden of the particular strain responsible for the epidemic, the adequacy of any public health response during the outbreak, and to inform responses in future outbreaks. However, such CSRs are challenging to directly observe, requiring therefore estimation.

Prospectively, estimation would require a cohort of cases, i.e. individuals with laboratory-confirmed influenza to be followed up over time. However, a representative sample of those who are infected is almost impossible to recruit, particularly as infections that are asymptomatic are less likely to be observed in health-care data than symptomatic infections. Even if it were possible, prospective estimation would have to account appropriately for censoring, as the end points of interest might take time to occur.

For retrospective estimation, censoring may not be an issue; however, differential probabilities of observing cases at different levels of severity (ascertainment/detection probabilities) may lead to biases [23]. "Multiplier" methods [26–28] therefore have been proposed when individual-level survival-type data are not available, combining aggregate case numbers at different levels of severity, for example. surveillance data on sero-prevalence (i.e., the proportion of blood samples testing positive for influenza), general practice [GP] consultations for influenza-like-illness [ILI]; hospital/ICU admissions, and mortality to obtain esti-

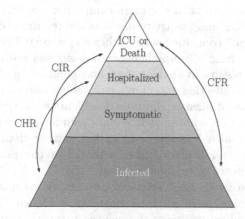

FIGURE 24.1
Severity of influenza as a "pyramid": infected individuals progress from asymptomatic infection ("I") to symptomatic infection ("S"), hospitalization ("H"), intensive care unit (ICU)-admission ("ICU") and/or death ("D"). Case-severity risks, that is, the case-hospitalization (CHR), case-ICU-admission (CIR), and case-fatality (CFR) risks, are defined as probabilities of a severe event given infection.

mates of the CSRs. These methods account for the ascertainment/detection biases suffered by aggregate surveillance data through multiplication by inverse proportions detected with informal uncertainty quantification using Monte Carlo forward simulation (e.g., [26, 27]).

Hybrid methods that combine hierarchical models with multiplier methods in different stages have appeared recently [28]. However, multiplier methods to estimate severity were first formalized using Bayesian evidence synthesis to simultaneously account for uncertainty, prior information on some ascertainment/detection biases, and censoring [15, 29, 30]. The uncertainty inherent in each data source, together with prior uncertainty, is propagated formally through to posterior estimates of the CSRs. The estimated CSRs are derived as products of probabilities of being at one severity level conditional on being at lower severity level (Figure 24.1).

Such an evidence synthesis is presented in [15], for the A/H1N1 pandemic in the UK during each of three waves experienced in summer 2009, the 2009/2010, and 2010/2011 seasons. The available data sources include (1) cross-sectional sero-prevalence data from laboratory-tested residual sera from patients after diagnostic testing for various (non-respiratory) conditions—these data, over time, inform changes in the proportion of the population exposed to influenza strains (i.e., the population level of immunity, and hence indirectly inform incidence), (2) estimates of numbers symptomatic based on potentially underascertained GP consultations for "influenza-like-illness" (ILI) and corresponding data on the proportion of nasopharyngeal swabs from individuals with ILI that test virologically positive for the A/H1N1pdm strain, (3) underascertained retrospective and prospective daily hospital admissions from 129 hospital trusts in the first two waves, and a sentinel set of 23 trusts in the third wave (Figure 24.2a), and (4) underascertained numbers of deaths occurring in individuals with confirmed A/H1N1 infection (Figure 24.2b). Each source poses a number of challenges in addition to the above-mentioned ascertainment/detection biases. The sero-prevalence data, although available for all three waves, in the second and third waves does not allow separation of individuals with antibodies in response to vaccination from infected individuals. Point estimates of the number symptomatic from the Health Protection Agency (HPA) are only available in the first two waves, with an informal "uncertainty range" from sensitivity analyses. For the third wave, such estimates are instead obtained from a joint regression model of the GP ILI and virological positivity data based on a much smaller sentinel set of general practices than the more comprehensive sentinel system used in the first two waves. Both the GP and positivity datasets are required to disentangle ILI consultations due to "background" consultations for other respiratory illness from actual influenza consultations. The switch from a comprehensive to a sentinel hospital system between the second and third waves results in sparser data and changes in the age groups recorded (Figure 24.3), particularly affecting the number of severe outcomes (ICU admissions and deaths) reported in the hospitalization data: no deaths are observed in the third wave. This sparsity requires the use of an additional ICU data source, which poses its own challenge. The system measures prevalent cases present in ICU rather than incident or cumulative incident ICU admissions, and hence requires a model of the process of admissions and discharges to obtain estimates of cumulative admissions.

None of the data sources on their own can provide an estimate of all CSRs of interest. However, by combining them all in a Bayesian evidence synthesis, the challenges just described can be resolved to derive the necessary severity estimates, as presented in Section 24.4.

24.2.2   Transmission

Understanding the dynamics of an infectious disease amounts to estimation of the rate at which it spreads and the factors that are contributing to its spread. To acquire such

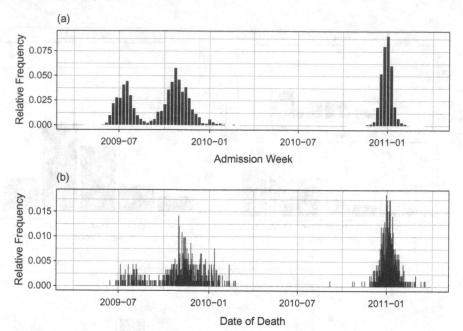

FIGURE 24.2
Frequency of observed severe events relative to the total number of events over the period April 2009-March 2011 of the three waves of infection among individuals with confirmed A/H1N1 pandemic influenza: (a) weekly hospitalizations by admission week; and (b) deaths by date of death.

knowledge, mechanistic transmission models are used [1], expressed by differential equations describing the disease dynamics resulting from the interaction between individuals at different disease stages. For example, in the susceptible-infectious-recovered (SIR) model new infections are generated through the contact between susceptible and infectious individuals (i.e., in state S and I, respectively). For influenza, and other respiratory infections, the relevant contact is between different age groups, since school-age children and their interactions with other children and with adults are known to be key drivers of transmission [31]. Historically, studies of influenza transmission have been carried out either by simulation [2] or by estimating the parameters of transmission models using direct information from a single time series of disease endpoints, such as confirmed cases (e.g., [31]).

However, in recent years the need and potential of combining data from multiple sources to infer latent characteristics of epidemics has been increasingly recognized. For influenza, in particular, since the 2009 A/H1N1 influenza pandemic, this recognition resulted in the development of a number of transmission models using data from either multiple surveillance time series (e.g., [20, 21, 32–35]) or a combination of surveillance and phylogenetic data (e.g., [36–38]). The integration of different sources of evidence can ensure identification of interpretable parameters in transmission models and a more comprehensive description of the evolution of an outbreak [22].

An example is given in [20] where, in the absence of a complete time series of confirmed influenza cases, various data sources are used to estimate retrospectively transmission during the first two waves of pandemic A/H1N1 influenza infection. Figure 24.4 shows the data for the London region: (a) GP consultations for ILI from May to December 2009, (b) a series of cross-sectional samples from sero-prevalence surveys (see Section 24.2.1),

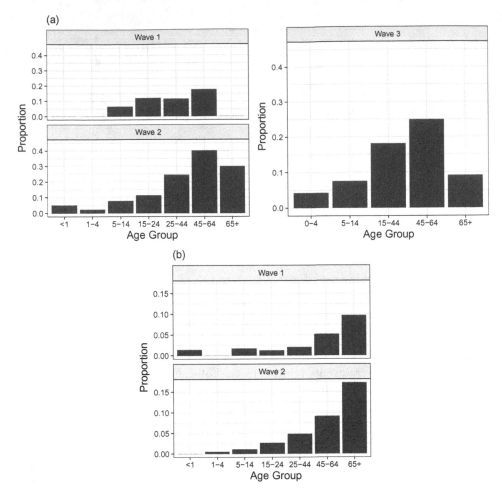

FIGURE 24.3
Proportion of observed individuals hospitalized with confirmed A/H1N1 pandemic influenza
who experienced severe events during the three waves of infection: (a) ICU admissions per
confirmed A/H1N1 hospitalization by age and wave and (b) deaths per confirmed A/H1N1
hospitalization by age and wave.

(c) virological data on nasopharyngeal positivity for A/H1N1 (again as in Section 24.2.1),
and (d) a limited time series of confirmed cases in the first few weeks of the outbreak, up
till June 2009, when contact tracing ceased. As in Section 24.2.1, GP consultation data are
contaminated by individuals experiencing non-A/H1N1-related ILI, whose health-care seeking behavior is highly influenced by governmental advice and media reporting. To reconstruct the underlying pattern of A/H1N1 infections, GP data had to be combined with
information on A/H1N1 virological positivity, on population immunity from the serological
surveys, knowledge on the natural history of A/H1N1, including the probability of developing symptoms and data on the propensity of patients with symptomatic infections to
consult a GP [39].

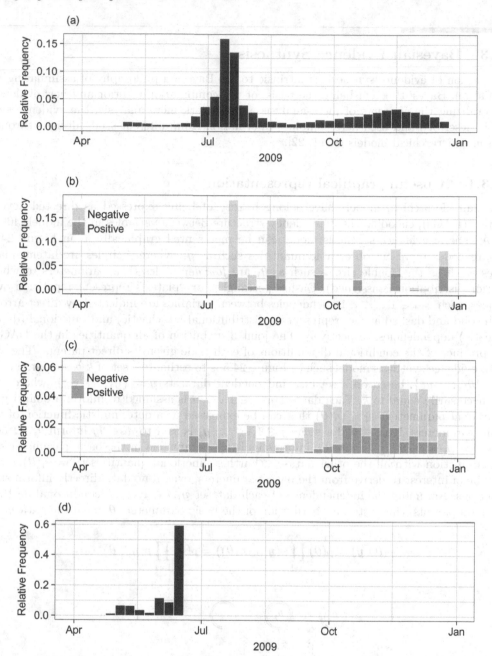

FIGURE 24.4
Four data streams used in the transmission model of [20]: (a) GP ILI consultations, (b) serological positivity, (c) virological positivity, and (d) confirmed cases. Each plot shows the frequency of events, (consultations per 100,000 population, positive and negative sera samples, positive and negative swabs, confirmed cases, respectively) relative to the total number of respective events over the period April 2009-December 2009 of the first two waves of infection.

24.3   Bayesian Evidence Synthesis

The notion of evidence synthesis is intrinsic to the Bayesian philosophy of assimilating information, Bayes' theorem being the basis for the combination of prior and new evidence. Generalizing the concepts of meta-analysis and network meta-analysis, the evidence synthesis described and used here combines information from different study designs through complex hierarchical models [8, 11, 22].

24.3.1   A useful graphical representation

Bayesian hierarchical models have a long history of being expressed as directed acyclic graphs (DAGs), encoding the dependency structure between variables in the model [40].

A generic evidence synthesis model can be represented graphically as in Figure 24.5. Square nodes represent observable quantities such as $\boldsymbol{y}_i$, whereas circles are latent quantities, such as ψ_i. Double circles such as θ_j are *founder* nodes (i.e., parameters to which a prior distribution is assigned). Dashed rectangles, or "plates," represent repetition over indices, such as $i \in 1, \ldots, n$. Dependencies between variables are indicated by direct arrows with solid and dashed arrows representing distributional (stochastic) and functional (deterministic) dependencies, respectively. The joint distribution of all quantities in the DAG is the product of the conditional distributions of each node given its direct parents. The aim of an evidence synthesis model such as Figure 24.5 is to estimate a set of k *basic* parameters $\boldsymbol{\theta} = \{\theta_1, \ldots, \theta_k\}$, based on a set of n independent datasets $\boldsymbol{y} = \{\boldsymbol{y}_1, \ldots, \boldsymbol{y}_n\}$, where n is not necessarily equal to k. Each dataset $\boldsymbol{y}_i, i \in 1, \ldots, n$ is assumed to inform a quantity (a *functional* parameter) $\psi_i = \psi_i(\boldsymbol{\theta})$ that can be expressed as a deterministic function of the basic parameters. If $\psi_i \equiv \theta_j$ for some $j \in 1, \ldots, k$, $\boldsymbol{y}_i$ is said to *directly* inform θ_j. Otherwise, for $\psi_i = \psi_i(\boldsymbol{\theta})$, $\boldsymbol{y}_i$ *indirectly* informs multiple parameters in the basic parameter set, in conjunction with all the other datasets. Further functional quantities $\psi_i = \psi_i(\boldsymbol{\theta}), i > n$ may be of interest to derive from the basic parameters, even if no data directly inform such functions. Assuming the independence of each dataset $\boldsymbol{y}_i, i \in 1, \ldots, n$ conditional on their common parents, the posterior distribution of the basic parameters $\boldsymbol{\theta}$ given the data $\boldsymbol{y}$ is

$$p(\boldsymbol{\theta} \mid \boldsymbol{y}) \propto p(\boldsymbol{\theta}) \prod_{i=1}^{n} p(\boldsymbol{y}_i \mid \psi_i(\boldsymbol{\theta})) = p(\boldsymbol{\theta}) \prod_{i=1}^{n} p(\boldsymbol{y}_i \mid \boldsymbol{\theta}).$$

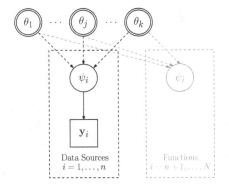

FIGURE 24.5
DAG of a generic evidence synthesis model.

Such an evidence synthesis model and DAG can clearly be extended both horizontally (more datasets) and vertically (hierarchical modelling).

Many evidence synthesis models used in the epidemic literature can be usefully represented graphically by DAGs [35, 41, 42]. Figure 24.6 is a generic DAG representation of a population-level multi-state disease transmission model where the vector-valued $\boldsymbol{X}(t) = (X_1(t), \ldots, X_K(t))$ corresponds to either the number or proportion of the population in each disease state $1, \ldots, K$ at time t. Movement between states is governed by transition rates $\boldsymbol{\lambda}(t)$, which are parameterized in terms of a collection of unknown basic parameters $\boldsymbol{\theta}(t)$, and the current state of the system $\boldsymbol{X}(t)$. If transmission is not explicitly modeled, the dependence of $\boldsymbol{\lambda}(t)$ on the states $\boldsymbol{X}(t)$, represented by the dashed arrow from $\boldsymbol{X}(t)$ to $\boldsymbol{\lambda}(t)$, is removed, and the model simplifies to a standard linear multi-state model. Typically, the $\boldsymbol{X}(t)$ and $\boldsymbol{\lambda}(t)$ are not directly observed. Instead, as in the simpler case of Figure 24.5, observations $\boldsymbol{y}_{t,i}, i = 1, \ldots, n_t$ are available at time t, with each $\boldsymbol{y}_{t,i}$ informing a functional parameter $\boldsymbol{\psi}_{t,i} = \boldsymbol{\psi}_{t,i}(\boldsymbol{X}(t), \boldsymbol{\lambda}(t)$. These relationships may be stochastic dependencies, or more usually, deterministic functions. Again assuming that the $\boldsymbol{y}_{t,i}$ for $i = 1, \ldots, n_t$ are independent conditional on their common parents, the likelihood of the data $\boldsymbol{y}_t = (\boldsymbol{y}_{t,i}, i = 1, \ldots, n_t)$ at time t is expressed as the product

$$L(\boldsymbol{y_t} \mid \boldsymbol{X}(t), \boldsymbol{\lambda}(t)) = \prod_{i=1}^{n_t} L(\boldsymbol{y}_{t,i} \mid \boldsymbol{\psi}_{t,i}(\boldsymbol{X}(t), \boldsymbol{\lambda}(t))).$$

When the data are also conditionally independent over time, the likelihood of all the data $\boldsymbol{y} = (\boldsymbol{y}_{0,1}, \ldots, \boldsymbol{y}_{t,n_t})$ given the basic parameters $\boldsymbol{\theta} = (\boldsymbol{\theta}_0, \ldots, \boldsymbol{\theta}_t, \ldots)$ is

$$L(\boldsymbol{y} \mid \boldsymbol{\theta}) = \prod_t \prod_{i=1}^{n_t} L(\boldsymbol{y}_{t,i} \mid \boldsymbol{\psi}_{t,i}(\boldsymbol{X}(t), \boldsymbol{\lambda}(t))) = \prod_t \prod_{i=1}^{n_t} L(\boldsymbol{y}_{t,i} \mid \boldsymbol{\theta}_t).$$

The posterior distribution of $\boldsymbol{\theta}$ given the data is then $p(\boldsymbol{\theta} \mid \boldsymbol{y}) \propto L(\boldsymbol{y} \mid \boldsymbol{\theta})p(\boldsymbol{\theta})$. Note that given the posterior distribution of the basic parameters and/or the states and transition rates, any function $\psi(\boldsymbol{\theta}, \boldsymbol{\lambda}, \boldsymbol{X})$, even if not directly observed, can be derived.

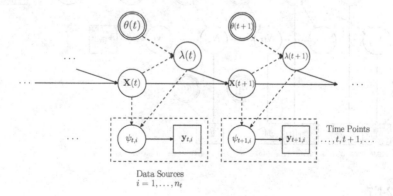

FIGURE 24.6
DAG of a multi-state model representing a transmission model embedded in an evidence synthesis.

24.4   Cross-Sectional Estimation: Severity

Static, cross-sectional models to estimate prevalence or cumulative incidence of (perhaps severe) disease are particular cases of the model in Figure 24.6. The influenza severity estimation of [15] can be seen as three cross-sectional analyses, one for each wave of infection, where severity is expressed in terms of ratios of cumulative incidence of infection at different levels of severity (Figure 24.1). The model is also stratified by age group $a \in \{< 1, 1-4, 5-14, 15-24, 25-44, 45-64, 65+\}$. The three timepoints $t \in \{0, 1, 2\}$ are not completely independent, as they share some parameters.

24.4.1   Model specification

24.4.1.1   First and second waves

Figure 24.7 displays the DAG corresponding to the first wave of infection, in summer 2009 ($t = 0$ in the notation of Figure 24.6). The disease states $\boldsymbol{X}(0)$ correspond to the numbers N_l of infections at each severity level $l = \{I,S,H,ICU,D\}$ (Figure 24.1). Note that age and wave/time indices have been omitted in the DAG and what follows, for brevity.

Functional parameters Ideally, we would assume a nested binomial structure for the states $N_l \sim \mathrm{Binomial}(N_m, p_{l|m})$ for a severity level m lower than l and for conditional probability $p_{l|m}$ of being a case at level l given infection at level m. However, for computational reasons, we instead assume a mean parameterization such that generically, the states N_l are deterministic functions

$$N_l = \lfloor p_{l|m} N_m \rfloor$$

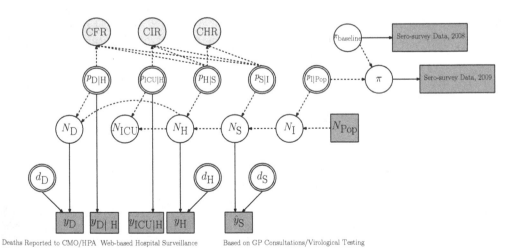

FIGURE 24.7
DAG representing the first wave of A/H1N1 pandemic influenza infection. (Adapted from Presanis et al. [15])

of the number N_m of infections at a lower level m of severity and the conditional probability $p_{l|m}$ of being a case at level l given infection at level m. The total population N_{Pop} is considered fixed. The CSRs of interest (i.e., the CHR, CIR, and CFR risks (Figure 24.1)), are products of component conditional probabilities:

$$\text{CHR} = p_{\text{H|I}} = p_{\text{H|S}} \times p_{\text{S|I}}$$
$$\text{CIR} = p_{\text{ICU|I}} = p_{\text{ICU|H}} \times \text{CHR}$$
$$\text{CFR} = p_{\text{D|I}} = p_{\text{D|H}} \times \text{CHR}.$$

The functional parameters ψ of Figure 24.6 are defined as the set $\psi = \{N_l, l \in \{\text{I,S,H,ICU,D}\}\}$ $\cup$ {CHR, CIR, CFR} of states and the corresponding CSRs.

Observational model The observations, $y_i, i = 1, \ldots, n$, where $n = 7$ per age group, are either reported numbers of infections at different levels of severity ($\hat{y}_\text{S}, y_\text{H}, y_\text{D}$ in Figure 24.7), reported numbers of hospitalizations that lead to severe events ($y_{\text{ICU|H}}, y_{\text{D|H}}$), or the cross-sectional sero-prevalence data before and after the first wave. Each observation is a realization of a binomial distribution with probability parameters representing either a detection probability d_l with size parameter the counts of the numbers of infections N_l at levels $l \in \{\text{S,H,D}\}$; a conditional probability $p_{\text{ICU|H}}$ or $p_{\text{D|H}}$ with size parameter the subset of observed hospitalizations y_H where the final outcome $y_{\text{ICU|H}}$ or $y_{\text{D|H}}$ or discharge was observed; or a sero-prevalence, either before the first wave (π_{baseline}) or after the first wave (π), with size parameter the number of sera samples tested. The latter sero-prevalence data inform, indirectly, the infection attack rate $p_{\text{I|Pop}}$ via their difference.

Basic parameters The basic parameters $\boldsymbol{\theta}$ of Figure 24.6 are the set $\boldsymbol{\theta} = \{p_{l|m}, l, m \in \{\text{I,S,H,ICU,D}\}\} \cup \{d_l, l \in \{\text{S,H,D}\}\}$ of conditional and detection probabilities in Figure 24.7. Each probability is given an independent flat prior, apart from the symptomatic CHR risk $p_{\text{H|S}}$ which is assigned an informative prior based on external data.

The second wave model is similar to that of the first wave excluding only the sero-prevalence data due to the challenges of disentangling vaccinated cases from true infections in the sero-samples in the absence of good data on vaccination in the dataset.

24.4.1.2 Third wave

The third wave model differs more substantially (Figure 24.8). Estimates of the number of symptomatic infections were derived from a joint Bayesian model of the GP consultation and virological positivity data from the smaller sentinel system, regressed on age group and time. This sub-model was fitted at a first stage, accounting for the probability of consulting a GP-given symptoms, and giving posterior mean (sd) estimates $\hat{y}_\text{S}$ ($\hat{\sigma}_\text{S}$) on a log scale. In contrast to the first two waves, these estimates are not considered underascertained. They are therefore incorporated in the third wave model, at a second stage, by a likelihood term, assuming $\hat{y}_\text{S} \sim \text{normal}(\log(N_\text{S}), \hat{\sigma}_\text{S})$. Finally, since the hospitalization data in the third wave (Figures 24.2 and 24.3) are sparse, they lead to uncertain and underascertained estimates of the numbers hospitalized and the proportion of hospitalizations leading to ICU admission. Extra prevalence-type data on the number $N_{t,\text{ILIC}}$ of suspected ILI cases present in all ICUs in the UK are therefore incorporated, through a sub-model for these data that assumes entrances at rate λ_t and exits at rate μ to/from ICU form an immigration-death stochastic process [15] (Figure 24.9). Note that this ICU sub-model is another example of a multi-state model as in Figure 24.6, where the state is $N_{t,\text{ILIC}}$. Since the observations are of ILI

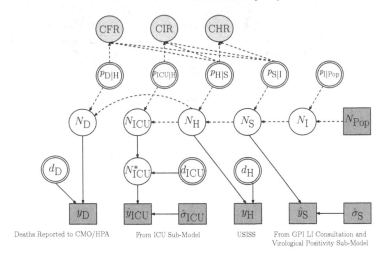

FIGURE 24.8
DAG representing the third wave of A/H1N1 pandemic influenza infection. (Adapted from
Presanis et al. [15])

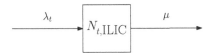

FIGURE 24.9
Immigration-death process model for ILI cases in ICU. λ_t is the daily rate of admissions
to ICU, $N_{t,\mathrm{ILIC}}$ the number of ILI cases present in ICU on day t, and μ the rate of exit
(discharges or deaths), so that the expected length of stay in ICU is $1/\mu$.

rather than confirmed influenza, estimates of the ILI admission rate λ_t are combined with
virological positivity data from secondary care to obtain estimates of the cumulative number
y_{ICU} of new ICU admissions for A/H1N1 influenza. The posterior mean (sd) estimates $\hat{y}_{\mathrm{ICU}}$
($\hat{\sigma}_{\mathrm{ICU}}$) from this sub-model, on a log scale, then are incorporated in the third wave model
by a contribution to the likelihood:

$$\hat{y}_{\mathrm{ICU}} \sim \mathrm{Normal}(\log(N_{\mathrm{ICU}}^*), \hat{\sigma}_{\mathrm{ICU}}) \tag{24.1}$$

where N_{ICU}^* is considered a lower bound for the total number of A/H1N1 ICU admissions,
N_{ICU}, since the prevalent ICU case data cover only a portion of the time period of the third
wave. This lower bound is implemented through a binomial assumption

$$N_{\mathrm{ICU}}^* \sim \mathrm{Binomial}(N_{\mathrm{ICU}}, d_{\mathrm{ICU}})$$

with probability parameter representing a detection probability d_{ICU}.

In contrast to the first two waves, priors for the conditional probabilities $p_{t=3,l|m}$ were
expressed hierarchically by centering these probabilities, on a logit scale, on their respective
second wave versions, $p_{t=2,l|m}$.

24.4.2 Results

Figure 24.10 and the left-hand side of Figure 24.11 give posterior summaries of the symptomatic CFR (sCFR = $p_{D|S}$), CFR and number of symptomatic infections N_S, by age and wave. Note that for the first two waves of infection, the model giving these results assumes that the HPA-provided estimates of N_S are underestimates, with detection probability d_S.

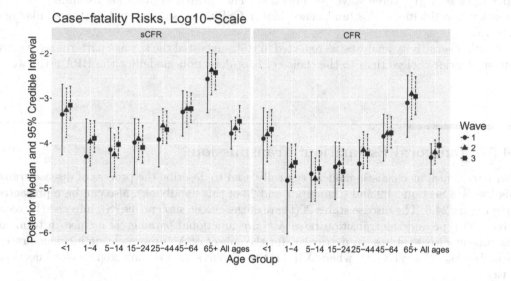

FIGURE 24.10
Posterior median and 95 percent credible intervals of symptomatic CFR and CFR by wave and age group, log-scale.

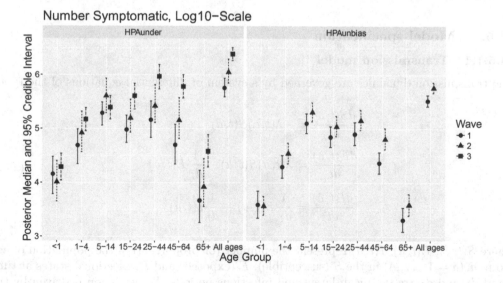

FIGURE 24.11
Left: Posterior median and 95 percent credible intervals of number of symptomatic infections by wave and age group, log-scale. Right: Same posterior summaries but for a sensitivity analysis assuming $d_S = 1$.

In [15], discussion of the assumptions about the potential under-estimation in HPA estimates of the number symptomatic led to a number of sensitivity analyses. An initial unpublished sensitivity analysis assumed the HPA estimates were unbiased, i.e., $d_S = 1$, giving the posterior estimates of N_S on the right-hand side of Figure 24.11 for waves 1 and 2 only.

Notable patterns include the "u"-shaped age distribution of the case-fatality risks and corresponding "n"-shaped age distribution of symptomatic cases; and an age shift towards older ages over the three waves of infection. The sensitivity analysis assuming $d_S = 1$ gives lower estimates of N_S (and hence higher CSRs, not shown), but with a similar age pattern.

Further sensitivity analyses, as reported in [15], suggested the key age patterns were more robust to prior choices than to the choice of bias/detection model for the HPA estimates.

24.5   Temporal Estimation: Transmission

Compartmental mechanistic models, typically used to describe the process of disease transmission (see Section 24.2 and Chapters 7 and 23 of this handbook), also can be represented as in Figure 24.6. The disease states $X(t)$ are of the classic susceptible (S), infected (I), recovered (R) type and the transition rates $\lambda(t)$ are functional parameters defined in terms of the current disease states. In particular, for the subset of $\lambda(t)$ representing incidence rates, we define $\lambda_{\text{Inc}}(t) = f(X_I(t))$ where $X_I(t)$ is the current size of the infected and/or infectious states.

In [20], the transmission of a novel pandemic A/H1N1 influenza strain among a fixed population stratified into A age groups is estimated through the combination of a deterministic age-structured transmission model with disease and reporting models, describing disease transmission, progression, and health-care seeking behavior of infected individuals, respectively.

24.5.1   Model specification

24.5.1.1   Transmission model

The transmission dynamics are governed by a system of differential equations of the type:

$$\frac{dS(t,a)}{dt} = -\lambda(t,a)S(t,a)$$

$$\frac{dE(t,a)}{dt} = \lambda(t,a)S(t,a) - \frac{1}{d_L}E(t,a) \qquad (24.2)$$

$$\frac{dI(t,a)}{dt} = \frac{1}{d_L}E(t,a) - \frac{1}{d_I}I(t,a)$$

where $S(t,a)$, $E(t,a)$, $I(t,a)$ represent the number (or proportion) of the population of age group $a, (a = 1, \ldots, A)$ in the S (susceptible), E (exposed) and I (infectious) states at time t and d_L and d_I are the mean latent and infectious periods. Transmission is driven by the time- and age-varying rate $\lambda(t,a)$ at which susceptible individuals become infected. The system in (24.2) is evaluated using an Euler approximation at times $t_k = k\delta t, k = 0, \ldots, K$, where the choice of $\delta t = 0.5$ days is sufficiently small that the probability of more than one change of state per period is negligible. Under this discretization, at time t_k the vector

$(S_{t_k,a}, E_{t_k,a}, I_{t_k,a})$ gives the number of individuals in each state with the number of new infections in $[t_{k-1}, t_k)$ being $\Delta_{t_k,a} = \lambda_{t_{k-1},a} S_{t_{k-1},a}$, where

$$\lambda_{t_k,a} = 1 - \prod_{b=1}^{A} \left\{ \left(1 - M_{t_k}^{(a,b)} R_0(\phi)/d_I \right)^{I_{t_k,b}} \right\} \delta t. \tag{24.3}$$

Here R_0 is the basic reproduction number, the expected number of secondary infections caused by a single primary infection in a fully susceptible population, often parameterized in terms of the epidemic growth rate ϕ [43]; and the time-varying mixing matrices $\boldsymbol{M}_{t_k}$, express the pattern of transmission between age groups, with the generic entry $M_{t_k}^{(a,b)}$ being the relative rate of effective contacts between individuals of each pair of age groups (a, b) at time t_k. The quantity $1 - M_{t_k}^{(a,b)} R_0(\phi)/d_I$ gives the probability of an individual in age group a not being infected by an infectious individual in age group b in the interval $k+1$. When raised to the power of all the infectious individuals in group b, the probability of not being infected by any individual in group b is obtained. Taking the product over all age groups gives the probability of not being infected at all. This expression for $\lambda_{t_k,a}$ is known as the Reed-Frost formulation [44]. The initial conditions of the system are determined by parameter I_0, the total number of infectious individuals across all age groups at time t_0; an assumed equilibrium distribution of infections over the age groups; and an assumption of initial exponential growth that determines the relationship between the numbers in the four disease states. The mean latent period d_L is taken as known, whereas the mean infectious period d_I is a parameter to be estimated. Therefore, the dynamics of the transmission model (24.2) depend on the *basic* parameter vector $\boldsymbol{\theta}_T = (\phi, I_0, d_I, \boldsymbol{m})$, where $\boldsymbol{m}$ parameterize the mixing matrices $\boldsymbol{M}_{t_k}$. The transmission model is represented schematically in DAG format in Figure 24.12. The dependency on age has been omitted in the DAG and in what follows for brevity.

24.5.1.2 Disease progression and health-care seeking

The newly infected individuals Δ_{t_k}, following an incubation time, develop ILI symptoms with probability p_{Sym} (Figure 24.12). With probability p_C, the symptomatic cases are virologically confirmed through contact tracing or hospitalization in the early phase of the epidemic; and with time-varying probability $p_{t,G}$, symptomatic patients choose to contact a primary care practitioner (GP). These processes result in the (latent) number of symptomatic cases $N_{t_s,\text{Sym}}$, confirmed cases $N_{t_u,C}$, and GP consultations $N_{t_v,G}$, which can each be expressed as a convolution of the new infections Δ_{t_k} with the distribution of the time delay between infection and the relevant health-care event. For instance, the number $N_{t_v,\text{GP}}$ of GP consultations in the interval $[t_{v-1}, t_v)$ is

$$N_{t_v,\text{GP}} = p_{\text{Sym}} p_{t_v,G} \sum_{k=0}^{v} \Delta_{t_k} f(v-k) \tag{24.4}$$

where the (discretized) delay probability mass function $f(\cdot)$ accounts for the time from infection to symptoms and the time from symptoms to GP consultation. The disease progression component of the model is specified by *basic* parameters $\boldsymbol{\theta}_D = (p_{\text{Sym}}, p_C, p_{t_v,G})$ (Figure 24.12) and, from equation (24.4), the quantities $N_{t_u,C}$ and $N_{t_v,G}$ are complex functions of both $\boldsymbol{\theta}_T$ and $\boldsymbol{\theta}_D$.

24.5.1.3 Observational model

The goal here is to estimate the rate of infections $\lambda_{t_{k-1}}$ over time and predict the resulting burden on health-care facilities, through the estimation of the basic parameters $\boldsymbol{\theta} = \boldsymbol{\theta}_T \cup \boldsymbol{\theta}_D$

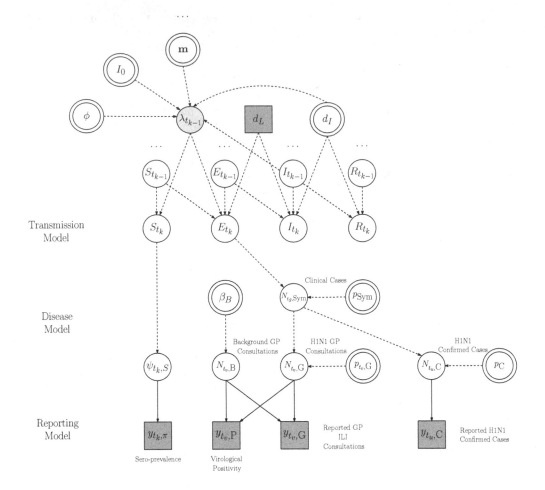

FIGURE 24.12
DAG representing the transmission model (From McDonald, S.A. et al., *BMC Infect. Dis.*, 14, 564, 2014.)

from observed data. As anticipated in Section 24.2.2, direct data on the number of new infections are not available. Therefore, a combination of a number of indirect evidence sources informing different aspects of the infection and disease processes needs to be used to estimate $\boldsymbol{\theta}$.

The observed data $\boldsymbol{y}_t = (y_{t_u,\mathrm{C}}, y_{t_v,\mathrm{G}}, y_{t_v,\mathrm{P}}, y_{t_k,\mathrm{S}})$ include $y_{t_u,\mathrm{C}}$, the counts of confirmed cases during the initial weeks of the outbreak (Figure 24.4d); $y_{t_v,\mathrm{G}}$, the number of primary care consultations for ILI, including the individuals attending for non-pandemic ILI (Figure 24.4a); $y_{t_v,\mathrm{P}}$, the complementary virological data on nasopharyngeal positivity for A/H1N1 (Figure 24.4c and Section 24.2.1); and $y_{t_k,\mathrm{S}}$, the cross-sectional sero-prevalence data (Figure 24.4b). Typically, there is some reporting delay between the disease diagnoses and their appearance in health-care surveillance, but for simplicity, here no such delay is assumed, so that $y_{t_i,i}$ is observed at the same time t_i as the disease endpoint $N_{t_i,i}$ for each i. Each item of data informs $\boldsymbol{\theta}$ through a probabilistic link.

More specifically, $y_{t_k,\mathrm{S}}$ is a realization of a binomial distribution,

$$y_{t_k,\mathrm{S}} \sim \mathrm{Binomial}\left(n_{t_k,\mathrm{S}}, \psi_{t_k,\mathrm{S}}\right),$$

with sample size $n_{t_k,\text{S}}$ and probability $\psi_{t_k,\text{S}} = 1 - \frac{S_{t_k}}{N}$. The sero-prevalence data $y_{t_k,\text{S}}$ therefore directly inform the number of susceptibles S_{t_k} and parameters $\boldsymbol{\theta}_T$ as $S_{t_k} = S_{t_k}(\boldsymbol{\theta}_T)$.

The counts of confirmed cases $y_{t_u,\text{C}}$ and ILI consultations $y_{t_v,\text{G}}$ are taken as realizations of negative binomial distributions, with means given by functional parameters $\psi_{t_u,\text{C}}$ and $\psi_{t_v,\text{G}}$, respectively, and time-varying over-dispersion parameter η_t,

$$y_{t_v,\text{G}} \sim \text{Negative Binomial}\left(\psi_{t_v,\text{G}}, \eta_{t_v}\right)$$

where

$$\psi_{t_u,\text{C}} = N_{t_u,\text{C}}$$

$$\psi_{t_v,\text{G}} = N_{t_v,\text{B}} + N_{t_v,\text{G}}$$

and are, therefore, functions defined by convolution equations of the type in (24.4).

To disentangle the GP ILI consultations due to the pandemic strain, $N_{t_v,\text{G}}$, from all other ILI consultations, $N_{t_v,\text{B}}$, information is needed on the proportion of all GP ILI consultations that result from the pandemic strain. This information is provided by virological positivity data, where observed positive samples $y_{t_v,\text{P}}$ are considered realizations of a binomial distribution,

$$y_{t_v,\text{P}} \sim \text{Binomial}\left(n_{t_v,\text{P}}, \psi_{t_v,\text{P}}\right),$$

with sample size (number of tests) $n_{t_v,\text{P}}$ and probability parameter $\psi_{t_v,\text{P}} = 1 - \frac{N_{t_v,\text{B}}}{N_{t_v,\text{B}}+N_{t_v,\text{G}}}$. The proportion positive, $\psi_{t_v,\text{P}}$, is expressed as a function of the disentangled counts $N_{t_v,\text{B}}$ and $N_{t_v,\text{G}}$. As in Section 24.4.1.2, the proportion positive $\psi_{t_v,\text{P}}$ and number of ILI consultations $\psi_{t_v,\text{G}}$ are jointly regressed on age and time, on logit and log scales, respectively. The background counts $N_{t_v,\text{B}}$ are therefore a function of the regression parameters $\boldsymbol{\beta}_B$ (Figure 24.12).

In each generic calendar time interval $[t_{j-1}, t_j]$, as indicated in Section 24.3.1, the likelihood of the data is the product

$$L(\boldsymbol{y}_{t_j} \mid \boldsymbol{\theta}) = \prod_{i \in \{\text{C,G,P,S}\}} L(y_{t_j,i} \mid \boldsymbol{\theta}) \tag{24.5}$$

of the contributions $L(y_{t_j,i} \mid \boldsymbol{\theta})$ of the four data streams, as these are considered to be independent conditional on their common parents. The posterior distribution then is obtained by combining the likelihood with the prior distribution $p(\boldsymbol{\theta})$.

24.5.2   Results

Figure 24.13 shows the posterior distribution for the number of new A/H1N1 infections by age group in London, revealing the two waves of infection in summer and autumn/winter 2009. The first wave of infection has a higher peak, whereas the second wave, particularly by age group, is spread over a longer period of time, resulting in a higher attack rate in the second wave. R_0 is estimated to be 1.65 (95% credible interval 1.56–1.75).

Figure 24.14 shows predictions forward in time based on the data up to days 83 and 192 of the epidemic, respectively. Note how the uncertainty in the predictions is progressively reduced as data accumulate.

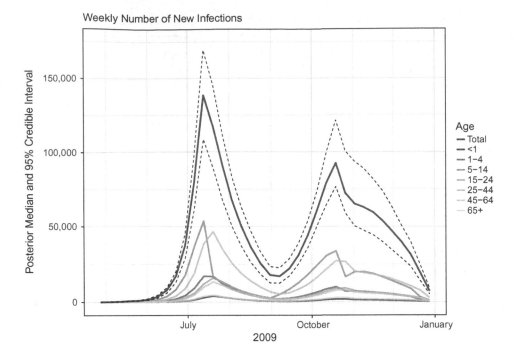

FIGURE 24.13
Posterior median (solid lines) and 95 percent credible interval (dashed) lines number of new
infections per week in London overall and by age group.

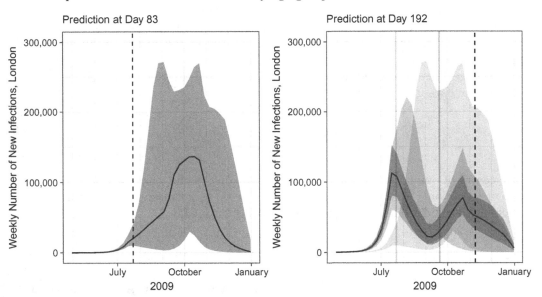

FIGURE 24.14
Predictions of the weekly number of new infections in London at days 83 and 192 of the
epidemic (vertical dashed lines): posterior median (black line) and 95 percent predictive
intervals (shaded areas). For the day 192 prediction, paler shaded areas represent the predictive intervals at two previous timepoints (days 83 and 143, respectively, shown by the
grey vertical lines).

24.6 Model Building, Inference and Criticism

The two influenza case studies just discussed, although relatively simple, have demonstrated how the combination of multiple sources can easily lead to complex probability models. This complexity can challenge standard inferential tools, motivating the development of novel approaches. In what follows, we continue to use the two influenza examples to illustrate such new approaches to model building, efficient inference, and model criticism.

24.6.1 Strategies for model building

There are two strategies to build a complex evidence synthesis model: (1) all the data are combined simultaneously, as in joint models (e.g., [45]); or (2) the model is assembled in stages, using subsets of the evidence initially, before combining the results in a second stage, as in standard meta-analysis [4]. When a model is complex, the latter strategy is sensible, to understand what might be inferred from each dataset in isolation. A staged approach is used in both the influenza examples of Sections 24.4 and 24.5. For example, in the severity model, a sub-model of a stochastic process describing entries to/exits from ICU is first fitted to the ICU prevalent case data in the third wave, before combining the results in the full evidence synthesis model. In the transmission model, a joint regression model of GP consultation and virological positivity data was fitted initially, before the results were incorporated in the transmission model to disentangle "background" non-influenza noise from the signal of influenza consultations.

To illustrate a two-stage process, we use the severity example. Figure 24.15 shows a simplified schematic DAG of the stages. In both the stage 1 and stage 2 models, the cumulative number of ICU admissions measured over the time period of the ICU prevalence data, N_I^*, has a prior model. The stage 1 prior is in terms of the parameters of the ICU entry/exit process, λ_t and μ; whereas the stage 2 prior is in terms of the parameters of the period-prevalence-type severity model (i.e., the conditional and detection probabilities described in Section 24.4).

The existence of two prior models poses the question of how to combine the two sources of information. In [15], the problem was solved using an approximate method, transferring

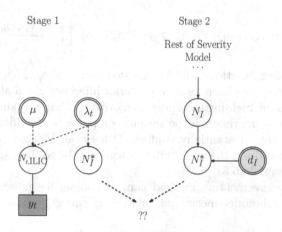

FIGURE 24.15
Two-stage modeling strategy for joining ICU sub-model with rest of severity model.

the posterior mean (sd) estimate of N_I^* from the stage 1 ICU sub-model to the stage 2 severity model by a likelihood term (equation (24.1) and Figure 24.8), such that the posterior of $\log(N_I^*)$ from the ICU sub-model is approximated by a normal distribution. This approximate approach is acceptable when the approximation is good (i.e., when the sample size in the stage 1 model is large enough to guarantee a Gaussian posterior distribution). If not, then in [46], an alternative, more general, exact method for joining (and splitting) models, "Markov melding," is proposed.

In general terms, suppose we have M probability submodels $p_m(\phi, \psi_m, Y_m)$, $m = 1, \ldots, M$, with parameters ϕ and ψ_m and observable random variables Y_m. Suppose further that ϕ is common to all modules, acting as a "link" between the submodels, and that the aim is to combine all modules into a single model $p_{comb}(\phi, \psi_1, \ldots, \psi_M, Y_1, \ldots, Y_M)$, so that the posterior distribution for the link parameter (ϕ) and the submodel-specific parameters ψ_m reflects all information and uncertainty. In some cases, such model joining is readily achievable using standard hierarchical modeling constructs. However, there are some contexts where this joining is not straightforward, in particular where (1) some sub-models may not be expressible conditional on the link parameter ϕ, particularly if ϕ is a non-invertible deterministic function of other parameters in a sub-model and (2) the prior marginal distributions $p_m(\phi)$ for ϕ differ in different submodels. Both of these situations arise in the severity estimation of Section 24.4 and Figure 24.15, where the link parameter ϕ is the cumulative number of ICU admissions N_I^*.

Markov melding [46] addresses model joining in these contexts by building on Markov combination [47–49] and Bayesian melding [50] ideas. Markov combination allows joining of sub-models under the restrictive constraint that the prior marginals $p_m(\phi)$ are identical for each m (i.e., the submodels $p_m(\phi, \psi_m, Y_m)$, $m = 1, \ldots, M$ are *consistent* in the link parameter ϕ: $p_m(\phi) = p(\phi)$ for all m). In practice, however, the marginal distributions $p_m(\phi)$ are usually *not* exactly identical, as in Figure 24.15. Markov melding therefore exploits the Bayesian melding approach [50] to replace each marginal with a pooled marginal distribution

$$p_{pool}(\phi) = g(p_1(\phi), \ldots, p_M(\phi)),$$

where g is a pooling function chosen such that $\int g(\phi)\, d\phi = 1$ and $p_{pool}(\phi)$ is an appropriate summary of the individual marginals. Since each replaced model is now consistent in ϕ, the Markov melded model can be obtained by a Markov combination of the replaced models:

$$p_{MM}(\phi, \psi_1, \ldots, \psi_M, Y_1, \ldots, Y_M) = p_{pool}(\phi) \prod_{m=1}^{M} \frac{p_m(\phi, \psi_m, Y_m)}{p_m(\phi)}.$$

Different possible pooling functions g for the melded marginal $p_{pool}(\phi)$ are discussed in [46]. After the new model p_{MM} has been formed, posterior inference given all the data $y_1, \ldots, y_M$ can be performed. Markov melding incorporates more data than any single submodel, and so will provide more precise inferences if the various components of evidence (priors and data) in each submodel do not substantially conflict. Otherwise, Markov melding may be misleading, so, before proceeding, the underlying reasons for the conflict should be investigated and resolved (see Section 24.6.3).

Note that the Markov melding method can, of course, be generalized to the case of multivariate link and submodel-specific parameters, $\boldsymbol{\phi}$ and $\boldsymbol{\psi}_m$ [46].

24.6.1.1   Markov melding in the influenza severity example

For the severity example, the use of Markov melding on the ICU and severity sub-model implied priors (Figure 24.16) results in greater posterior precision under different pooling

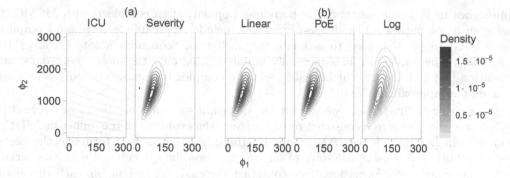

FIGURE 24.16

(a,b) Pooled prior marginal distributions under different pooling functions for the ICU and severity sub-models.

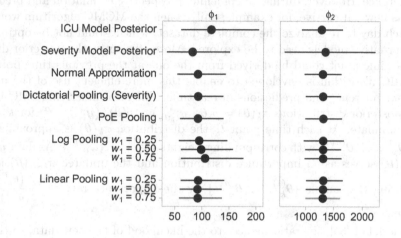

FIGURE 24.17

Posterior distributions (medians and 95% credible intervals) for the ICU and severity model parameters under the Markov melded model with different pooling functions in comparison to the separate sub-model posterior distributions.

functions, in comparison to both the sub-model posteriors alone and the normal approximation employed in [15] (Figure 24.17).

24.6.2 Computationally efficient inference

Markov chain Monte Carlo (MCMC) methods [51] have become standard tools in Bayesian inference to sample from posterior distributions. This sampling, in cross-sectional estimation problems of the type in Section 24.4 (e.g., [13]), can feasibly be carried out using available software implementing MCMC (e.g., [52]). On the other hand, inference for more complex models, such as transmission models similar to that of Section 24.5 (e.g., [21]), requires bespoke code and a tailored MCMC algorithm. However, classical MCMC often is not a computationally viable option in stochastic transmission models when the data structure is complex (e.g., [34]) and can become computationally inefficient even in inference for deterministic models, when inferences are required within a restricted time frame. Alternative approaches to Bayesian inference are becoming popular, often combined with MCMC, to tackle such computational challenges. Examples include Approximate Bayesian Computation (ABC) (e.g., [37]), used to estimate the likelihood; Sequential Monte Carlo (SMC) (e.g., [53]), where inference is sequentially updated using only the most recent data; and emulation [54] and history matching [55], where a complex transmission model is replaced by a simpler approximate model.

As a concrete illustration, we re-visit the deterministic transmission model of Section 24.5, where the goal is to reconstruct retrospectively the evolution of the influenza A/H1N1 epidemic. In [20], an adaptive Metropolis Hasting algorithm is used to derive the posterior distribution of $\boldsymbol{\theta}$ using 245 days of GP consultation data, combined with the various additional sources of information. To reconstruct the epidemic in London, each run of the MCMC algorithm requires around 7×10^5 iterations to reach convergence, taking more than 4 hours for a single MCMC chain The bottleneck is the evaluation of the likelihood in equation (24.5), which involves calculation of the computationally expensive convolutions in equation (24.4). This time is an acceptable computational burden in the case of retrospective inference. However, during an epidemic, prospective estimation and prediction will be needed as new data arrive, for example, daily. Then the MCMC algorithm would have to be rerun each day to re-analyze the complete dataset, which would not be optimal, particularly if alternative models need to be explored. More efficiently, the posterior distribution at each new time point could be derived from the one at the previous time point. In [35], a hybrid SMC algorithm is developed to enable this more efficient use of the information and carry out inference and predictions in real time. The idea underlying SMC is to derive sequential posterior distributions $\pi_k(\boldsymbol{\theta}) = p(\boldsymbol{\theta} \mid \boldsymbol{y}_{t_1:t_k}) \propto p(\boldsymbol{\theta})L(\boldsymbol{y}_{t_1:t_k} \mid \boldsymbol{\theta})$ for $k = 1, \ldots, K$ as data accumulate. At each time point t_k the distribution $\pi_k(\boldsymbol{\theta})$ is approximated by n_k particles $\{\boldsymbol{\theta}_k^{(1)}, \ldots, \boldsymbol{\theta}_k^{(n_k)}\}$ with corresponding weights $\{\omega_k^{(1)}, \ldots, \omega_k^{(n_k)}\}$. As data $\boldsymbol{y}_{t_{k+1}}$ arrive at t_{k+1}, $\pi_k(\boldsymbol{\theta})$ serves as an importance distribution and the updated $\pi_{k+1}(\boldsymbol{\theta})$ is obtained by re-weighting the sample $\{\boldsymbol{\theta}_k^{(1)}, \ldots, \boldsymbol{\theta}_k^{(n_k)}\}$ by the importance ratios $\dfrac{\pi_{k+1}\left(\boldsymbol{\theta}_k^{(j)}\right)}{\pi_k\left(\boldsymbol{\theta}_k^{(j)}\right)}$ for each $j \in 1, \ldots, n_k$.

In the model of [35] this ratio reduces to the likelihood of the new data, so that the jth particle has weight

$$\omega_{k+1}^j \propto \omega_k^j \frac{\pi_{k+1}\left(\boldsymbol{\theta}_k^{(j)}\right)}{\pi_k\left(\boldsymbol{\theta}_k^{(j)}\right)} = \omega_k^j L(\boldsymbol{y}_{k+1} \mid \boldsymbol{\theta}_k^{(j)}).$$

This simple SMC scheme works well when the data follow a stable pattern, as demonstrated in settings where only one data stream is available (e.g., [56]). However, in the specific application of [35], the challenge is not particularly posed by the multiplicity of data, but rather by the sudden change in the pattern of health-seeking behavior produced by a public health intervention (see Figure 24.4a). Such a change introduces a shock to the system and complicates dramatically the tracking of the sequential distributions $\pi_k(\cdot)$ over time. On arrival of a particularly informative new batch of data $\boldsymbol{y}_{t_{k+1}}$, the sample $\{\boldsymbol{\theta}_k^{(1)}, \ldots, \boldsymbol{\theta}_k^{(n_k)}\}$ degenerates to the few particles consistent with the new information, which, carrying large weights, give a misleading estimate of $\pi_{k+1}(\cdot)$. The naive SMC algorithm then is adapted to handle these highly informative observations by introducing resampling and MCMC jittering steps [57] to rejuvenate the sample and by sequentially including only fractions of the new data to minimize the divergence between posterior distributions at consecutive times [58, 59]. The result is a hybrid semi-automatic SMC algorithm that is more computationally efficient than the original MCMC, is highly parallelizable, and can deal with sudden shocks in the observational patterns.

24.6.3 Model criticism: Conflict and influence

Model criticism is crucial to any analysis. However, specific to the context of multiple source evidence synthesis are the potential for conflicting evidence, with such conflicts needing to be detected, quantified, and resolved, and the critical assessment of what the role and influence of different sources is.

In the influenza severity example of Section 24.4, the initial sensitivity analysis shown on the right-hand side of Figure 24.11 did not include a detection probability d_S for the HPA estimates $\hat{y}_S$ of the number symptomatic (i.e., with $d_S = 1$). However, this "naive" model led to high posterior mean deviances, as shown in Table 24.1, for "data" $\hat{y}_S$ on a log scale for the first wave. By comparison, the model assuming the HPA estimates are underestimates has much lower posterior mean deviances and DIC contributions (Table 24.2). The lack of fit in the "naive" model motivated a closer look at the consistency of the different sources of evidence about the denominators, or infections at lower levels of severity (asymptomatic and symptomatic), resulting in both the sensitivity analyses of [15] and more formal conflict assessment in [60].

24.6.3.1 Conflict assessment methods

Bayesian predictive diagnostics (e.g., [61–64]) have been used for a long time in model assessment, comparing observations to predictions from the model. Posterior predictive

TABLE 24.1
Deviance Summaries for "data" on number symptomatic in first wave, log-scale, by age group, for the "naive" model: HPA estimate ($\hat{y}_S$) and corresponding standard deviation ($\hat{\sigma}_S$); posterior mean estimate (N_S) and corresponding 95 percent credible interval (CrI); posterior mean deviance contributions ($\overline{D}$); plug-in deviance at posterior mean of parameters ($D(\overline{\theta})$); effective number of parameters (p_D); deviance information criterion (DIC)

Age	$\hat{y}_S$	$\hat{\sigma}_S$	N_S	95% CrI		$\overline{D}$	$D(\overline{\theta})$	p_D	DIC
< 1	8.11	0.30	8.27	7.70	8.85	1.32	0.32	1.01	2.33
1-4	7.81	0.26	9.89	9.42	10.38	66.72	65.80	0.92	67.65
5-14	9.78	0.28	11.75	11.32	12.16	49.16	48.58	0.58	49.74
15-24	10.23	0.26	11.17	10.74	11.62	14.05	13.30	0.76	14.81
25-44	11.46	0.29	11.30	10.83	11.80	1.03	0.30	0.73	1.75
45-64	12.03	0.26	10.06	9.61	10.52	59.17	58.36	0.81	59.98
65+	11.25	0.27	7.62	7.12	8.15	175.41	174.49	0.92	176.33

TABLE 24.2
Deviance summaries for "data" on number symptomatic in first wave, log-scale, by age group, for the model assuming HPA estimates are under-estimates

Age	$\hat{y}_S$	$\hat{\sigma}_S$	N_S	95% CrI		$\overline{D}$	$D(\overline{\theta})$	p_D	DIC
< 1	8.11	0.30	8.11	7.56	8.66	0.89	0.00	0.89	1.78
1-4	7.81	0.26	9.71	9.20	10.23	0.92	0.06	0.85	1.77
5-14	9.78	0.28	11.45	10.93	11.95	0.82	0.00	0.82	1.64
15-24	10.23	0.26	11.11	10.64	11.58	1.00	0.23	0.77	1.76
25-44	11.46	0.29	11.22	10.71	11.72	0.90	0.00	0.90	1.80
45-64	12.03	0.26	9.91	9.41	10.41	0.86	0.00	0.86	1.73
65+	11.25	0.27	7.56	7.03	8.10	0.92	0.00	0.92	1.84

tests [65] are known to be conservative, due to using the data both to fit the model and to compare to model predictions, so a variety of (computationally intensive) post-processing, approximate, or cross-validatory methods have been proposed instead (e.g., [63, 64, 66–69]). Typically, each of these methods has been used to assess models of a single dataset, rather than for an evidence synthesis.

"Conflict p-values" [60, 69–71] have been proposed as a generalization of Bayesian cross-validatory predictive p-values that compare not only subsets of data to predictions resulting from the rest of the data, but also whole sub-models, comprising data, model structure, and prior information, with predictions from the rest of the model. The key idea, known as "node-splitting," is to split a DAG $\mathcal{G}(\phi, \boldsymbol{\theta}_{\backslash\phi}, \boldsymbol{y})$, comprising data $\boldsymbol{y}$ and latent quantites $\boldsymbol{\theta} = (\phi, \boldsymbol{\theta}_{\backslash\phi})$, into two independent partitions at any "separator" node ϕ, $\mathcal{G}(\phi_a, \boldsymbol{\theta}_{a\backslash\phi}, \boldsymbol{y}_a)$ and $\mathcal{G}(\phi_b, \boldsymbol{\theta}_{b\backslash\phi}, \boldsymbol{y}_b)$. Two copies of the separator ϕ are created, ϕ_a and ϕ_b, that are each identifiable in partitions $\mathcal{G}(\phi_a, \boldsymbol{\theta}_{a\backslash\phi}, \boldsymbol{y}_a)$ and $\mathcal{G}(\phi_b, \boldsymbol{\theta}_{b\backslash\phi}, \boldsymbol{y}_b)$, respectively. The aim is to compare the posterior distributions from each partition, $p(\phi_a \mid \boldsymbol{y}_a)$ and $p(\phi_b \mid \boldsymbol{y}_b)$.

This comparison is achieved by defining a difference function $\delta = h(\phi_a) - h(\phi_b)$, on an appropriate scale $h(\cdot)$, and considering where 0 lies in the posterior distribution of the difference, $p_\delta(\delta \mid \boldsymbol{y}_a, \boldsymbol{y}_b)$. A two-sided conflict p-value corresponding to the hypothesis test $H_0 : \delta = 0$ is defined as $c = 2 \times \min[\Pr\{p_\delta(\delta \mid \boldsymbol{y}_a, \boldsymbol{y}_b) < p_\delta(0 \mid \boldsymbol{y}_a, \boldsymbol{y}_b)\}, 1 - \Pr\{p_\delta(\delta \mid \boldsymbol{y}_a, \boldsymbol{y}_b) < p_\delta(0 \mid \boldsymbol{y}_a, \boldsymbol{y}_b)\}]$, with different methods for evaluating c and one-sided variations given in [60, 70]. The conflict p-value has been demonstrated to be uniform under the null model in a range of models by [71]. This setup can be generalized to multiple partitions and multiple node-splits [72].

24.6.3.2 Conflict in the influenza severity example

To assess whether the lack of fit to the HPA estimates of the number symptomatic in the "naive" model (Table 24.1) could be due to conflicting evidence, the model for the first wave only is split into two partitions at N_{S}, as in Figure 24.18. The "parent" partition comprises the data and priors informing the parent nodes of N_{S} (i.e., the sero-prevalence data and an informative prior for the proportion of infections that are symptomatic, $p_{\mathrm{S|Inf}}$). The rest

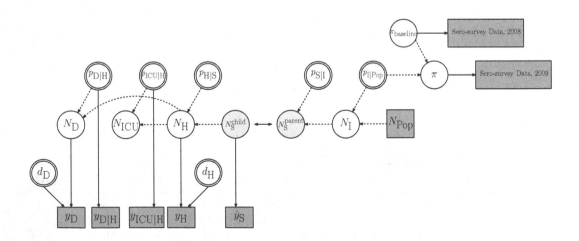

FIGURE 24.18
DAG showing node split at N_{S}. On the right is the "parent" model and on the left the "child" model. The double-headed arrow represents the comparison between the two.

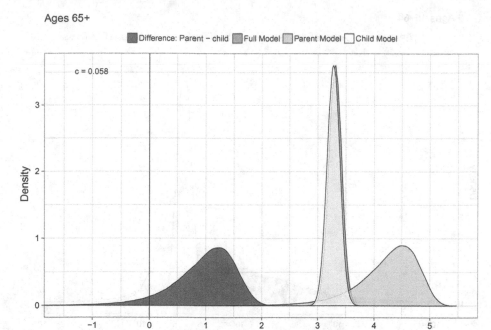

FIGURE 24.19

Conflict (posterior difference) at N_S between the parent and child models in age group 65+ in the first wave: difference function $\delta = \log_{10}(N_S^{\text{parent}}) - \log_{10}(N_S^{\text{child}})$ (dark grey); $\log_{10}(N_S)$ from full model (medium grey); $\log_{10}(N_S^{\text{parent}})$ from parent model (light grey); $\log_{10}(N_S^{\text{child}})$ from child model (ivory).

of the evidence (the severe case data and priors) comprises the "child" model. The test for conflict between the parent and child models demonstrated low posterior probabilities of no conflict, particularly for the youngest and oldest age groups [60]. The posterior difference function $\delta = \log_{10}(N_S^{\text{parent}}) - \log_{10}(N_S^{\text{child}})$ is plotted for the age group 65+ in Figure 24.19, together with the conflict p-value $c = 0.058$ and the corresponding posterior distributions for the two partitions and the full model. Note that the sero-prevalence data in the parent model imply a much higher, although also much more uncertain, number symptomatic than the severe case data in the child model. The lack of certainty in the sero-prevalence data means the severe case data and priors have more influence in the full model, so the full model posterior is much closer to the child model posterior than the parent one.

A similar investigation of conflict at a different node in the "naive" model, the number of hospitalizations N_H, leads to splitting the DAG into three partitions (not shown), based on the sero-prevalence data, the hospital data, and the mortality data, respectively. The influence of the evidence in the three partitions on the full model is shown in Figure 24.20. As in the previous example, the sero-prevalence (denominator) data in partition 1 are the most uncertain, with the hospital data in partition 2 having less uncertainty, and the mortality data in partition 3 even less uncertainty. The posterior distributions for all three partitions overlap substantially, however, so that conflict is not detectable. Instead, when the three partitions are combined in the full model, we obtain a much more precise estimate of the number hospitalized, which is a compromise between the three partitions, as would be expected.

Ages 45–64

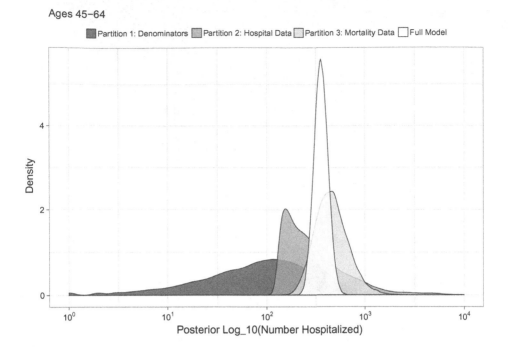

FIGURE 24.20
Influence and conflict at N_H between the three partitions in age group 45–64 in the first wave.

24.7   Discussion

This chapter has illustrated both the advantages and complexities of synthesizing multiple data sources to estimate various hidden characteristics of infectious disease, through the two examples of severity and transmission estimation for influenza. Section 24.6 introduced three sets of tools to approach the challenges of complex model building, computationally efficient inference and model criticism, respectively. However, these tools are a first step in resolving these challenges, with a number of questions remaining open.

Markov melding generalizes existing ideas that facilitate realistic evidence synthesis through a modular approach to model building. Some outstanding challenges include the choice of pooling function and the degree of heterogeneity between prior models that is acceptable for Markov melding to be appropriate – when does heterogeneity become conflict? Nevertheless, Markov melding is an important step in this era of big data, generalizing divide-and-conquer approaches [73].

Efficient inference for transmission models has been introduced using a sequential approach. Currently, the sequential approach is highly tailored to accommodate shocks to the system, so a question of interest is how to adapt a transmission model structure in real time to be able to generalize the SMC approach to any plausible epidemic scenario. The influenza model illustrated is deterministic in its dynamics, and the generic multi-state model description in Section 24.3.1 and Figure 24.6, while in theory accommodating stochastic dynamic transmission, is more focused on deterministic dynamics. An important area of research is to consider efficient, real-time, inference from multiple sources for stochastic epidemics, particularly in the early stages of an outbreak [3]. The influenza transmission model of [34] includes several levels of stochasticity and data, but is highly computationally intensive, and therefore not feasible in real time. How much stochasticity is therefore necessary to realistically model an emerging outbreak?

The illustration of conflict assessment in Section 24.6.3 is targeted, in that conflict was assessed at particular nodes in the DAG of the influenza severity model, following suspected biases in particular data sources. However, in some contexts, it may not be so clear where to look for potential conflict, in which case a systematic search throughout a DAG for conflict may be warranted. However, such systematic assessment entails multiple tests, either through a multivariate difference function (as in the example of Figure 24.20) or through fitting multiple node-split models. A framework for systematic assessment, accounting for the multiple tests and their correlation, has therefore been proposed [72]. Further open questions in this area include how to improve power to detect conflict and how to make such methods more accessible by improving the computational feasibility of systematic conflict assessment. As with any cross-validatory framework, multiple node-splitting can be computationally burdensome, so for hierarchical models, [74] have proposed an integrated nested Laplace approximation (INLA) approach to fast conflict diagnostics. A final area of open research related to understanding the influence of different, potentially conflicting, evidence sources on inference is the adaptation of value of information methods to evidence synthesis [75].

Acknowledgments

The authors would like to thank Robert Goudie and Paul Birrell for help with plots. Anne Presanis and Daniela De Angelis are supported by the Medical Research Council (Unit program number MC_UU_00002/11).

References

[1] R. M. Anderson and R. M. May. *Infectious Diseases of Humans: Dynamics and Control.* Oxford University Press, Oxford, UK, 1991.

[2] H. Heesterbeek, R. M. Anderson, V. Andreasen, S. Bansal, D. De Angelis, C. Dye, K. T. D. Eames et al. Modeling infectious disease dynamics in the complex landscape of global health. *Science*, 347(6227):aaa4339, 2015.

[3] P. J. Birrell, D. De Angelis, and A. M. Presanis. Evidence synthesis for stochastic epidemic models. *Statistical Science*, 33(1):34–43, 2018.

[4] M. Borenstein, L. V. Hedges, J. Higgins, and H. R. Rothstein. *Introduction to Meta-Analysis.* Wiley Online Library, Chichester, UK, 2009.

[5] D. M. Eddy, V. Hasselblad, and R. Shachter. *Meta-Analysis by the Confidence Profile Method.* Academic Press, London, UK, 1992.

[6] D. J. Spiegelhalter, K. R. Abrams, and J. P. Myles. *Bayesian Approaches to Clinical Trials and Health-Care Evaluation.* Statistics in Practice. Wiley, Chichester, UK, 2004.

[7] N. J. Welton, A. J. Sutton, N. J. Cooper, K. R. Abrams, and A. E. Ades. Evidence synthesis in a decision modelling framework. In *Evidence Synthesis for Decision Making in Healthcare*, pages 138–150. John Wiley & Sons, Hoboken, NJ, 2012.

[8] A. E. Ades and A. J. Sutton. Multiparameter evidence synthesis in epidemiology and medical decision-making: Current approaches. *Journal of the Royal Statistical Society: Series A (Statistics in Society)*, 169(1):5–35, 2006.

[9] M. C. Wheldon, A. E. Raftery, S. J. Clark, and P. Gerland. Bayesian reconstruction of two-sex populations by age: Estimating sex ratios at birth and sex ratios of mortality. *Journal of the Royal Statistical Society: Series A (Statistics in Society)*, 178(4):977–1007, 2015.

[10] J. S. Clark, D. Nemergut, B. Seyednasrollah, P. J. Turner, and S. Zhang. Generalized joint attribute modeling for biodiversity analysis: Median-zero, multivariate, multifarious data. *Ecological Monographs*, 87(1):34–56, 2017.

[11] D. De Angelis, A. M. Presanis, S. Conti, and A. E. Ades. Estimation of HIV burden through Bayesian evidence synthesis. *Statistical Science*, 29(1):9–17, 2014.

[12] R. J. Harris, M. Ramsay, V. D. Hope, L. Brant, M. Hickman, G. R. Foster, and D. De Angelis. Hepatitis C prevalence in England remains low and varies by ethnicity: An updated evidence synthesis. *European Journal of Public Health*, 22(2):187–192, 2011.

[13] S. A. McDonald, R. Mohamed, M. Dahlui, H. Naning, and A. Kamarulzaman. Bridging the data gaps in the epidemiology of hepatitis C virus infection in Malaysia using multi-parameter evidence synthesis. *BMC Infectious Diseases*, 14:564, 2014.

[14] I. Albert, E. Espié, H. De Valk, and J. B. Denis. A Bayesian evidence synthesis for estimating campylobacteriosis prevalence. *Risk Analysis*, 31(7):1141–1155, 2011.

[15] A. M. Presanis, R. G. Pebody, P. J. Birrell, B. D. M. Tom, H. K. Green, H. Durnall, D. Fleming, and D. De Angelis. Synthesising evidence to estimate pandemic (2009) A/H1N1 influenza severity in 2009–2011. *Annals of Applied Statistics*, 8(4):2378–2403, 2014.

[16] M. Shubin, M. Virtanen, S. Toikkanen, O. Lyytikäinen, and K. Auranen. Estimating the burden of A(H1N1) pdm09 influenza in Finland during two seasons. *Epidemiology and Infection*, 142(5):964–974, 2014.

[17] N. J. Welton and A. E. Ades. A model of toxoplasmosis incidence in the UK: Evidence synthesis and consistency of evidence. *Journal of the Royal Statistical Society. Series C: Applied Statistics*, 54(2):385–404, 2005.

[18] S. A. McDonald, A. M. Presanis, D. De Angelis, W. Van der Hoek, M. Hooiveld, G. Donker, and M. E. Kretzschmar. An evidence synthesis approach to estimating the incidence of seasonal influenza in the Netherlands. *Influenza and other Respiratory Viruses*, 8(1):33–41, 2014.

[19] S. A. Mcdonald, P. Teunis, N. van der Maas, S. de Greeff, H. de Melker, and M. E. Kretzschmar. An evidence synthesis approach to estimating the incidence of symptomatic pertussis infection in the Netherlands, 2005-2011. *BMC Infectious Diseases*, 15:588, 2015.

[20] P. J. Birrell, G. Ketsetzis, N. J. Gay, B. S. Cooper, A. M. Presanis, R. J. Harris, A. Charlett et al. Bayesian modeling to unmask and predict influenza A/H1N1pdm dynamics in London. *Proceedings of the National Academy of Sciences*, 108(45):18238–18243, 2011.

[21] I. Dorigatti, S. Cauchemez, and N. M. Ferguson. Increased transmissibility explains the third wave of infection by the 2009 H1N1 pandemic virus in England. *Proceedings of the National Academy of Sciences*, 110(33):13422–13427, 2013.

[22] D. De Angelis, A. M. Presanis, P. J. Birrell, G. S. Tomba, and T. House. Four key challenges in infectious disease modelling using data from multiple sources. *Epidemics*, 10:83–87, 2015.

[23] M. Lipsitch, S. Riley, S. Cauchemez, A. C. Ghani, and N. M. Ferguson. Managing and reducing uncertainty in an emerging influenza pandemic. *New England Journal of Medicine*, 361(2):112–115, 2009.

[24] A. J. Kucharski, S. Funk, R. M. Eggo, H.-P. Mallet, W. J. Edmunds, and E. J. Nilles. Transmission dynamics of Zika virus in island populations: A modelling analysis of the 2013–14 French Polynesia outbreak. *PLoS Neglected Tropical Diseases*, 10(5):e0004726, 2016.

[25] A. Camacho, R. M. Eggo, S. Funk, C. H. Watson, A. J. Kucharski, and W. J. Edmunds. Estimating the probability of demonstrating vaccine efficacy in the declining Ebola epidemic: A Bayesian modelling approach. *BMJ Open*, 5(12):e009346, 2015.

[26] C. Reed, F. J. Angulo, D. L. Swerdlow, M. Lipsitch, M. I. Meltzer, D. Jernigan, and L. Finelli. Estimates of the prevalence of pandemic (H1N1) 2009, United States, April-July 2009. *Emerging Infectious Diseases*, 15(12):2004–2007, 2009.

[27] S. S. Shrestha, D. L. Swerdlow, R. H. Borse, V. S. Prabhu, L. Finelli, C. Y. Atkins, K. Owusu-Edusei et al. Estimating the burden of 2009 pandemic influenza a (H1N1) in the United States (April 2009-April 2010). *Clinical Infectious Diseases*, 52(S1):75–82, 2011.

[28] C. Reed, S. S. Chaves, P. D. Kirley, R. Emerson, D. Aragon, E. B. Hancock, L. Butler et al. Estimating influenza disease burden from population-based surveillance data in the United States. *PLoS One*, 10(3):e0118369, 2015.

[29] A. M. Presanis, D. De Angelis, The New York City Swine Flu Investigation Team, A. Hagy, C. Reed, S. Riley, B. S. Cooper, L. Finelli, P. Biedrzycki, and M. Lipsitch. The severity of pandemic H1N1 influenza in the United States, from April to July 2009: A Bayesian analysis. *PLoS Medicine*, 6(12):e1000207+, 2009.

[30] A. M. Presanis, R. G. Pebody, B. J. Paterson, B. D. M. Tom, P. J. Birrell, A. Charlett, M. Lipsitch, and D. De Angelis. Changes in severity of 2009 pandemic A/H1N1 influenza in England: A Bayesian evidence synthesis. *BMJ*, 343(7824):d5408+, 2011.

[31] S. Cauchemez, A.-J. Valleron, P.-Y. Boelle, A. Flahault, and N. M. Ferguson. Estimating the impact of school closure on influenza transmission from sentinel data. *Nature*, 452(7188):750, 2008.

[32] M. Baguelin, S. Flasche, A. Camacho, N. Demiris, E. Miller, and W. J. Edmunds. Assessing optimal target populations for influenza vaccination programmes: An evidence synthesis and modelling study. *PLoS Medicine*, 10(10):e1001527+, 2013.

[33] D. E. Te Beest, P. J. Birrell, J. Wallinga, D. De Angelis, and M. van Boven. Joint modelling of serological and hospitalization data reveals that high levels of pre-existing immunity and school holidays shaped the influenza A pandemic of 2009 in the Netherlands. *Journal of the Royal Society, Interface / the Royal Society*, 12(103):20141244+, 2014.

[34] M. Shubin, A. Lebedev, O. Lyytikäinen, and K. Auranen. Revealing the true incidence of pandemic A(H1N1) pdm09 influenza in Finland during the first two seasons An analysis based on a dynamic transmission model. *PLoS Computational Biology*, 12(3):e1004803, 2016.

[35] P. J. Birrell, L. Wernisch, B. D. M. Tom, L. Held, G. O. Roberts, R. G. Pebody, and D. De Angelis. Efficient real-time monitoring of an emerging influenza epidemic: How feasible? *arXiv preprint arXiv:1608.05292*, 2016.

[36] R. J. F. Ypma, A. M. A. Bataille, A. Stegeman, G. Koch, J. Wallinga, and W. M. van Ballegooijen. Unravelling transmission trees of infectious diseases by combining genetic and epidemiological data. *Proceedings of the Royal Society B: Biological Sciences*, 279(1728):444–450, 2012.

[37] O. Ratmann, G. Donker, A. Meijer, C. Fraser, and K. Koelle. Phylodynamic inference and model assessment with approximate Bayesian computation: Influenza as a case study. *PLoS Computational Biology*, 8(12):e1002835, 2012.

[38] T. Jombart, A. Cori, X. Didelot, S. Cauchemez, C. Fraser, and N. Ferguson. Bayesian reconstruction of disease outbreaks by combining epidemiologic and genomic data. *PLoS Computational Biology*, 10(1):e1003457, 2014.

[39] E. Brooks-Pollock, N. Tilston, W. J. Edmunds, and K. T. D. Eames. Using an online survey of healthcare-seeking behaviour to estimate the magnitude and severity of the 2009 H1N1v influenza epidemic in England. *BMC Infectious Diseases*, 11:1–8, 2011.

[40] S. L. Lauritzen. *Graphical Models*. Clarendon Press, Oxford, UK, 1996.

[41] P. K. Andersen and N. Keiding. Multi-state models for event history analysis. *Statistical Methods in Medical Research*, 11(2):91–115, 2002.

[42] C. H. Jackson, M. Jit, L. D. Sharples, and D. De Angelis. Calibration of complex models through Bayesian evidence synthesis: A demonstration and tutorial. *Medical Decision Making*, 35(2):148–161, 2015.

[43] H. J. Wearing, P. Rohani, and M. J. Keeling. Appropriate models for the management of infectious diseases. *PLoS Medicine*, 2(7):e174, 2005.

[44] F. Ball. A threshold theorem for the Reed-Frost chain-binomial epidemic. *Journal of Applied Probability*, 20(1):153–157, 1983.

[45] D. Rizopoulos. *Joint Models for Longitudinal and Time-to-Event Data: with Applications in R*. CRC Press, Boca Raton, FL, 2012.

[46] R. J. B. Goudie, A. M. Presanis, D. Lunn, D. De Angelis, and L. Wernisch. Joining and splitting models with Markov melding. *Bayesian Analysis*, 14(1):81–109, 2019. doi:10.1214/18/BA1104.

[47] A. P. Dawid and S. L. Lauritzen. Hyper Markov laws in the statistical analysis of decomposable graphical models. *Annals of Statistics*, 21(3):1272–1317, 1993.

[48] M. S. Massa and S. L. Lauritzen. Combining statistical models. In M. A. G. Viana and H. P. Wynn, eds., *Contemporary Mathematics: Algebraic Methods in Statistics and Probability II*, pages 239–260. American Mathematical Society, Providence, RI, 2010. https://bookstore.ams.org/conm-516.

[49] M. S. Massa and E. Riccomagno. Algebraic representations of Gaussian Markov combinations. *Bernoulli*, 23(1):626–644, 2017.

[50] D. Poole and A. E. Raftery. Inference for deterministic simulation models: The Bayesian melding approach. *Journal of the American Statistical Association*, 95(452):1244–1255, 2000.

[51] D. Gamerman and H. F. Lopes. *Markov Chain Monte Carlo: Stochastic Simulation for Bayesian Inference*. CRC Press, Boca Raton, FL, 2006.

[52] D. Lunn, D. J. Spiegelhalter, A. Thomas, and N. Best. The BUGS project: Evolution, critique and future directions. *Statistics in Medicine*, 28(25):3049–3067, 2009.

[53] D. M. Sheinson, J. Niemi, and W. Meiring. Comparison of the performance of particle filter algorithms applied to tracking of a disease epidemic. *Mathematical Biosciences*, 255:21–32, 2014.

[54] M. Farah, P. J. Birrell, S. Conti, and D. De Angelis. Bayesian emulation and calibration of a dynamic epidemic model for A/H1N1 influenza. *Journal of the American Statistical Association*, 109(508):1398–1411, 2014.

[55] I. Andrianakis, N. McCreesh, I. Vernon, T. J. McKinley, J. E. Oakley, R. N. Nsubuga, M. Goldstein, and R. G. White. Efficient history matching of a high dimensional individual-based HIV transmission model. *SIAM/ASA Journal on Uncertainty Quantification*, 5(1):694–719, 2017.

[56] J. B. S. Ong, I. Mark, C. Chen, A. R. Cook, H. Chyi. Lee, V. J. Lee, R. T. P. Lin, P. A. Tambyah, and L. G. Goh. Real-time epidemic monitoring and forecasting of H1N1-2009 using influenza-like illness from general practice and family doctor clinics in Singapore. *PloS One*, 5(4):e10036, 2010.

[57] W. R. Gilks and C. Berzuini. Following a moving target: Monte Carlo inference for dynamic Bayesian models. *Journal of the Royal Statistical Society: Series B (Statistical Methodology)*, 63(1):127–146, 2001.

[58] P. Del Moral, A. Doucet, and A. Jasra. Sequential Monte Carlo samplers. *Journal of the Royal Statistical Society: Series B (Statistical Methodology)*, 68(3):411–436, 2006.

[59] R. M. Neal. Sampling from multimodal distributions using tempered transitions. *Statistics and Computing*, 6(4):353–366, 1996.

[60] A. M. Presanis, D. Ohlssen, D. J. Spiegelhalter, and D. De Angelis. Conflict diagnostics in directed acyclic graphs, with applications in Bayesian evidence synthesis. *Statistical Science*, 28(3):376–397, 2013.

[61] G. E. P. Box. Sampling and Bayes' inference in scientific modelling and robustness. *Journal of the Royal Statistical Society. Series A (General)*, 143(4):383–430, 1980.

[62] D. B. Rubin. Bayesianly justifiable and relevant frequency calculations for the applied statistician. *The Annals of Statistics*, 12(4):1151–1172, 1984.

[63] A. Gelman, X.-L. Meng, and H. Stern. Posterior predictive assessment of model fitness via realized discrepancies. *Statistica Sinica*, 6:733–807, 1996.

[64] M. J. Bayarri and M. E. Castellanos. Bayesian checking of the second levels of hierarchical models. *Statistical Science*, 22(3):322–343, 2007.

[65] A. Gelman, J. B. Carlin, H. S. Stern, and D. B. Rubin. *Bayesian Data Analysis*. Texts in Statistical Science. Chapman and Hall/CRC Press London, UK, 2nd ed., 2003.

[66] M. J. Bayarri and J. O. Berger. P-values for composite null models. *Journal of the American Statistical Association*, 95(452):1127–1142, 2000.

[67] N. L. Hjort, F. A. Dahl, and G. H. Steinbakk. Post-processing posterior predictive p-values. *Journal of the American Statistical Association*, 101(475):1157–1174, 2006.

[68] G. H. Steinbakk and G. O. Storvik. Posterior predictive p-values in Bayesian hierarchical models. *Scandinavian Journal of Statistics*, 36(2):320–336, 2009.

[69] E. C. Marshall and D. J. Spiegelhalter. Identifying outliers in Bayesian hierarchical models: A simulation-based approach. *Bayesian Analysis*, 2:409–444, 2007.

[70] J. Gåsemyr and B. Natvig. Extensions of a conflict measure of inconsistencies in Bayesian hierarchical models. *Scandinavian Journal of Statistics*, 36(4):822–838, 2009.

[71] J. Gåsemyr. Uniformity of node level conflict measures in Bayesian hierarchical models based on directed acyclic graphs. *Scandinavian Journal of Statistics*, 43(1):20–34, 2016.

[72] A. M. Presanis, D. Ohlssen, K. Cui, M.a Rosinska, and D. De Angelis. Conflict diagnostics for evidence synthesis in a multiple testing framework. *arXiv preprint arXiv:1702.07304*, 2017.

[73] R. Bardenet, A. Doucet, and C. Holmes. On Markov chain Monte Carlo methods for tall data. *The Journal of Machine Learning Research*, 18(1):1515–1557, 2017.

[74] E. Ferkingstad, L. Held, and H. Rue. Fast and accurate Bayesian model criticism and conflict diagnostics using R-INLA. *Stat*, 6(1):331–344, 2017.

[75] C. H. Jackson, A. M. Presanis, S. Conti, and D. De Angelis. Value of information: Sensitivity analysis and research design in Bayesian evidence synthesis. *Journal of the American Statistical Association*, 2019. doi:10.1080/01621459.2018.1562932.

25

Forecasting Based on Surveillance Data

Leonhard Held and Sebastian Meyer

CONTENTS

25.1 Introduction

Epidemic modelling has at least three distinct aims: (1) understanding the spread of infectious diseases, (2) identifying suitable measures to control the spread of an epidemic, for example through isolation or vaccination (Daley and Gani, 1999, Section 1.5), and (3) predicting the future course of an epidemic. Mathematical models often are used to better understand the dynamics of infectious disease spread and the effects of control measures (Keeling and Rohani, 2008, Section 1.5), but are less oriented towards predictions. In recent years, more emphasis has been placed on the development of predictive models and methods. The goal of this chapter is to review the literature in this area and to describe how general statistical principles from the forecasting literature can be applied to evaluate the quality of epidemic forecasts. The described methods will also be illustrated in two case studies, where we assess competing approaches to forecast time series of infectious disease counts.

25.1.1 The history of forecasting epidemics

Predicting the future course of epidemics has been a goal of mankind for a long time. Scientific forecasting based on mathematical models dates back to the pioneering work by Baroyan et al. (1971), who predicted the course of an influenza epidemic for the main cities in the Soviet Union. The rise of new infectious diseases, such as acquired Immunodeficiency syndrome (AIDS) and severe acute respiratory syndrome (SARS), has been a major trigger of novel forecasting methods (Daley and Gani, 1999; Hufnagel et al., 2004,

Section 25.2). Furthermore, meteorologic forecasting methods have been adopted in epidemiological research, including modeling (Viboud et al., 2003; Shaman and Karspeck, 2012) and assessment (Paul and Held, 2011; Held et al., 2017) techniques. Recent developments in influenza forecasting have focused on the integration of search logs from Google (Dukic et al., 2012; Shaman and Karspeck, 2012; Yang et al., 2015), social media data from Twitter (Paul et al., 2014), combinations thereof (Santillana et al., 2015), Wikipedia article views (Generous et al., 2014; Hickmann et al., 2015), or human mobility data (Pei et al., 2018). Compared to weather forecasting, epidemic forecasting is still in its infancy, and the human component makes it particularly challenging (World Health Organization, 2014; Moran et al., 2016).

25.1.2   Forecasting competitions

To develop better epidemic forecasting methods, the World Health Organization (WHO) has joined forces in an informal consultation with more than 130 global experts (World Health Organization, 2016), and the Centers for Disease Control and Prevention (CDC) in the USA have organized several seasonal forecasting competitions (Biggerstaff et al., 2016, 2018). Real-time influenza forecasts are now provided by Nicholas Reich and coworkers at the ReichLab (Tushar et al., 2017; see http://reichlab.io/flusight/). Other recent competitions include the Defense Advance Research Projects Agency (DARPA) challenge on forecasting chikungunya (Del Valle et al., 2018), the White House/Nation Oceanic and Atmospheric Administration (NOAA) challenge on forecasting dengue (Buczak et al., 2018), and the Research and Policy for Infectious Disease Dynamics (RAPIDD) ebola forecasting challenge (Viboud et al., 2018).

25.1.3   Forecasting targets

Several quantities are of interest in epidemic forecasting, such as timing of and incidence in the peak week (Ray et al., 2017), onset week (Pei et al., 2018), cumulative incidence (Lega and Brown, 2016), weekly incidence (Paul and Held, 2011; Reich et al., 2016a), outbreak size and duration (Farrington et al., 2003), and the epidemic curve (Jiang et al., 2009). Also of public health relevance are stratified forecasts of these quantities, for example, by region or by age group (Held et al., 2017). Forecasting targets for seasonal influenza epidemics in particular have been reviewed previously (Chretien et al., 2014; Nsoesie et al., 2014). More recently, the weekly proportion of doctor visits due to influenza-like illness (ILI) is becoming a popular forecasting target (Biggerstaff et al., 2018).

25.2   Evaluating Point Forecasts

A point forecast usually is made for a continuous or integer (often count) outcome, for example, the disease incidence in the next week, the number of newly confirmed cases in a certain time interval, or the timing of the peak week of an epidemic. Several measures have been proposed and used to evaluate the quality of a point forecast. Gneiting (2011) gives a comprehensive discussion of suitable measures for point predictions.

To introduce some notation, let $\hat{y}_i$ denote the point forecasts of the observations y_i, $i = 1, \ldots, n$. Given a suitable non-negative scoring function $S(\hat{y}_i, y_i)$, the overall predictive performance can be assessed with the mean score

$$\bar{S} = \frac{1}{n} \sum_{i=1}^{n} S(\hat{y}_i, y_i).$$

Scoring functions are usually negatively oriented, so the smaller a score, the better the forecast. Commonly used scoring functions are the *absolute error* (AE) $S(\hat{y}, y) = |\hat{y} - y|$, the *squared error* (SE) $S(\hat{y}, y) = (\hat{y} - y)^2$, the *absolute percentage error* $S(\hat{y}, y) = |\hat{y} - y|/y$, and the *relative error* $S(\hat{y}, y) = |\hat{y} - y|/\hat{y}$. Note that the latter two scoring functions require y and $\hat{y}$ to be positive, respectively. Other summary measures used in the infectious disease literature may be based on one of these scoring functions, for example the *root mean squared error* (RMSE) or the *relative mean absolute error* (Hyndman and Koehler, 2006; Reich et al., 2016b). The latter is defined as the ratio of the *mean absolute errors* of two competing forecasts and is not to be confused with the *mean relative absolute error* of one forecasting method.

The small simulation study reported by Gneiting (2011) reveals the key differences of these four scoring functions. It is based on a time series model commonly used in econometrics, but the results equally apply to other fields. A simple conditionally heteroscedastic Gaussian time series model is used to generate a non-negative time series $y_1, \ldots, y_n$. Model-based one-step-ahead point forecasts (based on the mean of the forecast distribution) then are compared to naive approaches, such as the so-called "fence-sitter forecast," a forecast with constant predictions. Quite surprisingly, one of the naive methods outperforms the model-based one-step-ahead forecasts under the *absolute error* and the *absolute percentage error* scoring functions.

Gneiting (2011) points out that the model-based forecast is only optimal under squared error loss but not necessarily for other loss functions, where other functions of the predictive distribution will be optimal. A scoring function is called consistent for a loss function, if the expected score is minimized when following this loss function. The *squared error* scoring function is consistent for the mean, and the *absolute error* scoring function for the median, both standard loss functions. However, the *mean absolute percentage error* commonly used in influenza forecasting (Chretien et al., 2014, Table 4) is consistent for a nonstandard and rather exotic functional. To quote Gneiting (2011), "it thus seems prudent that authors using this functional consider the intended or unintended consequences and reassess its suitability as a scoring function." Some scoring functions may be problematic *per se*, such as the commonly used correlation coefficient between predictions and observations. For example, point predictions always twice as large as the observations are obviously inappropriate, but the correlation coefficient between predictions and observations will be one.

25.3 Evaluating Probabilistic Forecasts

In many areas of science, researchers argue that forecasts should be probabilistic (Gneiting and Katzfuss, 2014) and this plea has recently been taken up in the infectious disease literature (Held et al., 2017; Funk et al., 2018).

Evaluating probabilistic forecasts requires suitable scores to quantify the "distance" between a cumulative distribution function F, the forecast, and the observation y that later realizes. Proper scoring rules play a key role, as they allow for a fair comparison of different probabilistic forecasting methods. In addition, the notions of calibration and sharpness are important. Calibration is a property of both the forecast and the observations, whereas sharpness is a property of the forecasts only. The paradigm of probabilistic forecasting is to "maximize sharpness subject to calibration" (Gneiting and Raftery, 2007).

Much of the literature on probabilistic forecasting focusses on continuous forecast distributions. However, in infectious disease epidemiology, the quantities to be predicted are often (incidence or prevalence) counts, which require suitable extensions of the assessment techniques (Czado et al., 2009; Held et al., 2017).

25.3.1 Calibration and sharpness

Calibration is defined as the statistical consistency of probabilistic forecasts and the observations (Gneiting et al., 2007). For continuous outcomes, calibration is usually assessed with the probability integral transform (PIT). Specifically, the PIT is $F(y)$, so will be uniformly distributed if the observation y is a realization from the forecast F. In practice we will compute PIT values for a series of forecasts and visually assess their distribution in a histogram. Modifications for count data exist (Czado et al., 2009).

For binary data, the calibration slope studies the association between the (logit-transformed) predicted probabilities with the binary outcomes in a logistic regression (Cox, 1958; Steyerberg, 2009). Calibration can also be visually assessed in a calibration curve (Gneiting and Katzfuss, 2014).

Statistical calibration tests are commonly employed to assess the evidence for miscalibration. Different methods exist for continuous outcomes (Mason et al., 2007; Held et al., 2010), count outcomes (Wei and Held, 2014) and binary outcomes (Spiegelhalter, 1986), but they may require certain distributional assumptions on the forecasts.

For continuous forecasts, sharpness is usually defined as the width of the associated prediction intervals. For multivariate forecasts, sharpness is defined based on the predictive covariance matrix, for example, its determinant (Gneiting et al., 2008).

25.3.2 Proper scoring rules

Proper scoring rules are summary measures of the predictive performance of probabilistic predictions $Y_i \sim F_i$, $i = 1, \ldots, n$, allowing for a joint assessment of calibration and sharpness (Gneiting and Katzfuss, 2014). As in Section 25.2 for point forecasts, the mean score across forecasts usually is reported and compared across different forecasting methods. For ease of presentation we drop the index i in this section and compare the probabilistic forecast $Y \sim F$ with the actual observation y.

The definition of propriety is mathematically somewhat demanding and we refer the interested reader to the review paper by Gneiting and Raftery (2007). Put simply, a proper scoring rule ensures that a forecaster reports his actual forecast and does not obtain a better score in expectation by digressing from his belief. Here we take scores to be negatively oriented penalties that forecasters wish to minimize, so the smaller a score, the better the forecast.

For forecasts of binary data $y \in \{0, 1\}$, commonly used scores are the *logarithmic score* (LS), i.e., the negative log-likelihood of the observation under the forecast distribution, and the *Brier score* (BS), also known as probability score. Specifically, let π denote the predicted probability of the observation $y = 1$, then

$$\mathrm{LS}(F, y) = -y \log(\pi) - (1 - y) \log(1 - \pi), \text{ and}$$

$$\mathrm{BS}(F, y) = (\pi - y)^2.$$

Both scores are proper, whereas the absolute score $\mathrm{AS}(F, y) = |\pi - y|$ can be shown to be improper (Held and Sabanés Bové, 2014, Chapter 9), so should not be used.

A probabilistic forecast for count data $y \in \{0, 1, 2, \ldots\}$ is represented by probabilities $\pi_k = \Pr(y = k)$, $k \in \{0, 1, 2, \ldots\}$, where $\sum_{k=1}^{\infty} \pi_k = 1$. The logarithmic score for the observation $y = j$ now simply reads $\mathrm{LS} = \log(\pi_j)$, where π_j is the probability of the observation $y = j$. An extension of the Brier score to forecasts of count data is the *ranked probability score*

$$\mathrm{RPS}(F, y) = \sum_{j=1}^{\infty} (P_j - \mathbf{1}\{y \le j\})^2,$$

where $P_j = \sum_{k=0}^{j} \pi_k$ and $\mathbf{1}$ denotes the indicator function. Probabilistic count forecasts often are summarized with the mean μ and the variance σ^2. A proper score that only uses these first two moments is the *Dawid-Sebastiani score* (DSS):

$$\mathrm{DSS}(F, y) = 2 \log \sigma + (y - \mu)^2 / \sigma^2.$$

This score can be generalized easily to multivariate predictions,

$$\mathrm{mDSS}(F, \boldsymbol{y}) = \log|\boldsymbol{\Sigma}| + (\boldsymbol{y} - \boldsymbol{\mu})^{\top} \boldsymbol{\Sigma}^{-1} (\boldsymbol{y} - \boldsymbol{\mu}), \tag{25.1}$$

which depends only on the mean vector $\boldsymbol{\mu}$ and the covariance matrix $\boldsymbol{\Sigma}$ of the predictive distribution. The first term $\log|\boldsymbol{\Sigma}|$ in equation (25.1) is called the log determinant sharpness (logDS) and is recommended as a (multivariate) measure of sharpness (Gneiting et al., 2008). To avoid unnecessarily large numbers it is common practice to report scaled versions of logDS and mDSS, obtained through division by $2d$ where d is the dimension of the observation $\boldsymbol{y}$. A possible alternative to mDSS is the *energy score*, a multivariate extension of the ranked probability score (Gneiting et al., 2008; Held et al., 2017).

The question arises about which scoring rule should be used in practice. The logarithmic score is known to be sensitive to outliers if π_j is close to zero. The ranked probability score is reported to be less sensitive to extreme observations (Gneiting and Raftery, 2007) and provides an attractive alternative. The DSS is particularly useful if the first two predictive moments are available but not the whole predictive distribution. It also has been argued that the choice of a scoring rule should take into account the costs of bad forecasts (Merkle and Steyvers, 2013). In practice, we recommend evaluation of several scores to obtain a more robust comparison of predictive performance.

The computation of the different scores depends on whether the forecast distributions are known analytically or derived from simulations. Care has to be taken with simulation-based forecasts as scores can become numerically instable; for example, the logarithmic score for count forecasts will be infinite if an observation $y = j$ has empirical frequency equal to zero in the forecast samples. A possible remedy is to apply a Rao-Blackwell/importance sampling scheme (Gelfand and Smith, 1990) and to average the conditional predictive distributions (see, also, Ray et al., 2017, Supp Mat Section 3.2). Alternatively, it is possible to use kernel density estimation as implemented in the R (R Core Team, 2018) package `scoringRules` (Jordan et al., 2019). The Dawid-Sebastiani score for multivariate forecasts can be numerically unstable if the predictive covariance matrix $\boldsymbol{\Sigma}$ is estimated from the empirical covariance matrix of Monte Carlo samples (Scheuerer and Hamill, 2015).

For independent forecasts, a simple paired t-test or a permutation test then can be used to assess the evidence for differences in predictive performance between two competing forecasting methods. If the forecasts are dependent as in a series of sequential k-step ahead forecasts, the Diebold-Mariano test can be used to account for the correlation between scores (Diebold and Mariano, 1995; Gneiting and Katzfuss, 2014).

25.4   Applications

We now describe two applications in which we compare the quality of forecasts provided by different models and methods. The data and code to reproduce these analyses are available in the R package `HIDDA.forecasting` (Meyer, 2018) at https://HIDDA.github.io/forecasting. The code is presented in several package vignettes that also give some additional results.

25.4.1   Univariate forecasting of influenza incidence

We consider a time series of weekly incidence counts on ILI in Switzerland from 2000 to 2016 (Figure 25.1). The last 213 weeks (starting from 2012-12-04) are used to assess 1-week-ahead forecasts. Four sets of 30-weeks-ahead long-term forecasts (shaded time periods in Figure 25.1) are computed for each of the last four seasons, conditional upon all data prior to the respective first week of December.

We have used five different methods to produce forecasts of influenza activity in Switzerland: an ARMA(2,2) time series model as estimated by `auto.arima()` from the `forecast` package (Hyndman and Khandakar, 2008), an observation-driven ARMA model for negative-binomial counts as implemented in the `glarma` package (Dunsmuir and Scott, 2015), the endemic-epidemic negative-binomial time-series model `hhh4` from the `surveillance` package (Meyer et al., 2017), Facebook's forecasting tool `prophet` (Taylor and Letham, 2018), as well as a recently proposed method based on kernel conditional density estimation (Ray et al., 2017), which we implemented following the code provided at https://github.com/reichlab/article-disease-pred-with-kcde. Note that forecasts from `arima` and `prophet` are

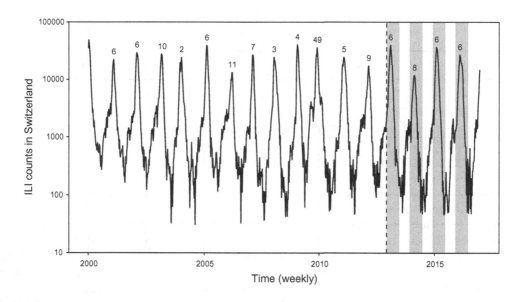

FIGURE 25.1

Surveillance of influenza-like illness (ILI) in Switzerland, 2000–2016. The last 213 weeks (to the right of the vertical dashed line) are used to assess 1-week-ahead forecasts. Long-term forecasts are assessed for the last four seasons starting in the first week of December (shaded time periods). The seasonal peaks are labelled with the corresponding ISO week. Note that the *y*-axis employs a log-scale for the ILI counts.

TABLE 25.1

Mean scores of the 213 1-week-ahead predictions (2012-W49 to 2016-W52) and of the long-term forecasts for the last four seasons of the Swiss ILI surveillance data

Method	1-Week-Ahead				Long-Term		
	RMSE	DSS	LS	Runtime	RMSE	DSS	LS
arima	2287	13.78	7.73	0.51	8471	16.43	8.88
glarma	2450	13.59	7.71	1.49	5558	19.61	9.12
hhh4	1769	13.58	7.71	0.02	8749	16.13	9.25
prophet	5614	15.00	8.03	3.01	7627	16.44	8.91
kcde	1963	13.79	7.80	1.30	—	—	—
naive	5010	14.90	8.06	0.00	6527	15.99	8.86

Note: Computing these long-term forecasts with the experimental kcde implementation was too cumbersome. The runtime for computing a single 1-week-ahead forecast is given in seconds. For hhh4 and glarma, the long-term results are based on 1000 simulations

generated on a log-scale. All models were configured to account for yearly seasonality. In the first three models, seasonality was represented by parametric sine-cosine regressors (Held and Paul, 2012) with frequency $2\pi/52.1775$ (derived from the average number of calendar weeks per year). For prophet and kcde, we followed the documented examples (see the supplementary vignettes for the exact model formulations). We also included a separate Christmas effect for calendar week 52 (not with kcde). For reference, we computed naive historical forecasts for the 213 weeks of the test period based on fitting log-normal distributions to the observed counts in the same calendar week of previous years.

We computed the RMSE and the mean DSS and LS for the 1-week-ahead forecasts and the long-term forecasts. The results are summarized in Table 25.1. As expected, the 1-week-ahead foreacasts have smaller (i.e., better) mean scores than the long-term forecasts for all methods considered. Note that we have not attempted to compute long-term forecasts with kcde due to excessively long runtimes. The time taken to compute a single 1-week-ahead forecast varied between 0.001 (naive) and 3 (prophet) seconds.

The best 1-week-ahead forecasts in terms of all scores are obtained with hhh4. Probabilistic forecasts with glarma achieve almost the same scores but the associated point forecasts have a larger RMSE of 2,450 cases. The second-best RMSE is obtained with kcde, but its probabilistic forecasts only rank fourth, after arima. The worst 1-week-ahead predictions are obtained from prophet, which achieves similar scores as the naive approach. Figure 25.2 shows the weekly forecasts and associated scores as well as the overall PIT histograms, which are computed based on the method for count data (Czado et al., 2009). There is no clear evidence for miscalibration of any of the 1-week-ahead forecasts, but the first three and the naive (not shown) forecasting methods have a distinct peak of the histogram in the first bin, indicating some evidence for biased or underdispersed predictions. The prophet and kcde (not shown) forecasts do not have this problem. PIT histograms for the kcde and naive forecasts can be found in the corresponding supplementary vignettes.

An interesting result is obtained from the long-term forecasts where the best scores are achieved by taking simple historical averages, except for RMSE where glarma is better. For the more sophisticated forecasts shown in Figure 25.3, the ranking is less clear. While hhh4 is the best model in terms of DSS, arima is the best model in terms of LS. Quite surprising is the large DSS value of the glarma method. Closer inspection of Figure 25.3 suggests this is caused by the excessively large uncertainty of the glarma long-term predictions, compared to the other three methods. From Figure 25.4 we can see that the prophet method has

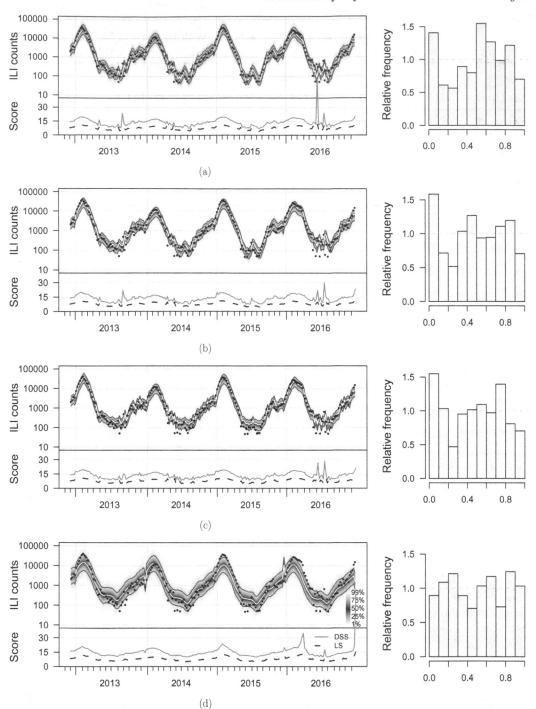

FIGURE 25.2

One-week-ahead forecasts of ILI counts in Switzerland for the last 213 weeks (2012-W49 to 2016-W52) of the available surveillance data. Predictive distributions are displayed as fan charts on a log-scale. The 10 percent and 90 percent quantiles and the mean are highlighted. The dots correspond to the observed counts and the lower panels show the associated weekly scores. The right-hand column shows the corresponding PIT histograms. Plots for `kcde` and naive forecasts can be found in the supplementary vignettes: (a) `arima`, (b) `glarma`, (c) `hhh4`, and (d) `prophet`.

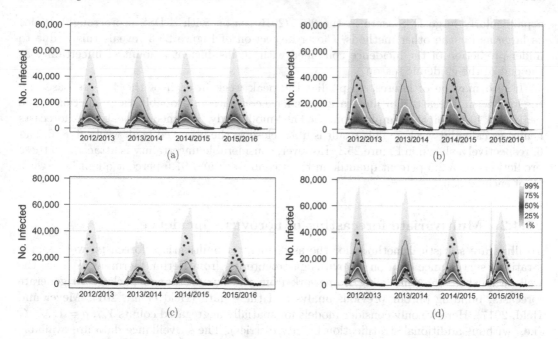

FIGURE 25.3

Long-term forecasts (30-weeks-ahead) of ILI counts in Switzerland for the last four seasons of the available surveillance data. Predictive distributions are displayed as fan charts, where the 10 percent and 90 percent quantiles and the mean are highlighted. The dots represent observed counts. In (b), quantiles above 95 percent are truncated around the peak weeks with the 99 percent quantile reaching seasonal maxima of between 251,000 and 325,000 cases: (a) `arima`, (b) `glarma`, (c) `hhh4`, and (d) `prophet`.

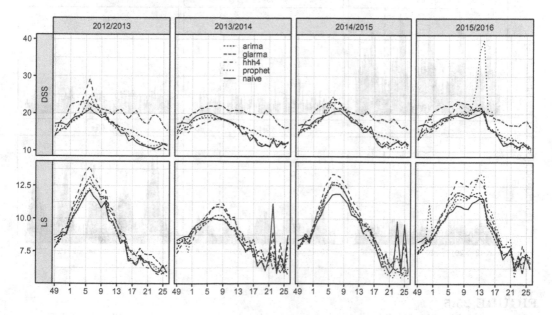

FIGURE 25.4

Weekly DSS (top) and LS (bottom) values of the different long-term forecasts of Swiss ILI counts displayed in Figure 25.3 and the naive forecasts.

a particularly large DSS score in the 2015/2016 season with a DSS score roughly twice as large as for the other methods. Closer inspection of Figure 25.3 reveals this is due to under-prediction of the incidence combined with an insufficient amount of uncertainty at the end of the epidemic season.

It also may be of interest to predict the peak week in each of the 4 years based on the long-term forecasts. For illustration, we have computed a probabilistic prediction of the peak week based on the samples from the hhh4 model only. The median peak week forecasts is always calendar week 5. This result is quite close to the observed peak weeks 6, 8, 6, and 6, respectively, shown in Figure 25.1. However, considerable uncertainty is attached to these predictions with 2.5 percent quantile in the second week and 97.5 percent quantile in week 16 of each season.

25.4.2   Multivariate forecasting of norovirus incidence

To illustrate statistical methods for the assessment of multivariate forecasts, we use age-stratified surveillance data on norovirus gastroenteritis from Berlin, Germany. We use the well-established hhh4 modeling framework from the surveillance package to generate forecasts, building on our previous analyses of these data (Held et al., 2017; Meyer and Held, 2017). Here we only consider models for spatially aggregated counts Y_{gt}, $g = 1, \ldots, G$ (i.e., without additional stratification by city district). The surveillance data are available from the package hhh4contacts (Meyer, 2017), cover five norovirus seasons from 2011-W27 to 2016-W26, and are stratified into $G = 6$ age groups: 0–4, 5–14, 15–24, 25–44, 45–64, and 65+ years of age. These groups reflect distinct social mixing of pre-school vs. school children, and intergenerational mixing. Figure 25.5 shows the age-specific incidence time series. Over the 5 years, the reported numbers of cases by age group were 2,783, 326, 553, 1,909, 2,530,

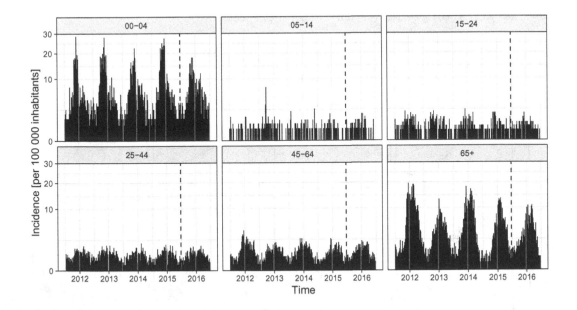

FIGURE 25.5
Age-stratified incidence of norovirus gastroenteritis in Berlin, Germany. The calendar weeks 52 and 1 (Christmas break period) are highlighted. The last 52 weeks (to the right of the vertical dashed line) are used to assess forecasts. Note that the y-axis employs a square-root scale.

and 8,335, respectively, corresponding to average yearly incidences of 346 (0–4), 24 (5–14), 30 (15–24), 36 (25–44), 52 (45–64), and 251 (65+) cases per 100,000 inhabitants.

Given the counts from the previous week, $Y_{g',t-1}$, $g' = 1, \ldots, G$, we assume Y_{gt} to follow a negative binomial distribution with a group-specific overdispersion parameter and mean

$$\mu_{gt} = \nu_{gt} + \phi_{gt} \sum_{g'} c_{g'g} Y_{g',t-1}.$$

The *endemic* log-linear predictor ν_{gt} contains group-specific intercepts, a Christmas break effect (via a simple indicator for the calendar weeks 52 and 1), and group-specific seasonal effects via $\sin(\omega t)$ and $\cos(\omega t)$ terms, $\omega = 2\pi/52$. The *epidemic* log-linear predictor ϕ_{gt} also contains group-specific intercepts, but shared seasonality and no Christmas break effect. The contact weights $c_{g'g}$ are estimated from the German subset of the POLYMOD survey (Mossong et al., 2008), taking into account the reciprocal nature of contacts (Wallinga et al., 2006). The resulting contact matrix (Figure 25.6) is subsequently row-normalized to a transition matrix, removing differences in group-specific overall contact rates.

The model described is the same as reference model 6 in Held et al. (2017, Section 3.3). As alternative models, we consider homogeneous mixing between age groups ($c_{g'g} = 1$), no mixing between age groups ($c_{g'g} = 1\{g' = g\}$), and a model where we estimate a power transformation C^κ of the contact matrix as described in Meyer and Held (2017). See the `vignette("BNV")` in the supplementary package `HIDDA.forecasting` for how to implement these models in R.

We have fitted the models to the first four seasons (2011-W27 to 2015-W26) and evaluated the quality of forecasts in the subsequent season (2015-W27 to 2016-W26). Figure 25.7 shows the fitted mean components from the Akaike information criterion (AIC)-optimal model with power-adjusted contact matrix. The proportion of the incidence that can be explained by the epidemic component varies between the age groups. The endemic-epidemic decomposition actually resembles Figure 4 in Meyer and Held (2017) quite well, which is based on a different model, additionally stratified by city district. Within the epidemic part, the incorporated social contact matrix results in predominant within-group reproduction of

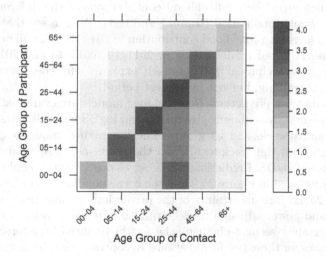

FIGURE 25.6
Age-structured social contact matrix estimated from the German POLYMOD sample. The entries refer to the mean number of contact persons per participant per day.

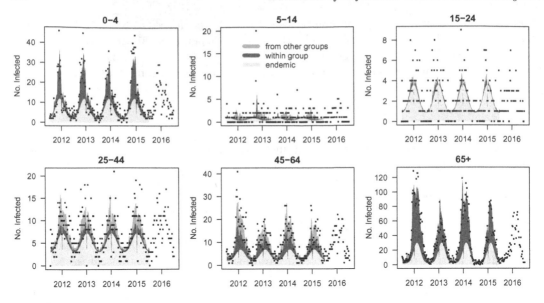

FIGURE 25.7

Estimated norovirus counts from the AIC-optimal `hhh4` model with power-adjusted contact matrix. The disease risk is additively decomposed into endemic and epidemic components. The dots show the observed counts.

the disease for the 0–4 and 65+ age groups, whereas the 25–44 and 45–64 year-old persons inherit a substantial proportion of cases from other age groups.

Turning to the predictive performance, Figure 25.8 shows the 1-week-ahead forecasts and associated scores during the last season for the power-adjusted contact model. Average scores of the different models are compared in Table 25.2. Although the power-adjusted model gives the best AIC score on the training data, it is outperformed by the "no mixing" model on the test season, both in terms of DSS and LS. This result can be explained by Table 25.3, which gives the log-likelihood contributions of the different models from a separate fit to the whole time period (training and test). We can see that the "no mixing" model has indeed a larger log-likelihood contribution in 2015/16 than all other three models. However, the power-adjusted model is best in 2011/12, 2013/14 and 2014/15 and second best in 2012/13 (after "reciprocal"). This result explains why the power-adjusted model performs best in the training, but not in the test period.

Multivariate long-term predictions from the four models are evaluated in Table 25.4 for the test period. The first two columns give mDSS and logDS for multivariate predictions (of dimension 6×52) across weeks and age groups. The "no mixing" model is again best in terms of mDSS, although both the "reciprocal" and the power-adjusted model provide sharper predictions in terms of logDS. Predictions of the age-stratified total number of cases (now of dimension 6) are displayed in Figure 25.9 and the corresponding scores listed in the last two columns of Table 25.4. More uncertainty of the predictions (in age group 65+) is visible for the "no mixing" and power-adjusted models, resulting in larger values of logDS. However, the increased uncertainty seems to be benificial for the quality of the forecasts, yielding the smallest mDSS scores for these two formulations. In contrast, the "homogeneous" prediction barely covers the observed count in age group 65+, resulting in a poor mDSS score. For comparison, a naive forecaster who independently fits negative binomial distributions to the age-stratified sizes of the past four seasons would reach mDSS = 4.084 (with logDS = 3.820), which is superior to the predictions from the homogeneous contact model.

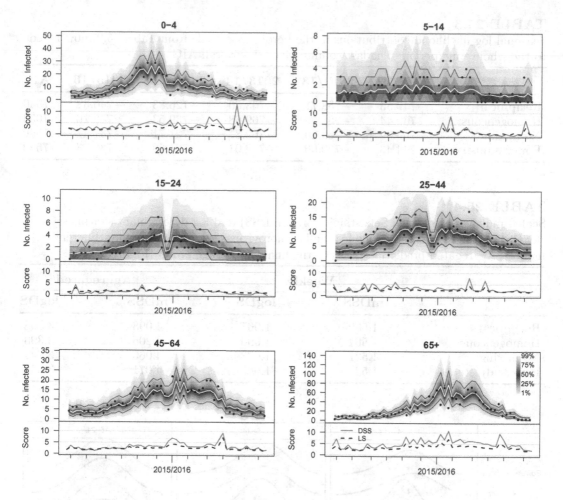

FIGURE 25.8

Age-stratified 1-week-ahead forecasts of norovirus counts in Berlin based on the power-adjusted contact model. The 10 percent and 90 percent quantiles and the means are highlighted within the fan charts. The dots represent observed counts. The bottom panels show weekly scores.

TABLE 25.2

Comparison of four `hhh4` models for the age-stratified norovirus time-series from Berlin, assuming different contact matrices. The table gives the number of parameters, the AIC for the training period, and average scores of the 6×52 1-week-ahead forecasts in the last season

	dim	AIC	DSS	LS
Reciprocal	33	6051	3.031	2.399
Homogeneous	33	6132	3.093	2.420
No mixing	33	6055	3.003	2.385
Power-adjusted	34	6035	3.012	2.391

TABLE 25.3
Seasonal log-likelihood contributions in the norovirus models from Table 25.2, now fitted to the whole time period. The last column gives the overall AIC

	2011/12	2012/13	2013/14	2014/15	2015/16	AIC
Reciprocal	−747.53	−758.71	−763.60	−726.83	−740.38	7540
Homogeneous	−762.44	−766.59	−769.68	−739.53	−745.16	7633
No mixing	−750.36	−763.29	−762.37	−721.71	−737.47	7536
Power-adjusted	−744.43	−759.06	−762.01	−721.68	−738.63	7520

TABLE 25.4
Scaled multivariate Dawid-Sebastiani scores (mDSS) and log determinant sharpness (logDS) of long-term predictions for the last norovirus season from the four different models. Aggregated predictions refer to the final size by age group (Figure 25.9)

	Weekly		Aggregated	
	mDSS	logDS	mDSS	logDS
Reciprocal	1.539	1.067	4.098	3.508
Homogeneous	1.564	1.096	4.205	3.393
No mixing	1.521	1.078	4.066	3.742
Power-adjusted	1.527	1.065	4.071	3.638

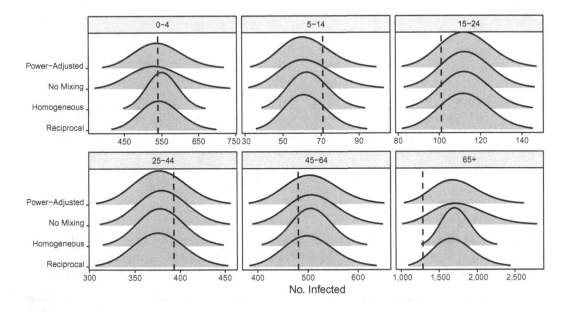

FIGURE 25.9
Forecast distributions of age-stratified sizes of the 2015/2016 norovirus epidemic from four different models. Shown are negative binomial approximations based on predictive moments, see Held et al. (2017, Appendix A) for details. The dashed vertical lines represent the observed counts.

25.5 Discussion

We have provided a non-comprehensive review of the literature on forecasting epidemics. We have focused on statistical methods to quantify the accuracy of predictions, distinguishing between point and probabilistic forecasts. Two applications show how the different techniques can be applied to uni- and multivariate forecasts.

Inspired by similar techniques in weather forecasting and other areas of science, recent work in this area has focused on model averaging and stacking in order to improve the predictive quality of single model forecasts (Ray and Reich, 2018). Perhaps the biggest challenge to epidemic forecasting is the incorporation of reporting delays and underreporting, as described in Chapter 22 of this handbook. A rigorous analysis requires surveillance and internet search data archived in a way where you can see actually what was available at a given time (McIver and Brownstein, 2014). Such real-time epidemiological data should become the standard in surveillance systems, facilitating the development of novel forecasting techniques.

Acknowledgments

We are grateful to the Swiss Federal Office of Public Health (BAG) for access to the data on influenza in Switzerland. We thank Nicholas Reich for helpful comments on a previous version of this chapter.

References

Baroyan, O. V., Rvachev, L. A., Basilevsky, U. V., Ermakov, V. V., Frank, K. D., Rvachev, M. A., and Shashkov, V. A. (1971). Computer modelling of influenza epidemics for the whole country (USSR). *Advances in Applied Probability*, 3(2):224–226.

Biggerstaff, M., Alper, D., Dredze, M., Fox, S., Fung, I. C.-H., Hickmann, K. S., Lewis, B. et al. (2016). Results from the centers for disease control and prevention's predict the 2013–2014 influenza season challenge. *BMC Infectious Diseases*, 16(1):357.

Biggerstaff, M., Johansson, M., Alper, D., Brooks, L. C., Chakraborty, P., Farrow, D. C., Hyun, S. et al. (2018). Results from the second year of a collaborative effort to forecast influenza seasons in the United States. *Epidemics*, 24:26–33.

Buczak, A. L., Baugher, B., Moniz, L. J., Bagley, T., Babin, S. M., and Guven, E. (2018). Ensemble method for dengue prediction. *PLoS One*, 13(1):e0189988.

Chretien, J. P., George, D., Shaman, J., Chitale, R. A., and McKenzie, F. E. (2014). Influenza forecasting in human populations: A scoping review. *PLoS One*, 9(4):e94130.

Cox, D. R. (1958). Two further applications of a model for binary regression. *Biometrika*, 45(3/4):562–565.

Czado, C., Gneiting, T., and Held, L. (2009). Predictive model assessment for count data. *Biometrics*, 65(4):1254–1261.

Daley, D. J., and Gani, J. (1999). *Epidemic Modelling: An Introduction*. Cambridge University Press, Cambridge, UK.

Del Valle, S. Y., McMahon, B. H., Asher, J., Hatchett, R., Lega, J. C., Brown, H. E., Leany, M. E. et al. (2018). Summary results of the 2014–2015 DARPA Chikungunya challenge. *BMC Infectious Diseases*, 18(1):245.

Diebold, F. X., and Mariano, R. S. (1995). Comparing predictive accuracy. *Journal of Business & Economic Statistics*, 13(3):253–263.

Dukic, V., Lopes, H. F., and Polson, N. G. (2012). Tracking epidemics with Google Flu Trends data and a state-space SEIR model. *Journal of the American Statistical Association*, 107(500):1410–1426.

Dunsmuir, W., and Scott, D. (2015). The `glarma` package for observation-driven time series regression of counts. *Journal of Statistical Software*, 67(1):1–36.

Farrington, C. P., Kanaan, M. N., and Gay, N. J. (2003). Branching process models for surveillance of infectious diseases controlled by mass vaccination. *Biostatistics*, 4(2): 279–295.

Funk, S., Camacho, A., Kucharski, A. J., Lowe, R., Eggo, R. M., and Edmunds, W. J. (2018). Assessing the performance of real-time epidemic forecasts: A case study of the 2013–16 Ebola epidemic. bioRxiv. doi:10.1101/177451.

Gelfand, A. E., and Smith, A. F. M. (1990). Sampling-based approaches to calculating marginal densities. *Journal of the American Statistical Association*, 85(410):398–409.

Generous, N., Fairchild, G., Deshpande, A., Del Valle, S. Y., and Priedhorsky, R. (2014). Global disease monitoring and forecasting with Wikipedia. *PLoS Computational Biology*, 10(11):1–16.

Gneiting, T. (2011). Making and evaluating point forecasts. *Journal of the American Statistical Association*, 106(494):746–762.

Gneiting, T., Balabdaoui, F., and Raftery, A. E. (2007). Probabilistic forecasts, calibration and sharpness. *Journal of the Royal Statistical Society. Series B (Methodological)*, 69(2):243–268.

Gneiting, T., and Katzfuss, M. (2014). Probabilistic forecasting. *Annual Review of Statistics and Its Application*, 1(1):125–151.

Gneiting, T., and Raftery, A. E. (2007). Strictly proper scoring rules, prediction, and estimation. *Journal of the American Statistical Association*, 102(477):359–378.

Gneiting, T., Stanberry, L. I., Grimit, E. P., Held, L., and Johnson, N. A. (2008). Assessing probabilistic forecasts of multivariate quantities, with an application to ensemble predictions of surface winds. *Test*, 17(2):211–235.

Held, L., Meyer, S., and Bracher, J. (2017). Probabilistic forecasting in infectious disease epidemiology: The 13th Armitage lecture. *Statistics in Medicine*, 36(22):3443–3460.

Held, L., and Paul, M. (2012). Modeling seasonality in space-time infectious disease surveillance data. *Biometrical Journal*, 54(6):824–843.

Held, L., Rufibach, K., and Balabdaoui, F. (2010). A score regression approach to assess calibration of continuous probabilistic predictions. *Biometrics*, 66(4):1295–1305.

Held, L., and Sabanés Bové, D. (2014). *Applied Statistical Inference: Likelihood and Bayes.* Springer, Berlin, Germany.

Hickmann, K. S., Fairchild, G., Priedhorsky, R., Generous, N., Hyman, J. M., Deshpande, A., and Del Valle, S. Y. (2015). Forecasting the 2013–2014 influenza season using Wikipedia. *PLoS Computational Biology*, 11(5):1–29.

Hufnagel, L., Brockmann, D., and Geisel, T. (2004). Forecast and control of epidemics in a globalized world. *Proceedings of the National Academy of Sciences of the United States of America*, 101:15124–15129.

Hyndman, R., and Khandakar, Y. (2008). Automatic time series forecasting: The `forecast` package for R. *Journal of Statistical Software*, 27(3):1–22.

Hyndman, R. J., and Koehler, A. B. (2006). Another look at measures of forecast accuracy. *International Journal of Forecasting*, 22(4):679–688.

Jiang, X., Wallstrom, G., Cooper, G. F., and Wagner, M. M. (2009). Bayesian prediction of an epidemic curve. *Journal of Biomedical Informatics*, 42(1):90–99.

Jordan, A., Krüger, F., and Lerch, S. (2019). Evaluating probabilistic forecasts with `scoringRules`. *Journal of Statistical Software*.

Keeling, M. J., and Rohani, P. (2008). *Modeling Infectious Diseases in Humans and Animals.* Princeton University Press, Princeton, NJ.

Lega, J., and Brown, H. E. (2016). Data-driven outbreak forecasting with a simple nonlinear growth model. *Epidemics*, 17:19–26.

Mason, S. J., Galpin, J. S., Goddard, L., Graham, N. E., and Rajartnam, B. (2007). Conditional exceedance probabilities. *Monthly Weather Review*, 135(2):363–372.

McIver, D. J., and Brownstein, J. S. (2014). Wikipedia usage estimates prevalence of influenza-like illness in the United States in near real-time. *PLoS Computational Biology*, 10(4):e1003581.

Merkle, E. C., and Steyvers, M. (2013). Choosing a strictly proper scoring rule. *Decision Analysis*, 10(4):292–304.

Meyer, S. (2017). `hhh4contacts`: *Age-structured spatio-temporal models for infectious disease counts.* R package version 0.13.0, https://CRAN.R-project.org/package=hhh4contacts. Accessed June 30, 2017.

Meyer, S. (2018). `HIDDA.forecasting`: *Forecasting based on surveillance data.* R package version 1.0.0, https://HIDDA.github.io/forecasting. Accessed September 3, 2018.

Meyer, S., and Held, L. (2017). Incorporating social contact data in spatio-temporal models for infectious disease spread. *Biostatistics*, 18(2):338–351.

Meyer, S., Held, L., and Höhle, M. (2017). Spatio-temporal analysis of epidemic phenomena using the R package `surveillance`. *Journal of Statistical Software*, 77(11):1–55.

Moran, K. R., Fairchild, G., Generous, N., Hickmann, K., Osthus, D., Priedhorsky, R., Hyman, J., and Del Valle, S. Y. (2016). Epidemic forecasting is messier than weather forecasting: The role of human behavior and internet data streams in epidemic forecast. *Journal of Infectious Diseases*, 214(suppl 4):S404–S408.

Mossong, J., Hens, N., Jit, M., Beutels, P., Auranen, K., Mikolajczyk, R., Massari, M. et al. (2008). Social contacts and mixing patterns relevant to the spread of infectious diseases. *PLoS Medicine*, 5(3):e74.

Nsoesie, E. O., Brownstein, J. S., Ramakrishnan, N., and Marathe, M. V. (2014). A systematic review of studies on forecasting the dynamics of influenza outbreaks. *Influenza and Other Respiratory Viruses*, 8(3):309–316.

Paul, M., and Held, L. (2011). Predictive assessment of a non-linear random effects model for multivariate time series of infectious disease counts. *Statistics in Medicine*, 30:1118–1136.

Paul, M. J., Dredze, M., and Broniatowski, D. (2014). Twitter improves influenza forecasting. *PLoS Currents Outbreaks*. doi:10.1371/currents.outbreaks.90b9ed0f59bae4ccaa 683a39865d9117.

Pei, S., Kandula, S., Yang, W., and Shaman, J. (2018). Forecasting the spatial transmission of influenza in the United States. *Proceedings of the National Academy of Sciences of the United States of America*, 115(11):2752–2757.

R Core Team (2018). *R: A Language and Environment for Statistical Computing*. R Foundation for Statistical Computing, Vienna, Austria.

Ray, E. L., and Reich, N. G. (2018). Prediction of infectious disease epidemics via weighted density ensembles. *PLoS Computational Biology*, 14(2):e1005910.

Ray, E. L., Sakrejda, K., Lauer, S. A., Johansson, M. A., and Reich, N. G. (2017). Infectious disease prediction with kernel conditional density estimation. *Statistics in Medicine*, 36(30):4908–4929.

Reich, N. G., Lauer, S. A., Sakrejda, K., Iamsirithaworn, S., Hinjoy, S., Suangtho, P., Suthachana, S. et al. (2016a). Challenges in real-time prediction of infectious disease: A case study of dengue in Thailand. *PLoS Neglected Tropical Diseases*, 10(6):e0004761.

Reich, N. G., Lessler, J., Sakrejda, K., Lauer, S. A., Iamsirithaworn, S., and Cummings, D. A. T. (2016b). Case study in evaluating time series prediction models using the relative mean absolute error. *The American Statistician*, 70(3):285–292.

Santillana, M., Nguyen, A. T., Dredze, M., Paul, M. J., Nsoesie, E. O., and Brownstein, J. S. (2015). Combining search, social media, and traditional data sources to improve influenza surveillance. *PLoS Computational Biology*, 11(10):e1004513.

Scheuerer, M., and Hamill, T. M. (2015). Variogram-based proper scoring rules for probabilistic forecasts of multivariate quantities. *Monthly Weather Review*, 143(4):1321–1334.

Shaman, J., and Karspeck, A. (2012). Forecasting seasonal outbreaks of influenza. *Proceedings of the National Academy of Sciences of the United States of America*, 109(50): 20425–20430.

Spiegelhalter, D. J. (1986). Probabilistic prediction in patient management and clinical trials. *Statistics in Medicine*, 5(5):421–433.

Steyerberg, E. (2009). *Clinical Prediction Models*. Springer, New York.

Taylor, S., and Letham, B. (2018). **prophet:** *Automatic forecasting procedure*. R package version 0.3.0.1, https://CRAN.R-project.org/package=prophet. Accessed June 15, 2018.

Tushar, A., Reich, N. G., Ray, E. L., and Smith, A. (2017). reichlab/flusight v2.0.0: Influenza forecasts visualizer. Zenodo. doi:10.5281/zenodo.888171. Accessed September 10, 2017.

Viboud, C., Boëlle, P.-Y., Carrat, F., Valleron, A.-J., and Flahault, A. (2003). Prediction of the spread of influenza epidemics by the method of analogues. *American Journal of Epidemiology*, 158(10):996–1006.

Viboud, C., Sun, K., Gaffey, R., Ajelli, M., Fumanelli, L., Merler, S., Zhang, Q., Chowell, G., Simonsen, L., and Vespignani, A. (2018). The RAPIDD ebola forecasting challenge: Synthesis and lessons learnt. *Epidemics*, 22:13–21.

Wallinga, J., Teunis, P., and Kretzschmar, M. (2006). Using data on social contacts to estimate age-specific transmission parameters for respiratory-spread infectious agents. *American Journal of Epidemiology*, 164(10):936–944.

Wei, W., and Held, L. (2014). Calibration tests for count data. *Test*, 23(4):787–805.

World Health Organization (2014). Anticipating epidemics. *Weekly Epidemiological Record*, 89(22):244.

World Health Organization, editor (2016). Anticipating Emerging Infectious Disease Epidemics: Meeting report of WHO informal consultation, number WHO/OHE/PED/ 2016.2, Geneva, Switzerland. WHO Press.

Yang, S., Santillana, M., and Kou, S. C. (2015). Accurate estimation of influenza epidemics using Google search data via ARGO. *Proceedings of the National Academy of Sciences of the United States of America*, 112(47):14473–14478.

26

Spatial Mapping of Infectious Disease Risk

Ewan Cameron

CONTENTS

26.1   A Case for High-Resolution, Infectious Disease Risk Maps

The continued uptake of electronic health information technologies across high- and low-resource settings alike [1, 2] reflects an increasing recognition of the valuable contributions of data-driven decision making throughout the healthcare sector. The wealth of spatially referenced disease data these systems provide, coupled with the ready availability of remote sensing image products and powerful geographical information system (GIS) packages for desktop computers, makes possible the production of high-resolution disease risk maps for use by multiple potential stakeholders. These include national disease control programs, responsible for resource allocation decisions and the assessment of past intervention efficacies within country; supra-national organizations (such as the World Health Organization (WHO) and the Global Fund), concerned with the same issues in the context of funding decisions made largely at the inter-country level; and individual citizens, interested in the performance of their local community health system or the risks of foreign travel. Corresponding examples from the field of malariology are the use of disease maps by national malaria control programs to guide the allocation of community health workers or to better target indoor residual spraying [3]; the evaluation of progress towards the United Nations (UN) Millennium Development Goal (6C) to 'halt by 2015 and begin to reverse the incidence of malaria' through cartographic disease burden estimation across sub-Saharan Africa [3, 4]; and the inclusion of detailed sub-national risk maps in government guidelines for travellers to malarious regions [6].

Though in many ways a "Big Data" problem, the disaggregation and interrogation of infectious disease data at fine spatial scales demands a formal statistical approach to account for the inherent stochasticity of the generating process—a product of randomness both in the governing transmission dynamics and in human behaviors towards treatment seeking and record keeping. Consequently, the resulting maps must be considered as fundamentally probabilistic in nature, with the understanding of their uncertainties being of central importance. In this Chapter, I describe a number of statistical challenges for the spatial mapping of infectious disease risk and review the contemporary approaches designed to address them. A focus throughout on low-resource settings and vector-borne diseases almost surely reflects the author's personal experience more so than the relative progress in this endeavor between disease research communities.

26.2   Data for Infectious Disease Risk Mapping

26.2.1   Georeferenced disease data

Identifying the nature of the available response data is the first step in any disease mapping exercise as different data types require different analysis approaches. In the Bayesian framework, determination of the appropriate likelihood function will guide many of the remaining model building decisions—a key consideration to this end is the degree of spatial precision in the response data. Data may be available either at point level, meaning that precise geographic coordinates are given for case locations and survey sites, or at areal level, meaning that observations are aggregated over spatial blocks of a non-negligible size. A further consideration for point level data is the geographic reporting precision. For example, cluster locations in Demographic Health Survey data releases are randomly displaced by up to 2 kilometers in urban areas and 5–10 km in rural areas to preserve respondent anonymity [7]. A distinction between modes of areal aggregation is also useful to identify whether the data are accumulated over well-defined geographic domains, such as specific provinces or districts, or whether there is also uncertainty in the unit boundaries, such as those of health facility catchments (as per the example in Figure 26.1a). Even in the former case, complications can arise when, for example, administrative boundaries are re-drawn within the sample collection period [8].

   Both point level and areal level observations may come in the form of prevalence or incidence data, which is another key factor in identifying the appropriate likelihood function. Prevalence data represent the observed proportion of individuals in a given population with some measurable disease characteristic at a particular time, such as the proportion of villagers having a microscopically patent blood density of malaria parasites. These data will usually come as a numerator and denominator pair reported for groups of test subjects (e.g., households, villages, and districts), although sometimes in the case of point level data no prior aggregation will have been conducted such that results are entered as zeros (negative) or ones (positive) for each individual. Incidence data represent the observed number of disease events experienced by a given population over a given period of time. Again, these data usually will come as a numerator and denominator pair, but with additional information on the temporal window of sampling. When dealing with surveillance-based incidence data from low-resource settings the case count (numerator) may have additional uncertainty due to suspected reporting incompleteness, while the population-at-risk (denominator) may be uncertain due to an absence of reliable, up-to-date census statistics. Recently, there has been increasing interest in risk mapping with "new" response data types, such as antibody titers from serological measurements [9], which may require a preliminary modeling step to reduce them to a prevalence form [10] or else motivate deeper hierarchical models beyond those of the routine disease mapping toolkit.

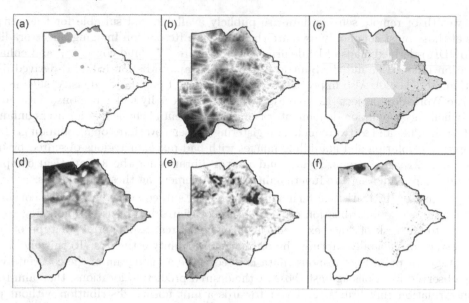

FIGURE 26.1
Components of an infectious disease risk mapping analysis for malaria in Botswana: (a) case incidence counts over a 2-year period (2015–2016) at a georeferenced health facilities (i.e., areal level data; uncertain catchment boundaries), (b) map of travel time to nearest health facility (derived from a 'friction surface' [11]), (c) WorldPop map of population density [12], (d) output posterior median risk map (incidence rate; pointwise median) (e) illustration of relative posterior uncertainties (pointwise interquartile range divided by posterior median map), and (f) posterior median incidence count map (population-weighted risk).

26.2.2 Spatial covariates

When examined at the finest granularity, for example, at the household or individual level, the factors shaping the transmission risk of any particular infectious disease may seem overwhelmingly complex; well beyond our ability to enumerate and measure. However, for risk mapping, our interest is in prediction at a coarser granularity—broadly, the community level, or more specifically at a pixel resolution level of order 1–5 km^2—at which the relevant factors operating "in mean" might be abstracted to a simpler set of social and environmental effects. For instance, in the case of diseases spread by night-time feeding, indoor-biting mosquitoes, the blood-seeking female depends on access to sleeping humans, which may be impeded by improved housing construction (e.g., screened windows and closed eaves [13]) and the use of well-maintained, insecticide-treated bed nets [14]. Although it may be infeasible to gather data on these factors across both the domain of the observations and our intended predictions, at the community level a wealth or development index, such as the intensity of night-time lights by remote sensing imagery [15], might serve as an effective proxy. In this spirit, it may be advantageous to seek to introduce a number of ancillary data products as spatial covariates to improve the predictive accuracy of the statistical map making process. Worth emphasizing is that neither the goal of map making (i.e., predictive accuracy) nor the design of data-model pairs for this purpose (i.e., harnessing covariates to observations across multiple spatial scales) is optimal for uncovering the fundamental drivers of a transmission process; the temptation for over-interpretation should be avoided, as epitomized by the "ecological fallacy" [16].

A wealth of remote sensing data are publicly available and suitable for this purpose. Some of those most commonly used are the Moderate Resolution Imaging Spectroradiometer (MODIS)-derived maps of land-surface temperature [17], land cover [18], and enhanced vegetation index [19], and the Shuttle Radar Topography Mission (SRTM)-derived digital elevation models [20]. Also important are digital maps of population density, such as those from the WorldPop project [12] (see Figure 26.1c)—especially so for response data on incidence when the population denominator is missing! Potential challenges for users unfamiliar with GIS formats and software include registering chosen covariates on a common grid of an appropriate resolution and gap-filling images with bad pixels or regions obscured by heavy cloud cover [21]. The `rgeos`, `rgdal`, and `raster` libraries for the R statistical computing environment provide the core functionalities for implementing these procedures.

Regardless of the statistical techniques to be used subsequently, it is worth considering a further step of standardization of the spatial covariates before use in modeling to limit exposure to the risk of "over-extrapolation" of linear regression terms—a type of model choice error not generally captured by ordinary uncertainty estimates. To this end a sensible strategy for point level response data is to compare a histogram of the covariate values at the observed locations against those at the desired prediction locations, then aim to find a transformation that brings the latter towards a unit normal distribution without pushing the bulk of the former outside the central 2σ (95%) interval. For areal level data the aim may be to do the same in comparison of the histogram of (population-weighted) areal means of the spatial covariates against those at the pixel level for the desired domain of prediction. For covariates that already take a roughly normal distribution the appropriate standardization procedure may simply be subtraction of the empirical mean and division by the empirical standard deviation; for roughly exponentially distributed covariates an additional logarithmic transformation may be required. Reporting of key quantiles of covariates for within-sample and out-of-sample pixels often reflects a diligent analysis (e.g. [22]).

A note on uncertainties in the data products used as spatial covariates. Certain products, particularly those, such as the WorldPop surfaces that are the outputs of statistical or machine learning models, may come with substantial uncertainties, which raises the question of whether (and if so, how) to incorporate these uncertainties into the downstream error budget. For example, the Bayesian statistician could treat the "true" covariate surface as a latent variable to be learned jointly during model fitting, or more crudely to place a "cut" in the analysis pipeline such that the covariate uncertainties are onwards propagated but are not informed in reverse by the new response data. Choosing between the two becomes a decision theoretic problem of statistical methodology [23]. In routine analyses, it is more common to simply ignore covariate uncertainty, perhaps with the implicit justification that allowance for covariate errors will be made in the scale of the residual error term in a sufficiently flexible map-making model. For this to be a reasonable assumption, the hope would be that the covariate uncertainties at observed locations are of a similar magnitude to those at the predicted locations: a point which can again be quickly assessed by a comparison of histograms.

26.3   Statistical Approaches to Infectious Disease Risk Mapping

26.3.1   Bayesian hierarchical models

Bayesian hierarchical models offer a powerful tool for probabilistic map making and have been the subject of extensive theoretical and methodological study within the field of 'model-based geostatistics' [24]. The core Bayesian geostatistical model is a generalized linear regression in which an appropriate transformation—the inverse logistic, inverse probit, or exponential—connects a latent surface formed from a linear combination of the spatial covariates, plus a Gaussian random field representing spatially correlated residuals, to the domain of the likelihood function for the observed data. The hierarchy is completed by introducing priors on the slope coefficients and the hyperparameters of the Gaussian random field. An example for the mapping of point prevalence data on podoconiosis in Cameroon [25] illustrates the standard form:

$$y_i \sim \text{binomial}(p_i, n_i) \text{ [the sampling distribution]}$$

$$\log\left(\frac{p_i}{1 - p_i}\right) = d(x_i)^{\mathsf{T}}\beta + S(x_i) + Z(x_i) \text{ [a non-linear transformation]}$$

$$S(\cdot) \sim \text{GaussianProcess}(0, \Sigma) \text{ [the random field]}$$

$$\Sigma_{jk} = \sigma^2 \exp\left(-\frac{\|x_j - x_k\|}{\phi}\right) \text{ [covariance of the random field]}$$

$$Z(x_i) \sim \text{Normal}(0, \tau^2) \text{ [an independent error term]}$$

$$\beta, \tau, \sigma, \phi \sim \Pi \text{ [unspecified additional priors]}.$$

For areal incidence data, the sampling distribution typically takes a Poisson form with expectation set equal to the sum of the (population-weighted) pixel level incidence predictions [26], while for point incidence data the sampling distribution becomes a Poisson process—that is, a distribution over the observable sets of case locations and total case counts [27].

The key strengths of the hierarchical Bayesian approach to probabilistic map making are its flexibility, with sophisticated models able to be constructed piecewise from a sequence of simple, tractable layers, and its potential to comprehensively represent the uncertainties of the inference process. However, two issues must be addressed for a successful application of this approach: (1) implementation of a posterior approximation strategy within the available time and computational budget and (2) the difficulties of effective model scrutiny and validation. The first of these I will discuss here, while the latter is addressed across the two subsequent sections.

Although the Markov Chain Monte Carlo (MCMC) revolution of the 1990s [28] and subsequent developments in user-friendly Hybrid Monte Carlo methods [29] have made posterior sampling of a large class of Bayesian hierarchical models a quick and straightforward procedure on standard computing facilities, fast posterior sampling methods for geostatistical models can be more difficult to achieve. This difficulty is due primarily to the computational burden of matrix operations associated with the Gaussian process, which scale poorly with the number of unique observation locations. Methods developed to overcome these difficulties have focused on producing sparse matrix structures approximating the original model [30] and developing fast posterior approximations to the resulting proxy models (e.g., integrated nested Laplace approximation (INLA) [31]; or the method of variational approximations with inducing points [32]); or on identifying situations in which fast Fourier transforms may be used to accelerate matrix inversion [33], allowing for Gibbs sampling from the exact posterior of certain model types (e.g., the lgcp package [34]). Note that both INLA and lgcp are freely available online and operate within the R statistical computing environment; see also PrevMap [35] for an implementation of the Bayesian hierarchical model for point prevalence data described above.

In the case of areal level data from health facilities with unknown catchment domains it becomes necessary to add an additional layer to the hierarchical model to estimate this missing information. Access to healthcare is often represented by versions of the "gravity model" (e.g., [36]) in which the probability to seek care at a particular facility is imagined to be inversely proportional to the distance from that facility. Importantly, it is possible to increasingly improve on simple Euclidean distances for this purpose thanks to the availability of new "friction surface" models of human movement from which travel time distances can be derived [11] (example in Figure 26.1b). While recent efforts have focused on computational issues regarding the addition of pre-fitted implementations of these catchment models to the hierarchical framework [37], there remains work to be done to explore the potential for joint inference of catchments in conjunction with the disease risk surface.

26.3.2   Assessing model performance

A key step in model scrutiny and model validation is to examine the performance of a chosen model. In mapping infectious disease risk our goals are two-fold: to achieve a high level of predictive accuracy and to produce well-calibrated representations of our uncertainties. A common metric for the first goal is mean squared error, which can be assessed by leave-n-out cross validation approaches; namely, reserving a portion of the response data for testing model-based predictions made using only the remainder as a training dataset. It is important to recognize that geospatial models will borrow strength from observations at nearby locations, so if the goal is to estimate the likely performance across the full predictive domain we must bear in mind that this may well constitute a higher proportion of locations distant from the observation sites than in the neighbor distance distribution of the response dataset. For this reason, it is recommended to produce test datasets having a neighbor distance distribution similar to that of the pixels across which predictions are sought; for example, perhaps choose to remove not just individual locations from the training dataset but all those within a given radius [38]. Interesting to note is that this is the same philosophy—that of attempting to reproduce the pattern of missingness over the predictive surface during cross-validation—used by the high-profile Global Burden of Diseases project [39], although in that case for the prediction of national-level disease burden estimates.

Cross-validation approaches may be extended to test the calibration of posterior uncertainties. A useful diagnostic is the posterior integral transform (PIT [40]), which is a histogram of the posterior predictive mass lying below the observed value of each response when held out from the others. In a well-calibrated model the expectation is that this histogram should be roughly uniform, while ∪-shaped and ∩-shaped histograms reflect over- and under-confident predictive intervals, respectively. Caution is needed when using this diagnostic for small sample, discrete response data, and for discrete multivariate responses [41].

As model fitting must be repeated on each constructed subset of the response data, cross-validation can be a computationally expensive process. Nevertheless, the value of model assessment by cross-validation is such that it should not be neglected if at all possible, and for this reason the disease mapping practitioner may often prefer to use a reduced, but faster, model structure over a more complex one—identifying the most effective and least damaging places to make simplifications and approximations is an important skill that develops with experience. For reference, the INLA software package offers an approximate construction of the PIT without the need for cross-validation [42], but again caution is needed in certain discrete data settings. One regime in which cross-validation techniques are of limited power is in the case of high-resolution map made from areal level data where no pixel level response data is available. In this case the predictive accuracy at the original areal scale can be assessed, and in some cases this will be the target of prediction—the fine-scale model only being adopted to by-pass limitations of artificial covariance structures across administrative polygons [43]. However, when high-resolution pixel level predictions are indeed desired from areal data alone, their accuracy may well be impossible to establish satisfactorily [44].

26.3.3   Thinking about shrinkage and hyperparameters

A helpful way to think about the Bayesian hierarchical framework for geospatial modelling is in terms of (Bayesian) "shrinkage" and regularization [45, 46]—broadly, shrinkage of estimates at the observed locations relative to all others to improve their net predictive accuracy locally, and regularization by prior choice and model structure to produce sensible extrapolations to out-of-sample locations. One direction this line of thinking may take is towards the refinement of classical survey-based prevalence estimates by Bayesian modeling [47], which is an interesting area of application. Another is towards a framework for decision making with regard to those priors acting on the slope coefficients of the linear terms in a geostatistical model and those acting on the hyperparameters of the random field component. "LASSO" and "elastic net" style shrinkages can be achieved in the Bayesian paradigm via Laplace and Normal priors with a scale parameter shared across covariates to be learned in the spirit of an "empirical Bayes" model during posterior sampling [48, 49]. With point level data, these methods can perform well to avoid over-fitting and to improve out of sample performance, albeit with caution required to ensure that posterior approximations or sampling methods are behaving properly. For the case of areal level data, there is much less power in the available observations to identify significant covariates and it may be seen that aggressive regularization procedures can overly reduce the effective set of spatial covariates [50, 51] upon which these models heavily rely for producing fine-scale structure in their predictions, potentially exposing the analyst to a false confidence due to the apparent stability of their outputs.

For both point level and areal level data types, it is also important to carefully consider the choice of prior on the hyper-parameters (typically range and scale) of the Gaussian random field term, since these frequently display a degenerate likelihood surface [52] and may have no hope of asymptotic concentration [53] in many geostatistical analysis scenarios. For this reason, the choice of prior plays an important role to regularize the posterior and should not be neglected. One direction of recent progress has been in the development of penalized-complexity priors for the hyperparameters of Gaussian random fields with Matérn covariance functions [54]. These priors may be specified intuitively by the choice of bound and exceedance probability pairs and have been included in recent releases of the INLA package. In any case, scrutiny of the posterior estimates of the hyperparameters and visual inspection of the contribution of the random field component to the predictive surface is to be advised, as is some degree of prior-sensitivity analysis.

26.3.4   Machine-learning tools

At present there is a (perhaps somewhat artificial) split in the modeling community between researchers using Bayesian hierarchical models for disease risk mapping and those using machine-learning tools. Examples of the latter include the use of boosted regression trees to map the geographic extent of dengue fever [55] and random forests for mapping tick-borne diseases [56]. A crude distinction between the two approaches is that Bayesian models (and statistical models in general) offer less flexibility to represent complex relationships between covariates and disease burden but a stronger representation of uncertainties, while machine learning approaches can produce richer relationships at the expense of a less satisfactory accounting of the relevant uncertainties. Specifically, machine-learning models come into their own when both the number of sampled locations and the sample sizes at those locations are large, such that the space of covariates is thoroughly probed and the response measurements are relatively noise free, which is not often the case for infectious disease datasets. Nevertheless, the power of machine-learning approaches should not be neglected and indeed recent efforts towards fusing these with Bayesian approaches in this field have proven fruitful [57].

26.4   Challenges for Utilizing and Improving Disease Risk Maps

Once the analyst is satisfied with the reliability of the probabilistic risk map created, there remains at least one further challenge: presenting the model outputs, including their uncertainties, effectively and efficiently to the target audience. A first step is generally to construct a pair of maps showing the pointwise (pixel-wise) posterior median in the output quantity of interest (e.g., disease prevalence or incidence rate) and an associated indication of uncertainty such as the standard deviation or interquartile range (again, pointwise; examples in Figure 26.1d & e). However, since pixels in the predictive surface will be highly correlated in a standard geostatistical model (due both to the Gaussian random field and the spatial covariates) the uncertainties in areal level summaries of the predictive surface cannot simply be computed as if they were the sum of independent random variables. For this reason it is often helpful to produce maps showing areal level averages and their uncertainties from the full posterior, anticipating the needs of end-users (e.g., aggregating to various levels of official administrative subdivisions). Another helpful way to represent uncertainty is by exceedance maps [58], which show the posterior probability that the prevalence or case incidence rate in a given pixel is above a policy-relevant threshold. Another potential pitfall in presenting outputs concerns the role of population in modulating the importance—and even meaning—of prevalence and incidence rate maps. While from a statistical perspective it may be perfectly reasonable to predict a high risk of infection over an unpopulated area of marshland between two highly endemic villages, it certainly doesn't make sense for a control program to consider sending community health workers there! For this reason, it is a good practice to generate population-weighted risk maps to present alongside the base model outputs (as shown in Figure 26.1f), and in some instances a judicious use of masking to remove unpopulated areas may be advised.

The response from end-users to delivery of a final set of maps and uncertainty illustrations is often (in my experience) 'thanks' followed by a series of new questions regarding onwards decision making. Many of these can be answered through straightforward computations on the posterior samples (e.g., how many community health workers are required to address the case burden in each administrative area?), while others may require deeper methodological techniques from the field of operations research or optimization theory (e.g., in which villages should we station the available community health workers to best access the potential patient pool [59]?). Another interesting area of research concerns the use of existing disease risk maps (with their associated uncertainties) to inform the design of future disease surveys [60].

Looking ahead there are two particular methodological issues that seem especially important to the development of improved disease risk maps. The first concerns the role of human movement in exposure to disease risk. In the previous paradigm, an individual's risk is treated as that predicted for their pixel of residence, despite the fact that at, for example, 1–5 square kilometers (km^2) resolution an individual is very likely to spend their time split between multiple adjacent pixels and perhaps some even further away. To a large extent the failure of the model to harness the power of potential covariate data from these additional pixels in which they spend time may simply result in more signal than necessary being picked up by the random field term. However, with digital technologies providing ever greater levels of information on population movements (such as through mobile phone cell tower logs [61]), it makes sense to explore methods for harnessing this additional data to the task of risk mapping. Recent efforts have shown the potential to sharpen the resolution of sources and sinks of malaria risk when movement models are applied *ex post facto* to existing risk maps [62], raising the question of how predictions could be improved by an integrated modeling approach.

The second methodological issue deserving further research concerns the treatment of temporal information at high resolution. Although I have restricted the previous discussion to purely spatial mapping of disease risk, many of the methods and approaches extend trivially to spatiotemporal modeling provided the number of time periods considered is relatively small (less than, for example, 15) and the space-time interaction term is treated with a separable, "Kronecker product" form [63]. Developing a framework for risk mapping that can efficiently and effectively harness the information content of response data with fine temporal resolution remains an ongoing challenge [64], as is the innovation of tractable, non-separable space-time kernels [65, 66].

References

[1] Ann W Hsing and John PA Ioannidis. Nationwide population science: Lessons from the Taiwan national health insurance research database. *JAMA Internal Medicine*, 175(9):1527–1529, 2015.

[2] Vincent Micheal Kiberu, Joseph KB Matovu, Fredrick Makumbi, Carol Kyozira, Eddie Mukooyo, and Rhoda K Wanyenze. Strengthening district-based health reporting through the district health management information software system: The Ugandan experience. *BMC Medical Informatics and Decision Making*, 14(1):40, 2014.

[3] Judy A Omumbo, Abdisalan M Noor, Ibrahima S Fall, and Robert W Snow. How well are malaria maps used to design and finance malaria control in Africa? *PLoS One*, 8(1):e53198, 2013.

[4] Samir Bhatt, DJ Weiss, E Cameron, D Bisanzio, B Mappin, U Dalrymple, KE Battle, CL Moyes, A Henry, PA Eckhoff et al. The effect of malaria control on Plasmodium falciparum in Africa between 2000 and 2015. *Nature*, 526(7572):207–211, 2015.

[5] World Health Organization. World malaria report 2015. Geneva, Switzerland: World Health Organization, 2016.

[6] PHE Advisory Committee for Malaria Prevention for UK Travellers. Guidelines for malaria prevention in travellers from the United Kingdom: 2017. *Public Health England*, 2017.

[7] Clara R Burgert, Josh Colston, Thea Roy, and Blake Zachary. Geographic displacement procedure and georeferenced data release policy for the Demographic and Health Surveys. 2013. https://dhsprogram.com/pubs/pdf/SAR7/SAR7.pdf

[8] Ricardo Andrade-Pacheco, Martin Mubangizi, John Quinn, and Neil D Lawrence. Consistent mapping of government malaria records across a changing territory delimitation. *Malaria Journal*, 13(1):P5, 2014.

[9] Patrick Corran, Paul Coleman, Eleanor Riley, and Chris Drakeley. Serology: A robust indicator of malaria transmission intensity? *Trends in Parasitology*, 23(12):575–582, 2007.

[10] Ruth A Ashton, Takele Kefyalew, Alison Rand, Heven Sime, Ashenafi Assefa, Addis Mekasha, Wasihun Edosa, Gezahegn Tesfaye, Jorge Cano, Hiwot Teka et al. Geostatistical modeling of malaria endemicity using serological indicators of exposure collected through school surveys. *The American Journal of Tropical Medicine and Hygiene*, 93(1):168–177, 2015.

[11] DJ Weiss, A Nelson, HS Gibson, W Temperley, S Peedell, A Lieber, M Hancher, E Po-yart, S Belchior, N Fullman et al. A global map of travel time to cities to assess inequalities in accessibility in 2015. *Nature*, 553(7688):333, 2018.

[12] Andrew J Tatem. WorldPop, open data for spatial demography. *Scientific Data*, 4:170004, 2017.

[13] Lucy S Tusting, Matthew M Ippolito, Barbara A Willey, Immo Kleinschmidt, Grant Dorsey, Roly D Gosling, and Steve W Lindsay. The evidence for improving housing to reduce malaria: A systematic review and meta-analysis. *Malaria Journal*, 14(1):209, 2015.

[14] Christian Lengeler. Insecticide-treated bed nets and curtains for preventing malaria. *The Cochrane Library*, 2:1–46, 2004.

[15] Christopher D Elvidge, Kimberley E Baugh, Eric A Kihn, Herbert W Kroehl, Ethan R Davis, and Chris W Davis. Relation between satellite observed visible-near infrared emissions, population, economic activity and electric power consumption. *International Journal of Remote Sensing*, 18(6):1373–1379, 1997.

[16] William S Robinson. Ecological correlations and the behavior of individuals. *International Journal of Epidemiology*, 38(2):337–341, 2009.

[17] Zhengming Wan, Yulin Zhang, Qincheng Zhang, and Zhao-liang Li. Validation of the land-surface temperature products retrieved from Terra Moderate Resolution Imaging Spectroradiometer data. *Remote Sensing of Environment*, 83(1):163–180, 2002.

[18] Mark A Friedl, Damien Sulla-Menashe, Bin Tan, Annemarie Schneider, Navin Ra-mankutty, Adam Sibley, and Xiaoman Huang. MODIS Collection 5 global land cover: Algorithm refinements and characterization of new datasets. *Remote Sensing of Environment*, 114(1):168–182, 2010.

[19] Alfredo Huete, Chris Justice, and Wim Van Leeuwen. MODIS vegetation index (MOD13). *Algorithm Theoretical Basis Document*, 3:213, 1999.

[20] Tom G Farr, Paul A Rosen, Edward Caro, Robert Crippen, Riley Duren, Scott Hensley, Michael Kobrick, Mimi Paller, Ernesto Rodriguez, Ladislav Roth et al. The shuttle radar topography mission. *Reviews of Geophysics*, 45(2)1–3, 2007.

[21] Daniel J Weiss, Peter M Atkinson, Samir Bhatt, Bonnie Mappin, Simon I Hay, and Peter W Gething. An effective approach for gap-filling continental scale remotely sensed time-series. *ISPRS Journal of Photogrammetry and Remote Sensing*, 98:106–118, 2014.

[22] Marina Antillón, Joshua L Warren, Forrest W Crawford, Daniel M Weinberger, Esra Kürüm, Gi Deok Pak, Florian Marks, and Virginia E Pitzer. The burden of typhoid fever in low-and middle-income countries: A meta-regression approach. *PLoS Neglected Tropical Diseases*, 11(2):e0005376, 2017.

[23] Pierre E. Jacob, Lawrence M. Murray, Chris C. Holmes, and Christian P. Robert. Better together? Statistical learning in models made of modules. *ArXiv e-prints*, August 2017.

[24] Peter J Diggle, Jonathan A Tawn, and Rana A Moyeed. Model-based geostatistics. *Journal of the Royal Statistical Society: Series C (Applied Statistics)*, 47(3):299–350, 1998.

[25] Deribe, Kebede, Amuam Andrew Beng, Jorge Cano, Abdel Jelil Njouendo, Jerome Fru-Cho, Abong Raphael Awah, Mathias Esum Eyong et al. Mapping the geographical distribution of podoconiosis in Cameroon using parasitological, serological, and clinical evidence to exclude other causes of lymphedema. *PLoS Neglected Tropical Diseases*, 12(1):e0006126, 2018.

[26] Katherine Wilson and Jon Wakefield. Pointless continuous spatial surface reconstruction. *arXiv preprint arXiv:1709.09659*, 2017.

[27] Peter J Diggle, Paula Moraga, Barry Rowlingson, and Benjamin M Taylor. Spatial and spatio-temporal log-Gaussian Cox processes: Extending the geostatistical paradigm. *Statistical Science*, 28(4):542–563, 2013.

[28] Walter R Gilks. Markov chain Monte Carlo. In P Armitage and T Colton (Eds.), *Encyclopedia of Biostatistics*, Chichester, UK: John Wiley & Sons, 2005.

[29] Matthew D Hoffman and Andrew Gelman. The no-u-turn sampler: Adaptively setting path lengths in Hamiltonian Monte Carlo. *Journal of Machine Learning Research*, 15(1):1593–1623, 2014.

[30] Finn Lindgren, Håvard Rue, and Johan Lindström. An explicit link between Gaussian fields and Gaussian Markov random fields: The stochastic partial differential equation approach. *Journal of the Royal Statistical Society: Series B (Statistical Methodology)*, 73(4):423–498, 2011.

[31] Håvard Rue, Sara Martino, and Nicolas Chopin. Approximate Bayesian inference for latent Gaussian models by using integrated nested Laplace approximations. *Journal of the Royal Statistical Society: Series B (Statistical Methodology)*, 71(2):319–392, 2009.

[32] James Hensman, Nicolo Fusi, and Neil D Lawrence. Gaussian processes for big data. *arXiv preprint arXiv:1309.6835*, 2013.

[33] Tilmann Gneiting, Hana Ševčíková, Donald B Percival, Martin Schlather, and Yindeng Jiang. Fast and exact simulation of large Gaussian lattice systems in R2: Exploring the limits. *Journal of Computational and Graphical Statistics*, 15(3):483–501, 2006.

[34] Benjamin M. Taylor, Tilman M. Davies, Barry S. Rowlingson, and Peter J. Diggle. lgcp: An R package for inference with spatial and spatio-temporal Log-Gaussian Cox processes. *Journal of Statistical Software*, 52(i04):1–40, 2013.

[35] Emanuele Giorgi and Peter John Diggle. PrevMap: An R package for prevalence mapping. *Journal of Statistical Software*, 78(8), 2017.

[36] Nicole White and Kerrie Mengersen. Predicting health programme participation: A gravity-based, hierarchical modelling approach. *Journal of the Royal Statistical Society: Series C (Applied Statistics)*, 65(1):145–166, 2016.

[37] Benjamin M Taylor, Ricardo Andrade-Pacheco, and Hugh JW Sturrock. Continuous inference for aggregated point process data. *arXiv preprint arXiv:1704.05627*, 2017.

[38] Kévin Le Rest, David Pinaud, Pascal Monestiez, Joël Chadoeuf, and Vincent Bretagnolle. Spatial leave-one-out cross-validation for variable selection in the presence of spatial autocorrelation. *Global Ecology and Biogeography*, 23(7):811–820, 2014.

[39] Kyle J Foreman, Rafael Lozano, Alan D Lopez, and Christopher JL Murray. Modeling causes of death: An integrated approach using CODEm. *Population Health Metrics*, 10(1):1, 2012.

[40] A Philip Dawid. Present position and potential developments: Some personal views: Statistical theory: The prequential approach. *Journal of the Royal Statistical Society. Series A (General)*, 147(2):278–290, 1984.

[41] David I Warton, Loïc Thibaut, and Yi Alice Wang. The pit-trap—a "model-free" bootstrap procedure for inference about regression models with discrete, multivariate responses. *PLoS One*, 12(7):e0181790, 2017.

[42] Leonhard Held, Birgit Schrödle, and Håvard Rue. Posterior and cross-validatory predictive checks: A comparison of MCMC and INLA. In T Kneib and G Tutz (Eds.), *Statistical Modelling and Regression Structures*, pages 91–110, 2010. Cham, Switzerland: Springer.

[43] Melanie M Wall. A close look at the spatial structure implied by the CAR and SAR models. *Journal of Statistical Planning and Inference*, 121(2):311–324, 2004.

[44] Jonathan Wakefield. Ecologic studies revisited. *Annual Review of Public Health*, 29: 75–90, 2008.

[45] Bradley Efron. Empirical bayes estimates for large-scale prediction problems. *Journal of the American Statistical Association*, 104(487):1015–1028, 2009.

[46] Andrew Gelman, Daniel Simpson, and Michael Betancourt. The prior can often only be understood in the context of the likelihood. *Entropy*, 19(10):555, 2017.

[47] Victor A Alegana, Jim Wright, Claudio Bosco, Emelda A Okiro, Peter M Atkinson, Robert W Snow, Andrew J Tatem, and Abdisalan M Noor. Malaria prevalence metrics in low-and middle-income countries: An assessment of precision in nationally-representative surveys. *Malaria Journal*, 16(1):475, 2017.

[48] Trevor Park and George Casella. The Bayesian lasso. *Journal of the American Statistical Association*, 103(482):681–686, 2008.

[49] Minjung Kyung, Jeff Gill, Malay Ghosh, George Casella et al. Penalized regression, standard errors, and Bayesian lassos. *Bayesian Analysis*, 5(2):369–411, 2010.

[50] Hugh JW Sturrock, Justin M Cohen, Petr Keil, Andrew J Tatem, Arnaud Le Menach, Nyasatu E Ntshalintshali, Michelle S Hsiang, and Roland D Gosling. Fine-scale malaria risk mapping from routine aggregated case data. *Malaria Journal*, 13(1):421, 2014.

[51] Victor A Alegana, Peter M Atkinson, Carla Pezzulo, Alessandro Sorichetta, D Weiss, T Bird, E Erbach-Schoenberg, and Andrew J Tatem. Fine resolution mapping of population age-structures for health and development applications. *Journal of The Royal Society Interface*, 12(105):20150073, 2015.

[52] JJ Warnes and BD Ripley. Problems with likelihood estimation of covariance functions of spatial Gaussian processes. *Biometrika*, 74(3):640–642, 1987.

[53] Hao Zhang. Inconsistent estimation and asymptotically equal interpolations in model-based geostatistics. *Journal of the American Statistical Association*, 99(465):250–261, 2004.

[54] Geir-Arne Fuglstad, Daniel Simpson, Finn Lindgren, and Håvard Rue. Constructing priors that penalize the complexity of Gaussian random fields. *Journal of the American Statistical Association*. doi:10.1080/01621459.2017.1415907, 2019.

[55] Samir Bhatt, Peter W Gething, Oliver J Brady, Jane P Messina, Andrew W Farlow, Catherine L Moyes, John M Drake, John S Brownstein, Anne G Hoen, Osman Sankoh et al. The global distribution and burden of dengue. *Nature*, 496(7446):504–507, 2013.

[56] Cesare Furlanello, Markus Neteler, Stefano Merler, Stefano Menegon, Steno Fontanari, Angela Donini, Annapaola Rizzoli, and C Chemini. GIS and the random forest predictor: Integration in R for tick-borne disease risk assessment. In K Hornik, F Leisch, A Zeileis (Eds.), *Proceedings of DSC*, page 2, 2003.

[57] Samir Bhatt, Ewan Cameron, Seth R Flaxman, Daniel J Weiss, David L Smith, and Peter W Gething. Improved prediction accuracy for disease risk mapping using Gaussian process stacked generalization. *Journal of the Royal Society Interface*, 14(134):20170520, 2017.

[58] Peter J Diggle and Emanuele Giorgi. Model-based geostatistics for prevalence mapping in low-resource settings. *Journal of the American Statistical Association*, 111(515):1096–1120, 2016.

[59] Barnett R Parker, Sally K Stansfield, Antoine Augustin, Reginald Boulos, and Jeanne S Newman. Optimization of task allocation for community health workers in Haiti. *Socio-Economic Planning Sciences*, 22(1):3–14, 1988.

[60] Michael G Chipeta, Dianne J Terlouw, Kamija S Phiri, and Peter J Diggle. Adaptive geostatistical design and analysis for prevalence surveys. *Spatial Statistics*, 15:70–84, 2016.

[61] Marta C Gonzalez, Cesar A Hidalgo, and Albert-Laszlo Barabasi. Understanding individual human mobility patterns. *Nature*, 453(7196):779–782, 2008.

[62] Nick W Ruktanonchai, Patrick DeLeenheer, Andrew J Tatem, Victor A Alegana, T Trevor Caughlin, Elisabeth zu Erbach-Schoenberg, Christopher Lourenço, Corrine W Ruktanonchai, and David L Smith. Identifying malaria transmission foci for elimination using human mobility data. *PLoS Computational Biology*, 12(4):e1004846, 2016.

[63] Marc G Genton. Separable approximations of space-time covariance matrices. *Environmetrics*, 18(7):681–695, 2007.

[64] Cici Bauer, Jon Wakefield, Håvard Rue, Steve Self, Zijian Feng, and Yu Wang. Bayesian penalized spline models for the analysis of spatio-temporal count data. *Statistics in Medicine*, 35(11):1848–1865, 2016.

[65] Tilmann Gneiting. Nonseparable, stationary covariance functions for space–time data. *Journal of the American Statistical Association*, 97(458):590–600, 2002.

[66] Fabio Sigrist, Hans R Künsch, and Werner A Stahel. Stochastic partial differential equation based modelling of large space–time data sets. *Journal of the Royal Statistical Society: Series B (Statistical Methodology)*, 77(1):3–33, 2015.

Index

Note: Page numbers in italic and bold refer to figures and tables, respectively.

Printed in the United States
by Baker & Taylor Publisher Services

Printed in the United States
by Baker & Taylor Publisher Services